Ocular Therapeutics Handbook

A Clinical Manual

Second Edition

Ocular Therapeutics Handbook
A Clinical Manual
Second Edition

BRUCE E. ONOFREY, RPh, OD, FAAO, FOGS

Vice-Chair Eye Services, Lovelace-Sandia Medical Center,
Albuquerque, New Mexico; Adjunct Assistant Professor,
Pacific University, Forest Grove, Oregon; and University of California,
Berkeley, California

LEONID SKORIN, JR., OD, DO, FAAO, FAOCO

Staff Ophthalmologist, Albert Lea Eye Clinic, Mayo Health System, Albert Lea,
Minnesota; Adjunct Assistant Professor of Ophthalmology, Chicago College of
Osteopathic Medicine, Midwestern University, Downers Grove, Illinois; Clinical
Assistant Professor, Department of Neurology and Ophthalmology, College of
Osteopathic Medicine, Michigan State University, East Lansing, Michigan; Clinical
Assistant Professor of Ophthalmology and Visual Sciences, University of Illinois Eye
and Ear Infirmary, Chicago, Illinois; Adjunct Clinical Professor, College of Optometry,
Pacific University, Forest Grove, Oregon

NICKY R. HOLDEMAN, OD, MD, FAAO

Associate Professor, Associate Dean for Clinical Education, Executive Director,
University Eye Institute, Chief of Medical Services, University of Houston College
of Optometry, Houston, Texas

LIPPINCOTT WILLIAMS & WILKINS
A **Wolters Kluwer** Company
Philadelphia • Baltimore • New York • London
Buenos Aires • Hong Kong • Sydney • Tokyo

Acquisitions Editor: Jonathan Pine
Developmental Editor: Nicole T. Dernoski
Production Editor: Fran Gunning
Manufacturing Manager: Ben Rivera
Marketing Manager: Adam Glazer
Compositor: TechBooks
Printer: Edwards Brothers

First Edition, 1998, Lippincott Raven Publishers

Library of Congress Cataloging-in-Publication Data

Ocular therapeutics handbook : a clinical manual / [edited by] Bruce E. Onofrey, Leonid Skorin Jr., Nicky R. Holdeman.— 2nd ed.
    p. ; cm.
    Includes index.
    ISBN 0-7817-4892-5 (alk. paper)
1. Therapeutics, Ophthalmological—Handbooks, manuals, etc.   2. Ocular pharmacology—Handbooks, manuals, etc.   3. Ophthalmic drugs—Handbooks, manuals, etc.   4. Eye—Diseases—Handbooks, manuals, etc.   I. Onofrey, Bruce E. II. Skorin, Leonid.   III. Holdeman, Nicky R.
    [DNLM: 1. Eye Diseases—drug therapy—Handbooks.   2. Eye—drug effects—Handbooks.   3. Eye Diseases—diagnosis—Handbooks.   WW 39 O21 2005]
    RE991.O32 2005   617.7'061—dc22

                                                                        2005000258

Care has been taken to confirm the accuracy of the information presented and to describe generally accepted practices. However, the authors, editors, and publisher are not responsible for errors or omissions or for any consequences from application of the information in this book and make no warranty, expressed or implied, with respect to the currency, completeness, or accuracy of the contents of the publication. Application of this information in a particular situation remains the professional responsibility of the practitioner.

The authors, editors, and publisher have exerted every effort to ensure that drug selection and dosage set forth in this text are in accordance with current recommendations and practice at the time of publication. However, in view of ongoing research, changes in government regulations, and the constant flow of information relating to drug therapy and drug reactions, the reader is urged to check the package insert for each drug for any change in indications and dosage and for added warnings and precautions. This is particularly important when the recommended agent is a new or infrequently employed drug.

Some drugs and medical devices presented in this publication have Food and Drug Administration (FDA) clearance for limited use in restricted research settings. It is the responsibility of the health care provider to ascertain the FDA status of each drug or device planned for use in their clinical practice.

10 9 8 7 6 5 4 3 2 1

To primary care practitioners, the hardworking individuals that form the backbone of healthcare delivery, and to our families, who have always supported and encouraged our endeavors

CONTRIBUTORS

Jill C. Autry, OD, RPh
Adjunct Associate Professor
Department of Pharmacology
University of Houston College of
  Optometry
Houston, Texas

G. Richard Bennett, MS, OD
Associate Professor
Clinical Sciences
Pennsylvania College of Optometry
Director
The Glaucoma Service
Specialty Ophthalmology
The Eye Institute
Philadelphia, Pennsylvania

Helmut Buettner, MD
Professor of Ophthalmology
Department of Ophthalmology
Mayo Clinic
Mayo Medical School
Rochester, Minnesota

Andrew R. Buzzelli, OD, MS
Associate Professor
The Eye Institute
Pennsylvania College of
  Optometry
Philadelphia, Pennsylvania

Michael B. Caplan, MD
Glaucoma Subspecialist
Berkeley Eye Center
Houston, Texas

Steve Charles, MD
Ophthalmologist
Charles Retina Institute
Memphis, Tennessee

Brian Chou, OD
Private Practice
Carmel Mountain Vision Care
San Diego, California

Laurance Freier, OD
Private Practice
Fairfax, Virginia

Milan R. Genge, DO
Resident
Department of Ophthalmology
Midwestern University
Resident
Department of Ophthalmology
St. James Hospital
Olympia Fields, Illinois

Geoffrey J. Gladstone, MD
Oculoplastic Surgery
Southfield, Michigan

James A. Goodwin, MD
Director
Neuro-Ophthalmology Service
Department of Ophthalmology
University of Illinois at Chicago
Chicago, Illinois

Deepak Gupta, OD
Clinical Director
The Center for Keratocones
Stamford Ophthalmology
Stamford, Connecticut

Nicky R. Holdeman, OD, MD
Executive Director
University Eye Institute
Chief of Medical Services
Associate Dean for Clinical Education
College of Optometry
University of Houston
Houston, Texas

Ryan M. Hogan, OD
Private Practice
Limerick, Maine

Gregory G. Hom, OD, MPH
Private Practice
San Diego, California

Alan G. Kabat, OD
Associate Professor
College of Optometry
Nova Southeastern University
Attending Optometric Physician
The Eye Institute
Fort Lauderdale, Florida

Barry J. Kaufman, DO
Associate Clinical Professor
Ophthalmology
Midwestern University
Downers Grove, Illinois
Department of Ophthalmology
St. James Hospital
Olympia Fields, Illinois

Thomas J. Kelly, Jr., DO, MPH
Ophthalmologist
Vice President of Medical affairs
Union Hospital
Dover, Ohio

W. Craig Lannin, OD, DO
Staff Ophthalmologist
Department of Surgery
Mercy Medical Center
Redding, California

Andrew Mick, OD
Clinical Faculty
School of Optometry
University of California
Berkeley, California
Staff Optometrist
Student Extern Director
VA Medical Center
San Francisco, California

Bruce G. Muchnick, OD
Associate Professor
Department of Basic Sciences
Pennsylvania College of Optometry
Philadelphia, Pennsylvania
Staff Optometrist
Department of Optometry
Coatesville Veterans
   Administration Hospital
Coatesville, Pennsylvania

Richard F. Multack, OD, DO
Clinical Professor of Pharmacology
Adjunct Clinical Professor of Family
   Medicine
Chief, Ophthalmology Section
Department of Surgery
Midwestern University
Chicago College of Osteopathic Medicine
Downers Grove, Illinois
Chief, Ophthalmology Section
Department of Surgery
Saint James Hospitals and Medical Centers
Chicago Heights and
   Olympia Falls, Illinois

Shoib Myint, DO
Clinical Assistant Professor
Department of Ophthalmology
Wayne State University Kresge Eye Institute
Detroit, Michigan
Co-Director
Oculoplastic Surgery
Department of Ophthalmology
William Beaumont Hospital
Royal Oak, Michigan

Bruce E. Onofrey, RPh, OD
Vice-Chair Eye Services
Lovelace-Sandia Medical Center
Albuquerque, New Mexico
Adjunct Assistant Professor of Clinical
   Optometry
Pacific University and University of
   California
Berkeley, California

Anastas F. Pass, OD, MS, JD
Associate Professor
Chief Privacy Officer
College of Optometry
University Eye Institute
University of Houston
Houston, Texas

Marcus Piccolo, OD
Associate Professor and Associate Dean
   for Professional Advancement
University of Houston
College of Optometry
Houston, Texas

Christopher Quinn, OD
President
Omni Eye Services
Iselin, New Jersey

Mohammad R. Rafieetary, OD
Optometrist
Charles Retina Institute
Memphis, Tennessee

Lawrence D. Robbins, MD
Assistant Professor of Neurology
Department of Neurology
Rush Medical College
Chicago, Illinois
Attending Physician
Highland Park Hospital
Highland Park, Illinois

Padhmalatha Segu, OD
Clinical Associate Professor
College of Optometry
University of Houston
Houston, Texas

Jerome Sherman, OD
Distinguished Teaching Professor
Clinical Sciences
SUNY Optometry
New York, New York

John D. Siddens, DO
Clinical Instructor
Oculoplastic Surgery
Department of Ophthalmology
University of South Carolina School
   of Medicine
Columbia, South Carolina

Leonid Skorin, Jr., OD, DO
Staff Ophthalmologist
Albert Lea Eye Clinic
Mayo Health System
Albert Lea, Minnesota

Joseph W. Sowka, OD
Professor
College of Optometry
Nova Southeastern University
Fort Lauderdale, Florida

Loretta Szczotka-Flynn, OD, MS
Associate Professor
Ophthalmology
Case Western Reserve University
Director
Contact Lens Service
University Hospitals of
   Cleveland
Cleveland, Ohio

Tammy P. Than, MS, OD
Director
Primary Eye Care Services
University of Alabama at
   Birmingham School of Optometry
Birmingham, Alabama

Michael J. Trad, OD
Private Practice
Sterling, Illinois

James W. Walters, PhD, OD
Associate Professor
Director of the Ocular Diagnostic Service
University of Houston
College of Optometry
Houston, Texas

Suzanne M. Wickum, OD
Clinical Associate Professor
College of Optometry
University of Houston
Houston, Texas

Christopher Willingham, MD
Ophthalmologist
Charles Retina Institute
Memphis, Tennessee

REVIEWERS

Walter E. Beebe, MD
Cornea Associates of Texas
Dallas, Texas

Linda Casser, OD
Associate Dean for Academic
 Programs
Professor
Pacific University College of
 Optometry
Forest Grove, Oregon

Vernon Farthing, MD
Internal Medicine
Private Practice
University Medical Center;
Vice President
Medical Staff
Texas Tech University
Lubbock, Texas

Hani S. Ghazi-Birry, MS, MD, OD, PhD
Assistant Professor
Curriculum and Implementation
The Eye Center
Clinical Faculty
Southern College of
 Optometry
Memphis, Tennessee

John Goosey, MD
Houston Eye Associates
Houston, Texas

Jeffrey N. Holtzman, DO
Residency Program Director
Department of Ophthalmology
Metropolitan Hospital
Grand Rapids, Michigan;
Clinical Professor
Neurology & Ophthalmology
Michigan State University
College of Osteopathic Medicine
East Lansing, Michigan

Lawrence M. Kaufman, MD, PhD
Associate Professor of Clinical
 Ophthalmology
Department of Ophthalmology and Visual
 Science
University of Illinois at Chicago
Chicago, Illinois

Richard London, OD, MA
Professor
Department of Optometry
Pacific University College of Optometry
Forest Grove, Oregon

Danica J. Marrelli, OD
Clinical Associate Professor
University of Houston College of
 Optometry
Houston, Texas

Dawn Pewitt, OD
Staff Optometrist
Veterans Affairs Medical Center
Eye Clinic
VA San Diego Healthcare System
San Diego, California

Melissa L. Rice, OD
Senior Associate Consultant
Instructor of Ophthalmology
Department of Ophthalmology
Mayo Clinic
Rochester, Minnesota

Rosa A. Tang, MD, MPH
Medical Director
Professor
Ophthalmology and Surgery
Director of Neuro-ophthalmology,
UTMB–John Seely
Galveston, Texas

William D. Townsend, OD
Adjunct Professor
University of Houston, College of Optometry
Houston, Texas

Prathibha Varkey, MD, MPH
Assistant Professor
Preventive Medicine and Internal
  Medicine
Mayo Clinic
Rochester, Minnesota

Lesley L. Walls, OD, MD
President
Southern California College of
  Optometry
Fullerton, California

John J. Woog, MD
Consultant
Department of Ophthalmology
Mayo Clinic
Associate Professor
Department of Ophthalmology
Mayo Clinic College of Medicine
Rochester, Minnesota

Fiaz Zaman, MD
Houston Eye Associates
Houston, Texas

PREFACE TO THE SECOND EDITION

The second edition of *Ocular Therapeutics Handbook: A Clinical Manual* provides an understanding of various disease entities as well as expert recommendations for diagnosis and treatment of conditions most commonly encountered by eyecare providers. This book was designed to bridge the gap of information between the encyclopedic details found in some ophthalmic texts to the minimal information provided in others. The authors feel that the second edition provides key, concise, and essential information required to build a foundation in eye and systemic disorders most relevant to optometrists, optometry students, ophthalmology residents, medical students, as well as primary care and emergency room physicians who encounter various ophthalmic conditions.

The design of the book permits easy, rapid access of relevant data. Because of our problem-oriented approach, repetition of some material was unavoidable. However, the standardized format for most conditions allows clinicians to obtain the information necessary to provide appropriate care in a time-efficient manner. (While every attempt was made to verify drug concentration and dosage, we recommend that all practitioners check with the manufacturer prior to administering any drug.)

The second edition is not only updated and greatly expanded in scope of material, but an added feature is the inclusion of ICD–9 and CPT codes, which can be most helpful in proper coding and billing.

Lastly, this book is a compilation of many people's efforts, including the contributing authors and the consultants who reviewed the topics; each one deserves special thanks for his or her time and dedication. We are truly indebted to these many individuals for their expertise, experience, and advice, without which this project would never have come to fruition. The authors would also like to thank the editorial and production staff at Lippincott Williams & Wilkins for their support and patience throughout this endeavor.

Bruce E. Onofrey, RPh, OD
Leonid Skorin Jr, OD, DO
Nicky R. Holdeman, OD, MD

PREFACE TO THE FIRST EDITION

Following the publication of *Clinical Optometric Pharmacology and Therapeutics*, it became clear that a transportable companion handbook, based loosely on the larger reference, would be useful to consolidate and summarize a significant body of information. For most practitioners, time is a luxury in short supply. *Ocular Therapeutics Handbook*, directed at the needs of optometric physicians, nurses, and primary care physicians, has been designed to provide succinct, rapid-access information for the most common problems encountered in a primary care setting.

Our *Handbook* is divided into three sections for speedy perusal: Quick Reference, Ocular Therapeutics, and Appendices. The Quick Reference portion encompasses topics such as ocular microbiology, laboratory tests and procedures, pharmaceutical agents, and side effects of systemic medications. The Ocular Therapeutics section discusses disease (isolated and systemic), disorders, traumatic injuries, ocular urgencies, and emergencies. Finally, the appendices provide important phone numbers, common abbreviations, and conversion and extended-range keratometry charts. We have also included a model Grand Rounds and Case Report Sheet for daily use. With the help of our esteemed colleagues, we have also provided you with extensive chapters on Glaucoma, Retinal and Vitreous Disease, and Neuroophthalmic Disease. Readers will also find informative and reliable data regarding glaucoma agents.

The chapters have been developed to serve as a snapshot, presenting the clinician with the most relevant information regarding the pathophysiology and etiology of diseases, patient demographics, signs and symptoms, laboratory tests, and recommended approaches to treatment. We designed the book to be succinct, thorough, and consistent. Most of all, we have designed it to be practical and both quick and easy to use. If this *Handbook* serves its purpose, soon it will be ragged from coming out and going back into your pocket all day.

Without a doubt, the most valuable asset of this text is the contributors' clinical experience and grounding in primary care. In addition to the Doctor of Optometry degree, we also bring to you the clinical experience of a pharmacist, internist, retinologist, and neuroopthalmologist. It was with this unique collection of experienced clinicians that we endeavored to produce a relevant and clinically useful test for our colleagues in primary care.

It is only appropriate that we thank Laurance Freier, Ron Melton, Randall Thomas, Marcus Piccolo, Michael Caplan, W. Craig Lannin, Michael Trad, and Anastas Pass, the individuals who assisted in the writing, editing, and production of this text. Without the help of these talented and dedicated people, this project would not have seen its fruition.

Bruce E. Onofrey, RPh, OD
Leonid Skorin, Jr, OD, DO
Nicky R. Holdeman, OD, MD

CONTENTS

Chapter 1

Ocular Microbiology

QUICK REFERENCE SECTION
Bruce E. Onofrey

PRACTICE MANAGEMENT INFORMATION REGARDING THE HIV-INFECTED PATIENT

This chapter has been designed to provide the primary care clinician with guidelines to quickly and accurately assess, diagnose, and treat ocular infection. Tables 1.1 to 1.16 provide a quick reference to accomplish this. HIV infection management and prevention is an important component of primary care practice. Tables 1.17 to 1.20 highlight prevention guidelines and patient management information for HIV-infected patients.

Use of this information not only prevents the spread of this devastating disease, but it also minimizes the spread of opportunistic infections in immunocompromised patients.

▎ **TABLE 1.1** In-Office Materials for Microbiological Testing Procedures

Lab manual*
Lab micro order forms
Marking pen for labeling samples
Ophthalmic anesthetic
Microscope slides†
Microscope†
Sterile dacron swabs
Methyl alcohol
Distilled water source
Kimura spatula
Alcohol lamp
Bacterial/viral culturettes
Culture media
    blood agar
    chocolate agar
Commercial chlamydia transport kits (nonrefrigerated type)
Gram stain materials
Diff-Quick stain materials

Clinical Manual of Ocular Microbiology and Cytology by Susan Haesert, St. Louis, MO: Mosby, 1993, is highly recommended by this author.
†Only needed if you do your own stains.

▶ **TABLE 1.2** Classification of Bacterial Organisms Having Ocular Significance

I. GRAM-POSITIVE ORGANISMS
   A. Staphylococci
      1. *Staphylococcus aureus*
      2. *Staphylococcus epidermidis*
   B. Streptococci
      1. α-Hemolytic streptococcus
      2. β-Hemolytic streptococcus
      3. *Streptococcus pneumoniae*
   C. Bacilli (rods)
      1. *Bacillus*
         a. *B. anthracis*
         b. *B. cereus*
         c. *B. subtilis*
      2. *Corynebacterium*
         a. *C. diphtheria*
         b. *C. xerosis*
         c. *C. pseudodiphtheriticum*
      3. *Listeria* species
      4. *Nocardia* species
      5. *Mycobacterium* species

II. GRAM-NEGATIVE ORGANISMS
   A. *Neisseria*
      1. *N. gonorrhoeae*
      2. *N. meningitidis*
   B. Bacilli
      1. Enterobacteriaceae
         a. *Escherichia coli*
         b. *Shigella sonnei* and *S. flexneri*
         c. *Klebsiella pneumoniae* and *K. oxytoca*
         d. *Serratia marcescens* and *S. liquefaciens*
         e. *Proteus mirabilis* and *P. vulgaris*
      2. *Moraxella*
         a. *M. lacunata*
         b. *M. nonliquefaciens*
         c. *M. bovis*
      3. *Haemophilus*
         a. *H. influenzae*
         b. *H. aegyptius*
      4. *Brucella*
         a. *B. abortus*
         b. *B. suis*
         c. *B. melitensis*
      5. *Pseudomonas*
         a. *P. aeruginosa*
         b. *P. cepacia*

▌ TABLE 1.3 Characteristics of Common Eyelid Bacteria

Characteristic	Staphylococcus	Streptococcus	Haemophilus
Morphology	Spheroids in clusters	Spheroids in chains	Pleomorphic
Gram Stain	Positive	Positive	Negative
Pathogenesis	Exotoxins, enzymes	Tissue invasion and multiplication, enzymes	Unknown
Exudate	Suppurative	Serous	Suppurative
Ocular Presentation	Blepharitis, dysfunction of glands	Blepharitis, cellulitis	Blepharitis, cellulitis
Antibiotic Sensitivity	Bacitracin,* gentamicin,* cephalosporins, erythromycin	Penicillin,* erythromycin*	Penicillin,* polymyxin B,* sulfonamides, erythromycin
Antibiotic	Wide variation, sulfonamides <15%	Aminoglycosides	

*Antibiotics of choice.

▌ TABLE 1.4 Comparison of Aerobic and Anaerobic Bacteria Isolated from 131 Patients with Inflamed Conjunctivae and 60 Normal Patients

	Organisms	Inflamed Conjunctivae No. Patients	% of Total	Normal No. Patients	% of Total
ANAEROBES	Peptococcus	7	5.4	2	3.2
	Peptostreptococcus	10	8		
	Propionibacterium	30	22.9	6	10.0
	Bacteroides melaninogenicus	3	2.3		
	Bacillus fragilis	1	0.76		
	Actinomyces	1	0.76		
	Bifidobacterium	1	0.76		
	Fusobacterium	1	0.76		
AEROBES	Staphylococcus epidermidis	65	49.6	25	42
	Staphylococcus aureus	23	17.5	2	3.3
	Viridans streptococcus	17	13.0	5	8.3
	Group D Streptococcus	4	3.0	5	8.3
	β-Hemolytic Streptococcus Group A	3	2.3		
	Streptococcus pneumoniae	4	3.0		
	Lactobacillus	5	3.8		
	Diphtheroids	24	18.3	15	25.0
	Haemophilus influenzae	9	6.9		
	Neisseria species	9	6.9	3	5
	Neisseria meningitidis	2	1.5		
	Acinetobacter	1	0.76	1	1.6
	Klebsiella pneumoniae	1	0.76	1	1.6
	Pseudomonas species	1	0.76	2	3.3
	Escherichia coli	2	1.5		
	Candida	1	0.76	3	5.0

(From: Brook I, Pettit TH, Martin WJ, Finegold SM. Anaerobic and aerobic bacteriology of acute conjunctivitis. *Ann Ophthalmol* 1979; 3:389.)

▶ TABLE 1.5 Common Microbiological Stains

Stain	Purpose
Gram stain	Differentiate gram (+) blue and gram (−) red organisms
Diff-Quick	Differentiates white blood cell types in eye disease; i.e.,
	Bacterial—neutrophils
	Viral—lymphocytes
	Allergic—eosinophils and basophils
	Vernal—mast cells/lymphocytes
Giemsa	Identifies cellular inclusion bodies in chlamydial infection
Calcofluor	Identification of *Acanthameoba*

▶ TABLE 1.6 Gram Stain Procedure

Fix smear in methanol for 5 min, then allow to air dry.
Flood with crystal gentian violet for 1 min.
Rinse with tap water.
Flood with Gram's iodine for 1 min.
Rinse with tap water.
Decolorize with acid alcohol until solvent flows clearly from the slide (10 to 20 s).
Rinse with tap water.
Counterstain with safranin, flood for 1 min.
Rinse with tap water.
Air dry or blot gently.

▶ TABLE 1.7 Diff-Quick Stain

Fix smear in methanol for 5 min, then air dry.
Dip slide in fixative 5 × −1 s each/then drain.
Dip slide in solution I 5 × −1 s each/then drain.
Dip slide in solution II 5 × −1 s each/then drain.
Rinse slide in distilled water.
Air dry or blot gently.

▶ TABLE 1.8 Giemsa Stain Procedure

Fix smear in methanol for 5 min.
Prepare fresh stain by adding 1 mL Giemsa stain and 2 mL Paragon buffer to 47 mL distilled water in Coplin jar.
Immerse slide in stain and incubate for 1 h.
Dip twice into ethyl alcohol to rinse.
Rinse with tap water.
Air dry.

▶ TABLE 1.9 Common Ophthalmic Culture Media and Usage

Media	Composition	Usage
Blood agar	Defibrinated sheep's blood	Detect hemolytic activity
Chocolate agar	Heat denaturalized sheep's blood + nutrients	Best medium for *Hemophilus* and *Neisseria*
Sabaroud's medium	Glucose/peptone and antibiotics	Fungal culture media
Thioglycolate broth	Sodium thioglycollate	General culture media/ improved anaerobe growth
Brain–heart infusion broth	Beef brain and heart/protease/dextrose/ neopeptone/gentamycin	Fungal growth media
Thayer Martin medium	Modified chocolate agar with nutrients and selected antibiotics	Best for *Neisseria*

▶ TABLE 1.10 Antibiotic Susceptibility of Various Pathogens *In Vitro*

	Ampicillin	Bactracin	Cefa-mandole
GRAM-POSITIVE COCCI			
S. epidermidis	+	+	+
S. aureus	−	+	
Methicillin resistant	−	+	+
Staphylococcus sp.			−
β-Hemolytic streptococci	+	+	+
β-Hemolytic streptococci	+	+	+
S. faecalis	+	+	−
S. pneumoniae	+	+	+
Anaerobic Streptococcus sp.	+	+	+
GRAM-POSITIVE BACILLI			
Bacillus anthracis	0	+	−+
Bacillus sp.	0	+	0
Clostridium sp.	0	−+	−+
Cornybacterium sp.	+	+	+
L. monocytogenes	+	0	0
GRAM-NEGATIVE COCCI			
N. gonorrhoeae	+	+	−+
N. meningitidis	+	+	−+
GRAM-NEGATIVE BACILLI			
Acinetobacter sp.	−	−	−
B. fragilis	−	0	−
Bacteroides sp.	+	0	+
Bordetella pertussis	0	0	0
Brucella sp.	0	0	0
Enterobacter sp.	+	0	−+
E. coli	+	0	+
Francisella tularensis	0	0	0
H. influenzae	+	+	−+
Klebsiella sp.	−	0	+
Moraxella sp.	+	0	−+
Pasturella multocida	0	0	0
Proteus mirabilis	+	−	−+
P. aeruginosa	−	−	−
Salmonella sp.	+	−	0
Serratia sp.	−	0	−
Shigella sp.	+	−	0
OTHERS			
Actinomyces sp.	+	+	−+
C. trachomatis	−	0	0
Mycobacterium fortuitum	0	0	0
Mycobacterium marinum	0	0	0
Nocardia sp.	+	0	0
Toxoplasma gondii	−	−	−

Cefa-zolin	Chloram-phenicol	Clinda-mycin	Erythro-mycin	Genta-micin	Methic-illin	Moxa-lactam
+	−+	−+	−+	+ +	+	+
+	−+	−+	−+	+	+	+
−	0	−	−	−	−	−
+	+	+	+	−	+	+
+	+	+	+	−+	+	+
−	0	−	−	−	−+	−
+	+	+	+	−	+	+
+	+	+	+	−	−+	+
−+	+	0	+	0	0	−+
−	+	0	+	+	0	0
−+	−+	−+	−+	−	0	−+
−	0	0	+	0	0	0
−	+	0	+	0	0	0
−	+	+	+	−+	−+	+
−	+	−|	+	−+	−+	0
−	0	0	−	+	−	0
−	+	+	−	−	−	−+
−	+	+	+	−	−	+
0	0	0	+	0	−	0
0	+	0	+	0	−	0
−	+	−	−	+	−	+
−+	+	−	−	+	−	+
0	+	0	0	0	−	0
−	+	+	−+	−+	−	+
−+	+	−	−	+	−	+
−+	0	0	+	−+	−	+
−	0	0	0	0	−	0
−+	−+	−	−	+	−	+
−	−	−	−	+	−	−+
−	+	0	−	+	−	+
−	−+	−	−	+	−	+
−	+	0	−	0	−	+
−+	+	+	0	−	0	0
0	+	0	+	−	−	0
0	0	0	+	0	0	0
0	0	0	0	0	0	0
0	0	0	0	0	0	0
−	−	+	−	−	−	−

(continued)

▶ **TABLE 1.10 Antibiotic Susceptibility of Various Pathogens
        *In Vitro (Continued)***

	Neomycin	Penicillin G	Polymyxin B
GRAM-POSITIVE COCCI			
S. epidermidis	−+	−+	−
S. aureus			
Methicillin resistant	−+	−	−
Staphylococcus sp.	0	−	−
α-Hemolytic streptococci	−	+	−
β-Hemolytic streptococci	−	+	−
S. faecalis	−	+	−
S. pneumoniae	−	+	−
Anaerobic Streptococcus sp.	−	+	0
GRAM-POSITIVE BACILLI			
Bacillus anthracis	0	+	−
Bacillus sp.	0	−+	−
Clostridium sp.	−	+	−
Cornybacterium sp.	0	+	−
L. monocytogenes	0	−+	−
GRAM-NEGATIVE COCCI			
N. gonorrhoeae	+	+	−
N. meningitidis	+	+	−
GRAM-NEGATIVE BACILLI			
Acinetobacter sp.	0	−	+
B. fragilis	−	−	−
Bacteroides sp.	−	+	−
Bordetella pertussis	0	0	0
Brucella sp.	0	0	0
Enterobacter sp.	−+	−	+
E. coli	+	−	+
Francisella tularensis	0	0	0
H. influenzae	−+	−+	−+
Klebsiella sp.	+	−	+
Moraxella sp.	+	+	+
Pasturella multocida	0	+	+
Proteus mirabilis	+	−	−
P. aeruginosa	−+	−	+
Salmonella sp.	0	−+	+
Serratia sp.	+	−	−
Shigella sp.	0	−+	+
OTHERS			
Actinomyces sp.	−	+	0
C. trachomatis	−	−	0
Mycobacterium fortuitum	0	0	0
Mycobacterium marinum	0	0	0
Nocardia sp.	0	0	0
Toxoplasma gondii	−	−	−

Rifampin	Sulfonamides	Tetracycline	Tobramycin	Trimethoprim/Sulfa	Vancomycin
−+	−+	−+	+	+	+
−+	−+	−+	+	+	+
+	0	0	−+	0	+
−	−+	−+	−	+	+
+	−	−+	−	+	+
0	−+	−+	−+	−+	+
+	−+	−+	−	+	+
0	0	−+	−	0	0
+	0	+	0	0	+
0	0	0	+	0	0
+	0	−+		0	+
+	0	0	0	0	+
0	0	+	0	0	0
+	−	+	−+	0	−
+	−	+	−+	0	−
0	0	−+	+	+	−
0	0	−	−	−	−
0	0	−+	−	−	−
0	0	0	0	+	−
0	+	+	0		−
0	−+	−+	+	+	−
−+	−+	−+	+	+	−
0	0	+	0	0	−
−+	−+	−+	−+	+	−
+	−	−+	+	+	−
0	+	0	−+	+	−
0	0	+	0	+	−
+	−	−	+	+	−
−+	−	−+	+	−	−
0	−	0	+	+	−
0	−	−	+	+	−
0	−	−+	0	+	−
0	+	−+	−	0	+
−+	+	+	−	+	−
−	−	−	0	0	−
+	−	−	0	+	−
0	+	+	0	+	0
0	−	−+	−	+	−

▶ **TABLE 1.11** **Management of Acute Conjunctivitis**

Thorough history and clinical examination
Bacterial and viral cultures
Consider chlamydial culture if sexually active
Gram and Diff-Quick stains
Suspect *Hemophilus* in children if history of URI or otitis media
Staphylococcus and *Streptococcus* most common in adults
Select appropriate antibiotic treatment and reevaluate after culture results returned

▶ **TABLE 1.12** **Management of Chronic Conjunctivitis**

Thorough history and evaluation
Discontinue ineffective therapies, i.e., antibiotic/steroid/decongestants
Consider trial with nonpreserved artifical tears
Cultures for:
    bacteria
    viral
    chlamydia (most common cause of chronic conjunctivitis)
Gram and Diff-Quick stains
Treatment based on cultures and clinical evaluation

▶ **TABLE 1.13 Clinical Documentation and Management of Bacterial Keratitis**

Thorough history and clinical examination
Drawing or photo of ulcer. Drawing should indicate:
  Size
  Depth
  Suppuration
  Anterior chamber reaction, i.e., is there a hypopion presence of neovascularization?
Gram stain
Take cultures from:
  Contact lenses if worn
  Conjunctiva (without anesthetic)
  Corneal scraping (delay scraping for 3–5 minutes after anesthetic instilled)
Plate samples on blood, chocolate, and Sabouraud's media
Initial therapy based on Gram stain results
If no Gram stain, then treat noncentral ulcers with ciprofloxacin or ofloxacin ophthalmic solution
  5 drops in 5 min, then every 15 min for 4 h, then every 1 h till bedtime, then every 2 h after bedtime
Polytrim with the fluoroquinolone—synergistic for *Pseudomonas*
If poor response or central, consider fortified antibiotic treatment (see fortified antibiotic
  preparation guide)
Cycloplegia prn anterior uveitis management
Monitor and manage increased IOP
Steroids when and if indicated

▶ **TABLE 1.14 General Time Course of Herpes Simplex Blepharoconjunctivitis**

Primary symptoms	2–3 wk
Lid lesion	2–3 wk
Follicular conjunctivitis	4–8 wk (persists 4–6 mo)
Papillary reaction (upper lid)	4–8 wk (persists 6 mo or more)
Overall disease	2–3 wk
	3–5 wk (severe)
Primary active disease	17.6 d (untreated)
	11 d (treated)
Recurrent active disease	28.4 d (untreated)
	22.1 d (treated)

▶ **TABLE 1.15 Differential Diagnosis of Herpes Simplex Blepharoconjunctivitis**

Disease	Pathogen	Age of Onset	Symptoms	Signs
Herpes simplex blepharoconjunctivitis	Herpes simplex virus	Childhood to adulthood	Malaise, fever, watery/mucoid discharge, photophobia, resp. infect.	Unilateral preauricular lymphadenopathy
Herpes zoster	Varicella	Middle-aged and older	Malaise, fever, nausea, lancing pain, hyperesthesia	Unilateral
Chickenpox	Varicella	Childhood	Malaise, fever, itching	Bilateral
Blepharitis	Staphylococcus	Childhood to adulthood	Grittiness, itching, tearing, burning	Bilateral
Epidemic keratoconjunctivitis	Adenovirus 8 or 19	Childhood	Fever, foreign body sensation, watery discharge	Starts unilateral, then bilateral
Pharyngoconjunctival fever	Adenovirus 3 or 7	Childhood	Fever, pharyngitis	Bilateral
Inclusion conjunctivitis	Chlamydia	Young adults	Watery/mucoid discharge, foreign body sensation, urethritis, cervicitis	Preauricular lymphadenopathy

Vesicles (Distribution)	Conjunctivitis	Cornea	Distinguishing Feature	Treatment
Random, single, lid area	Lower lid: follicular Upper lid: papillae, pseudomembrane	+ Infiltrates, decreased corneal sensation	Dendrite	Antiviral ointment or drops, observation
Follows path of nerve in groups, lid and upper face	Nonspecific	+	Neuralgia	Steroids, analgesics, antivirals (acyclovir)
Random, scalp and trunk	Papillary	+/−	Itching	Supportive
Ulceration, lid margin	Papillary	+ Infiltrates	Collarettes, madarosis	Antibiotics, lid scrubs and hygiene
	Follicular	+ Infiltrates, SPK	Time frame of signs	Supportive
	Follicular	+ SPK	Swimming pools	Supportive (cold compresses)
	Papillary and follicular	+ Infiltrates, SPK, keratitis	New sex partner	Oral antibiotics (tetracycline, erythromycin)

▶ **TABLE 1.16** Common Fungal Isolates in Keratomycosis

Moniliaceous Filamentous Fungi (Nonpigmented)	Dematiaceous Filamentous Fungi (Pigmented)	Yeasts
Acremonium sp. (Cephlosporium sp.)	Alternaria sp.	Candida albicans, C. parapsilosis, C. tropicalis*
Aspergillus flavus, A. fumigatus, A. niger*	Cladosporium sp.	
Fusarium solani, F. oxysporum, F. episphaeria, F. monilforme	Curvularia sp.	
Paecilomyces sp.	Drechslera sp. (Helminthosporium sp.)	
Penicillium sp.*	Phialophora sp.	
Pseudallescheria boydii (Petriellidum boydii; Allescheria boydii)		

*Commonly cultured from the eyelid.
(Data modified from Liesegang TJ, Forster RK. Spectrum of microbial keratitis in south Florida. *Am. J. Ophthalmol* 1980; 90:30; and O'Day DM. Fungal keratitis. In: Liebowitz HM, ed. *Corneal Disorders: Clinical Diagnosis and Management*. Philadelphia: WB Saunders, 1989, 420.)

▶ **TABLE 1.17** Universal Precautions

1. Gloves should be worn by all health-care workers coming into direct contact with blood and body fluids, mucous membranes, or nonintact skin and for handling objects contaminated with such. After the examination, hands should be thoroughly washed with soap and water.
2. Hands should be washed immediately and thoroughly if contaminated with blood or body fluids.
3. Masks may be worn by health-care workers who have direct or sustained contact with patients with AIDS, especially if the patient is coughing or when procedures are likely to generate droplets of blood or other body fluids.
4. Protective eyewear should be worn when procedures are likely to produce droplets of blood or body fluids.
5. Gowns or aprons should be worn during procedures likely to generate splashes of blood or body fluids.
6. Needles and syringes should be disposed of in rigid wall puncture-proof containers. Needles should not be bent or broken after use or resheathed or removed from disposable syringes.

▶ **TABLE 1.18** Disinfection Guidelines*

Instruments coming in direct contact with ocular surfaces should be cleaned and then disinfected with one of the following solutions:

1. 5- to 10-min exposure to fresh hydrogen peroxide (3%).
2. Fresh 1:10 dilution of common household bleach (5.25% sodium hypochlorite).
3. 70% ethanol.
4. 70% isopropanol; rinse and dry all instruments with tap water before reuse.

Contact lenses
1. Disinfect trial hard lenses with a commercially available hydrogen peroxide system or a standard heating unit for contact lenses.
2. Rigid gas-permeable lenses can be disinfected using a contact lens hydrogen peroxide solution.
3. Soft lenses can be disinfected using either heat or hydrogen peroxide.

*Data from *CDC update MMWR* 1986; 35:17.

▶ **TABLE 1.19** Nonocular Pathogens Reported Among AIDS Patients

Disease	Reported Cases (%)
Pneumocystis carinii pneumonia	63
Candida	14
Cytomegalovirus	7
Cryptococcus	7
Herpes simplex	4
Cryptosporidiosis	4
Toxoplasma gondii	3
Other	3

(From *CDC update MMWR* 1986; 35:17.)

▶ **TABLE 1.20** Differential Diagnosis of Cytomegalovirus (CMV) Infection Cotton Wool Spots

Feature	CMV Infection	Cotton Wool Spots
Appearance	Granular/feathery	Fluffy with diffuse edges
Course	Enlarge over time	Evanescent/decreased size
Blood	Present	Absent
Location	Deep retina/perivascular	Superficial retina
Number	One or two foci initially	Scattered/multiple
Color	Opaque at borders	Opaque throughout
Visual field defect	Absolute scotoma	No defect

Chapter 2

Common Laboratory Tests and Procedures

COMMON LABORATORY TESTS AND PROCEDURES

Laurance Freier and Bruce E. Onofrey

Laboratory tests can provide valuable information about the blood and many organ systems. They can be used to:

- Screen for certain diseases or conditions (infections, inflammatory processes, neoplasms, and so forth).
- Assess the function of a particular organ or system.
- Help with a differential diagnosis (e.g., in the case of a patient with chest pain, an acute myocardial infarction would show an elevated ESR test versus angina pectoris, in which the ESR would remain normal).
- Confirm a diagnosis (e.g., if a patient shows a positive VDRL test and a positive FTA-ABS test, a diagnosis of syphilis would be confirmed).
- Rule out diseases (e.g., if a patient shows a negative ANA test, systemic lupus erythematosus can almost certainly be ruled out).
- Follow the course of a disease and help monitor the effects of treatment (e.g., an ESR test will generally increase if a disease worsens and decrease as the disease improves).
- Determine compliance with medications.
- Determine whether a disease is in its active or dormant state.
- Check for drug toxicities and side effects of medications.
- Determine if a patient is in a risk group for a particular disease.
- Help identify systemic disorders that have ophthalmic manifestations.
- Determine whether a disease has spread systemically.
- Detect a disease that is otherwise not expected.

Knowledge of laboratory tests helps ensure appropriate patient care, facilitates communication with other health-care professionals, and assists in good patient education.

Every laboratory test has reference (or normal) values. Reference values are used as a general guide to help clinicians identify diseased patients. They can also be used to monitor the effects and course of therapy. Reference values, however, should not be considered as rigid dividers of normal from abnormal. Many factors can cause variations in laboratory test results, including the effects of medication; the presence of concurrent diseases; the effects of diet, age, sex, race, and emotional status; how the patient was prepared; patient posture; and intrapersonal differences (in a particular patient, the concentration of some substances may vary from day to day or even during the course of a day). Therefore, a definite diagnosis should not be made on the basis of a single test result. All laboratory tests should be evaluated in light of the patient's other clinical findings. Tests may have to be repeated, or a combination of test panels may be needed before a diagnosis can be confirmed. Reference values also vary from lab to lab because of differences in instrumentation and methodology. It is important, therefore, that the clinician only use reference values standardized by the laboratory that actually performed a particular test. Errors in interpretation can result if a clinician attempts to apply the reference values of one laboratory to the test results received from another laboratory. One common practice is to compare the patient's present laboratory results with the patient's previous values (these act as the patient's own reference values).

Clinicians should be aware of the possible effects of any medications a patient is taking on the results of a test. If a patient is taking a drug that is known to affect a particular test, the patient's physician should be consulted and the drug, if possible, should be discontinued or its initiation postponed until after the completion of the test. If this is not possible, any drugs the patient is taking should be noted on the laboratory request form.

The following sections describe some of the many laboratory tests that are available.

ANCA (ANTINEUTROPHIL CYTOPLASMIC ANTIBODY) TESTING
CPT: 86255

P-ANCA (Perinuclear antineutrophil cytoplasmic antibody)
C-ANCA (Cytoplasmic antineutrophil cytoplasmic antibody)

The antineutrophil cytoplasmic antibodies (ANCA) represent a group of antibodies directed against cytoplasmic components of neutrophil granulocytes and monocytes.

The gold standard of ANCA determination remains indirect immunofluorescence (IIF) on ethanol fixed neutrophils. Two main patterns can be distinguished: (a) a cytoplasmic pattern of course granular fluorescence with accentuation in the area of the nuclear lobes (cytoplasmic or C-ANCA; formerly termed "ACPA" for anticytoplasmic antibodies), and (b) a perinuclear pattern (P-ANCA). The specificity of this test depends on the ability of the laboratory personnel to distinguish these two patterns from a more diffuse cytoplasmic staining pattern and granulocyte-specific antinuclear antibody (GS-ANA) staining. In addition, without additional testing, determination of the P-ANCA pattern is not possible in most antinuclear antibody–positive sera. The P-ANCA staining pattern represents an artifact of ethanol fixation, which allows cationic proteins to move to the negatively charged nuclear membrane. This staining pattern reverts to a cytoplasmic fluorescence pattern if cross-linking fixatives such as formalin are used to prepare the neutrophil substrate. These formalin-fixed neutrophils can be used in special circumstances to allow the distinction of a true P-ANCA from an ANA (Table 2.1).

▶ **TABLE 2.1** The Target Antigens and Clinical Disease Associated with the P-ANCA and C-ANCA Tests

IFA-Pattern	Target Antigen	Associated Disease
P-ANCA	MPO	Churg-Strauss Syndrome
		Microscopic Polyangitis
	Lactoferrin	Lupus Erythematosus (SLE)
		Rheumatoid Arthritis
	Unknown antigens	Crohn's Disease
	Cathespin G	
	Unknown antigens	Ulcerative Colitis
	Unknown antigens	Chronic Hepatitis
C-ANCA	PR3	Wegener's Granulomatosis
		Microscopic Polyangiitis
	Unknown antigens	HIV

ANERGY PANEL
CPT: 83063

Reference Values

Reactive versus nonreactive

The anergy panel is used to verify a patient's ability to exhibit a delayed hypersensitivity response. It is commonly used in combination with the tuberculin PPD skin test as a control. This serves to validate a negative PPD test.

A common antigen such as mumps, candida, or trichophytin is injected intradermally at the same time as the PPD tuberculin test. An individual with a normal immune response would produce a localized reaction to the injection within 48 to 72 hours. A lack of reaction suggests that the patient's immune system is compromised and therefore the results of a negative PPD test would be less conclusive. Such an individual should undergo a chest x-ray and sputum testing.

ANGIOTENSIN-CONVERTING ENZYME (ACE) TEST
CPT: 82164

Reference Values

23–57 U/mL (Units = nanomoles per minute)

The ACE test is used to help diagnose and manage patients with sarcoidosis. Serum levels of ACE are increased in 85% of patients with active sarcoidosis. The ACE test is primarily used to evaluate the severity of the sarcoidosis and its response to therapy. Angiotensin converting enzyme is found in pulmonary epithelial cells. It converts angiotensin I to angiotensin II, a potent vasoconstrictor. The ACE test is therefore sometimes used to evaluate special cases of hypertension. Clinical disorders that may increase ACE levels include active histoplasmosis, amyloidosis, alcoholic cirrhosis, diabetes mellitus, Gaucher's disease (a familial disorder of fat metabolism), Hodgkin's disease, hyperthyroidism, leprosy, pulmonary embolism, idiopathic pulmonary fibrosis, scleroderma, and tuberculosis. ACE levels may be decreased in patients with sarcoidosis who are treated with prednisone. The ACE test is not done on patients <20 years old, because this age group normally has very high levels.

Procedure
- Five milliliters of venous blood is collected.
- The sample is taken to the lab.

ANTINUCLEAR ANTIBODY (ANA) TEST
CPT: 86038–86039

Reference Values

Negative—no ANA detected

ANAs are immunoglobulin protein antibodies (IgG, IgM, IgA) that react against the nuclear material in leukocytes. They act as antibodies against DNA, RNA, and other nucleoproteins. The ANA test was developed to assess tissue-antigen antibodies. It is often used to diagnose systemic lupus erythematosus (SLE), an autoimmune collagen disease. Patients with autoimmune diseases have many abnormal antibodies. Two antinuclear antibodies, anti-DNA and antideoxyribose nucleoprotein (anti-DNP), are almost always present in patients with SLE. The ANA test is quite sensitive in detecting SLE (approximately 95% of patients with SLE will show a positive ANA) but is not very specific, because many other disorders can cause a positive ANA. The ANA is therefore often used as a screening test for SLE. A negative ANA would suggest that it is unlikely that the patient has SLE. When a patient has a positive ANA, along with a positive LE (lupus erythematosus) prep, then SLE would be strongly suspected.

Other disorders that can cause a positive ANA include systemic sclerosis, scleroderma, rheumatoid arthritis, myasthenia gravis, leukemia, cirrhosis of the liver, ulcerative colitis, and infectious mononucleosis. Many drugs can also cause a positive ANA, including penicillin, tetracycline, acetazolamide, thiazides, and oral contraceptives.

Procedure
- Five to 7 milliliters of venous blood is collected in a red-top tube.
- The serum is then incubated with traumatized rat's liver to obtain the antinuclear immune complex.
- The mixture is then incubated with fluorescein-labeled antihuman serum (to tag any immune complex).
- The preparation is then examined under an ultraviolet microscope for fluorescent ANAs.
- The patient's serum is then serially diluted, and the ANA test is performed on each dilution (the most dilute serum in which the ANAs can be detected is called the *titer*).
- The test is considered positive if ANAs are detected in a titer with a dilution greater than 1:32.
- The pattern of nuclear fluorescence is also documented (this pattern is considered equally important in determining whether or not a patient has SLE or other autoimmune disease).
- A positive ANA should then be compared with other tests for SLE.

ANTICARDIOLIPIN PROFILE
CPT: 86147

Reference Values

<23 GPL (IgG phospholipid units)
<11 MPL (IgL phospholipid units)

This test is positive in some patients with SLE. The presence of this antibody places the patient at higher risk for "antiphospholipid syndrome" (venous or arterial thrombosis, thrombocytopenia, recurrent spontaneous abortions). This test is performed on those who test positive for SLE to identify those at risk for the aforementioned complications.

Interfering Factors
- Patients who have had syphilis can produce a false-positive on this test.
- Patients with infections, HIV-positive status, inflammatory disease, or cancer can produce false-negative results.
- The drugs chlorpromazine, procainamide, phenytoin, penicillin, hydralazine, and quinidine can produce false-positive results.

BLEEDING TIME
CPT: 85002

Reference Values

Normal range: 1–9 minutes
Critical value: >15 minutes

The bleeding time is a test to evaluate the vascular and platelet factors associated with hemostasis. When vascular injury occurs, the first hemostatic response is a spastic contraction of the injured microvessels. Next, platelets adhere to the injured area. Failure of either process results in prolonged bleeding time.

Procedure

A small, standardized incision is made in the forearm, and the time required for the bleeding to stop is recorded. Because vessel constriction and platelet adherence are not affected by coagulation (intrinsic and extrinsic), defects in this system will not affect this test. It should be noted that the bleeding time is only an indirect method of platelet function. A complete blood count (CBC) should be performed to identify this directly.

BLOOD UREA NITROGEN (BUN) TEST
CPT: 84520

Reference Values

Men: 10–25 mg/dL
Women: 8–20 mg/dL
Children: 5–20 mg/dL
Infants: 5–15 mg/dL

The BUN test is one of the most commonly ordered tests to assess kidney function. The BUN measures the amount of urea nitrogen found in the blood. Urea is formed in the liver as an end product of protein metabolism. It circulates in the blood and is excreted by the kidneys. The concentration of urea in the blood is directly related to how well the kidneys are excreting it. The BUN, therefore, is used as an indicator of kidney function.

Most renal diseases decrease the kidney's ability to excrete urea. The result is an increased BUN level. Other problems can also increase the BUN level. Dehydration from diarrhea, vomiting, or inadequate fluid intake can cause the BUN to elevate up to 50 mg/dL. The BUN should return to normal once the patient is rehydrated; if it does not, renal or prerenal failure should be suspected. Excessive protein intake causes the body to make large quantities of urea. The kidneys may become overloaded and be unable to excrete the excess urea. The BUN level will then rise. Gastrointestinal bleeding, diabetes, renal insufficiency because of shock, and sepsis can all cause increased BUN levels. Many drugs can also elevate the BUN, including diuretics; antibiotics such as bacitracin, gentamicin, and neomycin; antihypertensive agents; sulfonamides; and salicylates. Older patients may also show an increased BUN, because the amount of nephrons tends to decrease with age. Because urea is formed in the liver, decreased BUN levels are seen in patients with severe liver damage. Low BUN levels may also indicate overhydration, malnutrition, or a low-protein diet. Pregnancy, which causes an increase in fluid volumes, also reduces the BUN. Phenothiazines can also reduce the BUN.

Procedure

- Five to 7 milliliters of venous blood is collected in a gray-top tube.
- The sample is sent to the chemistry lab. A multifunctional analysis machine determines the BUN.
- Some labs prefer that the patient has not eaten for 8 hours before the test.

CHLAMYDIA TESTING
CPT: 86631–86632, 87270, 87320, 87110

Reference Values

Negative versus positive

There are several traditional and more advanced methods of testing for chlamydia. The methods are as follows:

Enzyme-linked immunosorbent assay (ELISA, EIA). This common, rapid test detects substances (chlamydia antigens) that trigger the immune system to fight a chlamydia infection. EIA testing is done by taking a sample of secretions from the potentially affected area.
Direct fluorescent antibody test (DFA). This common, rapid test detects chlamydia antigens. DFA testing is done by taking a sample of secretions from the potentially affected area.
Nucleic acid amplification tests (NAAT). These tests detect the genetic material (DNA) of chlamydia bacteria. Testing can be done on either a urine specimen or a sample of secretions from the potentially affected area. Polymerase chain reaction (PCR) and ligase chain reaction (LCR) testing are examples of nucleic acid amplification tests.

Nucleic acid hybridization tests (DNA probe testing). Probe testing also detects chlamydia DNA. Probe testing is very accurate and can be done by taking a sample of secretions from the potentially affected area. DNA probe testing is not as sensitive as nucleic acid amplification tests.

Chlamydia culture. A culture provides the right environment for chlamydia bacteria to grow. This test is expensive and not commonly done. It requires high technical skills and results take 5 to 7 days. The chlamydia culture test is usually done when the number of bacteria is very low, when child sexual abuse is suspected, or when treatment for infection has failed.

CHOLESTEROL SERUM
CPT: 82465

Reference Values

Adults: Less than 200 mg/dL - Desirable 200–239 mg/dL - Borderline greater than or equal to 240 mg/dL - High
Children: 120–240 mg/dL
Infants: 70–175 mg/dL

Serum cholesterol levels are used in the diagnosis and management of atherosclerosis and coronary artery disease. They can also be used as an indicator of liver function because cholesterol is synthesized by the liver.

Cholesterol is a blood lipid. It is found in red blood cells, cell membranes, and muscle. Approximately 70% of cholesterol is in an esterified form (i.e., combined with fatty acids) and 30% is in the free form. Plasma cholesterol can be fractionated into high-density lipoprotein cholesterol (HDL-C), which makes up approximately 25% of the total cholesterol and normally ranges from 40 to 60 mg/dL, low-density lipoprotein cholesterol (LDL-C), and very-low-density lipoprotein cholesterol (VLDL-C). The body uses cholesterol to form bile salts for fat digestion and to form hormones made in the adrenal glands, testes, and ovaries. Hypercholesterolemia can lead to the formation of plaques in the coronary and carotid arteries. Elevated cholesterol levels (>250 mg/dL) may be seen in atherosclerosis, acute myocardial infarction (MI), hypothyroidism, biliary obstruction, uncontrolled diabetes mellitus, familial hypercholesterolemia, type II hyperlipoproteinemia, high-stress periods, high-cholesterol diet (animal fats), and pregnancy. Decreased cholesterol levels may be associated with hyperthyroidism, Cushing's syndrome (adrenal hormone excess), anemias, acute infections, and malabsorption. Drugs that may decrease the serum cholesterol include the antibiotics neomycin and tetracycline, corticosteroids such as cortisone, estrogens, glucagon, hypoglycemic agents, thyroxine, heparin, nicotinic acid, and aspirin. Drugs that may elevate the serum cholesterol include epinephrine, norepinephrine, steroids, androgens, oral contraceptives, sulfonamides, Thorazine, vitamins A and D, and aspirin.

Procedure

- The patient is kept NPO (no food, fluids, or medications) for 12 hours. Water is permitted. (Patient should have had a normal diet for at least 2 weeks before the test.)

If possible, lipid-lowering drugs, steroidal contraceptives, and thyroid medication should be avoided for at least 3 weeks.

- Five to 10 milliliters of venous blood is collected in a red-top tube.
- The blood sample is taken to the lab.
- Any drugs that are not withheld should be listed.

CBC WITH DIFFERENTIAL
CPT: 85025–85027

The CBC with differential is a group of tests that can provide a great deal of information about the condition of the blood and many organ systems. It is often used because it is inexpensive and easily performed. The test includes six components: (a) a red blood cell (RBC) count; (b) hemoglobin (Hb or Hgb); (c) hematocrit (Hct); (d) red blood cell characteristics (mean corpuscular volume [MCV], mean corpuscular hemoglobin [MCH], and mean corpuscular hemoglobin concentration [MCHC]); (e) a white blood cell (WBC) count; and (f) a differential WBC.

Procedure

- Peripheral venipuncture is performed using a 20-gauge needle.
- Seven milliliters of blood is obtained in an oxalate-containing Vacutainer (lavender top).
- The blood tube is tilted up and down several times to ensure adequate mixing of blood and the anticoagulant oxalate.
- The specimen is then sent to the hematology lab for analysis.
- A differential count is performed by examination of 1 mm^3 of a blood smear under a microscope. Each type of leukocyte is identified by morphology and counted and its percentage recorded.
- RBC, Hb, Hct, MCV, MCH, MCHC, and WBC are measured automatically by machine.

RED BLOOD CELL COUNT
CPT: 85032–85041

Reference Values

Men: 4.7–6.1 million/mm^3
Women: 4.2–5.4 million/mm^3
Children: 3.8–5.5 million/mm^3
Newborns: 4.8–7.1 million/mm^3

The red blood cell count represents the number of circulating RBCs in 1 mm^3 of blood. Reference values vary according to age and sex. A patient is said to be anemic if his or her RBC count is decreased by more than 10% of this expected reference value. There are many causes for low counts, including hemorrhage, anemias, chronic infections, chronic renal failure, dietary deficiencies, leukemia, overhydration, and pregnancy. An RBC count can also be greater than normal. Causes include cardiovascular disease, high altitude, and polycythemia vera.

HEMOGLOBIN
CPT: 85018

Reference Values

Men: 14–18 g/dL
Women: 12–16 g/dL
Children: 11–16 g/dL
Infants: 10–15 g/dL
Newborns: 14–24 g/dL

The hemoglobin test measures the total amount of Hb found in the blood. Hemoglobin is a pigment found in red blood cells that carries oxygen. Most factors that affect the RBC count also affect the Hb concentration.

The Hb concentration, however, is more sensitive to fluid (plasma) volume changes. Abnormally high hemoglobin levels may result from dehydration. Overhydration may cause a low hemoglobin concentration. Clinical problems that may cause a decreased Hb level include anemias, cancers, sarcoidosis, and pregnancy. An elevated Hb may be caused by chronic obstructive pulmonary disease (COPD), congestive heart failure (CHF), polycythemia, and dehydration.

GLYCOSYLATED HEMOGLOBIN (HB A_{LC})

Nicky R. Holdeman

CPT: 83036

Glycosylated hemoglobin is produced by nonenzymatic condensation of glucose molecules on the globin component of hemoglobin. The major form of glycohemoglobin is termed hemoglobin A_{1c}, which normally comprises only 4%–6% of the total hemoglobin. However, glucose passes freely on to erythrocytes and the rate of HbA_{1c} formation is directly proportional to the concentration of free glucose (Table 2.2). Because the normal erythrocyte (red blood cell) has a life span of about 8 to 12 weeks, the

▶ **TABLE 2.2 Hemoglobin A_{1c} Relative to Average Daily Blood Glucose Ranges**

Hemoglobin A_{1c} Level	Average Blood Glucose Range for Last 3 Months
4.0–6.0%	60 to 120 mg/dL
6.1–7.0%	121 to 150 mg/dL
7.1–8.0%	151 to 180 mg/dL
8.1–9.0%	181 to 210 mg/dL
9.1–10.0%	211 to 240 mg/dL
10.1–11.0%	241 to 270 mg/dL
11.1–12.0%	271 to 300 mg/dL
12.1–13.0%	301 to 330 mg/dL
13.1–14.0%	331 to 360 mg/dL
greater than 14.0%	greater than 360 mg/dL

HbA_{1c} measurement provides an excellent index of the average blood glucose level for approximately the preceding 2 to 3 months.

It should be noted that HbA_{1c} measurements are *not* recommended for the initial diagnosis of diabetes, but are a critical supplement to home–blood glucose testing. HbA_{1c} measurements should be obtained in patients with either type 1 or type 2 diabetes mellitus at 3–4-month intervals, so that adjustments to therapy can be made if glycohemoglobin is either subnormal or if it is more than 2% above the upper limits of normal.

Several large clinical trials have demonstrated that both type 1 (DCCT) and type 2 (UKPDS) diabetes had less risk of developing long-term complications if the HbA_{1c} was kept close to normal. The UKDPS data showed that for every percentage point decrease in HbA_{1c}, there was a 35% overall reduction in risk of complications (i.e., a 25% reduction in diabetes-related deaths, a 7% reduction in all causes of mortality, and an 18% reduction in combined fatal and nonfatal myocardial infarction).

Normal HbA_{1c} for people without DM is <6%.
Good HbA_{1c} for people with DM is <7%.
For additional action suggested if the HbA_{1c} is >8%, see Table 2.2.

HEMATOCRIT (Hct)
CPT: 85014

Reference Values

Men: 42%–52%
Women: 37%–47%
Children: 31%–43%
Infants: 30%–40%
Newborns: 44%–64%

This is a measure of the percentage of red blood cells in the total blood volume. The Hct is the volume (in milliliters) of RBCs found in 100 mL of blood, expressed as a percentage. If 45 mL of RBCs were found in 100 mL of blood, the hematocrit would be 45%.

Factors that affect the RBC count and Hb concentration also affect the Hct. Clinical problems that may cause a decreased Hct include anemias, blood loss, leukemias, neoplasms, pregnancy, rheumatoid arthritis (especially juvenile), and vitamin deficiencies. An elevated Hct may be caused by dehydration, polycythemia, diabetic acidosis, and transient cerebral ischemia.

MEAN CORPUSCULAR VOLUME (MCV)
Reference Values

Adults: 80–98 Cu μm
Children: 82–92 Cu μm
Newborns: 96–108 Cu μm

The mean corpuscular volume is a measure of the average volume or size of a single RBC. The MCV and the other RBC indices (MCH and MCHC) are used to help identify types of anemias. The MCV value is calculated by dividing the hematocrit by the total RBC count. Reference values vary according to age and sex. If the MCV becomes abnormally large, the red blood cells are termed *macrocytic*. Macrocytic RBCs are most frequently associated with megaloblastic anemias (vitamin B_{12} or folic acid deficiency) or pernicious anemia. *Microcytic* RBCs (i.e., when the MCV value is abnormally small) are associated with iron deficiency anemia, malignancies, rheumatoid arthritis, sickle-cell anemia, and thalassemia. If the MCV value is within the reference value range, the RBCs are termed *normocytic*.

MEAN CORPUSCULAR HEMOGLOBIN (MCH)

Reference Values

Adults: 27–31 μg/dL
Children: 27–31 μg/dL
Newborns: 32–34 μg/dL

The MCH is a measure of the average amount of Hb (by weight) within an RBC. The value is derived by dividing 10 times the total Hb concentration by the number of RBCs:

$$MCH = Hb \times 10/RBC \text{ count}$$

Because larger (macrocytic) cells generally contain more Hb than smaller (microcytic) cells, those factors that affect the MCV usually have similar effects on the MCH. The MCH value can be accurately determined with the new Coulter counter.

MEAN CORPUSCULAR HEMOGLOBIN CONCENTRATION (MCHC)

The MCHC is a measure of the average concentration (weight per volume) or the percentage of Hb within a single RBC. It can be calculated from the MCV and MCH:

$$MCHC = MCH/MCV \times 100 \text{ or } MCHC = Hb \times 100/HCt$$

It can also be derived by dividing the total Hb concentration times 100 by the hematocrit. If the MCHC value becomes abnormally low, RBCs are deficient in their concentration of Hb and are termed *hypochromic*. This condition is frequently seen with iron deficiency anemia and thalassemia. Elevated MCHC values do not occur because red blood cells can only hold a physiologically limited amount of Hb.

WHITE BLOOD CELL (WBC) COUNT (TOTAL LEUKOCYTES)
CPT: 85032, 85048, 89055

Reference Values (Total WBCs)

Adults and children more than 2 years old: 5,000–10,000/mm^3
Children 2 years old and younger: 6,000–17,000/mm^3
Newborns: 9,000–30,000/mm^3

The WBC count measures the total number of WBCs (leukocytes) in 1 mm^3 of blood. WBCs can be divided into two groups: mononuclear leukocytes (monocytes and lymphocytes) and polymorphonuclear leukocytes (basophils, eosinophils, and neutrophils). WBCs are an important component of the body's defense system and respond immediately to foreign invasion. The total WBC count has a wide normal range, but many diseases can significantly decrease or increase the count. An increase in WBCs to more than 10,000/mm^3 is called leukocytosis. This condition usually suggests infection or a *leukemia*. Stress, trauma, and tissue necrosis can also increase the total WBC count. A decrease in WBCs to less than 5000/mm^3 is called *leukopenia*. Diseases associated with this situation include aplastic anemia, pernicious anemia, overwhelming infections, bone marrow failure, autoimmune diseases, and dietary deficiencies. Many drugs can also affect the WBC count. Drugs causing a decreased count include acetaminophen, barbiturates, chloramphenicol, penicillins, sulfonamides, Lasix, Valium, and Librium. Drugs that can cause an increased count include ampicillin, erythromycin, tetracycline, salicylates, and atropine (in children).

DIFFERENTIAL WHITE BLOOD CELL COUNT
CPT: 85004–85007, 85009

Reference Values

Adults:

Neutrophils: 50%–70% (of total WBC)
Segmented neutrophils: 50%–65%
Band neutrophils: 0%–5%
Eosinophils: 0%–4%
Basophils: 0.5%–3%
Lymphocytes: 20%–40%
Monocytes: 2%–8%

Children (2 weeks to 12 years old):
Neutrophils: 29%–47%
Eosinophils: 0%–3%
Basophils: 1%–3%
Lymphocytes: 38%–63%
Monocytes: 4%–9%

The differential WBC count measures each type of leukocyte as a percentage of the total number of leukocytes. The leukocyte types observed on a peripheral blood smear are identified by their morphology. Neutrophils make up the largest percentage of leukocytes. They are the most important leukocyte (because of their ability to use phagocytosis) in the body's defense against infection and rapidly respond to both acute infection and inflammatory disease. Eosinophils increase during allergic reactions and parasite infestation. Basophils prevent blood clotting during an inflammation. They contain granules of heparin and histamine. Lymphocytes make up the second largest group of leukocytes. They are seen to increase in conditions such as chronic bacterial infection, viral infection, infectious mononucleosis, lymphocytic leukemia, and multiple myeloma. Their numbers decrease as a result of immune deficiency diseases, steroid therapy, excess hormone production, or sepsis. Monocytes act as a second line of defense against infection. They respond more slowly than neutrophils to acute infection and inflammation, but once in action, they operate as powerful macrophages that continue into the chronic phase, ingesting dead tissue and debris and clearing the tissue for healing. Diseases in which monocytes increase include collagen diseases, rheumatoid arthritis, sickle-cell anemia, viral diseases, herpes zoster, tuberculosis, toxoplasmosis, and cancers. The elevation, then, of any one type of leukocyte may serve as an important clue in the diagnosis of disease.

COMPUTERIZED TOMOGRAPHY (CT) SCAN

CPT: 70450 CT, head or brain; without contrast material
CPT: 70460 CT, head or brain; with contrast material(s)
CPT: 70480 CT, orbit, sella, or posterior fossa without contrast material
CPT: 70481 CT, orbit, sella, or posterior fossa with contrast material(s)

Normal Values

Normal tissue
No evidence of a pathologic condition

The CT scan can be used to detect diseases of the brain or orbit. The CT scanner produces a narrow x-ray beam that can examine the body from many different angles. A CT scan of the brain consists of a sequence of tomographic x-ray films taken of the brain tissue at successive layers. The films are subjected to a computerized analysis that builds up the shots into a three-dimensional picture. The CT x-ray image produced is a view of the head as if one were looking down through its top. Each type of tissue has its own density and each permits the x-ray beam to penetrate only so far. An attached computer calculates the amount of x-ray penetration of each tissue. It displays this as varying shades of gray. The x-ray image appears on a television screen and is photographed. The denser the tissue, the lighter it appears in the image. The densest tissue appears white and less-dense tissue appears in progressively darker shades of gray. The result is an actual anatomic picture of a coronal section of the brain. The CT scan can be performed with or without iodine contrast dye. The iodine in the contrast dye causes a greater tissue absorption. This is referred to as contrast enhancement. A small tumor may not be observed if contrast enhancement is not used.

CT scans can be used to detect intracranial neoplasms, cerebral aneurysms, intracranial hemorrhages or hematomas, cerebral infarctions, cortical atrophy, arteriovenous (AV) malformations, or ventricular enlargement or displacement. CT scans can be repeated to monitor the progress of a disease or to monitor the effects of treatment. One advantage of the CT is that it has eliminated the need for more invasive procedures such as cerebral arteriography and pneumoencephalography.

Procedure

- The patient is kept NPO for 3 to 4 hours before the test. If contrast enhancement is not to be performed, the patient need not be restricted from food or fluids. Contrast dye can cause nausea and vomiting.
- Jewelry, hairpins, clips, and so forth are removed from the patient's head.
- Steroids or antihistamines may be ordered several days prior to the test if the patient has a known allergy to iodine or contrast dye. Emergency equipment should be available to treat any severe allergic reaction, such as anaphylactic shock.
- The patient lies supine on the examining table with the head resting in a snug-fitting rubber cap within a water-filled box. A rubberized strap is wrapped around the head to keep it immobilized during the test.

- The patient's head is moved into a circular scanner. The scanner passes a small x-ray beam through the brain from one side to the other. The machine then rotates 1°. The process is repeated at each degree through a 180° arc. The procedure takes approximately 45 to 60 minutes (filming 3 to 7 planes).
- If contrast enhancement is needed, an iodine contrast dye is injected intravenously over a period of 2 minutes. The patient may feel warm and flushed and experience a salty or metallic taste. Nausea may occur. These symptoms usually last only about a minute.
- A mild sedative may be ordered for a restless patient, or an analgesic for a patient with neck or back pains.

CREATININE (SERUM)
CPT: 82565

Reference Values

Adults: 0.6–1.2 mg/dL; 53–106 pmol/liter (SI units)
Infants to 6 years old: 0.3–0.6 mg/dL; 27–54 pmol/liter (SI units)
Older children: 0.4–1.2 mg/dL; 36–106 pmol/liter (SI units)

The serum creatinine test and the BUN are the tests most commonly used to assess kidney function. Creatinine is a by-product of muscle catabolism. It is derived from creatine phosphate, which is used in skeletal muscle contraction. The amount of creatinine produced daily is proportional to the amount of muscle mass. Creatinine circulates in the blood and is excreted by the kidneys. The concentration of creatinine in the blood is directly related to how well the kidneys are functioning. The serum creatinine level, then, can be used as an indicator of kidney function. It is considered to be a more specific and sensitive indicator of renal disease than the BUN. It is not influenced by diet or fluid intake, and rises more slowly than the BUN. A small rise in the BUN may indicate dehydration, GI bleeding, or malnutrition; a serum creatinine of 2.5 mg/dL could indicate renal disease. When the BUN level rises but serum creatinine remains normal, dehydration is suspected. When both rise, the patient should be assessed for kidney disease. Clinical problems that can cause the serum creatinine level to rise include acute and chronic renal failure, hypertension, diabetic nephropathy, cancer, SLE, and a diet high in creatinine (lots of beef, poultry, and fish). Drugs that can elevate serum creatinine include antibiotics such as gentamicin and cephalosporin, barbiturates, and ascorbic acid. High intake of glucose or protein can also elevate serum creatinine. A decreased serum creatinine may be seen during pregnancy.

Procedure

- Seven to 10 milliliters of venous blood is collected in a red-top tube.
- The sample is sent to the chemistry lab with a list of any drugs the patient is taking that could elevate the serum level.
- A multifunctional analysis machine is used to determine the serum creatinine level.

ERYTHROCYTE SEDIMENTATION RATE (ESR); SEDIMENTATION (SED) RATE
CPT: 85651

Reference Values (Westergren Method)

Men <50 years old: 0–15 mm per hour
Men >50 years old: 0–20 mm per hour
Women <50 years old: 0–20 mm per hour
Women >50 years old: 0–30 mm per hour
Children 4–14 years old: 3–13 mm per hour
or
Men: Patient's age/2
Women: Patient's (age + 10)/2

The ESR test is used to detect inflammatory conditions, infections, neoplasms, and necrotic processes. It measures the rate at which the red blood cells in a sample of anticoagulated blood settle to the bottom of a narrow-bore tube in a 1-hour period. The ESR is a nonspecific test and is not diagnostic for any specific disease or injury. The test can detect inflammatory processes, but the ESR can also be increased by acute and chronic infections, rheumatoid collagen diseases, neoplasms, pneumonia, syphilis, tissue necrosis, pregnancy, and general physiologic stress. All these conditions can cause an increase in the amount of protein (mainly fibrinogen and globulins) in the plasma. As a result, the repellent forces between adjacent red blood cells begin to break down and RBCs tend to stack on top of one another (rouleaux), increasing their weight and causing them to sediment faster than single cells. The ESR is therefore increased.

Decreased ESR values can also occur. Causes include congestive heart failure, polycythemia vera, sickle-cell anemia, and hypofibrinogenemia. Some clinicians think the ESR is not that useful because it is so nonspecific and because it is affected by so many physiologic factors. The C-reactive protein (CRP) test is sometimes preferred because CRP tends to increase more rapidly during an acute inflammatory process and return more quickly to normal than an ESR. The ESR, however, is a fairly reliable indicator for following the course of a disease. It is, therefore, used to monitor the effects of therapy. Generally, the ESR will increase if a disease worsens and decrease as the disease improves. The ESR is also sometimes used to help with a differential diagnosis (e.g., rheumatoid arthritis versus osteoarthritis; or, in the case of a patient with chest pain, acute myocardial infarction, which would show an increased ESR, versus angina pectoris, in which the ESR would remain normal). One of the most important roles for the ESR in eye care is in the diagnosis and management of giant cell arteritis. In the majority of affected patients, the ESR will be significantly raised. Usually, the higher the value, the more active the disease is. Two methods, the Westergren and the Wintrobe, are commonly used to determine ESRs. The Westergren method is generally preferred.

Procedure

- Seven to 10 milliliters of venous blood is collected in a lavender-top tube containing EDTA or an oxalate (to keep the blood from coagulating).

- The specimen is taken immediately to the hematology lab. The blood should not be allowed to stand, because this may affect the SED rate. Therefore, the test should be performed within 2 to 3 hours after the specimen has been obtained. If refrigerated, the blood should be allowed to return to room temperature before testing.
- The blood is drawn into the Westergren tube, placed in a vertical rack, and left undisturbed.
- At the end of 1 hour, the height of the clear plasma above the red cell column is measured. This height, the distance the RBCs settle in 1 hour, is a measure of the rate of fall of the red cells.

FASTING BLOOD SUGAR (FBS); SERUM GLUCOSE
CPT: 82947

Reference Values

Adults:
Serum: 70–115 mg/dL
Whole blood: 60–100 mg/dL
Children: 60–100 mg/dL
Newborns: 30–80 mg/dL

Glucose is derived from dietary carbohydrates. It is stored in the liver and in skeletal muscle in the form of glycogen. Blood glucose levels are controlled by two hormones, insulin and glucagon, both produced by the pancreas. Insulin is necessary in order for glucose to enter cells. Glucagon helps the liver convert glycogen back into glucose.

An increased blood glucose level (hyperglycemia) occurs when there is an insufficiency of insulin. This condition indicates diabetes mellitus. An FBS greater than 120 mg/dL is usually considered diagnostic for diabetes. However, there are other possible causes of an elevated blood sugar, including adrenal gland hyperfunction (Cushing's syndrome), an acute stress response, acute MI, infections, renal failure, hyperthyroidism, and drugs such as diuretics and corticosteroids.

Decreased blood glucose (hypoglycemia) also has many causes. The most common cause is insulin overdose. Other problems that can cause a decreased blood glucose level include hypothyroidism, Addison's disease, cancer, extensive liver disease, malnutrition, and strenuous exercise.

Procedure
- The patient should have had no food for 8 to 12 hours (water is permitted).
- Peripheral venipuncture is performed and 5 to 10 milliliters of blood is collected in a gray-top tube containing sodium fluoride (to diminish glycolysis). Blood should be collected before insulin or any hypoglycemic agent is administered.
- The blood sample is taken to the chemistry lab. The most frequently used method of analysis involves enzyme reactions (hexokinase and glucose oxidase).

2-HOUR POSTPRANDIAL BLOOD SUGAR (PPBS); 2-HOUR POSTPRANDIAL GLUCOSE TEST (2-HOUR PPG)
CPT: 82950

Reference Values

Adults:
  Serum: <140 mg/dL at 2 hours
  Whole blood: <120 mg/dL at 2 hours
Older Adults:
  Serum: <160 mg/dL at 2 hours
  Whole blood: <140 mg/dL at 2 hours

This test measures the amount of glucose in a patient's blood 2 hours after a meal (postprandial). The PPBS is used as a screening test for diabetes and is often ordered if a fasting blood sugar test comes out high-normal or slightly elevated. A blood glucose level >120 mg/dL or a serum glucose >140 mg/dL is considered abnormal. A glucose tolerance test may then be ordered to confirm the diagnosis.

The PPBS tests a patient's response to high carbohydrate intake 2 hours after a meal. In normal patients, insulin is secreted immediately after a meal in response to elevated blood glucose levels. The insulin brings the blood sugar level back to its premeal range within 2 hours. In diabetic patients, there is insufficient insulin and the glucose level is usually found to be still elevated 2 hours after a meal.

Procedure

- A high-carbohydrate meal (consisting of at least 75 g of carbohydrate) is taken at breakfast or lunch.
- Two hours after the meal, 7 to 10 milliliters of venous blood is collected into a gray- or red-top tube.
- The tube is taken to the chemistry lab for a glucose determination.
- Food is restricted for 8 hours before the meal. Water is permitted.

GLUCOSE TOLERANCE TEST (GTT); ORAL GLUCOSE TOLERANCE TEST (OGTT)
CPT: 82951

Reference Values

Adults: See Table 2.3
Children: Varies with child's age. Infants normally have a lower blood sugar level.
  Children age 6 or older have GTT values similar to adults.

The glucose tolerance test is the most specific and sensitive test for diabetes. It measures a patient's ability to handle a standard oral glucose load. Blood and urine samples are collected at specific times (before glucose administration, 30 minutes after, 1 hour after, 2 hours after, 3 hours after, and sometimes 4 hours after) and checked for their glucose levels. Normal patients handle the glucose dose easily and show only a minimal, transient rise in their blood glucose levels within 1 hour, and there is no glucose spillover

▶ **TABLE 2.3** Adult Reference Values for GTT

Time	Serum (mg/dL)	Whole Blood (mg/dL)
Fasting	70–115	60–100
30 min	<200	<180
1 h	<200	<180
2 h	<140	<120
3 h	70–115 (fasting level)	60–100
4 h	70–115	60–100

into their urine. Diabetics are deficient in insulin and therefore have difficulty tolerating the standard glucose load. Their blood glucose levels will increase significantly between 1 and 5 hours, and glucose will usually be detected in their urine.

A GTT is often ordered if a patient shows a high-normal or slightly elevated fasting blood sugar. Other possible indications for this test include a family history of diabetes, obesity, extensive surgery, or injury, and women having babies weighing ≥10 lb. The GTT is contraindicated if the fasting blood sugar is over 200 mg/dL, or if the patient has a serious concurrent illness, endocrine disorder, or infection (because a glucose intolerance will probably be observed even if the patient is not diabetic).

The peak glucose level for an oral GTT is usually observed within 30 minutes to 1 hour after ingestion of the standard dose. If the patient is normal, blood sugar should return to fasting level in 3 hours. Patients older than age 60 often have a blood glucose level 10 to 30 mg/dL higher than the "normal range."

There are other causes of glucose intolerance besides diabetes. Elevated GTT values may be seen in patients with hyperthyroidism, Cushing's syndrome, hyperlipoproteinemia, cancer, duodenal ulcer, stress, infection, acute MI, and alcoholism. Elevations may also be seen in pregnant or obese patients. Certain drugs can also lead to increased GTT values, including corticosteroids, thiazide diuretics, salicylates, and oral contraceptives. Decreased GTT levels (<70 mg/dL at 3 hours) can also occur. Causes include hyperinsulinism, adrenal gland insufficiency, protein malnutrition, and malabsorption.

Procedure

- High-carbohydrate diet (at least 200—300 g of carbohydrate daily) for at least 3 days before the test.
- Patient remains NPO (nothing by mouth) for 12 hours before the test, except for water (no food, no smoking, no caffeine, and no medications).
- Five milliliters of venous blood is collected in a gray-top tube for an FBS. A fasting urine specimen is also collected.
- The patient is given a 100-g glucose load. This comes in various forms: an orange- or lemon-flavored solution; a cherry-flavored gelatin (Gel-a-dex); Glucola, a carbonated sugar beverage (many patients have difficulty keeping this down); or 100 g of glucose dissolved in water and flavored with lemon juice. Some clinicians give glucose according to body weight (1.75 g/kg, or 1 g/lb for children weighing less than 100 lb). The patient must ingest the entire glucose load because GTT values are based on a standard 100-g glucose load.

- Blood and urine specimens are obtained at 30 minutes, 1 hour, 2 hours, 3 hours, and 4 hours after glucose ingestion, and their glucose levels determined.
- During testing, no food, caffeine, or smoking is permitted. The patient is encouraged to drink water to facilitate the obtaining of urine specimens. The patient should also be at rest, because exercise (including walking) can affect glucose levels.
- During testing, the patient is checked for any dizziness, sweating, weakness, or giddiness.
- No insulin or oral hypoglycemics should be taken during testing.

FLUORESCENT TREPONEMAL ANTIBODY ABSORPTION TEST (FTA-ABS)
CPT: 86592

Reference Values

Negative or nonreactive

The FTA-ABS test is used to determine whether a patient has or has not had systemic syphilis. It is the most sensitive and specific test for diagnosing any stage of the disease and is the test of choice for confirming a diagnosis. Once the test shows positive, it tends to remain positive indefinitely (even after treatment) in 95% of patients. Therefore, this test cannot be used to establish the activity of syphilis, how recently it was incurred, or how effective any treatment has been.

The FTA-ABS is usually ordered in combination with an RPR or VDRL test to determine if the disease is active. If a patient has a positive FTA-ABS but shows a nonreactive RPR or VDRL, this indicates that the patient was exposed to *Treponema pallidum* (the causative agent for syphilis) sometime in the past but does not currently have the active disease. A positive FTA-ABS and a positive RPR or VDRL suggest that the patient has active syphilis. A negative FTA-ABS and a positive RPR or VDRL suggest a false-positive RPR or a laboratory error.

False-positive FTA-ABS tests occur in about 1% to 2% of normals and may also occur in patients with collagen disease (e.g., SLE), but stained preparations from patients with SLE usually show an atypical beaded appearance not usually seen with syphilis.

Procedure
- Five to 7 milliliters of venous blood is collected in a red-top tube.
- The patient's serum is placed on a slide that contains fixed *T. pallidum* organisms. If antibodies are present, the organisms become coated.
- A fluorescent antibody against human globulin is then added to the slide. This combines with any coated organisms, causing a fluorescence.
- The slide is rinsed and observed under an ultraviolet microscope. If fluorescence is present, the test is positive. If no fluorescence is seen, the test is negative.

Two newer tests for syphilis are the microhemagglutination assay for antibodies to *T. pallidum* (MHA-TP) and the hemagglutination treponemal test for syphilis (HATTS). Both tests compare well with the FTA-ABS in terms of sensitivity and specificity (although the MHA-TP is less sensitive in primary syphilis). Their interpretation and use are also similar to that of the FTA-ABS.

HLA-B27 ANTIGEN
CPT: 86812

Reference Values

No antigen present

The major histocompatibility locus antigens (HLAs) are extremely important in tissue recognition. Genes that regulate the HLAs are located on chromosome 6 at the HLA region. This region is composed of four closely linked genetic loci: HLA-A, HLAB, HLA-C, and HLA-D. Each person possesses two genes (one maternal gene and one paternal gene) at each of the four loci; this is because both mother and father contribute a complete haplotype of their HLA genes to each child. These eight genes together make up a person's complete HLA phenotype. Antigens are named by giving them a letter representing their locus and a number that is unique for each antigen.

There are many HLAs, but the one with the most clinical significance is HLA-B27. Approximately 5% to 8% of normal White patients and a smaller percentage of normal Black patients possess the HLA-B27 antigen. In Whites, HLA-B27 is found in more than 90% of the patients with ankylosing spondylitis, 75% to 85% of patients with Reiter's syndrome, 60% or fewer in those with psoriatic arthritis, and 20% to 50% of patients with acute uveitis regardless of cause. In Blacks with the same diseases, HLA-B27 is found to be about one-half as prevalent. HLA-B27 has also been associated with inflammatory bowel disease. The HLA-B27 antigen, then, can be used to help detect and diagnose some of these diseases, especially ankylosing spondylitis and Reiter's syndrome.

Procedure

- At least 10 milliliters of venous blood is obtained in a heparinized solution.
- Anti-HLA-B27 cytotoxic antibody is then incubated with lymphocytes taken from the patient. If HLA-B27 antigen is present, a complex will form on the cell surface. Serum complement is then added to the mixture; this kills the lymphocytes and recognizes the titer of HLA-B27.

HOMOCYSTEINE (PLASMA)
CPT: 83090

Reference Values

<10 mmole/L

Elevated homocysteine is associated with an increased risk of heart attack and stroke. It has also been associated with an increased risk of retinal vein occlusion.

Homocysteine is an amino acid that is produced as a by-product of meat consumption. Normally it is converted to methionine and cysteine with the help of folic acid, B12, and B6. A shortage of these compounds can contribute to elevated levels of homocysteine. Elevated homocysteine levels have been associated with an increased risk of atherosclerotic vessel disease. Treatment includes folic acid and B vitamin supplementation.

INR (INTERNATIONAL NORMALIZED RATIO)
CPT: 85610

Reference Values

Normal: 1
Warfarin patient: 2–3

The INR is a system established by the World Health Organization (WHO) and the International Committee on Thrombosis and Hemostasis for reporting the results of blood coagulation tests. All results are standardized using the international sensitivity index for the particular thromboplastin reagent and instrument combination utilized to perform the test. It is a standardized version of the prothrombin time or PT test.

For example, a person taking the anticoagulant warfarin might optimally maintain a prothrombin time (PT) of 2 to 3 INR. No matter what laboratory checks the test time, the result should be the same even if different thromboplastins and instruments are used. This international standardization permits the patient on warfarin to travel and still obtain comparable test results.

LIPIDS (SERUM)
CPT: 80061

Reference Values

Total lipids: 400–1000 mg/dL (depending on the laboratory)
Cholesterol: 150–250 mg/dL
Triglycerides: 10–190 mg/dL
Phospholipids: 150–380 mg/dL
Cholesterol lipoproteins:
  HDL
    Men: 45 mg/dL
    Women: 55 mg/dL
  LDL
    60–180 mg/dL
  VLDL
    25%–50%

Serum lipid levels are used to help diagnose and manage atherosclerotic disease. When lipids (cholesterol, triglycerides, phospholipids) are transported in the blood, they are combined with proteins and called *lipoproteins*. There are two major classes of lipoproteins: α and β. These can be separated by electrophoresis. The α fraction is the high-density lipoprotein (HDL). It is made up mostly of protein with small amounts of cholesterol, triglycerides, and phospholipids. The β fraction is low-density lipoprotein (LDL). It is made up of small amounts of protein plus varying amounts of cholesterol, triglycerides, and phospholipids. The β fraction has three subgroups: chylomicrons, LDL (low-density lipoprotein, also known as β-lipoprotein), and VLDL (very-low-density lipoprotein, or pre-β). LDLs have a strong association with atherosclerosis and coronary artery disease. HDLs are known as the "good" lipoproteins. They are associated with a

▶ **TABLE 2.4 Types of Hyperlipoproteinemia**

Type	Major Lipoprotein Elevation	Major Lipid Elevation
I	Chylomicrons	Triglycerides
IIa	LDL	Cholesterol
IIb	LDL and VLDL	Cholesterol and triglycerides
III	Remnants	Triglycerides and cholesterol
IV	VLDL	Triglycerides
V	VLDL and chylomicrons	Triglycerides and cholesterol

decreased risk of coronary artery disease. HDLs seem to have a protective function. When there are increased levels of lipoproteins in the blood, the condition is called *hyperlipidemia* or *hyperlipoproteinemia*. There are six types of hyperlipoproteinemia, classified according to the major lipoprotein elevation and the major lipid elevation (Table 2.4). Types II and IV are the most common and most prevalent in atherosclerosis and coronary artery disease.

Lipoprotein electrophoresis can be used to assign "risk factors" for cardiovascular disease. It can also be used for screening and diagnosis.

Clinical problems associated with increased lipid levels include type II hyperlipoproteinemia, hypothyroidism, diabetes, and a high-saturated fat diet. Decreased lipid levels may be associated with COPD and β-lipoproteinemia.

Procedure

- The patient is not allowed food, medication, or fluids (except water) for 12 to 14 hours prior to the test.
- The patient should have eaten a normal diet for at least 2 weeks.
- Ten milliliters of venous blood is collected in a red-top tube.
- The lipoproteins are fractionated by electrophoresis.

PARTIAL THROMBOPLASTIN TIME (PTT); ACTIVATED PARTIAL THROMBOPLASTIN TIME (APTT)
CPT: 85730

Reference Values (vary according to the laboratory)

PTT: 60–70 seconds
APTT: 20–35 seconds

The PTT test is a screening test for coagulation disorders. It is used to detect any defects in the intrinsic coagulation system and common pathway and to assess any deficiencies in clotting factors II, V, VIII, IX, XI, and XII. A deficiency in any one of these factors would cause an increased PTT. The PTT is more sensitive than the prothrombin time (PT) test in detecting minor deficiencies, but it is not as sensitive as an APTT. The APTT is similar to the PTT except that activators (celite or kaolin) for identifying deficient factors are added to the PTT test reagents. This shortens the clotting time and allows detection of minor clotting defects.

The APTT (or PTT) is often used to monitor heparin therapy. It is also frequently used to detect factor VIII and IX deficiencies (which together make up approximately 95% of all clotting factor deficiencies). Clinical problems that can increase the APTT (or PTT) include hemophilia (factors V and VIII are deficient), cirrhosis of the liver, hepatocellular disease, vitamin K deficiency, leukemias, malaria, and prothrombin deficiency. Drugs that increase the APTT include heparin and salicylates. A decreased APTT may occur with extensive cancer.

Procedure
- Seven to 10 milliliters of venous blood is collected in a blue-top tube containing the anticoagulant sodium citrate. The tube should be filled to capacity.
- The blood sample is packed in ice and taken to the lab immediately.
- An activated thromboplastin mixture (thromboplastin reagent plus an activator such as kaolin) is added to the patient sample and to a control sample.
- A small amount of calcium chloride solution is added. A timer is started and stopped when clotting begins.
- All tests are performed in duplicate and should agree to within 1 to 1.5 seconds.

POLYMERASE CHAIN REACTION (PCR)

The PCR provides an extremely sensitive means of amplifying small quantities of DNA. The development of this technique resulted in an explosion of new techniques in molecular biology (and a Nobel Prize for Kary Mullins in 1993) as more and more applications of the method were published. The technique was made possible by the discovery of Taq polymerase, the DNA polymerase that is used by the bacterium *Thermus auquaticus* that was discovered in hot springs. This DNA polymerase is stable at the high temperatures needed to perform the amplification, whereas other DNA polymerases become denatured.

Because this technique involves amplification of DNA, the most obvious application of the method is in the detection of minuscule amounts of specific DNAs. This is important in the detection of low-level bacterial infections or rapid changes in transcription at the single-cell level as well as the detection of a specific individual's DNA in forensic science (like in the O. J. Simpson trial). It can also be used in DNA sequencing, screening for genetic disorders, site-specific mutation of DNA, or cloning or subcloning of cDNAs.

These processes have allowed for improved identification for a host of disorders that include gonorrhea, chlamydia, and tuberculosis.

PROTEIN (SERUM)
CPT: 84155

Reference Values

Total protein (adult): 6.0–8.0 g/dL
Albumin (adult): 3.2–5.0 g/dL
Globulin (adult): 2.3–3.4 g/dL

A serum protein test can be used to assess the function of the liver. Serum proteins are made up of albumin and globulins. Albumin, the smallest of the protein molecules, makes up the largest percentage of the total protein. Albumin is formed in the liver; however, if the liver becomes diseased, it loses its ability to synthesize albumin and the serum albumin level drops significantly. The half-life of albumin is 12 to 18 days; decreased albumin production will not be recognized until after this period.

The total protein (albumin plus globulins) level is of limited value unless a serum albumin, albumin/globulin (A/G) ratio, or protein electrophoresis test is also performed. For example, although serum albumin may become decreased because of severe liver disease, globulins (made in many organs) may be increased. The result will be a normal total serum protein level. An A/G ratio determination, however, would reveal a reversal in the normal A/G ratio (liver disease showing a decrease in albumin with the increase in globulins). If a clinician only looked at the total protein level, an incorrect assessment of normal liver function could have been made.

Albumin levels may show a decrease in chronic liver disease, chronic renal failure, malnutrition, malabsorption syndromes, hyperthyroidism, neoplasms, leukemia, nephrotic syndrome, SLE, congestive heart failure, and pregnancy. Increased albumin levels may occur in cases of dehydration or with exercise. Decreased globulin levels may be seen in emphysema, hypocholesterolemia, hemolytic anemia, severe liver disease, lymphocytic leukemia, and nephrotic syndrome. Many diseases can cause increased globulin levels, including acute infection, acute MI, collagen disease, Cushing's disease, diabetes, Hodgkin's disease, kidney nephtosis, lupus erythematosus, liver disease, neoplasms, malignant hypertension, rheumatoid arthritis, and hypothyroidism. Pregnancy can also cause increased globulin levels.

Procedure

- Five to 10 milliliters of venous blood is collected in a red-top tube.
- Some labs require the patient to be kept without food for 8 hours preceding the test. Water is permitted.

PROTHROMBIN TIME (PT)
CPT: 85610

Reference Values

11–15 seconds (depending on the method reagents used)
70%–100%

The PT test is used as a screening test to evaluate the adequacy of the extrinsic system and the common pathway of clot formation. This includes fibrinogen and clotting factors II, V, VII, and X. When any of these factors exist in deficient quantities, the prothrombin time will be prolonged. Many diseases can cause a deficiency in one or more of the factors and increase the PT. These include liver diseases (cirrhosis, hepatitis, neoplasm), which can produce deficiencies in factors II, VII, IX, and X. The liver produces these factors. If disease is severe, their synthesis will not occur. Obstructive biliary disease prevents vitamin K absorption. Factors II, VII, IX, and X depend on vitamin K and will therefore not be adequately produced and the PT will increase. Leukemias and congestive heart failure can also prolong the PT. Drugs that can increase the PT include penicillin, streptomycin, neomycin, tetracycline, anticoagulants, Librium, Thorazine, sulfonamides, and aspirin. Decreased prothrombin times are associated with myocardial infarction, pulmonary embolism, and thrombophlebitis. Drugs that can shorten the PT include barbiturates, diuretics, Benadryl, vitamin K, rifampin, and oral contraceptives.

PT test results are reported in seconds or as a percentage of normal activity (the patient's PT is compared with a curve representing a normal clotting time). Prothrombin time tests are also used to screen for anticoagulants and to monitor sodium warfarin anticoagulant therapy.

Procedure

- Seven to 10 milliliters of venous blood is collected in a blue-top tube containing the anticoagulant sodium citrate. The tube should be filled to capacity (to prevent an artificially prolonged PT because of extra citrate in the tube).
- The blood is transported on ice to the lab to be tested as soon as possible. Testing should be within 4 hours to prevent inactivation of some of the clotting factors.
- The blood is mixed with calcium chloride and thromboplastin, circumventing the intrinsic system of clotting.
- The time required for clotting is recorded.
- Tests should be run in duplicate. Agreement between tests should be within 1 second. If it is not, a third test must be run.
- The PT test results are given, along with a control value.

PURIFIED PROTEIN DERIVATIVE (PPD; TUBERCULIN SKIN TEST)
CPT: 86580

Normal Values

Negative results
Reaction <5 mm

The PPD test is used to determine whether a person has been infected by the tubercle bacillus. It cannot indicate whether an infection is active or dormant. The test consists of injecting a PPD of the tubercle bacillus intradermally. There are several different strengths of PPD. An intermediate strength (5 tuberculin units or 0.1 mL) is usually used unless a patient is known to be hypersensitive to skin tests. A patient should not receive PPD if there is a history of a positive test. The test is read in 48 to 72 hours. If the patient is infected with tuberculosis (whether active or dormant), lymphocytes will recognize the PPD antigen and cause a local reaction. If there has been no infection by tuberculosis, no reaction will occur. If the test is negative but tuberculosis is strongly suspected, a second test can be performed with a higher strength PPD (100 or 250 tuberculin units). If this test is also negative, tuberculosis can usually be ruled out.

As with all tests, the PPD test should be interpreted only in light of the overall clinical picture. A positive PPD reaction does not necessarily mean that active tuberculosis is the cause of a patient's complaints. It may only mean that the patient was exposed to tuberculosis in the past, that it is now dormant, and that it is not the cause of any current problems.

The PPD test can also be used to assess a patient's immune system. A series of skin tests is performed. If a patient is immunoincompetent because of a chronic illness (e.g., infection or neoplasm) or poor nutrition, the PPD test will show negative, even though the patient has had an active or dormant tuberculosis infection.

Procedure

- The inner aspect of the forearm is cleansed with alcohol and allowed to dry.
- PPD (0.1 mL) is injected intradermally with a tuberculin syringe.
- The test is read 48 to 72 hours later.
- The test site is examined for hardening (induration). The hardened area (not the reddened area) is marked and measured.
- A thickened, swollen area measuring >10 mm is considered a positive test. Measurements between 5 and 10 mm are considered doubtful. A reaction of <5 mm is labeled negative.

Contraindications

- The PPD test is contraindicated in a patient with a known, active tuberculosis infection.
- PPD is contraindicated in a patient who has received a bacille Calmette-Guerin (BCG) immunization against PPD, because a positive reaction to the PPD vaccination will be demonstrated even though the patient has never had a tuberculosis infection.

RAPID PLASMA REAGIN (RPR)
CPT: 86592

Reference Values

Nonreactive or negative

The RPR test is used as a rapid screening test for syphilis. It detects a nontreponemal antibody (reagin) directed against a lipoidal antigen that results from infection by *T. pallidum*, the causative agent of syphilis. The test is relatively nonspecific and has a high false-positive rate. False-positives can occur as a result of acute bacterial and viral infections, tuberculosis, pneumonia, subacute bacterial endocarditis, chicken pox, malaria, rheumatoid arthritis, SLE, hepatitis, and pregnancy. False-negatives can occur in the early primary and tertiary stages of syphilis. The RPR is more sensitive but less specific than the VDRL test. If the RPR is positive, the diagnosis should be confirmed with an FTA-ABS test.

Procedure

- Five to 7 milliliters of venous blood is collected in a red-top tube.

- The patient's serum is added to a synthetic lipoid antigen and observed for flocculation (a positive test).
- Patients should have no alcohol intake for 24 hours before the test. Some labs require that the patient not have eaten for 8 hours before the test.

RHEUMATOID FACTOR (RF)
CPT: 86430–86431

Reference Values

<1:20 titer is normal
1:20–1:80 titer is positive for rheumatoid arthritis and other diseases
>1:80 titer is positive for rheumatoid arthritis

The RF test is a screening test used to detect antibodies to antigenic determinants on abnormal IgG molecules. The test is used to help diagnose rheumatoid arthritis (RA). Other diseases may also cause a positive RF test. Elevated levels of rheumatoid factor may be seen in SLE, scleroderma, tuberculosis, infectious mononucleosis, chronic hepatitis, sarcoidosis, syphilis, leukemia, chronic infections, cirrhosis of the liver, and older patients. The presence of rheumatoid factor is therefore nonspecific.

RA is a chronic inflammatory disease that causes lymphocytes to produce abnormal IgG antibody in the synovial membranes of joints. This abnormal IgG then acts as an antigen, which reacts with IgG and IgM antibodies and forms immune complexes. The immune complexes activate complement and other inflammatory processes, causing joint damage. The reactive IgM immunoglobulin antibody is the rheumatoid factor. RF tests are designed to detect this IgM antibody.

RF tests are not particularly sensitive. Only approximately 80% of patients with rheumatoid arthritis will show a positive RF titer. There are several techniques for detecting rheumatoid factors. The most common agglutination test is the latex fixation method for RA. It is considered the most specific of the RF tests because it shows the lowest percentage of positives (1%) in normals. The technique detects RF in approximately 76% of RA patients. The Waaler-Rose method is the second most common RF test. It shows positive RF results in approximately 64% of RA patients and in 5.6% of normals. The Hyland RA slide test shows a positive RF in 82% of RA patients, but shows the largest percentage of false-positives (8%–10%) in normals. A large number of laboratories use nephelometry because this procedure can be automated.

RF found in titers >1:80 is considered positive for RA. If the titer is <1:80, other diseases should be considered (but RA cannot be ruled out).

Procedure
- Five to 10 milliliters of venous blood is collected in a red-top tube.
- The Waaler-Rose method uses sensitized sheep RBCs. Rabbit IgG is placed on sheep RBCs. This is mixed with a serial dilution of the patient's blood. Visual agglutination will occur if RF is present.
- In the latex fixation method, human IgG is placed on a latex particle and mixed with a serial dilution of the patient's blood. Again, visual agglutination occurs if RF is present.

SERUM TRIIODOTHYRONINE (T_3) TEST
CPT: 84480

Reference Values

Adults: 80–200 ng/dL
Children 6 to 12 years old: 115–190 ng/dL
Newborns: 90–170 ng/dL

The serum triiodothyronine (T_3) test is an accurate measure of thyroid function. T_3 is one of the thyroid hormones. It is present in the blood in small quantities. T_3 is less stable but more potent than thyroxine (T_4). T_3 and T_4 have similar actions in the body. When blood levels of T_3 and T_4 fall, thyroid-releasing hormone (TRH) is secreted by the hypothalamus. The TRH stimulates the anterior pituitary gland to secrete thyroid-stimulating hormone (TSH). When blood levels of T_3 and T_4 return to normal, the secretion of TRH is inhibited by a negative feedback mechanism. In a patient with a normal, functioning thyroid regulation system, increased levels of TRH and TSH should be seen when T_3 and T_4 levels are decreased (unless the pituitary is not functioning). When T_3 and T_4 levels are increased, TRH and TSH levels should be decreased. In a patient with a thyroid adenoma or carcinoma, thyroid regulation is lost and the tumors will secrete thyroid hormone irrespective of the levels of TRH, TSH, T_3, or T_4.

Serum T_3 is measured by radioimmunoassay (RIA), which measures both bound and free T_3. The T_3 determination is clinically important in a patient who shows a T_4 in the normal range, but who has symptoms of hyperthyroidism. The T_3 may identify T_3 thyrotoxicosis. The T_3 test may not be reliable for diagnosing hypothyroidism, because T_3 may remain in the normal range. Elevated T_3 levels, may be seen in T_3 thyrotoxicosis, toxic adenoma, and Hashimoto's thyroiditis. Estrogen, methadone, and progestins may raise the T_3. Decreased levels of T_3 may be caused by severe acute illness, trauma, or malnutrition. Drugs that may lower T_3 include propranolol, reserpine, lithium, aspirin, steroids, and sulfonamides.

Procedure
- Five to 10 milliliters of venous blood is collected in a red-top tube.
- The sample is sent to the laboratory as soon as possible.
- An RIA technique is used. Antibodies to T_3 are produced by injecting a test animal with T_3. The antibodies are tagged with a radioactive tracer and added to the patient's serum. The tagged antibodies bind to the T_3. All T_3-bound antibodies are then separated out. They are measured and compared with a standard curve. The amount of T_3 in the patient's serum can be accurately determined.
- Drugs that may affect this test should be withheld for 24 hours, if possible.

SERUM THYROXINE (T_4) TEST
CPT: 84436

Reference Values

Adults:
6.0–11.8 μg/dL (Murphy-Pattee)

4.5–11.5 μg/dL (T$_4$ by column)
5.0–12 μg/dL (T$_4$ RIA)
1.0–2.3 μg/dL (Free T$_4$)
Reported as thyroxine iodine:
4.0–7.8 μg/dL (Murphy-Pattee)
3.2–7.2 μg/dL (T$_4$ by column)
Children:
1 to 6 years old: 5.5–13.5 μg/dL
6 to 10 years old: 5–12.5 μg/dL
Newborns:
11–23 μg/dL

The serum thyroxine (T$_4$) test is a direct measurement of the total amount of T$_4$ present in a patient's blood. It is a very reliable test of thyroid function. T$_4$ is the major hormone secreted by the thyroid gland. The ratio of T$_4$ to T$_3$ in the serum is approximately 20:1. Most of the T$_4$ (and some T$_3$) becomes bound to thyroid-binding globulin (TBG) and thyroid-binding prealbumin (TBPA). Therefore, any increase in these serum thyroid-binding proteins (as occurs during pregnancy and in women taking oral contraceptives) will cause T$_4$ levels to increase. The levels of these proteins must be considered when interpreting T$_4$ test results. They can be measured by a T$_3$ resin uptake test.

Decreased levels of T$_4$ are seen in hypothyroidism (cretinism, myxedema, surgical removal of the thyroid, radioactive iodine ablation of the thyroid, autoimmune destruction of the thyroid), anterior pituitary hypofunction, protein malnutrition, and strenuous exercise. Drugs that may decrease T$_4$ include cortisone, heparin, lithium, sulfonamides, Dilantin, testosterone, and Thorazine. Elevated T$_4$ levels occur with hyperthyroidism (the most common cause of which is Graves' disease), thyroid adenoma or carcinoma, nodular toxic goiter, acute thyroiditis, myasthenia gravis, viral hepatitis, and pregnancy. Oral contraceptives and estrogens can also elevate the T$_4$.

Procedure

- For the Murphy-Pattee method, 5 milliliters of venous blood is collected in a red-top tube. The patient's serum (containing T$_4$) is mixed with a solution containing a known amount of labeled T$_4$. TBG is then added. The labeled T$_4$ and the patient's T$_4$ compete for uptake by the TBG-binding protein. The higher the level of T$_4$ in the patient's serum, the smaller the amount of labeled T$_4$ that can bind to TBG. The amount of free, labeled T$_4$ is measured and compared with a standard curve. The level of T$_4$ in the patient's serum can then be accurately estimated.
- The RIA method is more accurate. Antibodies to T$_4$ are produced by injection of T$_4$ into a test animal. The antibodies are tagged with radioactive tracer and then added to the patient's serum (where they bind to the patient's T$_4$). All T$_4$-bound antibodies are then separated out, measured, and compared with a standard curve. An accurate estimation of the level of T$_4$ in the patient's blood can be determined.

THYROID-STIMULATING HORMONE (TSH)
CPT: 84443

Reference Values

Adults: 0.1–4.0 μIU/mL
Newborns: <25 μIU/ml by 3 days of age

The TSH test can be used to help differentiate a primary from a secondary hypothyroidism. TSH is secreted by the anterior pituitary gland in response to stimulation by TRH, which is secreted by the hypothalamus. In turn, low levels of thyroid hormones T_3 and T_4 cause secretion of TRH. Therefore, in patients with a primary hypothyroid condition (e.g., surgical or radioactive thyroid ablation; congenital cretinism) or patients taking antithyroid medications, there should be compensatory increased TRH and TSH levels. In a secondary hypothyroidism, either the hypothalamus or the pituitary does not function properly because of a tumor, trauma, or infarction. TSH and TRH cannot be secreted and their plasma levels drop to near zero.

TSH and T_4 levels are also measured to differentiate pituitary from thyroid dysfunction. A decreased T_4 level and a normal or elevated TSH suggests a thyroid disorder. A decreased T_4 with a decreased TSH suggests a pituitary disorder.

Clinical problems associated with an increased TSH level include primary hypothyroidism, Hashimoto's disease, autoimmune thyroiditis, and cirrhosis of the liver. Decreased TSH levels are caused by secondary hypothyroidism and anterior pituitary hypofunction.

Procedure
- Five milliliters of venous blood is collected in a red-top tube.
- An RIA procedure is used.

TRIGLYCERIDES (SERUM)
CPT: 84478

Reference Values

Adults: 10–190 mg/dL
Children: 10–140 mg/dL
Infants: 5–40 mg/dL

Triglyceride levels are important when studying conditions involving fat metabolism, including atherosclerosis, coronary artery disease, and diabetes. Triglycerides are blood lipids. They are formed by the esterification of glycerol and three fatty acids. When triglycerides travel in the bloodstream, they are combined with proteins as lipoproteins. Fatty acids in the diet are processed into triglycerides by the intestines and then transported in the blood as chylomicrons (emulsifications of fat covered with protein). The liver also produces triglycerides, but these triglycerides do not form chylomicrons. Most of the triglycerides are stored in adipose tissue as lipids. One function of triglycerides is to provide energy to the heart and skeletal muscles.

Clinical problems associated with increased triglyceride levels include hyperlipoproteinemia, acute MI, arteriosclerosis, cerebral thrombosis, diabetes mellitus, hypothyroidism, liver diseases, hypertension, alcoholism, nephrotic syndrome, Down syndrome, high-carbohydrate diets, stress, and pregnancy. Drugs that can elevate the triglyceride level include estrogen and oral contraceptives. Decreased triglyceride levels are seen in congenital β-lipoproteinemia, hyperthyroidism, chronic obstructive lung disease, hyperparathyroidism, and protein malnutrition as well as with intense exercise and high doses of ascorbic acid.

Procedure
- The patient should have no food, drink, or medication for 12 to 14 hours before the test. Water is permitted.
- The patient should have been consuming a normal diet for at least 2 weeks prior to the test.
- Alcohol should be avoided because it causes the triglyceride level to rise and remain elevated for several hours.
- If possible, thyroid medication, lipid-lowering drugs, and steroidal contraceptives should be avoided for at least 3 weeks prior to the test.
- Five milliliters of venous blood is collected in a red-top tube.
- The sample is taken to the laboratory.

VENEREAL DISEASE RESEARCH LABORATORY (VDRL) TEST
CPT: 86592

Reference Values

Nonreactive or negative

The VDRL is a routine screening test for syphilis. It is used to detect nontreponemal antibodies (reagins) whose formation is stimulated by the presence of the spirochete *T. pallidum,* the causative agent of syphilis. The test is useful for detecting primary syphilis 1 to 3 weeks after the appearance of a primary lesion and for detecting secondary syphilis. The VDRL is relatively nonspecific and has a high false-positive rate. Biologic false-positives can be caused by diseases such as tuberculosis, pneumonia, malaria, infectious mononucleosis, RA, SLE, hepatitis, and chicken pox and by pregnancy. False-negatives may appear in early primary-stage syphilis and tertiary syphilis. If the VDRL test shows positive, the diagnosis should be confirmed by an FTA-ABS test.

Procedure
- No alcohol should be consumed for 24 hours before the test. Some laboratories also require that the patient have no food for 8 to 10 hours before the test.
- Five to 7 milliliters of venous blood is collected in a red-top tube.
- The patient's serum is added to a synthetic lipid antigen. If nontreponemal antibodies are present, they will react with the antigen, causing a flocculation reaction. This indicates a positive or reactive VDRL test.

- A high titer (>1:16) usually indicates active disease. A titer >1:32 can indicate secondary-stage syphilis. A low titer (≤1:8) usually suggests a biologic false-positive but may indicate active disease.

MAGNETIC RESONANCE IMAGING (MRI)

Deepak Gupta

CPT: 70540-MR

CPT: 70542-MR

CPT: 70551-MR

CPT: 70552-MR

Normal Values

Normal tissue
No evidence of pathological condition

MR is a diagnostic exam used to image many types of soft tissue. When it was first introduced, it was mainly used to image the brain and spinal column, but now it can be used to image virtually any part of the body, including checking for injuries of the joints (elbow, wrist), blood vessels (carotid arteries, renal arteries, peripheral leg arteries), breast, as well as abdominal and pelvic organs such as the liver or male and female reproductive organs. Advances in MR technology allow it to contrast detail between different tissues with very similar densities. MR imaging is used in the detection, diagnosis, and treatment of heart disease, heart attack, acute stroke, and vascular diseases that can lead to stroke. MR imaging is a vital part of diagnosing and treating sports injuries and has an increasing role in the diagnosis of breast and other forms of cancer.

MR uses magnetic energy and radio waves to create cross-sectional images or "slices" of the human body. The main component of most MR systems is a large cylindrical shaped tube that functions on metric units called "Tesla." Most modern-day MR imaging devices feature a strength between 0.5 and 1.5 Tesla, where the upper limit is equivalent to a magnetic field 30,000 times stronger than the pull of gravity on the earth's surface.

Medical images taken of the human body are acquired or displayed in three main orientations: coronal, sagittal, or axial. Also possible are oblique views featuring any combination of these three orientations.

A benefit of MR is that, unlike conventional x-ray or CT imaging, it does not use x-ray radiation. MR imaging is noninvasive and provides exquisite images with excellent contrast detail of soft tissue and anatomic structures. One nice feature of MR imaging is that it can create detailed images of blood vessels *without* the use of contrast media (although there is a recent trend toward the use of gadolinium contrast media when imaging the vessels as well as soft tissue like the brain).

Procedure

- To begin the MR examination, the patient is positioned on a special table and positioned inside the MR system opening where the magnetic field is created by the magnet.

- People who cannot safely be scanned with MR include those with pacemakers, those who are too obese to fit into the tube, and patients who are extremely claustrophobic. The patient must stay still for 20 minutes to 90 minutes or more. Even very slight movement of the tissue being scanned can cause much-distorted images and the procedure will have to be repeated. In addition, orthopedic hardware (screws, plates, artificial joints) in the area of a scan can cause severe artifacts on the images.
- A mild sedative may be necessary for an extremely anxious patient.
- Each total MR examination typically is comprised of a series of two to six sequences, with each sequence anywhere from 2 to 15 minutes. An "MR sequence" is defined as an acquisition of data that yields a specific image orientation and a specific type of image.
- During the examination, a radio signal is turned on and off, causing the resultant energy to be absorbed by different atoms in the body. This signal is echoed or reflected back out of the body. The MR scanner monitors these echoes and then a digital computer reconstructs these echoes into images of the body.

MAGNETIC RESONANCE ANGIOGRAPHY (MRA)

Deepak Gupta

CPT: 70544-MRA
CPT: 70545-MRA

Normal Values

The blood vessels appear normal and there is no significant impairment of the blood flow through them
No blood clots or significant plaque buildup is seen
Blood vessel walls are normal with no aneurysms present

MRA is a basically an MR study of the blood vessels. It utilizes MR technology to detect, diagnose, and aid the treatment of heart disorders, stroke, and blood vessel diseases. The procedure is painless, and the magnetic field does not appear to cause any tissue damage. In many cases, MRA can provide information that cannot be obtained from an x-ray, ultrasound, or CT scan.

MRA has found widespread acceptance as a diagnostic tool in patients with diseased intracranial vessels, so that only those with positive findings will need to have a more invasive catheter study. It is also used to detect disease in the aorta and in blood vessels supplying the kidneys, lungs, and legs. Specifically, it can detect an aneurysm, a clot, or the buildup of fat and calcium deposits in the blood vessels leading to the brain, legs, or kidneys as well as evaluate clots in the deep veins of the legs.

The test works by emitting radio waves in a strong magnetic field, which is transformed by a computer into images of tissue slices that may be viewed in any plane or from any direction. Specifically, the magnetic field lines up atomic particles called protons in the tissues, which are then spun by a beam of radio waves and produce signals that are picked up by a receiver in the scanner. The images created by this process are very sharp and detailed, so they can help detect tiny changes from the normal pattern that are caused by disease or injury. Information from an MRA can be saved and stored on a computer for further study. Photographs of selected views can also be made.

Procedure

- The patient is placed on a special table and positioned inside the opening of the MR unit.
- Patients with a pacemaker, artificial limb, any metal pins or metal fragments in their body, metal heart valves, metal clips in the brain, tattooed eyeliner, or any other implanted or prosthetic medical devices may not be candidates.
- In addition, all metal objects (such as hearing aids, dentures, jewelry, watches, and hairpins) will have to be removed.
- During the test, the patient typically lies on his or her back on the part of the table with the MR scanner. In many cases, his or her head, chest, and arms may be held with straps to help the patient remain still.
- Once properly positioned, the table will slide into a space that contains the magnet. Depending on the part of the body to be analyzed, the patient's head, limbs, or entire body may be moved into the center of the magnet. Some MR machines (open MR) are now made so that the magnet does not totally surround the person being tested.
- When contrast material (gadolinium) is needed, it is given by IV injection during one of the imaging sequences. This material highlights blood vessels, making them stand out from surrounding tissues.
- A typical exam consists of two to six imaging sequences, each taking 2 to 15 minutes. Each sequence provides a specific image orientation and a specified degree of image clarity or contrast. Therefore, total testing time can be anywhere from 10 minutes to several hours.

CEREBRAL ARTERIOGRAPHY

Deepak Gupta

CPT: 75671

Normal Values

Normal tissue
No evidence of pathological condition

This procedure is also called a cerebral angiogram, neuroangiography, or a neuroangiogram. It is an imaging test used to diagnose problems with the arteries or veins principally in the neck and brain. This test involves the use of catheters, an x-ray machine, and a TV system. It may be ordered for patients with an injury to the neck or face, a brain tumor, cerebral aneurysm, a fracture of the skull or neck, or other head injury, or for someone with a history of epilepsy or a stroke.

In this test, a contrast agent is injected into a catheter and enters the arteries. This allows the arteries to be seen more clearly. The x-ray machine is used to take several pictures as the contrast agent travels through the arteries. These images are projected onto a TV or video screen so that the doctor can visualize the arteries during the test. In most cases, several pictures of arteries filled with contrast agent from different angles and positions are taken, which usually requires several injections of the contrast agent.

Procedure

- This test requires that a person lie on a flat platform in room set up with the appropriate cameras, TV screens, and x-ray devices. An artery in the right groin, called the femoral artery, is usually used for catheter placement.
- A brief physical exam is done to evaluate pulses in the groin and legs. If a person has a weak pulse in the groin, a different artery will be used to insert the catheter. Before the test, the person's blood is tested to check for any bleeding tendency and to check kidney function. A woman of childbearing age will be screened for pregnancy, usually with a urine or blood pregnancy test.
- In some centers, general anesthesia is used for this procedure.
- The person cannot eat or drink anything for 6 to 8 hours before the test. Dentures, eyeglasses, and jewelry, such as a necklace or earrings, should be removed before the exam.
- Once the catheter is in place in the artery, the doctor will advance it into the largest artery in the body, the aorta, which connects directly to the heart. An x-ray machine is used to help guide this catheter into proper position.
- The standard test will typically take less than an hour. In more complex cases, the exam may last for several hours.

DUPLEX ULTRASONOGRAPHY

Deepak Gupta

CPT: 93880

Normal Values

Normal tissue
No evidence of pathological conditions

This diagnostic technique involves applying the Doppler effect combined with real-time ultrasonography. The real-time image is created by rapid movement of the ultrasound beam. The major advantage of this technique is the ability to estimate the velocity of flow from the Doppler shift frequency. Carotid, vertebral, transcranial, and orbital Duplex imaging have been utilized to examine directly vessel patency, blood flow, and pulsation. The Doppler principle is based on the shift in frequency that happens when ultrasound waves are reflected from flowing blood vessels. This change in frequency can be converted into conventional B-mode ultrasound images to help localize the vessel and investigate flow information. The visual display is derived from a spectrum analyzer, which is an instrument that determines the strength of echoes in the Doppler signal that fall into each of several frequency bands during a specific time interval. It also allows for measurement of vessel size and pinpoints irregularities such as plaque or narrowing in the vessel.

Recently, color flow imaging has been created that allows for simultaneous 2-D and color flowing imaging. In this method, flow toward the transducer is usually marked red while flow away from it is blue.

Procedure

- Duplex ultrasonography enables physicians to assess a patient's vascular status without x-rays or puncturing the skin. The test is performed by a technologist using a hand-held Doppler, which emits sound waves.
- A gel is usually applied over the skin of the area to be examined, which functions as a medium to transmit the sound into a patient to receive the images.
- Generally, no medications or injections are needed.

OPHTHALMODYNAMOMETRY (ODM)

Deepak Gupta

CPT: 92260

Normal Values

> 30–50 mm Hg for diastolic arterial reading
> 60–85 mm Hg for systolic arterial reading

Abnormal readings are a greater than 20% decrease from the expected or a greater than 15% difference between the two eyes.

ODM is a procedure that allows the examiner to measure the relative ophthalmic artery pressure. It can be used in conjunction with other tests (such as auscultation, angiography, and Doppler studies) to obtain an accurate profile of carotid artery insufficiency.

During ODM, the arterial tree at the optic disc is examined while external pressure is applied to the sclera, leading to a rise in intraocular pressure (IOP). When the IOP exceeds the arteries' diastolic pressure but is less than the systolic pressure, an arterial pulse is observed. Clinically this is seen as the vessel collapsing and reopening. The first arterial pulse indicates the diastolic pressure, and the loss of this pulse indicates the systolic pressure.

There are two general methods of ODM, compression and suction, but compression ODM is by far the most commonly used in clinical practice. The ODM instrument itself has either a linear or dial scale, both of which work via a spring tension. The dial type has two indicators, one active and the other passive. The passive indicator stays at the highest scale reading after pressure is released or the instrument is removed from the patient's eye. The linear type consists of a spring-loaded sliding rod with graduated markings along a cylinder. The movement of the rod, scale, and footplate is controlled by a button that is pushed to permit their movement. Either a direct or binocular indirect ophthalmoscope may be used to observe the retinal arteries during the procedure.

Procedure

- The intraocular pressure and bilateral brachial blood pressure readings are usually taken prior to performing ODM.
- The procedure itself is begun once the pupils are dilated and a drop of topical anesthetic has been instilled in each eye.
- Room illumination is kept moderate so the scale on the ophthalmodynamometer is visible.

- The ophthalmodynamometer is held like a pencil alongside the eye being examined and the major artery around the optic disc is located.
- With the patient sitting erect in the examination chair and fixating straight ahead, pressure is applied with the ODM at a rate of approximately 20 grams per second.
- This pressure is stopped as soon as the first initial pulse (diastole) is seen and the value is read directly from the instrument.
- Once the index pointer has been zeroed or the linear scale has been reset, more pressure is applied to get past the initial pulse. Pressure is applied until the pulse stops and the vessel collapses (systole). This reading is also noted.
- Repeated measurements may be taken so that a mean may be obtained for greater accuracy.

FLUORESCEIN ANGIOGRAPHY (FA)

Jerome Sherman

CPT: 92235

Normal Values

Fluorescein limited to all retinal vessels without leakage

Visual inspection of the fundus of the eye is an integral part of any visual examination. The direct ophthalmoscope (resolving power about 70 microns and a magnification about 15x) and the indirect ophthalmoscope (resolving power about 200 microns and a magnification about 5x) are the two most commonly employed methods of fundus viewing. More than 40 years ago, Novotny and Alvis suggested a somewhat more sophisticated method of inspection that was capable of far improved resolution. They cleverly utilized the fluorescent properties of sodium fluorescein in combination with the fine optics of the modern fundus camera. This technique, commonly referred to today as *fundus fluorescein angiography* or just *fluorescein angiography*, is a clinical procedure in which, immediately following an intravenous injection of sodium fluorescein, a series of fundus photos are obtained. Fluorescein is a vegetable dye, which is an inexpensive, nontoxic, and highly fluorescent compound that can be used safely in the vast majority of patients. Because fluorescein absorbs blue light and emits yellow light, only minor modifications of the standard fundus camera are required. Specifically selected excitation and emission filters are utilized that document the flow of fluorescein through the fundus of the eye. Minimal overlap of the filters is desired to obtain high-quality images.

The procedure is used to aid the clinician in the evaluation of select choroidal, retinal, and optic nerve abnormalities. Under ideal conditions, optical resolution of approximately 5 microns is a clinical reality. Essentially all retinal blood vessels, including the finest capillary plexus, are clinically discernible. Moreover, this technique provides us with the opportunity for detecting early permeability defects of retinal arterioles, venules, and capillaries. Fluorescein angiography often yields information not obtainable with either direct or indirect ophthalmoscopy.

Fluorescein angiography is helpful in the diagnosis and treatment of myriad disorders of the retina and choroid. These include common disorders such as age-related macular degeneration, choroidal neovascularization, central serous choroidopathy, diabetic retinopathy, and central and branch retinal and vein occlusions. Rare disorders in which a fluorescein angiogram should be considered include choroidal melanoma, idiopathic polypoidal choroidal vasculopathy, retinal arteriolar macroaneurysm, idiopathic retinal vasculitis with macroaneurysms and neuroretinitis (IRVAN), and Coat's disease.

Procedure

- The patient, who is fully dilated, sits upright and comfortably in front of a fundus camera. One forearm is extended and exposed.
- An emergency tray is kept in close proximity to the patient.
- Pre-injection images are obtained.
- Appropriate filters in the fundus camera, barrier and exciter, are dialed into place.
- A qualified individual administers an injection of sodium fluorescein, typically into the antecubital vein.
- The timer on the fundus camera is triggered at the time of injection.
- One or two photos are taken in the first 10 to 13 seconds. The fluorescein first reaches the eye at about 13 seconds after injection. The choroid lights up in a patchy manner and then images are obtained every second or so thereafter for about 10 seconds.
- Based on the condition, late phase images are obtained for the next several minutes with the last few being acquired as late as one-half hour following injection.
- The patient is monitored for 30 to 60 minutes following the procedure for any adverse reactions.

The images are developed (if film was used) and then later reviewed or immediately analyzed (if a digital camera was utilized).

INDOCYANINE GREEN ANGIOGRAPHY (ICG)

Jerome Sherman

CPT: 92240

Normal Values

Quite variable among normal eyes

ICG fluorescence angiography was first introduced and demonstrated 30 years ago by Flower and Hochheimer but widespread clinical utilization is still in its infancy. This technique provides images of the retinal and choroidal vasculature through mildly thick blood, serous fluid, and hypertrophied retinal pigment epithelial cells. ICG yields better images of deeper structures than does fluorescein because the near infrared wavelengths of light emitted by the dye penetrates through pigmented tissue more easily than does the visible light associated with FA. Unlike fluorescein, ICG molecules accumulate in choroidal vessels and tend not to extravasate into the surrounding tissues. Hence, choroidal vessels are better defined with ICG than with FA. Although the clinical utilization of FA is far greater at the present time than ICG angiography, the more recently introduced ICG technique has several distinct advantages. In FA, retinal vessels are visualized with much greater detail than are the deeper choroidal vessels but with ICG angiography the choroidal vessels are generally better visualized than the retinal vessels, even in patients with dark fundi. Choroidal neovascularization, even occult choroidal vessels, can be imaged effectively. Several rare conditions sometimes require ICG rather than FA. One example is idiopathic polypoidal choroidal vasculopathy in which polyp-like vascular lesions at the level of the choroid leak and cause massive lipid deposition and hemorrhages. These polyp-shaped dilations are much better visualized with ICG than with FA.

Procedure

- The patient, who is fully dilated, sits upright and comfortably in front of a fundus camera. One forearm is extended and exposed.
- An emergency tray is kept in close proximity to the patient.
- Preinjection, baseline near-infrared images, which show the important landmarks, are obtained.
- Appropriate filters in the fundus camera, excitation and emission, are dialed into place.
- A qualified individual administers an intravenous injection, typically into the antecubital vein, of indocyanine green. (The technique of dye administration varies according to whether late-phase or early transit images are desired.)
- Care is taken to prevent extravasation into adjacent tissue.
- The timer on the fundus camera is triggered at the time of injection.
- Images are obtained over the course of 30 minutes, although images obtained as late as 60 minutes following injection are sometimes informative in investigating choroidal neovascularization.
- The patient is monitored for 30 to 60 minutes following the procedure for any adverse reactions.

OPHTHALMIC ULTRASONOGRAPHY

Jerome Sherman

Sound can be used advantageously as an alternative to light in the examination of the eye under two conditions. When the tissues are translucent or opaque to light, sound can penetrate and reflect a fairly regular image to provide information not available using light. Second, the relatively slow speed of sound can be used for making distance and thickness measurements.

A-SCAN

CPT: 76511

Normal Values

Normal tissue
No evidence of a pathologic condition

In the A-mode, also referred to as *time amplitude ultrasonography*, each tissue boundary is displayed graphically as a function of distance along a selected axis. It is a one-dimensional display because only one axis is displayed at a time. The amplitude of the echoes on the display is proportional to the sound energy reflected at a specific tissue boundary. The A-mode display is frequently used because of the popularity of intraocular lenses. The axial length of the eyes is one of the primary determinants of intraocular lens power and is best measured using the A-mode display. In ocular disease diagnosis, however, A-mode is not the preferred display because it is one-dimensional. The term *A-scan* is often used to describe this mode, but it is not an appropriate term because the transducer is fixed in one position during biometric procedures and is not scanning. In clinical practice today, the primary reason for obtaining A-scan ultrasound is to measure the axial length of the eye (defined as the distance from the cornea to the retina) in order to properly calculate the necessary intraocular lens power prior to cataract surgery. Various programs exist that allow the calculation of the IOL power for a desired postoperative refractive error by simply entering the keratometry reading and axial length measurement.

Procedure

- The cornea is anesthetized and the patient is given a distant fixation spot.
- The appropriately cleaned tip of a small hand-held probe is brought into contact with the cornea.
- Many commercially available A-scans today only yield measurements once the probe is aligned properly to the cornea.
- Usually several measurements are obtained and averaged.

The axial length is then obtained and this data along with a standard keratometric reading are used for the IOL power calculation.

B-SCAN

CPT: 76512

Normal Values

Normal tissue with normal size and shape
No evidence of a pathologic condition

Unlike the one-dimensional A-mode display, the B-mode display presents a cross-sectional or two-dimensional image of the eye and the orbit. The transducer undergoes a scanning motion in one plane to produce a two-dimensional display. Because the transducer scans over the globe in this mode, the term *B-scan* is usually used. The circular structure of the globe can be visualized in this mode, unlike in the A-mode, which simply processes reflections along a single axis. The B-mode image is composed of many spots, and the greater the sound energy reflected by a particular tissue boundary, the brighter a particular spot or group of spots will be.

This type of B-mode is also called *intensity-modulated ultrasonography*, and the relative brightness of a particular area of B-scan comparative to another area is referred to as the *gray scale*. In a gray scale, there are many gradations of gray, ranging from black to white. This is important, because the relative brightness of a displayed image or echo helps to identify certain tissue. More recently, some systems have capabilities of producing B-scan in color, which may enhance tissue differentiation. In the B-scan mode, the examiner mentally assembles many two-dimensional images into a three-dimensional percept, although recent advances allow computers to assemble this three-dimensional image. This is considerably easier to do than to assemble all the complex one-dimensional images of the A-mode to form the same three-dimensional picture.

In a similar fashion to light, sound energy can be focused. In standard B-scan, the sound is focused at about 25 mm. Structures resolved at this distance include the retina, optic nerve head, the optic nerve, and the orbital fat pads. Anterior structures such as the cornea, lens, iris, and ciliary body are poorly visualized. Because there is always a trade-off in ultrasound, high-resolution systems (such as the UBM) penetrate poorly. The probe used in most ophthalmic B-scan systems fails to yield high resolution of anterior segment structures. It yields adequate detail in most cases of retinal and optic nerve head structures but also fails to penetrate to the apex of the orbit.

B-scan ultrasound is most helpful in those cases of dense media opacities such as opaque corneas, advanced cataracts, and vitreal hemorrhages. The single most important clinical application is perhaps the identification of a retinal detachment in an eye with opaque media. B-scan is also particularly valuable in demonstrating a mass lesion, such as a choroidal melanoma in an eye with a nonrhegmatogenous retinal detachment. A well-trained and experienced ultrasonographer can generally differentiate between retinal detachment, retinoschisis, choroidal detachment, and a dense posterior hyaloid based on membrane thickness, movement characteristics, and position relative to the optic nerve head.

B-scan ultrasonography should be performed at various sensitivity levels. Reflections still present at low sensitivity levels could represent bone, calcification, or a metallic foreign body. Hence, buried disc drusen, which are often calcified, can be found within the optic nerve head at low sensitivity settings. An osseous choristoma of the choroid will similarly persist at low sensitivity levels and appear as a plaque-like lesion deep to the retina. Retinal detachments most often persist longer as sensitivity is reduced than do vitreal membranes.

Just as B-scan can penetrate through opaque media, sound will penetrate through the entire globe and allow visualization of orbital structures. Patients with proptosis or choroidal folds can benefit from an orbital B-scan to either confirm or rule out the presence of an orbital mass. Not all masses can be detected with orbital ultrasound, especially those confined to the apex of the orbit. Proptosis can also be because of heavily infiltrated rectus muscles. B-scan can document such muscle enlargement. On rare occasion, B-scan can confirm end-stage cupping in a blind eye with opaque media. B-scan may reveal a large round mass in the inferior vitreal cavity that at first glance appears to be a melanoma but careful assessment often reveals no connection to the choroid. Slit lamp may reveal the absence of the crystalline lens and the patient denies eye surgery. The diagnosis: Dislocated crystalline lens located in the inferior vitreous because of gravity!

Procedure

- The patient usually sits upright in an ophthalmic chair and is told to gently close his or her eyes.
- A viscous substance such as gonioscopic prism solution is applied to the probe tip that has been appropriately cleaned. The probe is then gently brought into contact with the closed lid.

- The examiner depresses a foot pedal and the transducer in the probe tip undergoes a scanning motion in one plane. The examiner views the cross section on a monitor.
- In some systems, the scan can be frozen, then saved and later printed.
- The examiner then moves the probe to a different location on the closed lid with the goal of obtaining representative slices of the entire globe and orbit.
- Some experienced ultrasonographers are capable of mentally assembling the multiple two-dimensional images into a three-dimensional percept.
- Slices through the optic nerve, which appears as a sonolucent structure (one that does not reflect sound), are important to obtain and analyze. Does a membrane in the sonolucent vitreous attach back to the optic nerve head? Such a membrane may be a retinal detachment.
- While the examiner views the various cross sections, the patient is asked to move his or her eye under the closed lid.
- The eye not being scanned can be open and the patient can be instructed to look up, look down, left, right, and so on.
- A fresh retinal detachment will demonstrate an undulating movement such as a slow-motion video of a flag in a breeze. Long-standing retinal detachments, in contrast, are rather fixed in position by glial tissue proliferation.
- While performing the examination, the ultrasonographer should explore the scans at various sensitivity levels. Bone, metallic structures, and calcium persist at all sensitivity levels. A membrane that disappears at low sensitivity is more likely a posterior hyaloid rather than a retinal detachment.

ULTRASOUND BIOMICROSCOPY (UBM)

Jerome Sherman

CPT: 76513

Normal Values

Normal tissue with normal size and shape
No evidence of a pathologic condition

The UBM operates on the same principles as conventional diagnostic ultrasound although the operating frequencies and resolving capacities are different. In ultrasound in general, there is always a trade-off between resolution and penetration. In standard B-scan or B-mode ultrasonography, penetration to the retina and even beyond to the orbit is imperative and hence resolution is sacrificed. Rather than using a 10-MHz probe as in B-scan, the UBM uses a transducer frequency of 50 MHz, which makes it ideal for very high resolution but limits the penetration. Whereas the B-scan generates cross sections of posterior vitreous, the retina, and the orbit, the UBM yields cross sections of tissue close to the probe head.

The UBM is the ideal diagnostic instrument for viewing anterior segment structures such as the filtration angle, the iris, the crystalline lens, and the ciliary body. The angle formed by the cornea and iris can easily be visualized and even measured if desired. The UBM can confirm the presence of a plateau iris and demonstrate the change in angle configuration before and after a laser peripheral iridotomy (LPI). In narrow angles, the UBM will typically demonstrate a deepening of the angle following an LPI whereas in pigmentary glaucoma, the UBM often reveals a shallower and normal angle configuration following an LPI.

Localized iris elevations are of great concern to the ophthalmic clinician because ciliary body tumors are often impossible to visualize with standard procedures. Most localized iris elevations are because of an iris cyst or a ciliary body cyst but some are because of ciliary body malignant melanomas. The UBM is the preferred procedure and often the only technique available to differentiate between solid and cystic tumors in the vicinity of the ciliary body. The UBM is also occasionally helpful to demonstrate an angle recession and/or a cyclodialysis cleft because of trauma and to document a malpositioned intraocular lens. Because the UBM uses sound and not light to depict structure, scans can be obtained in both light and dark conditions.

Procedure

- The patient lies flat on an ophthalmic chair or table and looks at various fixation spots on the ceiling.
- The eye is anesthetized and a watertight device akin to an eyecup is inserted and then filled with balanced saline solution (BSS). The examiner manipulates the probe, makes contact with the BSS, and then obtains various cross sections of the anterior segment.
- The patient is instructed to change fixation in order to scan all desired areas. The procedure is generally performed initially with room lights on and hence the initial scans are obtained through a somewhat constricted pupil. Room lights are then turned off, the pupil dilates, and additional scans are obtained.
- Some patients with apparent open angles with room lights on demonstrate very narrow angles once the pupil dilates.
- By obtaining the same section with room lights on and off, the examiner can often differentiate between peripheral anterior synechiae, which are independent of room illumination and appositional closure, or iris-corneal touch, which is increased in the dark and hence not yet a permanent adhesion.

CORNEAL TOPOGRAPHY

Loretta Szczotka-Flynn

Corneal topography, or more formally computerized videokeratoscopy (CVK), is commonly used as an ancillary test for the detection and treatment of corneal irregularity associated with corneal disease. Other common uses of this procedure are for contact lens fitting and follow-up (including managing modern orthokeratology procedures) and refractive surgery screening and postoperative management.

The Technology

The most common measuring system in CVK technology utilizes a reflective placido-based device that utilizes the corneal tear film as convex mirror to reflect a series of illuminated annular rings. Placido devices measure rate of change of the corneal slope and can only acquire information from the anterior corneal surface. There are at least a dozen manufacturers of purely placido-based systems on the market today, and they are the most common instruments in clinical practice. An enhancement to a placido-based system is the addition of slit scanning device that enables the acquisition of elevation topography from the anterior and posterior corneal surfaces (as well as from the anterior surface of the crystalline lens). The Orbscan II system (Bausch & Lomb, Rochester, NY) is currently the only commercially available example of this combination technology. Light slits are projected at 45-degree angles to the cornea, which allows calculation of the anterior and posterior corneal surface elevations by comparison to a precalibrated known spatial position. This allows for the computation of corneal thickness, which can then be determined by the difference in elevation from the anterior and posterior corneal surfaces.

Data Displays

When interpreting the CVK map, a critical first step is to understand and utilize the appropriate data display. Data display options include various color scales, curvature maps, and elevation or refractive maps.

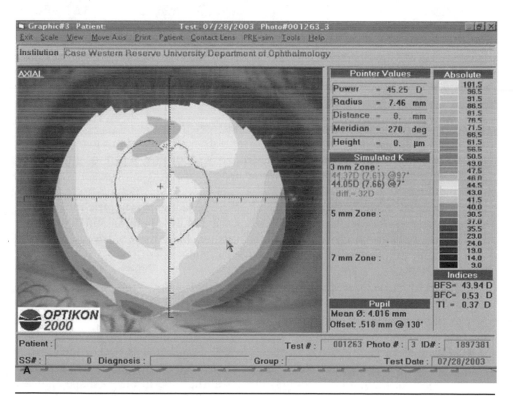

FIGURE 2.1a. Absolute map from a placido device of a corneal scar, showing very subtle irregularity in the superior nasal quadrant.

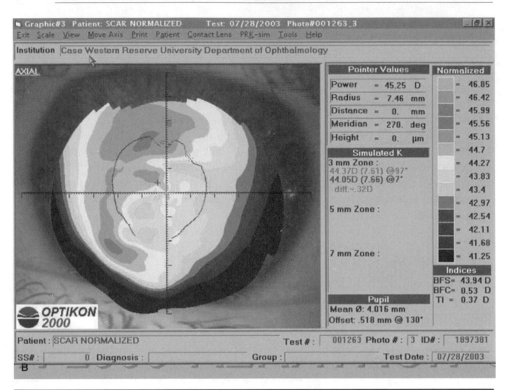

FIGURE 2.1b. Normalized map of same eye in Figure 1a, highlighting the corneal irregularity from the scar.

1. Color Scales
    - Absolute scales consistently assign the same dioptric interval to a given color. Use the absolute map to get a global view of the eye; however, it can mask subtle differences and irregularity. (Also referred to as "Standard Scale" on some systems.) (Figure 2.1a)
    - Normalized color scales adjust to a given eye based on the dioptric range of curvatures present. Smaller intervals will provide more definition and allow subtle irregularities to be viewed compared to the absolute map. (Also referred to as "Color or Autosize Scale" on some systems.) (Figure 2.1b)
2. Curvature Maps
    - The axial "curvature" is a reference distance that refers to the distance along the normal from the corneal surface to the optic axis. The axial algorithm effectively averages curvatures radially, resulting in insensitivity to abrupt curvature changes. (Also referred to as "Sagittal, Color, or Default Map" on some systems.)
    - Tangential curvature is a derivative of axial data, but it is proportional to the local curvature and is axis independent. In diseased or surgically altered corneas, a tangential map more accurately depicts abrupt and localized shape changes. These are the best curvature maps to detect subtle changes of topography, such

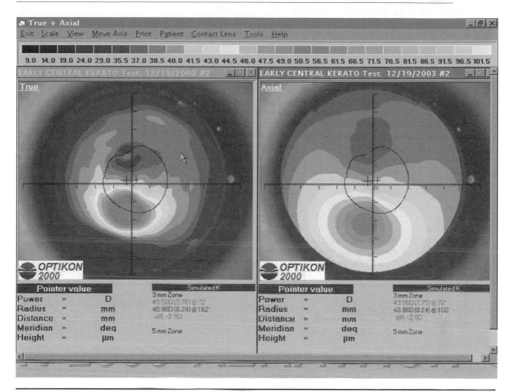

FIGURE 2.2. Central keratoconus outlined on the tangential display (left) compared to the axial algorithm display (right).

as refractive surgery outcomes and corneal disease such as keratoconus. (Also referred to as "Instantaneous, Local, or True Map" on some systems.) (Figure 2.2)

3. Elevation or Refractive Maps
   - Elevation maps depict relative height differences from a computer-selected best-fit reference sphere. Warmer colors (toward reds) identify areas above the reference sphere and cooler colors (toward blues) denote areas of the cornea that are lower than the specified reference sphere (Figure 2.3).

Detecting Pathology with Corneal Topography

CVK is the best diagnostic tool to detect subtle and global corneal irregularity associated with visual disturbances in corneal pathology. Most irregular cornea conditions are best treated with rigid gas-permeable contact lenses utilizing the underlying corneal shape determined by CVK.

Corneal Dystrophies
- **Keratoconus.** The topographic shape is that of an irregular prolate ellipse. The cone type can be classified as either a central (nipple) cone or a sagging (oval) cone. In a

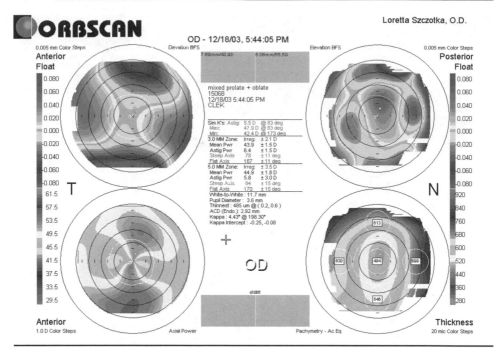

FIGURE 2.3. Orbscan II quad map depicting high (mixed) astigmatism after penetrating keratoplasty. The upper left map is the anterior surface elevation, the upper right map is the posterior corneal elevation, the lower left map is the anterior axial curvature, and the lower right map is the corneal thickness. Note the cornea is steeper vertically, and the elevation in the steep meridian is lower then the reference sphere.

central cone, a small area of elevation or unusually steep curvature is located near the visual axis and is surrounded by (normal) corneal flattening (Figure 2.2). A sagging cone is characterized by a larger area of steepening or elevation typically located infero-temporal to the visual axis. Symptoms and signs include decreased spectacle acuity, increased regular and irregular corneal astigmatism, deposition of iron in a ring or segment in the corneal epithelium surrounding the base of the cone (Fleisher's ring), (Vogt's) striae in the posterior corneal stroma, and possibly central corneal scarring.

- **Pellucid Marginal Degeneration.** The topographic shape is characterized by a narrow, arcuate band of corneal thinning usually located between 4 o'clock and 8 o'clock in the peripheral cornea. A "butterfly shaped" curvature map is produced with central horizontal steepening and vertical flattening. The central cornea is of normal thickness and protrudes forward creating the irregular and against-the-rule astigmatism (Figure 2.4).
- **Epithelial Basement Membrane Dystrophy** presents with focal or diffuse epithelial and/or stromal areas of corneal irregularity.
- **Corneal Stromal Dystrophies** can also result in corneal opacity and secondary surface irregularities.

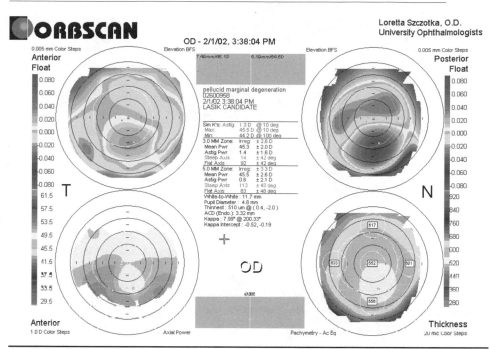

FIGURE 2.4. Orbscan II quad map of pellucid marginal degeneration. The upper left map is the anterior surface elevation, the upper right map is the posterior corneal elevation, the lower left map is the anterior axial curvature showing a classic butterfly appearance, and the lower right map is the corneal thickness.

Corneal Degenerations

- **Salzmann's Nodular Degeneration** is characterized by elevated subepithelial nodules. Irregular astigmatism results adjacent to the nodules and can extend into the visual axis.
- **Terrien's Marginal Degeneration** is characterized by progressive thinning of the peripheral cornea resulting in irregular (and regular) central astigmatism.

Surgically Induced Conditions

- **Penetrating Keratoplasty.** After penetrating keratoplasty, one of five classic corneal shapes can be produced: (a) prolate, (b) oblate, (c) mixed prolate and oblate (Figure 2.3), (d) asymmetric (Figure 2.5), and (e) steep to flat graft tilt. The asymmetric and steep to flat patterns have the highest rate of corneal irregularity resulting in visual loss.
- **Complications of Keratorefractive Procedures.** The predominant shape after a keratorefractive procedure is oblate (for a pre-operative myope) or prolate for a (pre-operative hyperope). In rare cases, postoperative ectasia can result in an abnormal area of elevation (and steepening) similar to keratoconus (Figure 2.6).

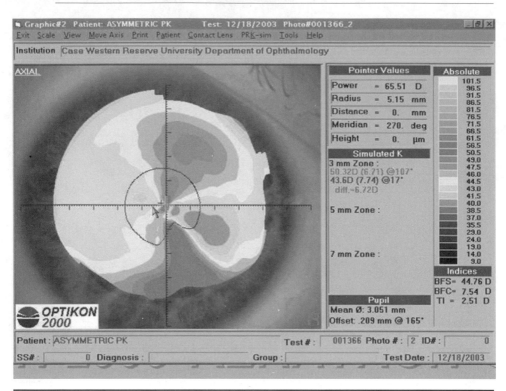

FIGURE 2.5. Asymmetric astigmatism graft shape on an absolute color scale after penetrating kerato-plasty.

Other Corneal Pathology

- **Corneal Trauma.** Corneal lacerations and subsequent repair produce corneal irregularity at the site of the injury (or suture scars) and immediately adjacent to it. Healed lacerations will usually create a raised flattened area over the scar, and an adjacent corneal depression (Figure 2.1a–b).
- **Herpes Keratitis.** Scarred herpetic keratitis often leaves residual (flattened) depressions over the scar.
- **Pterygium.** This fibrovascular connective tissue overgrowth of bulbar conjunctiva onto the nasal corneal surface can result in induced regular and irregular astigmatism, most commonly asymmetric with-the-rule astigmatism caused by flattening of the cornea in the direction of the pterygium.
- **Permanent Contact Lens–Induced Warpage.** The topographic pattern is a reversal of the classic prolate pattern, and an area of central flattening is produced with peripheral steepening. Alternatively, inferior corneal steepening (but no thinning) is observed, which mimics early keratoconus.

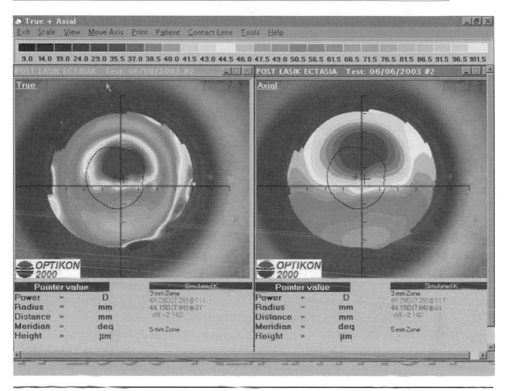

FIGURE 2.6. Axial and tangential maps of the same eye with postoperative corneal ectasia after LASIK.

ELECTROPHYSIOLOGICAL TESTING

James W. Walters

CPT: 92275-Electroretinography
CPT: 92270-Electro-Oculography
CPT: 95930-Visual-evoked potential

Introduction

There are three electrophysiological tests of visual system function that are of clinical value. These are the electroretinogram (ERG); the visual-evoked potential (VEP), sometimes called the visual-evoked response (VER); and the electro-oculogram (EOG). These tests came into widely accepted clinical use in the latter half of the 20th century. Of these, the ERG and VEP are the most useful. The EOG has limited diagnostic value and is discussed only briefly. For a more detailed and continuously updated introduction to electrodiagnostic testing, the reader is referred to the official web site of the International Society for Clinical Electrophysiology of Vision (ISCEV) at <www.iscev.org>.

The Electroretinogram

The ERG is a graphical representation of a change of voltage as a function of time measured at the cornea and referenced to the back of the eye. This voltage change is the result of light-induced massed ion motion in retinal cells with a front to back orientation. As such, the ERG is an artifact produced by light-induced cellular activity. The clinical (flash) ERG is produced by a stroboscopic flash presented in a (Ganzfield) bowl much like a bowl perimeter. Stimulus rate, intensity, color, and background illumination are varied to separate scotopic and photopic responses. The flash ERG is particularly valuable in the early identification of inherited and acquired retinal dystrophies affecting the retinal pigment epithelium (RPE), the photoreceptors (rods and cones), and/or the inner retinal layers. A number of variations and innovations have been introduced into clinical ERG testing with the purpose of enhancing its diagnostic value. The pattern ERG uses a pattern stimulus (usually a checkerboard) with equal areas of light and dark undergoing simultaneous substitution (i.e., the black checks turn white at the same moment that the white checks turn black). Such a configuration is thought to emphasize a ganglion contribution in the ERG, which can be useful in the evaluation of ganglion cell function. The latest innovation in electroretinography is the multifocal ERG (mfERG). In this form of ERG testing, the stimulus is a cathode ray tube (CRT monitor), which displays a "honeycomb"-patterned stimulus comprised of radially oriented hexagons, with the more peripheral hexagons being larger to compensate for changes in cone density. Roughly 50% of the hexagons are illuminated at any given time with the illumination pattern being rotated in a pseudo-random order. This pattern array produces a corresponding array of mini-ERGs that can be displayed much like an automated visual field printout. Such a display has the advantage of revealing localized areas of retinal disfunction. The mfERG is a particularly promising recent development; however, the mainstay of clinical electroretinography is still the flash ERG (Figures 2.7 and 2.8).

Indications for ERG Testing

An ERG is indicated whenever a patient presents with what appears to be a retinal disease that can't be explained or adequately diagnosed by normal clinical means (e.g., ophthalmoscopy, visual fields, color vision, etc.). Examples would include:

1. Symptoms suggestive of known retinal disease, which require confirmation of the diagnosis (e.g., retinitis pigmentosa, x-linked retinoschisis, rod monochromacy, juvenile macular degeneration, siderosis, and central retinal artery occlusion to name a few).
2. Reduced visual function in children or any patient unable to fully participate in subjective testing.
3. Media opacities, which interfere with other clinical procedures.
4. Suspected disease or carrier state of inherited visual disorders prior to the development of other signs or symptoms (e.g., parents or siblings with an inherited retinal degeneration).

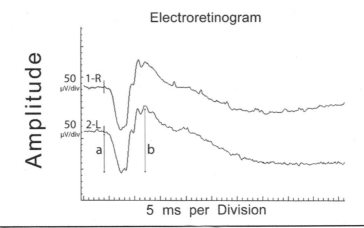

FIGURE 2.7. The flash ERG is a complex waveform. It is the product of the mass movement of ions, toward or away from the cornea, in radially oriented retinal cells. Depicted here are normal ERGs taken from the left and right eye of the same individual. The stimulus is a bright (Ganzfield) flash on a dark background. This waveform is the product of both rod and cone, inner and outer layer cell activity. The ERG produced by a normal retina a very predictable. Changes in ERG shape and/or amplitude are frequently the earliest sign of retinal disease.

5. Objective assessment of the progress of a retinal disease where subjective tests such as visual fields are not a viable option.
6. Differentiating between clinically similar disease entities early in the disease processes (e.g., Stargardt's, cone rod dystrophy, x-linked retinoschisis, etc.).
7. Assessment of retinal function following trauma (e.g., metallic intraocular foreign body).

FIGURE 2.8. The multifocal ERG (mfERG) can be considered as a series of localized flash ERGs. Advanced statistical analysis can be applied to the data; however, they are often "read" clinically like the printed gray scale of an automated perimeter. Care must be taken in doing this as the relative amplitudes at any given locus varies with the size of the retinal area stimulated. The mfERG is particularly valuable in identifying localized retinal disease where normal and abnormal retina are present in the same eye.

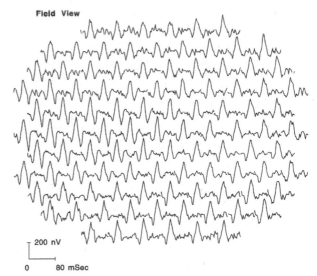

The Visual-Evoked Potential

The visual-evoked potential, like the ERG, is a graphical representation of a voltage change as a function of time following the introduction of a stimulus. Unlike the flash ERG, which for the most part is recorded in real time, the VEP must rely on "signal averaging" in order for the VEP response to be separated from the ongoing but unrelated other brain activity. Like the ERG, the VEP is an artifact of normal brain activity. The voltage changes seen in the VEP are produced by mass ion movement toward or away from the scalp electrode in response to repetitive visual stimulation. The amplitude of the VEP can be quite variable from one subject to the next. Children often give the best amplitude followed by women, then men. Because of the variability in amplitude between patients, relative amplitudes become very important. Therefore, when assessing VEP amplitude, it helps if the patient has one "good eye" that can be used as a control. The implicit time of the VEP wave (the time for stimulus onset to a VEP peak or trough) is much more stable across subjects. Because of cortical magnification and the placement of the macular projections in the cortex, the VEP is predominantly the result of central retinal stimulation. Where media opacities exist, a flash VEP can be performed to get a rough estimate of the integrity of the eye to cortex pathway. Because the shape and timing of the flash VEP show considerable variability across subjects, the flash VEP's diagnostic usefulness is limited. For the pattern reversal VEP (PVEP), a checkerboard pattern is used. The checkerboard is made to undergo simultaneous substitution (i.e., black checks turn white while white checks simultaneously turn black). In this manner, the average luminance remains constant. This testing paradigm has the effect of minimizing but not totally eliminating the luminance response, while simultaneously enhancing the "pattern response." When performing this test, it is important to provide the best possible refraction for the testing distance and to ensure accurate and steady fixation. This latter point becomes particularly critical when assessing the vision of someone thought to be malingering or unable to cooperate by attentively fixating.

Recently, a multifocal VEP (mfVEP) technology has been introduced. The stimulus array is basically the same as that used in the mfERG. The analysis software is much more complex, however, and not yet widely available. In addition, the variability of the VEP response across subjects is further compounded when trying to delineate local VEP responses. Nevertheless, this newest VEP procedure holds the promise that, sometime in the future, simultaneous recording of both the mfERG and mfVEP could be accomplished in one testing session. This would make it possible to differentiate outer retinal disease (before the retinal ganglion cells) from ganglion cell and optic nerve disease with the spacial spasticity of a visual field test (Figure 2.9).

Indications for VEP Testing

VEP testing first came into clinical use in the late 1960s and early 1970s. At that time, considerable focus was placed on using it for objective refraction, especially in the young and in those who were otherwise unable to fully participate in subjective refractive testing. It was and still is used to roughly approximate visual acuity in infants, the mentally

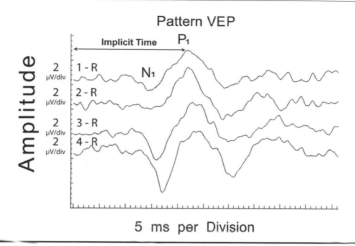

FIGURE 2.9. The pattern reversal VEP most presents as a multiphasic waveform that begins with a negative directed response followed by a positive response. These are called the N_1 and P_1 respectively. The P_1 is sometimes called the P_{100} because it occurs approximately 100 milliseconds from the time of a pattern reversal. In a demyelinating disease, these response times can be lengthened by as much as 40 milliseconds or more. The term *implicit time* refers to the time to a peak or trough and is much easier to measure than *latency*, which refers to the place where a waveform just begins to change.

compromised, and those with emotional or volitional factors that bear on visual function. The most common use presently is of the assessment of optic nerve disease, especially demyelinating optic neuritis. Optic neuritis goes through several stages. During the active stage, it frequently depresses acuity and the VEP becomes nonrecordable. If the neuritis goes into remission and the acuity returns, the implicit time may return to normal or become prolonged, indicating the presence of demyelination. Examples of where VEP testing might be warranted include:

1. Suspected malingering and/or conversion reactions.
2. Confirmation of optic neuritis.
3. Differentiating demyelinating and nondemyelinating forms of optic neuritis.
4. Reduced visual acuity without fundus changes.
5. Gross assessment of visual acuity in a nonverbal patient.
6. Assessments of optic nerve function before and after neurosurgery of the brain.

The Electro-Oculogram

In a steady state, the eye presents electrophysiologically as a corneal-positive dipole. This is to say that if one were able to place an electrode on the cornea and another on the back of the eye, it would look like a weak, corneal-positive battery. This standing potential is largely generated by the transepithelial potential across the retinal pigment epithelium (RPE). The clinical EOG assesses the integrity of the RPE by measuring the change in the standing potential, which occurs in an eye going from a dark to a light adapted state. For a variety of reasons, this potential is very difficult to record directly. Instead, patients are required to follow an alternating fixation target to generate consistent saccades. By this procedure, relative values measured at the inner and outer canthus are obtained and a ratio of the potential in the light (L) and the dark (D) can be established. An L/D ratio of 1:8 or more is usually considered normal. Because repetitive and accurate fixation is required, infants, small children, patients with central scatomas, and uncooperative subjects cannot be tested by this method. There are very few conditions where in the EOG is abnormal and the ERG is normal. Best's autosomal dominant (vitelliform) macular degeneration is frequently sighted as an example of such a condition. Even in this condition, however, the EOG is an inconsistent indicator of retinal disease and of little additional value to the experienced clinician with ERG data at his disposal.

Summary

The ERG and the VEP are special tests that can be used singly or in concert to aid in the diagnosis of a variety of retinal and optic nerve diseases. The EOG has relatively less value.

EXOPHTHALMOMETRY

Anastas F. Pass

Procedure

Exophthalmometry is a noninvasive procedure used to measure the "exophthalmos" or "proptosis" (degree of globe protrusion from the orbit). The exophthalmometer also can identify "enophthalmos" (degree of retraction of the globe into the orbit), as this may be a relative finding, such as in orbital blow-out fracture or neoplasms that may undermine the integrity of the bony orbit. The exophthalmometer is the device that measures the degree of protrusion typically through the use of prisms mounted on carriers. The lower prisms reflect cornea profile, while upper prisms reflect a scale for direct measurements.

The use of an exophthalmometer may provide objective diagnostic data in patients that present with systemic disorders that affect the ocular structure (e.g., thyroid eye disease) but will also be useful in patients that present with proptosis secondary to inflammatory, vascular, or infectious disorders (e.g., Wegener's granulomatosis and orbital cellulitis). Other causes include neoplasms such as cavernous hemangiomas, lymphangiomas, and lymphomas. Patients with sudden changes in facial eye/orbit position (insidious or by trauma) or presentation of acquired strabismus should also be evaluated with exophthalmometry.

There are several types of exophthalmometers, but they all function to measure the distance of the corneal apex from the level of the lateral orbital canthus, or by simply providing a relative difference between each eye.

Hertel Exophthalmometer

- The most common form of exophthalmometry, the Hertel exophthalmometer position, is fixed at the lateral orbital canthus. This position determines the "base" measure that should always be used for future measurements on that same patient.
- In a brightly lit examination room, the patient should direct his or her gaze forward. Using parallax viewing for alignment, the corneal apex is viewed in the prism above a scale, and the degree of globe protrusion is read directly.
- If a patient presents with an orbital (zygomatic) fracture, the use of the Hertel exophthalmometer in the assessment of relative enophthalmos or exophthalmos may be complicated because the lateral orbital rim, which is displaced in most zygomatic complex fractures, serves as a reference point for this instrument. Consideration should be given to the use of the Naugle exophthalmometer in these cases.
- Hertel exophthalmometry is an "absolute" form of exophthalmometry; that is, though it compares the degree of difference in proptosis between the two eyes, it is also an absolute measure based on anatomical presentation.

Naugle Exophthalmometer

- Rather than stabilizing this device on the lateral orbital canthus, the Naugle instrument uses fixation points slightly above and below the superior and inferior orbital rims.
- This unit employs pupillary position as a mechanism for alignment of the patient with the exophthalmometer. It also relies on interpupillary distance as a base measure.
- In a brightly lit examination room, the patient should direct his or her gaze forward. Parallax (similar to that of Hertel exophthalmometer) is used to determine the degree of proptosis.
- Naugle exophthalmometry is a "comparative" form of exophthalmometry; that is, it compares the degree of difference in proptosis between the two eyes over serial measurements rather than an absolute measure based on anatomical presentation as with the Hertel method.

Luedde Exophthalmometer

- The Luedde exophthalmometer is a single clear acrylic bar-ruler-prism that utilizes direct measurement without the use of parallax. The eye is seen through the lower half of the scale, and the scale is seen through the upper half. In a brightly lit examination room, the patient should direct his or her gaze forward.
- The base of the transparent ruler is placed directly against the external orbital canthus. The ruler must be tilted slightly upward in order to obtain the highest reading of the apex of the cornea. By sighting the corneal apex at right angles through the device, the clinician measures the amount of protrusion of the eye from its orbit.
- The norm for this method is the other eye.

Normative Values

- Racial-based facial configurations allow for varying "averages" of exophthalmometry findings. The most important measure is the difference between the two eyes. It has

▶ **TABLE 2.5 Normative Exophthalmometry Demographic Data— Globe Protrusion (An Average of Averages)***

Race	Male	Female
African/American	18.24 mm	17.42 mm
Asian	15.50 mm	13.50 mm
Caucasian	16.22 mm	15.98 mm
Hispanic	15.18 mm	14.82 mm

*This table represents the average of several averages that have been published for exophthalmometry norms. The general standard deviation from the average norm reported was approximately 2.0 mm, with the upper limit of the normal range within a given group to be approximately 2.0 standard deviations from the norm. It should be noted that these are guidelines and that each patient should be evaluated in context with their overall history and review of systems.

been universally reported that a difference of greater than 2.0 mm is significant and indicative of clinical proptosis in (at least) the eye with the greater measure.

The clinician should be aware of individual facial configuration variation for each patient. Though >2.0 mm of difference is significant across a population, it may not be so in a given individual.

- Average (Hertel exophthalmometry) readings across various race-based populations are from 15 mm to 18 mm for adults with normal ranges of 12 mm to 24 mm. Repeated exophthalmometry readings should not vary more than 1 mm.
- Normal "base" ranges for the Hertel are reported to vary from 89.0 mm to 104.0 mm (Table 2.5).

SCANNING LASER IMAGING
James W. Walters
CPT: 92135

Introduction

There are three scanning laser devices widely used for imaging the retina and optic nerve. These are the Heidelberg Retina Tomograph (HRT II), the Laser Diagnostic Technologies GDx VCC, and the Carl Zeiss Meditec OCT (Stratus OCT 3). These are all scanning laser devices, but they function in different ways. The HRT II and the GDx VCC are used primarily for the evaluation of the optic nerve and nerve fiber layer, though the HRT has a function that measures macular topography as well. The OCT's first strength lies in its ability to provide cross-sectional views of the retina, but this third-generation instrument has been adapted to evaluate the topography of the optic nerve and to measure nerve fiber layer thickness.

Scanning Laser Devices in Clinical Practice

The role of each of these instruments is to provide information on the existence and/or the progression of disease. The regions of highest concern are the optic nerve, the nerve fiber layer, and the macula. Two questions may be answered: Does disease exist (e.g., are structures so abnormal that disease is apparent with a single measurement)? And are there changes over time that suggest the onset or progression of disease (e.g., glaucoma, or macular disease)? When evaluating the optic nerve, the wide variation in normal subjects has always made assessment of abnormal difficult. Consequently, while it is useful to look at the initial readings and compare them with normative data, often only serial imaging (which corroborates disease progression or documents the lack of structural changes over time) will clarify the diagnosis.

The Heidelberg Retina Tomograph (HRT II)

The Heidelberg Retina Tomograph is a confocal laser ophthalmoscope that scans the retina in 32 successive focal planes. These successive, highly focused images are "stacked" in order to produce a pseudo 3-D topographic image. In other words, it is a confocal scanning laser topographer. This topographic image can be viewed by the operator and provides for the qualitative assessment of the retinal topography similar to ophthalmoscopy but with much more parallax. The HRT is relatively easy to use. Dilation is not required. The spherical correction is dialed in while watching an image of the optic nerve for best focus. Cylinder corrections are compensated for in 1-diopter steps by placing a correcting lens over the front lens of the HRT. The absolute values assigned to the nerve head analysis are dependent on the operator's ability to subjectively identify the outer limits of the nerve head in the two images made available for this purpose. This step can be difficult, especially where the neural rim is not marked by a change in height or when it is confounded by anatomical anomalies of the rim/retina transition. An important feature of the change analysis is that the chosen rim markers are carried forward from one examination to the next, which eliminate it as a source of variance.

The standard printout incorporates a colored "picture" of the nerve as well a multicolored coded drawing of the nerve and cup. The optic nerve head and the optic cup are quantified by a variety of measurements. These include disc area, cup area, rim area, rim volume, cup/disc area ratio, linear cup/disc ratio, and more. A number of studies have been published showing that the HRT does well at identifying optic nerve parameters when compared with "expert" observers. The parameters that appear to show particular promise in the prediction of glaucoma are rim area, rim volume, cup shape measurement, height variation contour, and mean retinal nerve fiber layer (RNFL) thickness. These parameters and others have been subject to multivariant analysis and have been shown to be more predictive than the present instrument resident analysis. Longitudinal studies are in progress to further identify the most predictive statistical approach.

When evaluating a patient printout, the clinician should first note the topography standard values for reliability and image quality. A value <20 is considered good, and a value between 20–40 is marginal quality. It can also be helpful to review the normal values from a database provided by Heidelberg as shown in Table 2.6. It should be observed that the disc area is constant for the four groups of patients. The highlighted parameters are potentially the most predictive.

The strengths of this instrument are that it provides a quick and reproducible description of the optic nerve and to a lesser degree the nerve fiber layer, in a reliable, repeatable, and easily executed procedure through an undilated pupil. Following a

▶ **TABLE 2.6** Normal Values for the HRT II

Parameter	Normal	Early	Moderate	Advanced
disc area [mm²]	2.257 ± 0.563	2.346 ± 0.569	2.310 ± 0.554	2.261 ± 0.416
cup area [mm²]	0.768 ± 0.505	0.953 ± 0.594	1.051 ± 0.647	1.445 ± 0.562
rim area [mm²]	**1.489 ± 0.291**	**1.393 ± 0.340**	**1.260 ± 0.415**	**0.817 ± 0.334**
cup volume [mm³]	0.240 ± 0.245	0.294 ± 0.270	0.334 ± 0.318	0.543 ± 0.425
rim volume [mm³]	**0.362 ± 0.124**	**0.323 ± 0.156**	**0.262 ± 0.139**	**0.128 ± 0.096**
cup/disk area ratio	0.314 ± 0.152	0.380 ± 0.179	0.430 ± 0.203	0.621 ± 0.189
horizontal cup/disk ratio	0.567 ± 0.200	0.623 ± 0.221	0.658 ± 0.226	0.808 ± 0.185
vertical cup/disk ratio	0.460 ± 0.206	0.538 ± 0.214	0.573 ± 0.226	0.756 ± 0.194
mean cup depth [mm]	0.262 ± 0.118	0.279 ± 0.115	0.289 ± 0.130	0.366 ± 0.182
maximum cup depth [mm]	0.679 ± 0.223	0.680 ± 0.210	0.674 ± 0.249	0.720 ± 0.276
cup shape measurement	**−0.181 ± 0.092**	**−0.147 ± 0.098**	**−0.122 ± 0.095**	**−0.036 ± 0.096**
height variation contour [mm]	**0.384 ± 0.087**	**0.364 ± 0.100**	**0.330 ± 0.108**	**0.256 ± 0.090**
mean RNFL thickness [mm]	**0.244 ± 0.063**	**0.217 ± 0.076**	**0.182 ± 0.086**	**0.130 ± 0.061**
RNFL cross-sectional area [mm²]	1.282 ± 0.328	1.155 ± 0.396	0.957 ± 0.440	0.679 ± 0.302

Reinhard O.W. Burk, Heidelberg, 2000. Reprinted by permission from Heidelberg Eng.
The data for table 1 was derived from the following data base.
  HRT—examination of 743 eyes:
  349 with normal visual fields
  192 with early glaucomatous visual field defects (2–5 dB)
  97 with moderate glaucomatous visual field defects (5–10 dB)
  105 with advanced glaucomatous visual field defects (>10 dB)
  The ± values are for one standard deviation (STD). In a normally distributed population ± 1 STD
    encompasses 68% and ± 2 STD encompasses 95% of the population.

reliable baseline reading, sequential readings can be obtained in 9 to 12 months; a 10% deviation from baseline data is considered clinically significant. Its weaknesses include the need for a larger race- and age-specific normative database and more advanced statistical analysis. Its main weakness may be its reliance on optic nerve and retinal topography for the assessment of nerve fiber layer status. This is a common approach but one that fails in early glaucoma as well as end-stage glaucoma. It is also subject to the same classic difficulties that are induced by nerve size (very large and very small nerves), the hypoplastic nerve, and the tilted nerve, which clinicians encounter with direct, subjective assessment.

The Laser Diagnostic Technologies GDx VCC

The Laser Diagnostic Technologies GDx VCC is a third-generation scanning laser polarimeter that quantifies the retinal nerve fiber layer (NFL) by measuring the retardation of a polarized laser beam and equating it to nerve fiber layer thickness. By measuring the NFL more or less directly, it has the potential for avoiding some of the classic problems of inferring nerve fiber layer health by assessing at the optic disc. The nerve fiber layer is not the only structure in the eye that polarizes light; the cornea does as well. The first- and second-generation instruments (the GDx and the GDx Access) used a fixed corneal compensator to neutralize the corneal contribution, which worked well with many, but not all, patients. The new GDx VCC (variable corneal compensator) appears to more accurately compensate for corneal birefringence. When reviewing the literature on this instrument, the reader should be aware that the reports on the first- and second-generation GDx are not applicable to the GDx VCC.

The GDx VCC is also more fully automated than its predecessors. On a new patient, the GDx VCC will automatically default to setting the corneal compensation prior to analyzing the nerve fiber layer. Each step is subject to operator review, and validity scores are provided on a 1 to 10 scale, with 10 indicating the best quality and reliability. On successive patient examinations, the prior corneal compensation setting is used. The graphical data generated by the GDx is very intuitive. These include a colored "picture" of the nerve, a color-coded depiction of the nerve fiber layer, and a probability plot of any nerve fiber layer deficit. In addition, a TSNIT plot is provided. This plot is a graphical representation of the nerve fiber layer thickness at a fixed distance from the neural rim starting at the **T**emporal side and then progressing to the **S**uperior, **N**asal, **I**nferior and then back to the **T**emporal side. All of the GDx instruments employ a "neural network" (i.e., artificial intelligence that has been "trained" to differentiate between glaucomatous and nonglaucomatous patients). In the older-model GDx instruments, the summary "value" was called "the number." In the GDx VCC, it is called the nerve fiber indicator, or NFI. The NFI scale ranges from 1 to 100 where 1 represents no nerve fiber anomaly and 100 represents a very anomalous NFL. For the GDx VCC, the average NFI for the normal database is 18.5, an NFI of 31 is at the 95th percentile, and an NFI of 48 is at the 99th percentile. For clinical purposes, remember an NFI of $18 = 50\%$; an NFI of $30 \geq 5\%$ ($P = .05$); and an NFI of $50 \geq 1\%$ ($P = .01$). This indicator should not be considered the sole determinant of nerve fiber layer status; however, it correlates as well or better with the clinically determined NFL status as many of the other individual parameters. The numbers cited above are for the GDx VCC only. The older values had a broader range, perhaps because of the contamination of uncorrected corneal birefringence. The strengths of this instrument are that it provides a quickly obtained assessment of the NFL in an undilated pupil. These measures have been made more accurate by the adoption of variable corneal compensation. By assessing the NFL directly, it avoids many of the problems induced by nerve size and tilt that potentially confound the HRT. Some of the weaknesses are that scleral crescents, peripapillary degeneration, and even very "blond" fundi produce heightened reflectivity that interferes with the measurement of modulation depth. The lack of an alternate binocular fixation device can prohibit its use in an eye with poor central fixation.

The Carl Zeiss Meditec OCT (Stratus OCT 3)

The Zeiss Optical Coherence Tomographer (OCT 3) is a third-generation confocal scanning laser interferometer that produces cross-sectional images of the retina including the nerve fiber layer and the optic nerve. It is a very versatile instrument and, perhaps because of this, it is more technically challenging to operate than the HRT or GDx VCC. The cross-sectional views of the retina have a reported resolution of 10μm and are very illustrative of anomalies in the retinal anatomy (e.g., retinal detachment, retinoschisis, macular holes, etc.). In addition, this instrument does a credible job of providing estimates of nerve fiber layer thickness with a TSNIT analysis that looks much like the analysis provided by the GDx VCC. A statistical analysis of a variety of parameters is provided, but without the neural net analysis that the GDx VCC provides. The nerve topography function on the OCT does not provide the 3-D plot of the HRT but rather a series of cross sections. These data are rapidly acquired but the analysis is done one cross section at a time and sometimes involving difficult judgments about the nerve-retina boundary. No statistical analysis is provided for the topography data, a fact that probably reflects Zeiss Meditec's preference for the direct measures of the NFL rather than inferring NFL status from topographical measures of the optic nerve. In summary, the OCT is a very vestal and powerful instrument. Its major strength is its ability to image cross sections of the retina, providing an invaluable view of these structures. It has also been adapted to furnish information about NFL thickness and optic nerve topography similar to the GDx VCC and HRT respectively. Its weakness is that, perhaps because it does so much, it is more difficult to use and it is best performed through a dilated pupil. The data produced by this instrument appears reliable and reproducible though there is some concern about the variability in glaucoma patients for the faster sampling techniques.

Summary

Each of these instruments has strengths and weaknesses. None of them will perform well all of the time. All three manufacturers will need to pursue software and hardware upgrades in order to maintain market share.

PACHYMETRY

Anastas F. Pass

CPT: 76514

Procedure

Pachymetry (or pachometry) is a method of determining the thickness of the cornea (at any given point on the cornea). Though ultrasound, pachymetry may be the gold standard for measuring central corneal thickness (CCT), other pachymetry forms exist, such as optical pachymetry and slit-scan pachymetry (Orbscan®). One study has demonstrated that the Orbscan® system (an optical coherence tomographic method) is the most repeatable technique for measuring corneal thickness but shows a significant bias toward greater corneal thickness measures than both ultrasound and optical pachymetry. Another study failed to demonstrate a significant difference between these three types of pachymetry, noting that the measurements of the three methods showed significant linear correlations with one another and that all of the methods provided an acceptable repeatability of measurements. The clinician should be aware of the advantages and limitations of each instrument and of possible differences in the CCT measurements.

Ultrasound Pachymeter
- Anesthetize the patient with a topical anesthetic.
- Place the pachymeter probe so that it just touches the cornea with the propagated ultrasonic wave directed perpendicular to the corneal plane. Many devices will prompt

the clinician with a tone or synthesized voice audio output of the corneal measurement.
- Several measures of corneal thickness should be generated for each point of the cornea desired.

Optical Pachymeter
- This is a noncontact procedure and requires no patient preparation other than instruction for fixation control.
- Used in conjunction with a biomicroscope, the optical pachymeter typically relies on alignment of, or manipulation of, images of the corneal cross section. Readings can be read off by the user or collected digitally.
- Several measures of corneal thickness should be generated for each point of the cornea desired.

Orbscan® Slit-scan Pachymeter
- This is a noncontact procedure and requires no patient preparation other than instruction for fixation control.
- Data acquisition is mediated by software control of a scanning slit beam. Corneal thickness data is digitally acquired along with other corneal and anterior segment parameters.

Normative Values
- Normative values for CCT vary. It can be said conservatively that a normal cornea can range in thickness from 475 μm to 650 μm.
- The mean CCT in the non-Black population is approximately 550 μm. It has been reported that the mean CCT in the Black population is from 530 μm to 540 μm.
- The Ocular Hypertension Treatment Study (OHTS) has brought focus of attention to the importance of CCT measurement. The study determined that CCT can be a risk factor in the development of glaucoma.

   The OHTS has demonstrated that a central corneal thickness of 555 μm or less had a threefold greater risk of developing POAG than those with a central corneal thickness of 588 μm or greater.
- Goldmann applanation tonometry was developed for accuracy with a reference CCT of 520 μm. However, different investigators found that a variation of 70 μm in thickness or thinness from that reference CCT resulted in an applanation tonometry reading that differed from 3.5 mmHg to 5 mmHg from the true IOP. Other studies have reported that for every 25 μm of change in CCT from a mean of 530μm resulted in an overestimation or an underestimation of IOP by 1 mmHg. While the exact conversion or compensation varies slightly, it is well known that the thicker cornea overestimates the true IOP and that the thinner cornea underestimates the true IOP.
- CCT is one of the critical measurements in corneal refractive procedures. LASIK requires a minimum of 250 μm corneal stromal residuum. The amount of dioptric change will then be limited (at least) by CCT. A thicker cornea will have more potential power change than that of a thinner cornea.

ABBREVIATIONS FOR LABORATORY AND DIAGNOSTIC TESTS

Laurance Freier and Bruce E. Onofrey

ACE: Angiotensin-converting enzyme
ACP: Acid phosphatase
A/G ratio: Albumin/globulin ratio
ALP: Alkaline phosphatase
ALT: Alanine aminotransferase (formerly SGPT)
ANA: Antinuclear antibodies
APTT: Activated partial thromboplastin time
AST: Aspartate aminotransferase (formerly SGOT)
BP: Blood pressure
BUN: Blood urea nitrogen
C: Complement
Ca: Calcium
CAT: Computerized axial tomography
CBC: Complete blood count
CEA: Carcinoembryonic antigen
CHO: Carbohydrate
Cl: Chloride
Cp: Ceruloplasmin
Cr: Creatinine
CRP: C-reactive protein
CSF: Cerebrospinal fluid
CT: Coagulation time
CT: Computerized tomography
CTT: Computerized transaxial tomography
Cu: Copper
ECG (EKG): Electrocardiogram
EEG: Electroencephalogram
ELISA: Enzyme-linked immunosorbent assay
EMG: Electromyography
EOG: Electro-oculogram
ERG: Electroretinogram
ESR: Erythrocyte sedimentation rate
FBS: Fasting blood sugar
FTA-ABS: Fluorescent treponemal antibody absorption
G-6-PD: Glucose-6-phosphate dehydrogenase
GGTP or GTP: γ-glutamyl (transferase) transpeptidase
GTT: Glucose tolerance test
HAA: Hepatitis-associated antigen
HAI or HI: Hemagglutination inhibition
Hb or Hgb: Hemoglobin

HBcAb: Hepatitis B core antibody
HBsAb: Hepatitis B surface antibody
HBsAg: Hepatitis B surface antigen
Hct: Hematocrit
HDL: High-density lipoprotein
HTLV-III: Human T-lymphotropic virus-III
IBC: Iron-binding capacity
Ig: Immunoglobulin
IVP: Intravenous pyelography
K: Potassium
LAP: Leucine aminopeptidase
LAV: Lymphadenopathy-associated virus
LDH (LD): Lactic dehydrogenase
LDL: Low-density lipoprotein
MCH: Mean corpuscular hemoglobin
MCHC: Mean corpuscular hemoglobin concentration
MCV: Mean corpuscular volume
Mg: Magnesium
MHA-TP: Microhemagglutination assay-*Treponema pallidum*
MRI: Magnetic resonance imaging
MRA: Magnetic resonance angiography
5'N: 5' Nucleotidase
Na: Sodium
P: Phosphorus
PPBS: Postprandial blood sugar (feasting blood sugar)
PPD: Purified protein derivative (tuberculin skin test)
PT: Prothrombin time
PTH: Parathyroid hormone
PTT: Partial thromboplastin time
RAIU: Radioactive iodine uptake
RBC: Red blood cell
RF: Rheumatoid factor
RIA: Radioimmunoassay
RPR: Rapid plasma reagin
SGOT: Serum glutamic oxaloacetic transaminase (now AST)
SGPT: Serum glutamic pyruvic transaminase (now ALT)
T_3: Triiodothyronine
T_4: Thyroxine
TA: Thyroid antibodies
TBG: Thyroxine-binding globulin
TIBC: Total iron-binding capacity
TRH: Thyrotropin-releasing hormone
T_3RU: T_3 resin uptake
TSH: Thyroid-stimulating hormone
UA: Urinalysis

VDRL: Venereal Disease Research Laboratory
VEP: Visual-evoked potential
VER: Visual-evoked response
VLDL: Very-low-density lipoprotein
VMA: Vanillylmandelic acid
VS: Vital signs
WBC: White blood cell (leukocyte)

Chapter 3

Ophthalmologic Laboratory and Diagnostic Tests

SELECTED LABORATORY TESTS IN OCULAR DISEASE
Laurance Freier

SELECTED LABORATORY TESTS IN OCULAR DISEASE

This section lists suggested laboratory and diagnostic tests for ocular disorders and systemic diseases that may have ophthalmic manifestations. These lists are not meant to be exhaustive, nor should every test listed be done in every case. In general, diagnostic tests are ordered only when their results will have a direct bearing on the management of the patient.

For the abbreviations of tests used in the lists, see Chapter 2, "Common Laboratory Tests and Procedures." Asterisks (*) indicate a nonspecific, initial group of tests. If the patient's history, signs, or symptoms suggest a particular etiology, additional tests should be done as indicated. See tests listed under individual etiologies. For systemic diseases associated with anterior uveitis, see Table 3.1.

Acanthamoeba
- Gram stain
- Giemsa stain (to help distinguish from herpes simplex)
- Calcofluor white stain
- Culture: Non-nutrient agar with *Escherichia coli* overlay
- Corneal biopsy (if stains and cultures are all negative and condition does not improve)

Acute Retinal Necrosis (ARN)
- CBC with differential
- ESR
- RPR and FTA-ABS
- Chest x-ray
- PPD with anergy panel
- CT scan of the orbit or B-scan ultrasound (to check for an enlarged optic nerve)
- Consider a fluorescein angiogram

▶ **TABLE 3.1 Systemic Diseases Associated with Anterior Uveitis**

Anklylosing spondylitis
Behçet's disease
Inflammatory bowel disease (Crohn's disease)
Juvenile rheumatoid arthritis (chronic iridocyclitis in children)
Lyme disease
Reiter's syndrome
Sarcoidosis
Syphilis
Tuberculosis
Fuch's heterochromic iridocyclitis
Glaucomatocyclitic crisis
Psoriatic arthritis
Uveitis, glaucoma, hyphema syndrome

- Consider urine studies for cytomegalovirus (especially if patient is immunocompromised)
- Consider toxoplasmosis enzyme-linked immunosorbent assay and serum titers for herpes simplex and varicella zoster
- HIV test if patient is from a high-risk group for AIDS

Amaurosis Fugax
- Immediate ESR, Westergren method (if giant cell arteritis is suspected)
- FBS and GTT (to rule out diabetes)
- CBC with differential and platelet count (to rule out polycythemia and thrombocytosis)
- Lipid profile (to rule out hyperlipidemia)
- Serum cholesterol
- Hemoglobin, Hct
- Carotid artery evaluation (duplex scan-Doppler and ultrasound)
- Two-dimensional echocardiogram
- Holter monitor
- ECG
- Digital subtraction angiogram
- CT scan or MRI
- Carotid arteriogram (only if carotid surgery is planned)
- Consider a fluorescein angiogram (may show focal staining at the site of the embolus)

Angioid Streaks
- Skin biopsy (if pseudoxanthoma elasticum is suspected)
- Cardiovascular exam to rule out aortic aneurysm
- Skull x-ray to rule out Paget's disease

- Serum alkaline phosphatase and urine calcium level if Paget's disease is suspected
- Sickle-cell prep and hemoglobin electrophoresis (to rule out homozygous sickle-cell disease) if patient is Black or has Mediterranean background
- PO_4 levels (to rule out hyperphosphatemia)
- Fluorescein angiogram to check for neovascular membrane

Aniridia
- Consider renal ultrasound (if Wilms' tumor is suspected)
- Consider intravenous pyelography (if ultrasound suggests possibility of Wilms' tumor)
- Consider chromosomal karyotype (deletion of the short arm of chromosome II suggests an increased chance of a Wilms' tumor)

Ankylosing Spondylitis
- Men: x-ray of sacroiliac joints; CT scan
- Women: x-ray of shoulders
- ESR
- HLA-B27

Anterior Uveitis; Iritis/Iridocyclitis*
- ANA
- CBC
- ESR
- RPR or VDRL and FTA-ABS
- Chest x-ray (to rule out sarcoidosis and tuberculosis)
- PPD and anergy panel
- In endemic areas, lab tests for Lyme disease

Arcus Senilis (in a patient <50 years old)
- Serum cholesterol
- Lipoprotein electrophoresis
- Serum triglycerides (to rule out type II or V hyperlipoproteinemia)
- FBS (to rule out adult onset diabetes mellitus)

Argyll Robertson Pupil
- RPR or VDRL
- FTA-ABS or MHA-TP
- Consider a lumbar puncture (if diagnosis of syphilis is established)

Band Keratopathy
- Albumin
- BUN
- Creatinine

- Magnesium
- Phosphorus level
- Serum calcium
- Uric acid level (if gout is suspected)
- ANA, ESR, RF, x-rays of the knees (if juvenile rheumatoid arthritis is suspected)
- Other tests directed toward a specific, suspected etiology (e.g., sarcoidosis)

Behçet's Disease
- Behçet's skin puncture test
- HLA-B27 or HLA-B5
- Medicine or rheumatology consult

Blind Infant
- ERG
- Visual-evoked potential
- Consider a CT scan and/or MRI of the brain

Blow-Out Fracture of the Orbit
- CT scan (axial and coronal views) of the orbits and brain if surgery is planned or if the diagnosis is uncertain

Branch Retinal Artery Occlusion (BRAO)
- Carotid artery evaluation (Doppler and ultrasound)
- FBS (3-hour GTT if findings are negative)
- Immediate ESR, Westergren method (to rule out giant cell arteritis if patient is ≥55 years old)
- Greater superficial temporal artery biopsy if giant cell arteritis is suspected because of symptoms or ESR findings
- Echocardiogram
- Holter monitor
- Blood tests: ANA, CBC with differential and platelets, FTA-ABS, lipid profile, PT or PTT, and RF
- Hct and hemoglobin electrophoresis
- Serum protein electrophoresis

Branch Retinal Vein Occlusion (BRVO)
- FBS
- CBC with differential and platelets
- ANA
- ESR
- PT or PTT
- RF
- Fluorescein angiogram

- Chest x-ray
- Internal medicine consult (to check for cardiovascular disease)

Canaliculitis

- Cultures of material expressed from the punctum
- Blood agar
- Chocolate agar
- Sabouraud's medium
- Thioglycolate broth
- Gram stain
- Giemsa stain

Candidiasis

- BUN
- CBC
- Creatinine
- Liver function tests (see list under "Postoperative Endophthalmitis")
- Blood and urine cultures for *Candida*
- Vitreous cultures (when there is a significant amount of vitreous involvement) can be used to confirm a diagnosis and to test sensitivity to antifungal agents
- Consider HIV tests

Cavernous Sinus Syndrome: Multiple Ocular Motor Palsies

- CT scan (axial and coronal views) or MRI of the brain, orbit, and sinuses
- If the CT scan and MRI are normal, consider:
  1. ANA, CBC with differential, ESR, and RF (to rule out infection, malignancy, or a systemic vasculitis)
  2. A blind nasopharyngeal biopsy (to rule out a nasopharyngeal carcinoma)
  3. Chest x-ray
  4. Lumbar puncture (three times; to rule out carcinomatous meningitis)
  5. Lymph node biopsy (if a lymphadenopathy is present)
  6. A repeat CT scan or MRI if the cavernous sinus was not well visualized
  7. A cerebral arteriogram to rule out an aneurysm or arteriovenous fistula (but these are usually seen on the CT scan)
- Blood cultures (three times) plus a culture of the presumed primary source of infection if a cavernous thrombosis is suspected

Central Retinal Artery Occlusion (CRAO)

- Immediate ESR, Westergren method (to rule out giant cell arteritis if patient is ≥55 years old)
- Greater superficial temporal artery biopsy if giant cell arteritis is suspected because of symptoms or ESR findings
- Carotid artery evaluation (Doppler and ultrasound)
- FBS (3-hour GTT if findings are negative)

- Echocardiogram
- Holter monitor
- Blood tests: ANA, CBC with differential and platelets, lipid profile, FTA-ABS, PT or PTT, and RF
- Hct and hemoglobin electrophoresis
- Serum protein electrophoresis
- Consider ERG or fluorescein angiogram to help confirm diagnosis

Central Retinal Vein Occlusion (CRVO)
- CBC with differential and platelets
- FBS
- Lipid profile
- VDRL and FTA-ABS
- Serum protein electrophoresis
- ANA
- Cryoglobulins
- ESR
- Hemoglobin electrophoresis
- PT or PTT
- Fluorescein angiogram (to rule out diabetic retinopathy)
- Ophthalmodynamometry or oculopneumoplethysmography (to help distinguish a CRVO from carotid artery disease; ophthalmic artery pressure is usually normal or elevated in a CRVO, but is usually low in carotid disease)
- Chest x-ray (to rule out an underlying medical problem)

Chlamydial Inclusion Conjunctivitis
- Giemsa stain of conjunctival scraping (will show inclusion bodies within epithelial cells, lymphocytes, and polymorphonuclear leukocytes)
- Chlamydial immunofluorescence test

Choroidal Detachment
- B-scan ultrasonography if melanoma is suspected

Congenital Cataract
- B-scan ultrasound if fundus view is obscured
- RBC galactokinase activity and RBC galactose-l-phosphate-uridyltransferase activity (to rule out galactosemia)
- Serum calcium (to rule out hypocalcemia or hypoparathyroidism)
- Serum glucose (to check for diabetes mellitus and hypoglycemia)
- Urine copper level (to check for Wilson's disease)
- Urine amino acid content (to check for Lowe's syndrome)
- Urine protein and blood quantitation (to check for Alport's syndrome)
- Urine sodium nitroprusside test (to rule out homocystinuria)
- Rubella antibody detection test

Conjunctival Laceration
- B-scan ultrasound
- CT scan of the orbit (axial and coronal views) to rule out an intraorbital or intraocular foreign body or a ruptured globe

Hyperacute Conjunctivitis
- Gram stain
- Cultures:
  1. Blood agar (supports growth of most bacteria)
  2. Chocolate agar (enhances isolation of Hemophilus, Moraxella, and Neisseria)
  3. Thayer-Martin plate (isolates *Neisseria*)
- Antibiotic sensitivity testing

Cornea: Central Crystalline Dystrophy
- Fasting serum cholesterol
- Serum triglycerides (to check for hypercholesterolemia and hyperlipidemia)

Corneal Thinning
- CBC with differential, ESR, RF, and ANA (to rule out collagen vascular disease)
- Cultures (if infection is suspected):
  1. Blood agar
  2. Chocolate agar
  3. Sabouraud's agar
  4. Thioglycolate agar
  5. Gram stain
  6. Giemsa stain
- If a scleritis is present:
  1. RPR and PTA-ABS
  2. Uric acid
  3. FBS
  4. Serum protein electrophoresis and circulating immune complexes (if connective tissue disease is suspected)
  5. C-reactive protein
  6. B-scan ultrasound (to detect posterior scleritis)
  7. CT scan or MRI, if indicated
  8. Chest x-ray
  9. PPD with anergy panel
  10. X-rays of joints
  11. X-ray of sacroiliac joints
- Internal medicine consult if collagen vascular disease or leukemia is suspected

Infectious Corneal Ulcers
- Smears and cultures:
  1. Blood agar
  2. Chocolate agar

3. Sabouraud's medium
4. Thioglycolate broth
5. Gram stain
6. Giemsa stain
- Other stains:
  1. Methenamine silver (if fungal infection)
  2. Potassium hydroxide preparation and periodic acid-Schiff (PAS) stains (useful in identifying fungi)
  3. Papanicolaou's stain (to rule out intranuclear inclusions)
  4. Acid-fast (when *Mycobacterium* or *Nocardia* is suspected)
  5. Calcofluor white (when *Acanthamoeba* is suspected)
- Other media:
  1. Lowenstein-Jensen agar (if *Mycobacterium* or *Nocardia* are suspected)
  2. Thayer-Martin agar (to isolate *Neisseria*)
  3. Brain-heart infusion broth (useful in patients with fastidious bacteria or fungi, or those already on antibiotics)
  4. Non-nutrient agar with *E. coli* overlay (if *Acanthamoeba* is suspected)

Cortical Blindness
- CT or MRI scan of the brain
- CBC (to rule out polycythemia)
- Neurologic consult to evaluate risk of stroke

Cystoid Macular Edema (CME)
- Fluorescein angiography (may show classic "flower petal" pattern)
- When indicated:
  1. FBS
  2. GTT
  3. CRVO lab tests
  4. BRVO lab tests
  5. ERG (retinitis pigmentosa); other lab tests indicated by suspected etiology

Cytomegalovirus Retinopathy (CMV)
- Urine studies for CMV
- ESR
- Consider fluorescein angiography
- Complement fixation test
- Internal medicine consult
- Consider HIV tests

Dacryoadenitis

Acute Infectious
- Cultures of any discharge:
  1. Blood agar

2. Chocolate agar
3. Sabouraud's medium
4. Thioglycolate broth
5. Gram stain
- CBC with differential (if patient is febrile)
- CT scan (axial and coronal views) of the orbit and brain (if a mass is suspected, if there is a motility restriction, or if there is a proptosis)

Chronic
- CBC with differential
- ESR
- ACE
- PPD with anergy panel
- Chest x-ray (to help detect sarcoidosis or TB)
- RPR or VDRL and FTA-ABS
- CT scan (axial and coronal views) of the orbit
- Lacrimal gland biopsy (if a malignant tumor is suspected or if the diagnosis is uncertain)
- If a lymphoma is suspected:
  1. Bone marrow biopsy
  2. CT scan of the abdomen
  3. CT scan of the brain
  4. Serum protein electrophoresis
  5. Internal medicine or oncology consult

Dacryocystitis
- Cultures of material expressed from punctum:
  1. Blood agar
  2. Chocolate agar
  3. Sabouraud's medium
  4. Thioglycolate broth
  5. Gram stain
- CT scan (axial and coronal views) of the orbit and paranasal sinuses (if condition does not improve, or in atypical cases)

Diabetic Retinopathy
- FBS
- GTT
- Fluorescein angiogram if neovascularization or macular edema is suspected
- Consider blood tests for hyperlipidemia if much exudate is found

Episcleritis
- ANA
- ESR
- RF and CBC with differential (if collagen vascular disease is suspected)

- Serum uric acid (if gout is suspected)
- RPR or VDRL and FTA-ABS (if syphilis is suspected)

Eyelid Laceration
- Consider CT scan (axial and coronal views) of the orbit and brain (to rule out an intraorbital foreign body, or a ruptured globe, or in cases of significant orbital trauma)

Malignant Tumors of the Eyelid
- Incisional biopsy
- Excisional biopsy (preferable for malignant melanoma)
- Internal medicine consult for metastatic workup if sebaceous cell carcinoma is confirmed
- Oil red-O stain of frozen or nonfixed tissue if sebaceous-cell carcinoma is suspected

Foreign Body (Corneal, Conjunctival, Subconjunctival)
- Consider a B-scan ultrasound (to rule out an intraocular foreign body, especially if there is a history of hammering or striking on metal)
- Consider a CT scan of the orbit (axial and coronal views) to rule out an intraorbital or intraocular foreign body or a ruptured globe
- An MRI is contraindicated if a metal foreign body is suspected or cannot be ruled out

Fourth-Nerve Palsy
- FBS or GTT (especially if there is a sudden onset) to check for diabetes
- Tensilon test (edrophonium chloride) if myasthenia gravis is suspected
- CT scan (axial and coronal views) or MRI of the brain if the fourth-nerve palsy is accompanied by an additional cranial nerve or neurologic abnormality or the patient is a child with a symptomatic fourth-nerve palsy

Fungal Keratitis
- Giemsa stain
- Methenamine silver stain
- Periodic acid-Schiff stain
- Corneal biopsy (if all cultures are negative but an infectious etiology is still suspected)

Giant Cell Arteritis (GCA): Arteritic Ischemic Optic Neuropathy
- Stat ESR (Westergren method; may be normal)
- Greater superficial temporal artery biopsy (if the biopsy is normal and symptoms persist, take a biopsy of the other side)
- If the biopsy is positive, the patient is kept on systemic steroids and monitored with an ESR 2 weeks after starting therapy. The steroids may then be tapered slowly according

to the ESRs. If the ESR increases or symptoms start to return, dosages must be increased again.

Graves' Ophthalmopathy: Thyroid Eye Disease
- Thyroid function tests (T_3, T_4, TSH)
- Tensilon test (edrophonium chloride) if myasthenia gravis is suspected
- CT scan (axial and coronal views) of the orbit if diagnosis is uncertain or surgery is planned

Gyrate Atrophy
- Plasma ornithine levels (hyperornithemic type of gyrate atrophy will typically show ornithine levels 6 to 10 times higher than normal; nonhyperornithemic gyrate atrophy shows normal ornithine levels)
- Amino acid levels
- ERG
- Consider a fluorescein angiogram if ornithine level is not significantly elevated

Headache
- Carotid flow studies (Doppler and ultrasound) if ocular ischemic syndrome is suspected
- CT scan (axial and coronal views) or MRI of the brain if an intracranial lesion is suspected
- Stat ESR and greater superficial temporal artery biopsy if giant cell arteritis is suspected
- Lumbar puncture if meningitis or subarachnoid hemorrhage is suspected
- Neurology consult if indicated
- Consider a Paredrine (hydroxyamphetamine) test if Horner's syndrome is suspected

Herpes Simplex Virus (HSV)
- Giemsa stain of corneal scrapings (multinucleated giant cells may be seen)
- Papanicolaou's stain (will show intranuclear eosinophilic inclusion bodies)

Herpes Zoster Virus (HZV)
- Medical tests to determine if patient is immunocompromised (when the patient is <40 years old or if an immunodeficiency is suspected based on the patient's history)

Horner's Syndrome
- CT scan of the chest (adult); chest MRI (children)
- CT scan (axial and coronal views) or MRI of the brain
- Radiographic studies:
    1. Apical spine series
    2. Laminogram or lordotic x-ray views of the chest
    3. Stereo x-rays of base of skull, giving special attention to fissures and foramina

- CBC with differential
- Lymph node biopsy if lymphadenopathy is present

Hypertensive Retinopathy
- Internal medicine consult
- Refer to the emergency room of a hospital if the diastolic blood pressure is >110 to 120 mm Hg or if the patient has chest pain, difficulty breathing, headache, or blurred vision with disc edema
- Consider FBS (to check for diabetes)

Hyphema
- B-scan ultrasound if fundus view is obscured (to rule out a retinal detachment)
- CT scan (axial and coronal views) of the orbits and brain, if indicated

Hypotony (Bilateral)
- BUN
- Creatinine
- Glucose
- B-scan ultrasound if fundus cannot be seen
- Internal medicine consult (to check for conditions that may cause blood hypertonicity)

Inflammatory Bowel Disease (Crohn's Disease)
- ESR
- Barium enema
- Rectal biopsy
- Sigmoidoscopy
- Consider HLA-B27
- GI or internal medicine

Interstitial Keratitis (IK)
- RPR or VDRL and FTA-ABS or MHA-TP
- ANA
- CBC
- ESR
- RF
- PPD with anergy panel
- Chest x-ray (if positive PPD or negative FTA-ABS)
- Consider audiogram (if Cogan's syndrome suspected)

Intraorbital or Intraocular Foreign Body

- CT scan (axial and coronal views) of the brain, globe, and orbit (to rule out optic nerve or CNS involvement, to determine the location of the foreign body, and to check for a ruptured globe)
- B-scan ultrasound of the globe and orbit (if a foreign body is suspected but is not detected by a CT scan)
- An MRI is contraindicated if a metallic foreign body is suspected or cannot be ruled out
- Cultures: If infection is a possibility, attempt to culture the source of the foreign body and any wound sites

Juvenile Rheumatoid Arthritis (JRA)

- ANA
- ESR
- RF
- X rays of arthritic joints (if no arthritic joints, then x-rays of the knees)
- Pediatric or rheumatology consult

Dislocated or Subluxated Lens

- RPR or VDRL and FTA-ABS
- Echocardiogram (to rule out Marfan's syndrome)
- Urine sodium nitroprusside test (to rule out homocystinuria)
- Internal medicine consult

Leukocoria (Table 3.2)

- B-scan ultrasound (in cases of congenital cataract, persistent hyperplastic primary vitreous, or suspected retinoblastoma)
- CT scan or MRI of the brain and orbit (if retinoblastoma is suspected, especially if the condition is bilateral or there is a positive family history)

▌ **TABLE 3.2 Differential Diagnosis of Leukocoria**

Retinoblastoma
Persistent hyperplastic primary vitreous
Retinopathy of prematurity
Toxocara
Toxoplasma gondii
Coats' disease
Cataracts
Corneal scarring
Large coloboma
Retinal astrocytoma, choristoma, or hamartoma
Retinal detachment

- Fluorescein angiogram (in suspected cases of Coats' disease, retinoblastoma, or retinopathy of prematurity)
- ELISA antibody for *Toxocara*

Louis-Bar Syndrome (Ataxia Telangiectasia)
- CBC
- Chest x-ray
- MRI of the brain

Low-Tension Glaucoma
- CBC with differential (to check for anemia or polycythemia)
- ESR
- ANA
- RPR or VDRL and FTA-ABS
- CT scan (axial and coronal views) or MRI of the brain and orbit (if neurologic signs or symptoms are present, if visual fields are uncharacteristic or appear to have a neurologic etiology, if the patient is young, or if the case is otherwise atypical)
- Carotid artery ultrasonography

Lyme Disease*
- Immunofluorescence assay or ELISA to check serum Ab levels against *Borrelia burgdorferi*
- RPR and FTA-ABS
- Consider HLA-DR2
- Consider a lumbar puncture (if neurologic abnormalities appear or meningitis is suspected)

Malignant Melanoma of the Choroid
- A-scan ultrasound (to document thickness)
- B-scan ultrasound
- CT scan or MRI of the brain and orbit
- Fine-needle aspiration biopsy
- Phosphorus-32 test
- If a malignant melanoma is confirmed:
    1. Liver enzyme tests: ALP, ALT, AST, GGT or GGTP, LAP, LDH
    2. Liver scan (to rule out liver metastasis if liver enzymes are found to be elevated)
    3. Chest x-ray
- Consider a CEA if a choroidal metastasis is suspected

Myasthenia Gravis
- Tensilon test (edrophonium chloride; this should be done in the emergency room of a hospital because cardiovascular collapse is possible)
- ANA, RF, and thyroid function tests (T_3, T_4, TSH) to rule out other immunologic disorders
- Chest x-ray or CT scan of the chest (to rule out a thymoma)

- Blood test for acetylcholine receptor antibodies
- Blood sugar level
- CBC
- Consider electromyography

Neonatal Ophthalmia

Conjunctival Scrapings for:

- Chlamydial immunofluorescent antibody test
- Cultures:
  1. Blood agar
  2. Chocolate agar
  3. Sabouraud's agar
  4. Thayer-Martin agar (designed to isolate *Neisseria*)
  5. Thioglycolate broth
  6. Viral transport medium
- Gram stain and Giemsa stain (chlamydia shows basophilic staining, intracytoplasmic inclusion bodies in epithelial cells, polymorphonuclear leukocytes, and lymphocytes)

Neurofibromatosis (Von Recklinghausen's Syndrome)

- CBC
- Chest x-ray
- CT scan (axial and coronal views) or MRI of the brain
- CT scan of the abdomen
- ECG
- EEG
- Serum electrolytes

Neurotrophic Keratopathy

- CT scan (axial and coronal views) of the brain if a CNS lesion is suspected

Nonarteritic Ischemic Optic Neuropathy

- Stat ESR (Westergren method)
- If giant cell arteritis is suspected because of symptoms or ESR findings, a greater superficial temporal artery biopsy is necessary
- Internal medicine consult to rule out diabetes, cardiovascular disease, or hypertension

Acquired Nystagmus

- Consider a CT scan (axial and coronal views) or MRI
- Consider testing the urine and serum for any drug, nutritional, or toxin abnormality
- Consider Tensilon test to rule out myasthenia gravis

Congenital Nystagmus

- Consider a CT scan (axial and coronal views) or MRI of the brain to rule out organic pathology, especially if patient demonstrates symptoms of spasmus nutans (unilateral or bilateral head turn and head nodding with a horizontal, vertical, or torsional nystagmus; this usually appears between 6 months and 3 years of age and resolves between ages 2 and 8). A CT scan is necessary to rule out a glioma of the optic chiasm.
- Measure urinary VMA and consider an abdominal CT scan when an opsoclonus (repetitive, irregular, multidirectional eye movements associated with brainstem or cerebellar disease, neuroblastoma, or postviral encephalitis) is suspected

Ocular Ischemic Syndrome

- Carotid artery evaluation (Doppler and ultrasound)
- Consider fluorescein angiography
- Consider ophthalmodynamometry (to help distinguish carotid occlusive disease from a CRVO; ophthalmic artery pressure is usually low in carotid disease, but normal or elevated with a CRVO)
- Carotid arteriogram (only if carotid surgery is planned)
- Cardiology consult
- Consider FBS, serum cholesterol, lipid profile, and FTA-ABS

Chronic Progressive External Ophthalmoplegia (CPEO)

- Tensilon test (edrophonium chloride) to rule out myasthenia gravis (caution: some patients with CPEO are supersensitive to Tensilon)
- Consider electromyography
- Annual EKG if Kearns-Sayre syndrome is suspected
- Consider a lumbar puncture if Kearns-Sayre syndrome is suspected
- Lipoprotein electrophoresis and a peripheral blood smear if abetalipoproteinemia is suspected (to check for acanthocytes)
- Serum phytanic acid level if Refsum's disease is suspected

Internuclear Ophthalmoplegia (INO)

- MRI of the brainstem and midbrain
- Tensilon test (edrophonium chloride) if myasthenia gravis cannot be ruled out
- Neurologic evaluation for stroke

Binocular Internuclear Ophthalmoplegia (BINO)

- MRI scan
- An evaluation of the cerebrospinal fluid using electrophoresis (including check of protein and γ-globulin levels and cell count)

Optic Nerve Hypoplasia in Children

- CT scan (axial and coronal views) or MRI of the brain (if there is an associated neuro-ophthalmic abnormality)

- Endocrine evaluation (if child is of small stature or has a history of failure to thrive or developmental delay)

Optic Neuritis
- CBC
- ESR
- RPR, FTA-ABS
- ANA
- Chest x-ray
- CT or MRI scan of the brain and orbits
- Consider an evaluation of the CSF using electrophoresis (including a check of protein and γ-globulin levels and cell count)

Optic Neuropathy
- ESR
- FTA-ABS
- RPR or VDRL
- Skull films

Optic Neuropathy Because of Trauma
- CT scan* (axial and coronal views) of the head and orbit (to rule out an intraorbital foreign body)
- B-scan ultrasound of the orbit (if a foreign body is suspected but is not detected by a CT scan)

Diseases of the Orbit
- ANA
- BUN
- CBC with differential
- Creatinine
- ESR
- FBS
- Thyroid function tests (T_3, T_4, TSH)
- CT scan (axial and coronal views) of the orbit
- B-scan ultrasound of the orbit
- MRI (if diagnosis is uncertain)
- Orbital biopsy (if indicated)

Orbital Cellulitis
- Blood cultures
- CBC with differential
- CT scan (axial and coronal views, with and without contrast) of the orbits and sinuses

- Cultures of any wound or drainage:
  1. Blood agar
  2. Chocolate agar
  3. Sabouraud's medium
  4. Thioglycolate broth
  5. Gram stain
- Lumbar puncture (if meningitis is suspected)

Nonspecific Orbital Inflammation

- CBC with differential
- ANA
- BUN
- Creatinine
- ESR
- FBS
- CT scan (axial and coronal views) of the orbit(s)
- Incisional (or fine-needle aspiration) biopsy of the orbit (if there is a history of cancer, if an acute case does not respond to systemic steroids within a few days, if the case is atypical, or if the diagnosis is uncertain).

Tumors of the Orbit

In Adults

- CT scan (axial and coronal views) of the brain and orbit
- B-scan ultrasound of the orbit
- MRI (if indicated)
- Orbital biopsy (incisional or fine-needle aspiration) if metastasis is suspected
- Chest x-ray
- Estrogen receptor assay (if breast cancer is suspected)
- Mammogram (if indicated)
- If a lymphoma is suspected:
  1. Bone marrow biopsy
  2. CBC with differential
  3. CT scan of the abdomen
  4. CT scan of the brain
  5. Serum protein electrophoresis
  6. Incisional biopsy (if workup is negative)
  7. Fine-needle biopsy (to confirm diagnosis)

In Children

- CT scan (axial and coronal views) of the brain and orbit
- B-scan ultrasound of the orbit
- MRI of the orbit (if indicated)
- Incisional biopsy (in cases of acute onset and rapid progression, to rule out rhabdomyosarcoma or other aggressive malignancy)

- If leukemia is suspected:
  1. CBC with differential
  2. Bone marrow studies
- If neuroblastoma is suspected:
  1. CT scan of the abdomen
  2. Check urine for vanilyllmandelic acid
- If rhabdomyosarcoma is suspected:
  1. Bone marrow aspiration
  2. Bone x-rays
  3. Chest x-rays
  4. Liver function studies
  5. Lumbar puncture

Papilledema

- CT scan (axial and coronal views) or MRI of the head and orbit
- Lumbar puncture (if the CT scan does not reveal a cause for the papilledema)

Parinaud's Oculoglandular Conjunctivitis

- CBC
- ESR
- Cultures:
  1. Blood agar
  2. Chocolate agar
  3. Cystine-glucose blood agar
  4. Lowenstein-Jensen agar (isolates *Mycobacterium*)
  5. Sabouraud's medium
  6. Thioglycolate broth
- Stains of conjunctival scrapings:
  1. Gram stain
  2. Giemsa stain
  3. Acid-fast stain (used to detect *Mycobacterium*)
- Conjunctival biopsy
- PPD with anergy panel
- Chest x-ray
- RPR or VDRL and FTA-ABS
- Agglutination test for tularemia antibodies (if tularemia is suspected)

Conjunctival or Corneal Phlyctenule

- PPD with anergy panel (to check for TB)
- Chest x-ray (if TB is suspected)
- ESR
- Cultures (if an infectious ulcer is suspected)

Posterior Uveitis*

- ACE level
- Chest x-ray

- RPR or VDRL and FTA-ABS
- ANA
- ESR
- B-scan ultrasound (to rule out intraocular foreign body or malignant melanoma)
- ERG (to rule out retinitis pigmentosa)
- CT scan of the globe (e.g., to rule out an intraocular foreign body or a retinoblastoma in young children)
- PPD and anergy panel
- Toxoplasmosis antibody titer test
- *Toxocara* ELISA antibody test
- HLA-B5 (if Behçet's disease is suspected)
- HLA-A29 (if birdshot [vitiliginous] retinochoroidopathy is suspected)
- Lyme disease immunofluorescent assay or ELISA
- If patient is immunocompromised:
  1. Microscopic viral studies of urine for CMV
  2. Titers for herpes simplex and varicella zoster
- Blood culture if an infectious etiology is suspected
- Lumbar puncture and CT scan of the brain if a reticulum-cell sarcoma is suspected
- In newborns, consider titer for rubella virus

Postoperative Endophthalmitis

Acute
- CBC with differential
- Serum electrolytes
- Vitreous cultures:
  1. Blood agar
  2. Chocolate agar
  3. Sabouraud's medium
  4. Thioglycolate broth
  5. Giemsa stain
  6. Gram stain
- Consider a B-scan ultrasound (to check for vitreous cells)

Delayed-Onset (Onset 1 Week to 4 Months after Surgery)
- CBC with differential
- Serum electrolytes
- Liver function tests (may include):
  1. Liver enzyme tests (ALP, ALT, AST, 5'N, GGTP, LAP, LD/LDH)
  2. Ammonia (plasma, blood)
  3. Serum bilirubin
  4. Serum cholesterol
  5. Serum protein, protein electrophoresis

6. PT
7. Urine bilirubin
8. Urine urobilinogen
9. HBsAg
10. HBsAb/anti-HBs
11. HBcAb/anti-HBc
12. Vitreous cultures (especially for *Propionibacterium acnes*)
13. Blood agar
14. Chocolate agar
15. Sabouraud's medium
16. Thioglycolate broth
17. Anaerobic cultures (e.g., *Brucella*)

Postoperative Uveitis (Atypical)

- Vitreous culture for *P. acnes* if an infectious endophthalmitis is suspected
- B scan ultrasound if fundus view is obscured

Preseptal Cellulitis

- CBC with differential (severe case or if fever is present)
- Cultures of conjunctival scrapings (especially if *Hemophilus influenzae* is suspected):
  1. Blood agar
  2. Chocolate agar
  3. Sabouraud's medium
  4. Thioglycolate broth
  5. Gram stain
- Cultures (as above) of any drainage or open wound
- CT scan (axial and coronal views) of the orbits and brain (if an intraorbital or intraocular foreign body, a cancer, cavernous sinus thrombosis, or an orbital cellulitis are suspected, or if the patient fails to respond to antibiotic therapy)

Presumed Ocular Histoplasmosis Syndrome

- Histoplasmin skin test
- HLA-B27
- ESR

Progressive Visual Loss and Optic Nerve Dysfunction

- CT scan (coronal and axial views) or MRI of the brain and orbit

Pseudotumor Cerebri

- CT scan (axial and coronal views) or MRI of the brain and orbit
- Lumbar puncture (if CT scan is normal)
- Neuroophthalmology consult
- Endocrinology consult

Racemose Hemangiomatosis (Wyburn-Mason Syndrome)

- EEG
- MRI of the brain

Reiter's Syndrome

- Conjunctival, urethral, and prostatic cultures (if indicated)
- ESR
- WBC counts
- Joint x-rays
- HLA-B27
- Medicine or rheumatology consult

Reticulum-Cell Sarcoma

- CT scan (axial and coronal views), with and without contrast, or MRI of the head and orbit
- Lumbar puncture for:
  1. Culture
  2. Cell count
  3. Cytology
  4. Glucose
  5. Gram stain
  6. Methenamine silver stain
  7. Protein
  8. VDRL
- Biopsy of any suspicious lymph nodes
- Bone marrow biopsy (if indicated)
- CT scan of the body (if indicated)
- Diagnostic vitrectomy for cytologic and immunohistologic studies (if indicated)

Retinitis Pigmentosa (RP)

- ERG (to help confirm diagnosis and rule out congenital rubella)
- FTA-ABS (to rule out syphilis)
- Fasting serum phytanic acid level (to rule out Refsum's disease) if patient has ataxia, deafness, or other neurologic abnormalities or has shown a progressive restriction of ocular motility or a progressive weakening of distal extremities
- Serum cholesterol and triglyceride levels if hereditary abetalipoproteinemia is suspected (low levels are usually found)
- Serum protein and lipoprotein electrophoresis if hereditary abetalipoproteinemia is suspected (a lipoprotein deficiency would be found)
- Peripheral blood smears (with previous two tests); an acanthocytosis would be found
- Cardiology consult with sequential electrocardiograms if Kearns-Sayre syndrome is suspected

Retrobulbar Hemorrhage Because of Trauma
- CT scan (axial and coronal views) of the orbit (to check for orbital fracture or ruptured globe)

Ruptured Globe
- B-scan ultrasound
- CT scan (axial and coronal views) of the orbits and of the brain (to determine the location of the rupture and to rule out any intraorbital or intraocular foreign bodies)

Sarcoidosis
- ACE* (>43 is considered positive)
- Blind conjunctival biopsy (look for noncaseating granuloma)
- Chest x-ray (potato lesion)
- Limited gallium scan* (head and neck)
- Immunoglobulin levels (look for elevation)
- Kveim-Siltzback skin-antigen test
- PPD and anergy panel (to rule out TB)
- Serum calcium
- Serum lysozyme (>12 is considered positive)
- Skin lesion biopsy
- RPR and FTA-ABS (to rule out syphilis)
- ESR

Scleritis
- ANA
- CBC
- ESR
- RF
- Serum uric acid (if gout is suspected)
- FBS
- PPD with anergy panel
- Chest x-ray
- B-scan ultrasound (to detect posterior scleritis)
- CT scan or MRI (if indicated)
- X-rays of joints (hands, feet, hips)
- X-rays of sacroiliac
- Serum protein electrophoresis, C-reactive protein, and circulating immune complexes (if connective tissue disease is suspected)

Sickle Cell Disease
- Sickle cell prep and hemoglobin electrophoresis (patients with sickle cell trait or sickle cell hemoglobin C disease may show a negative sickle cell prep)
- Consider fluorescein angiogram

Sixth-Nerve Palsy
- FBS
- CBC
- ESR (usually done only if patient is <50 years old)
- CT scan (axial and coronal views) or MRI of the brain if (a) the sixth-nerve palsy is accompanied by an additional cranial nerve or neurologic abnormality; (b) there is severe pain; (c) the patient is a child; (d) any neurologic signs or symptoms develop during follow-up (patient is re-examined every 6 weeks until the palsy resolves); (e) ocular motility becomes even more restricted; or (f) the palsy does not resolve in 3 to 6 months

Stevens-Johnson Syndrome (Erythema Multiforme)
- CBC
- Serum electrolytes
- Cultures from conjunctival and corneal scrapings if infection is suspected:
  1. Blood agar
  2. Chocolate agar
  3. Sabouraud's medium
  4. Thioglycolate broth
  5. Gram stain
  6. Giemsa stain

Strabismus

Esotropia in Children
- CT scan (axial and coronal views) or MRI of the brain (if a divergence insufficiency or paralysis is present, to rule out an intracranial mass; if an isolated sixth-nerve palsy is suspected; or if abduction is limited and the esodeviation appears incomitant, varying with the direction of gaze)
- Neurology consult (if above)

Exodeviations in Children
- Tensilon test (edrophonium chloride) if myasthenia gravis is suspected
- CT scan (axial and coronal views) or MRI of the brain and orbit (if indicated; e.g., suspected orbital tumor, third-nerve palsy, or convergence paralysis)
- CBC with differential (if third-nerve palsy is suspected)

Sturge-Weber Syndrome
- CT scan (axial and coronal views) or MRI of the brain
- EEG

Recurrent Subconjunctival Hemorrhages
- Bleeding time test
- CBC
- Platelet count

- PT
- PTT

Superior Limbic Keratoconjunctivitis (SLK)
- Thyroid function tests (T_3, T_4, TSH; to rule out associated thyroid disease)

Sympathetic Ophthalmia
- CBC
- RPR and FTA-ABS
- ACE (if sarcoidosis is suspected)
- Chest x-ray (to rule out sarcoidosis)
- Consider B-scan ultrasonograph or fluorescein angiogram (to help confirm diagnosis)

Syphilis

Acquired
- RPR or VDRL
- FTA-ABS or MHA-TP
- CBC
- ESR
- Consider lumbar puncture
- Consider HIV tests

Congenital
- RPR or VDRL
- FTA-ABS or MHA-TP
- Consider titers for herpes simplex, zoster, rubella, toxoplasmosis, and CMV if diagnosis is uncertain
- Consider B-scan ultrasound if no view of the fundus is obtained (to rule out a mass or retinal detachment)

Systemic Lupus Erythematosus (SLE)
- ANA
- ESR
- Immunoglobulin electrophoresis
- Lupus erythematosus cell prep
- Serum complement

Third-Nerve Palsy
- Immediate CT scan (axial and coronal views) or MRI of the brain if:
  1. The pupil is involved
  2. The pupil is spared but (a) the patient has an additional cranial nerve or neurologic abnormality; (b) the palsy is >2 to 3 months old but has not improved; (c) the

patient is <50 years old (unless there is a history of long-standing diabetes or hypertension); or (d) the patient has an incomplete third-nerve palsy, for example, some sparing of muscle function
- The patient develops an aberrant regeneration (except for a regeneration following a traumatic third-nerve palsy)
- CBC with differential (especially in children)
- FBS
- ESR
- Cerebral angiogram in all patients <20 years old whose CT scan or MRI showed normal, but who fit one of the criteria listed earlier
- Tensilon test if the pupil is spared and there is no improvement in ocular motility (to rule out myasthenia gravis)
- Neurology consult

Toxic-Nutritional Disease
- CBC (to check for macrocytic anemia associated with alcoholism)
- Serum vitamin B_{12} (consider a GI consult if the vitamin B_{12} level is found to be low)
- Serum folate (<3 mg/ml is abnormal)
- Consider a screening for heavy metal toxicity (e.g., lead)

Toxoplasma Gondii*
- Complement fixation test (will show a positive result in active disease)
- Sabin-Feldman dye test
- Indirect fluorescent antibody test or ELISA antibody
- ESR
- HIV test in atypical cases or when the patient is from a high-risk group for AIDS
- If the diagnosis is uncertain:
  1. FTA-ABS
  2. PPD and anergy panel
  3. Chest x-ray
  4. *Toxocara* ELISA
- Fluorescein angiogram if a choroidal neovascular membrane is suspected

Trachoma
- Giemsa stain (will show intracytoplasmic inclusions within epithelial cells, lymphocytes, and polymorphonuclear leukocytes)
- Chlamydial immunofluorescence test

Tuberculosis
- PPD and anergy panel
- Chest x-ray
- ESR
- Medicine consult

Vertebral-Basilar Insufficiency
- CBC (to rule out anemia and polycythemia)
- ESR (to rule out giant cell arteritis)
- Consider noninvasive carotid flow studies
- Consider EKG and Holter monitor for 24 hours (to check for a ventricular ectopy or sick sinus syndrome)
- Consider x-rays of the cervical spine (to rule out compressive cervical spine disease)

Vision Loss Not Accounted for by Ocular Findings
- CT or MRI scan of the brain
- ERG (to check for cone-rod dystrophy)
- Fluorescein angiogram
- VEP

Vogt-Koyanagi-Harada (VKH) Syndrome
- CBC
- RPR and FTA-ABS
- ACE
- Chest x-ray
- PPD with anergy panel
- Audiogram
- Lumbar puncture for:
  1. Cell count with differential
  2. Glucose
  3. Gram stain
  4. Methenamine silver stain
  5. Protein
  6. VDRL
  7. Culture (This is done during an attack with meningeal symptoms. VKH often shows a lymphocytosis.)
- CT scan with and without contrast or MRI of the brain if patient demonstrates neurologic abnormalities
- Consider fluorescein angiogram

Von Hippel-Lindau Syndrome
- CBC
- Serum electrolytes
- Urine epinephrine and norepinephrine levels
- CT scan of the abdomen
- MRI of the brain
- Fluorescein angiogram (if treatment is planned)

Wilson's Disease

- Serum ceruloplasmin
- Serum copper
- Serum protein electrophoresis
- Urine copper
- Internal medicine consult
- Neurology consult

Chapter 4

Ocular Side Effects of Systemic Medications

OCULAR SIDE EFFECTS OF SYSTEMIC MEDICATIONS

Bruce E. Onofrey

Drug toxicity is not an infrequent occurrence. Systemic medications have the potential, under certain circumstances, to produce undesirable adverse effects. The eye is not immune to these problems.

Because of its extensive neurological and vascular components, the eye can be affected in a variety of ways by systemically administered medications. The following tables will illustrate some of the more frequent drug–eye interactions (Tables 4.1 through 4.12).

▶ TABLE 4.1 Drugs That Cause Dry-Eye

Drug	Indication
Oral retinoids	Cystic acne
Antihistamines	Allergic rhinitis/sinusitis
Anticholinergics	Parkinson's disease
Anticholinergic effect	Psychoses, anxiety
Diuretics	Hypertension

▶ TABLE 4.2 Drugs That Cause Blepharoconjunctivitis

Drug	Indication
Isoretinoin	Cystic acne
Etretinate	Cystic acne
Amiodarone	Cardiac arrhythmia
Gold salts	Arthritis
Methotrexate	Neoplastic disease/arthritis
Potassium penicillin	Antibiotic
Rifampin	Tuberculosis

▶ **TABLE 4.3 Corneal Toxicity from Systemic Drugs**

Drug	Corneal Response
Chloroquine/hydroxychloroquine	Whorl-like epithelial deposits below the horizontal midline
Phenothiazines	Endothelial dusting
Amiodarone	Whorl-like epithelial deposits greater in the periphery
Gold salts	Ocular chrysiasis

▶ **TABLE 4.4 Systemically Administered Medications Most Likely to Induce Relative Pupil-Block Glaucoma**

Drug	Indication
Benztropine mesylate	Movement disorders
Diazepam	Anxiety
Chlorpheniramine	Antihistamine
Tricyclic antidepressants	Depression
Diphenoxylate	Antidiarrheal
Chlordiazepoxide	Anxiety
Amphetamine derivatives	Appetite suppression
Scopolamine	Motion sickness

▶ **TABLE 4.5 Commonly Prescribed Systemic β-Blockers**

Generic Identification	Proprietary Identification
Propranolol	Inderal
Atenolol	Tenormin
Metoprolol	Lopressor
Nadolol	Corgard
Labetalol	Trandate

▶ TABLE 4.6 Anterior Segment Side Effects of Systemic Medications

Miosis	Cycloplegia	Diplopia/ Nystagmus	Iritis
Heroin	Phenothiazines	Carbamazepine	Opiates
Opium	Tricyclic antidepressants	Tricyclic antidepressants	Carbonic anhydrase inhibitors
Marijuana	Benzodiazepines	Phenothiazines	Gold salts
Hashish	Butyrophenones	Oral hypoglycemics	Radioactive iodides
Codeine	Lithium carbonate	Antihistamines	Pralidoxime
Morphine	Loxapine	Ethanol	
Nitrous oxide	Meprobamate	Corticosteroids	
	Hashish	Marijuana	
	Marijuana	Phenytoin	
	LSD		
	Psilocybin		
	Mescaline		

▶ TABLE 4.7 Drugs That Induce Changes in Refractive Error

Drug	Refractive Change
Corticosteroids	Myopia
Acetazolamide	Myopia
Oral hypoglycemics	Hyperopia
Hydrochlorothiazide	Myopia
Oral contraceptives	Myopia
NSAIAs	Myopia
Oral retinoids	Myopia

▶ TABLE 4.8 Drugs That Alter Color Perception

Drug	Color Anomaly
Digitalis glycosides	Xanthopsia
Amiodarone	Colored halos
Ethambutol	Red-green defect
Isoniazid	Red-green defect
Indomethacin	Tritan defect
Chloroquine	Tritan defect
Thioridazine	Tritan defect
LSD/mescaline/psilocybin	Variable

▶ TABLE 4.9 Drugs That Induce Retinal Changes

Drug	Retinal Change
Phenothiazines	Pigmentary retinopathy
Chloroquine/hydroxychloroquine	Bull's-eye maculopathy
Indomethacin	Pigmentary retinopathy
Quinine	Vessel attenuation
Oral retinoids	Decreased retinal function
Antineoplastics	Whitish exudates in posterior pole
Talc	Refractile bodies in posterior pole
NSAID's	Retinal hemorrhages
Oral contraceptives	Retinal signs of vascular occlusive disease

▶ TABLE 4.10 Differential Diagnosis of Chloroquine
or Hydroxychloroquine Retinopathy

Age-related maculopathy
Best's vitelliform disease
Serous detachment of the macula
Lamellar hole of the macula
Stargardt's disease
Kuhnt-Junius macular disease
Retinitis pigmentosa
Rubella retinopathy

▶ TABLE 4.11 Differential Diagnosis of
Phenothiazine Retinopathy

Reticular degeneration
Age-related maculopathy
Chloroquine retinopathy
Hydroxychloroquine retinopathy
Syphilis
Vitelleruptive changes

▶ TABLE 4.12 Drugs That Induce Optic
Nerve Changes

Drug	Optic Nerve Change
Ethambutol	Optic neuritis
Isoniazid	Optic neuritis
Rifampin	Optic neuritis
Lithium	Papilledema
Oral contraceptives	Papilledema
Ethanol	Toxic neuropathy
Amiodarone	Papilledema
Estrogen therapy	Papilledema

Chapter 5

Pharmaceutical Agents

THE PRESCRIPTION/PATIENT COMPLIANCE
Jill C. Autry

THE PRESCRIPTION DOS AND DON'TS: PRESCRIBING GUIDELINES (See Figures 5.1 to 5.3 and Tables 5.1 to 5.2)

1. *Do* write legibly.
2. *Do* check drug spelling; many drug names look alike.
3. *Do* include dosage form, quantity, and strength of medication.
4. *Do* specify length of treatment on acute care prescriptions.
5. *Do* use the most economical size package on chronic care prescriptions.
6. *Do* make sure the patient understands all special instructions, for example:
   - Refrigeration
   - Shake suspensions
   - Proper instillation techniques
7. *Do* specify the symptoms that require "as needed" treatment, for example:
   - Itch
   - Pain
   - Redness
8. *Do* use only metric measurement. DO NOT use household or apothecary measurement systems.
9. *Do not* pre-print your DEA number on your prescription pad.
10. *Do* use carbonless copy prescription pads to ensure that a duplicate record of prescription is in your possession.
11. *Do not* leave prescription pads unattended on counter tops.

Patient _____   Date _____

Procedure _____   Time _____

Administered By _____

Pharmaceutical(s)—Percentage (Concentration) and Name

_____

_____

Dosage (No. of Drops) and Time(s) Administered

_____

_____

Adverse Reactions

_____

Steps Taken _____

Current Medications _____

Precautions/Warnings

_____

Comments

_____

_____

_____

FIGURE 5.1. Sample drug record—diagnostic.

Patient _____   Date _____

Pharmaceutical(s) Prescribed—Concentration, Dosage

_____

Precautions/Warnings

_____

Adverse Reactions

_____

Steps Taken _____   Refills _____

Not Refillable _____   Current Medications _____

Comments _____

Return Visit(s) _____

FIGURE 5.2. Sample drug record—therapeutic.

Patient _____   Date _____

      I have had the following diagnostic/therapeutic procedure explained to me, and have been informed of the risks, benefits, and alternative methods of treatment.

Procedure _____

I authorize or refuse treatment, as indicated below.

           AUTHORIZE _____

           REFUSE   _____

Signature _____

(Patient/Guardian/Conservator)

Witness _____   Date _____

FIGURE 5.3. Sample consent form.

▶ **TABLE 5.1** Latin Abbreviations Commonly Used in Ophthalmic
Prescription Writing

Latin	Abbreviation	Meaning
Ad	Ad	Up to, to
Admove	Admov.	Apply
Alternis horis	Alt. hor.	Every other hour
Ante	A	Before
Ante cibos	ac	Before meals
Bis in di'e	bid	Twice a day
Capsula	caps	Capsule
Cum	c̄	With
Diebus alternis	Dieb. alt.	Every other day
Gram	g, gm	Gram
Gutta	gt, gtt	A drop
Hora	h	An hour
Hora somni	hs	At bedtime
Nocte	noct.	At night
Oculo utro	O.U.	Each eye
Oculus dexter	O.D.	Right eye
Oculus sinister	O.S.	Left eye
Per os	po	By mouth
Pro re nata	prn	When needed
Quaque	q	Each, every
Quaque hora	qh	Every hour
Quater in di'e	qid	Four times a day
Recipe	Rx	Take, you take
Signatura	Sig.	Write, you write
Sine	s̄	Without
Solutio	Sol.	Solution
Tabella	tab	Tablet
Ter in di'e	tid	Three times a day
Unguentum	ung.	Ointment
Ut dictum	Ut dict.	As directed
Unus	i	One
Duo	ii	Two
Tres	iii	Three
Quattour	iv	Four
Quinque	v	Five

▶ **TABLE 5.2   A "Minimum List" of Dangerous Abbreviations, Acronyms, and Symbols Has Been Approved by Joint Commission. (Beginning January 1, 2004, the Following Items Must Be Included on Each Accredited Organization's "Do Not Use" List.)**

Set	Item	Abbreviation	Potential Problem	Preferred Term
1.	1.	U (for unit)	Mistaken as zero, four or cc	Write "unit"
2.	2.	IU (for international unit)	Mistaken as IV (intravenous) or 10 (ten)	Write "international unit"
3.	3.	QD,	Mistaken for each other. The	Write "daily" and "every
	4.	QOD	period after the Q can be	other day"
		(Latin abbreviation for once daily and every other day)	mistaken for an "I" and the "O" can be mistaken for "I."	
4.	5.	Trailing zero (X.0 mg)	Decimal point is missed.	Never write a zero by
	6.	[Note: Prohibited only for medication-related notations];		itself after a decimal point (X mg), and always use a zero before a
		Lack of leading zero (.X mg)		decimal point (0.X mg).
5.	7.	MS	Confused for one another.	Write "morphine sulfate"
	8.	MSO₄	Can mean morphine sulfate	or "magnesium sulfate.
	9.	MgSO₄	or magnesium sulfate.	

Effective April 1, 2004 (if your organization does not already have additional "do not use" items in place), each organization must identify and apply at least another three "do not use" abbreviations, acronyms, or symbols of its own choosing. [Revised 11/3/03]

IMPROVING PATIENT COMPLIANCE

One of the most difficult things that any physician faces in managing the patient with chronic disease, be it systemic hypertension, elevated cholesterol, diabetes, or as in this case, glaucoma, is patient compliance with drug therapy.

Use the following recording and education sheets to assist your patient to utilize their medications more effectively (Figures 5.4 to 5.6).

Eye Medication Instructions

Eyedrop #1 _____

Instill one drop _____ times daily every _____ hours in the RIGHT, LEFT, BOTH eye(s)

Eyedrop #2 _____

Instill one drop _____ times daily every _____ hours in the RIGHT, LEFT, BOTH eye(s)

Eyedrop #3 _____

Instill one drop _____ times daily every _____ hours in the RIGHT, LEFT, BOTH eye(s)

FIGURE 5.4. Patient medication instruction sheet.

Patient _____

Medication _____

Pharmacy _____

Pharmacy phone # _____

Reason for refill _____

Date of last visit _____

Date of last refill _____

May refill 0   1   2   3   4   PRN

(circle one)

FIGURE 5.5. Medication refill request form.

Missed Appointment

Date of Appointment _____

Time of Appointment _____

_____ No Answer

_____ Patient Will Return Call

_____ Left Message with _____

_____ Other _____
                    (Check one)

Patient rescheduled _____ YES _____ NO

New Appointment Date _____ _____

File Chart _____ YES _____ NO

FIGURE 5.6. Missed appointment record sheet.

OPHTHALMIC DYES
Jill C. Autry

Ophthalmic dyes are among the most useful diagnostic agents used in the management and detection of disorders of the visual system. The most common uses of these agents and their properties are listed in Tables 5.3 to 5.8 and Figure 5.7.

▶ **TABLE 5.3 Common Uses of Ophthalmic Dyes**

FLUORESCEIN
Lacrimal testing (TBUT, Jones test)
Detection of corneal epithelial defects
Detection of penetration of globe (Seidel's sign)
Applanation tonometry
Contact lens/corneal fitting relationship
Retinal angiography

LISSAMINE GREEN
Dry eye evaluation

FLUOREXON
Evaluation of soft contact lens fit

ROSE BENGAL
Dry eye evaluation
Herpes simplex keratitis

INDOCYANINE GREEN
Angiography

▶ **TABLE 5.4 Properties and Characteristics of Fluorescein**

CHEMICAL PROPERTIES
$C_2H_{12}O_5Na$
Molecular weight $= 376.27$
Orange-red powder
Yellow in solution
Fluorescence
   Yellow-green with blue light in weak alkali solution
   Peak absorption: 465–490 nm
   Peak emission: 520–530 nm
   Fluorescence increases with greater concentrations up to 0.001%
Fluorescence increases with greater pH up to pH 8
At very high concentrations:
   Quenching occurs
   It dimerizes and polymerizes
   Emission shifts to longer wavelengths

CLINICAL CHARACTERISTICS
Stains epithelial defects bright green
Diffuses into intercellular spaces
Will not stain devitalized cells nor mucus
Tear film appears yellow-orange
Can exhibit:
   Pseudoflare
   Fisher-Schweizer mosaic
   Negative staining
Promotes growth of *Pseudomonas* in solution
Will stain soft contact lenses

▶ **TABLE 5.5** **Characteristics of Fluorexon**

N_1 N-bis (carboxymethyl)-aminoethyl-fluorescein tetra-sodium salt
Molecular weight = 710
Stains epithelial defects, devitalized cells, and mucin (less than
  fluorescein or rose bengal)
Fluorescence
  Less brilliant than fluorescein
  Does not increase linearly with increasing concentration
Does not stain most soft contact lenses
May stain high water (greater than 60%) contact lenses
Promotes the growth of *Pseudomonas*

▶ **TABLE 5.6** **Characteristics of Rose Bengal**

4,5,6,7-tetrachloro-2',4',5',7'-tetraiodofluorescein sodium
Stains devitalized cells and mucin a brilliant red
Stains the nucleus more than cytoplasm
Higher concentrations stain more distinctly and highlight more subtle defects
Stings upon instillation
Antiviral properties
Stains a line along the ciliary margin on conjunctival tarsus in normal eyes

▶ **TABLE 5.7** **Comparative Staining Characteristics of Fluorescein, Rose Bengal, and Fluorexon**

	Epithelial Defects	Devitalized Cells	Mucin
Fluorescein	++	0	+
Rose Bengal	0	++	++
Fluorexon	+	+	+
Lissamine Green	0	++	+

▶ **TABLE 5.8** **Topical Products**

Product	Concentration	How Supplied
FLUORESCEIN		
Fluorescein (Alcon, Iolab)	2%	1, 2, and 15 mL
Fluorocaine (Akorn)	0.25% fluorescein sodium, 0.1% proparacaine hydrochloride, 0.01% thimerosal preservative	5 mL
Flucaine (Pharmafair, Inc)	0.25% fluorescein sodium, 0.50% proparacaine hydrochloride, 0.01% thimerosal preservative (povidone, boric acid polysorbate 80)	5 mL
Fluress (Sola/Barnes-Hind)	0.25% fluorescein sodium, 0.4% benoxinate hydrochloride, 1% chlorbutanol, povidone buffers	5 mL
Ful-Glo (Sola/Barnes-Hind)	0.6-mg strips	300 strips
Fluor-1-Strip (Wyeth-Ayerst)	9-mg strips (boric acid polysorbate 80, 0.5% chlorbutanol)	300 strips
Fluor-1-Strip AT (Wyeth-Ayerst)	1-mg strips (boric acid polysorbate 80, 0.5% chlorbutanol)	300 strips
Fluorets (Akorn)	1-mg strips	100–1300 strips
FLUOREXON		
Floresoft (Holles)	0.35%	0.5-mL pipettes
LISSAMINE GREEN	1-mg strips	100 strips
ROSE BENGAL		
Rose Bengal 1% (Akorn) Americil	1% solution (povidone, sodium borate, PEG P-isoc tylphenolio, 0.01% thimerosal)	5 mL
Rose Bengal (Sola/ Barnes-Hind)	1.3-mg strip	100 strips
Rosets (Smith & Nephew)	1.3-mg strip	100 strips

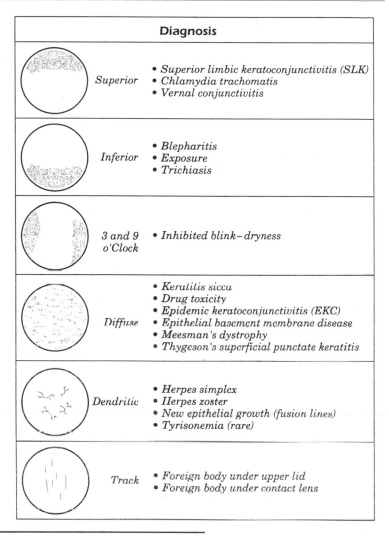

FIGURE 5.7. Common corneal fluorescein patterns.

ANESTHETIC AGENTS

Jill C. Autry

Clinical procedures that may induce patient discomfort should always include the use of an appropriate anesthetic agent. These drugs can vary in their ability to decrease pain, duration of effect, and potential to induce allergic and toxic reactions. It is important to select the most appropriate agent with adequate efficacy and minimal adverse effects (Tables 5.9 to 5.13).

▶ TABLE 5.9 Physiochemical and Pharmacologic Properties of the Injectable Local Anesthetics

Agent (Trade Name)	Physiochemical Properties				Pharmacologic Properties			
	pK_a (25°)	Partition Coefficient*	Percent Protein Binding (%)	Onset (min†)	Relative Potency	Duration (hr†)	Concentration (%)
ESTERS							
Procaine (Novocain)	8.9	0.02	6	Slow (15–25)	1	Short (0.5–1)	1–2
Tetracaine (Pontocaine)	8.5	4.1	76	Slow (20–30)	8	Long (3–5)	0.25
AMIDES							
Prilocaine (Citanest)	7.9	0.9	55	Fast (5–15)	2	Moderate (1–3)	1–3
Lidocaine (Xylocaine)	7.9	2.9	64	Fast (5–15)	2	Moderate (1–3)	0.5–2
Mepivacaine (Carbocaine)	7.6	0.8	78	Fast (5–15)	2	Moderate (1–3)	1–2
Bupivacaine (Marcaine)	8.1	27.5	96	Moderate (10–20)	8	Long (3–5)	0.25–0.75
Etidocaine (Duranest)	7.7	141	94	Fast (5–15)	6	Long (3–5)	0.5–1

*Partition coefficient is a measure of lipid solubility.
†Onset and duration times seen with epidural injection.
(Modified from Covino BG. Pharmacology of local anesthetics. Ration Drug Ther 1987; 21:1–9, and Local anesthetics. In: Facts and Comparisons, St. Louis: Lippincott, 1990: 691–694.

▶ **TABLE 5.10 Commonly Used Topical Ocular Anesthetics**

Drug (Trade Name)	Concentration (%)	Onset (sec)	Duration (min)	Maximum Dose* (drops[†])
Benoxinate (Fluress)[‡]	0.4	20	10	
Cocaine[§]	1.0–10	30	12	20 mg (about 5 drops to each eye of a 4% solution)
Proparacaine (various) (Fluoracaine)[‡] (I-Parescein)[‡]	0.5	15	14	10 mg (about 20 drops to each of a 0.5% solution)
Tetracaine (various) (Pontocaine Eye)[∥]	0.5	20	10	5 mg (about 10 drops to each eye of a 0.5% solution)

*Suggested maximum total topical doses. (Based on theoretical calculations from Lyle WM, Page C. Possible adverse effects from local anesthetics and the treatment of these reactions. *Am J Optom Physiol Opt* 1975; 52:736.)
[†]Assumes approximately 20 drops per mL of solution.
[‡]Combined with 0.25% fluorescein sodium.
[§]Must be prepared from a powder.
[∥]Ointment, 0.5%.

▶ **TABLE 5.11 Central Nervous System Toxicities of Local Anesthetics**

EARLY EXCITATORY EFFECTS
Restlessness
Anxiety
Dizziness
Tinnitus
Miosis
Tremors
Convulsions

DEPRESSIVE EFFECTS
 (MAY OR MAY NOT BE PRECEDED BY THE EXCITATORY SYMPTOMS)
Drowsiness
Sedation
Generalized CNS depression
Unconsciousness
*Coma
Apnea and respiratory depression
Death from respiratory arrest

▶ **TABLE 5.12 Cardiovascular Symptoms of Toxicity from Local Anesthetics**

Hypertension and tachycardia (associated with the CNS excitatory phase)
Myocardial depression
Decreased cardiac output
Peripheral vasodilation
Hypotension
Bradycardia
Methemoglobinemia (seen only with prilocaine)
Heart block
Ventricular arrhythmias
Circulatory collapse

▶ **TABLE 5.13 Ocular Toxicity from Acute Administration of Topical Ocular Anesthetics**

Mild stinging, burning
Vasodilation
Shortening of the tear break-up time
Decreased reflex tearing
Decreased blinking
Corneal edema
Decreased epithelial mitosis and migration
Slowed epithelial healing
Punctate epithelial keratitis
Epithelial desquamation
Allergic reactions of the lids and conjunctiva

DILATING AGENTS AND PROCEDURES
Jill C. Autry

Of all the tests that we, as primary eyecare providers, perform to assess the ocular health of our patients, there is probably no more important test than the dilated fundus examination.

This section provides a quick reference to the procedures and medications that will improve the efficiency of this all-important procedure (Tables 5.14 and 5.15).

Prior to dilation, the clinician must assess the potential for angle closure. This can be done by gonioscopy or by the slit-lamp estimation procedure as seen in Table 5.16. See also Tables 5.17 and 5.18.

▶ **TABLE 5.14** Indications for Dilation

1. Any new patient
2. Established patient every 2–4 y
3. Any patient with flashes or floaters
4. Unexplained vision loss
5. Any patient with progressive retinal disease (e.g., macular degeneration, diabetic retinopathy)
6. Any patient with systemic disorders that can affect the eye (e.g., systemic hypertension)
7. History of ocular trauma
8. History of chronic uveitis
9. Any child under 6 y (with cycloplegia—see section on cycloplegic refraction)
10. Once yearly if history of ocular surgery
11. Moderate to high myopia:
    a. 3 D to 7 D of myopia—at least every 2 y
    b. >8 D of myopia—at least yearly
12. Any patient with history of peripheral retinal degeneration
13. Any patient with developing cataract
14. All hyperopes or anisometropes (include cycloplegic refraction)

▶ **TABLE 5.15** Mydriatic Pharmaceuticals

Drug	Maximal Dilation	Duration
PARASYMPATHOLYTIC AGENTS		
Tropicamide		
0.5%	20–40 min	4–8 h
1.0%		6–8 h
Cyclopentolate		
0.5%	30–60 min	12–24 h
1.0%		12–36 h
Homatropine		
2.0%	40–60 min	24–72 h
5.0%		36–72 h
Scopolamine		
0.25%	20–30 min	3–7 d
Atropine		
1.0%	30–40 min	7–10 d
SYMPATHOMIMETIC AGENTS		
Phenylephrine		
2.5%	20–30 min	4–6 h
10%		
Hydroxyamphetamine		
1%	25–35 min	4–6 h

▌TABLE 5.16 Van Herick Filtration Estimation Guide

A/C Depth at Limbus Compared to Corneal Thickness at Limbus	Estimated Grade of Angle
1/2–1	Grade 4
1/4–1/2	Grade 3
= 1/4	Grade 2
<1/4	Grade 1
CLOSED	Grade 0

▌TABLE 5.17 Examination Procedures in Relation to the DFE

I. Perform these procedures *prior to* dilation
  1. Case history
  2. Best corrected acuity
  3. Extraocular muscle assessment
  4. Near point accommodation and steropsis
  5. External evaluation and pupil testing
  6. Biomicroscopy
  7. Tonometry
  8. Gonioscopy if indicated
II. Perform these procedures *during* dilation
  1. Color vision
  2. Visual field
  3. Frame selection
  4. Patient education
III. Perform these procedures *after* dilation
  1. Repeat retinoscopy and subjective to R/O latent hyperopia
  2. Binocular indirect opthalmoscopy
  3. Slit lamp of lens and vitreous chamber with 60, 78 or 90 diopter lens

▶ **TABLE 5.18 Example of the "Round Robin" Approach to Patient Scheduling for Dilation**

Morning Schedule*	Procedure
8:30–8:55 AM	Predilation examination of new patient A
8:55–9:20 AM	Predilation examination of new patient B
9:20–9:30 AM	Dilated exam and dismissal of patient A
9:30–9:40 AM	Brief follow-up examination of patient C (e.g., contact or glaucoma IOP recheck)
9:40–9:50 AM	Dilated exam and dismissal of patient B
9:50–10:15 AM	Predilation examination of new patient D
10:15–10:40 AM	Predilation examination of new patient E
10:40–10:50 AM	Dilated exam and dismissal of patient D
10:50–11:00 AM	Follow-up examination of patient F
11:00–11:10 AM	Dilated exam and dismissal of patient E
11:10–11:35 AM	Predilation examination of new patient G
11:35–11:50 AM	Follow-up examinations as needed and return morning phone calls
11:50–noon	Dilated exam and dismissal of patient G

*Afternoon schedule may repeat morning or use for specialty appointments. Examination times may vary from doctor to doctor. Delegation of tests and an adequate number of examination rooms is necessary to follow this type of scheduling.

DIAGNOSTIC AGENTS AND PROCEDURES FOR THE MANAGEMENT OF ACCOMMODATIVE DISORDERS

Jill C. Autry

The use of diagnostic pharmaceuticals during the examination procedure is necessary in a number of situations. This section provides information regarding the appropriate use of pharmaceutical agents for the diagnosis of accommodative disorders (Tables 5.19 to 5.24 and Figure 5.8) and accommodative esotropia (Table 5.25 and Figure 5.9).

▶ **TABLE 5.19 Indications for Cycloplegic Refraction**

1. Strabismus (particularly esotropia)
2. Amblyopia
3. Anisometropia
4. Pseudomyopia
5. Hyperopia associated with esophoria or a lag of accommodation
6. Unstable end point on static retinoscopy
7. For the uncooperative child during static retinoscopy

▶ **TABLE 5.20** Comparison of Cycloplegic Agents

Drug	Dosage	Onset of Cyclopelgia	Duration of Cycloplegia
Tropicamide 1%	1 drop, repeat after 5 min	20–30 min	4–8 hr
Cyclopentolate 0.5% and 1.0%	1 drop, repeat after 5 min	20–45 min	8–24 hr
Homatropine 5%	1 drop, repeat after 5 min	30–60 min	24–48 hr
Scopolamine 0.25%	1 drop, repeat after 20 min	30–60 min	5–7 d
Atropine			
0.5% ointment	1/4″ ointment at bedtime for 3 days prior to exam	30–60 min	10–14 d
1.0% solution	1 drop tid × 1 d prior to exam		

▶ **TABLE 5.21** Efficiency of Cycloplegics

Drug	% Efficiency
1% Atropine	100
1% Cyclopentolate	92
1% Tropicamide	80
5% Homatropine	54

▶ **TABLE 5.22** Ocular Side Effects of Cycloplegic Agents

Allergic contact dermatitis
Angle-closure glaucoma
Elevation of IOP with open angles

▶ **TABLE 5.23** Dose-related Systemic Side Effects of Atropine

Dose	Effects
0.5–2 mg (1–4 drops 1% solution)	Tachycardia
	Dry mouth
	Mydriasis/cycloplegia
5 mg (10 drops 1% solution)	The above plus:
	Speech disturbance
	Restlessness
	Confusion
	Hot, dry skin
	Decreased GI motility
	Urinary retention
>10 mg (over 20 drops 1% solution)	The above plus:
	Ataxia
	Hyperexcitability
	Hallucination
	Coma
	Convulsion
	Death

▶ **TABLE 5.24** **Side Effects Associated with Topical Cholinesterase Inhibitors**

OCULAR
Ciliary body
  Accommodative spasm*
  Anterior movement of the lens–iris diaphragm
  Breakdown of the blood-aqueous barrier
  Decreased anterior chamber depth
Conjunctiva
  Drug-induced cicatrizing conjunctivitis
  Hyperemia
Corneal toxicity
Increased intraocular pressure (paradoxical)
Lens
  Cataract formation[†] (particularly anterior subcapsular cataracts)
Lids
  Allergic blepharoconjunctivitis
  Depigmentation of the skin (reversible)
  Twitching of orbicularis oculi
Pupil
  Iris cysts*
  Miosis
Retina
  Increased peripheral vitreoretinal traction

SYSTEMIC
Cardiac
  Arrhythmia
  Bradycardia
Gastrointestinal*
  Abdominal cramps
  Diarrhea
  Nausea
Headache
Pulmonary
  Bronchospasm
  Upper respiratory congestion
Lacrimation
Reduced plasma cholinesterase levels
  Reduced breakdown of succinylcholine, procaine, and tetracaine
Rhinorrhea
Urinary incontinence

*More common in children.
[†]More common in elderly.

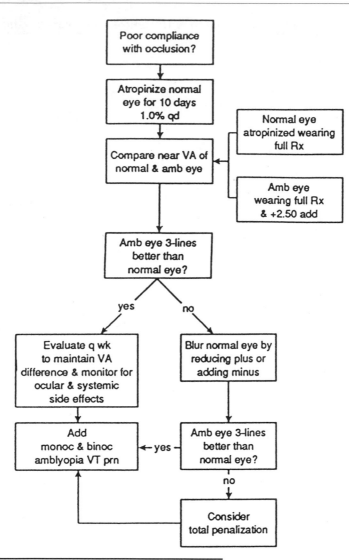

FIGURE 5.8. Management of amblyopia with penalization.

▶ **TABLE 5.25 Characteristics of Accommodative Esotropia**

1. Type of onset: Gradual and intermittent
2. Time of onset: Typically 2.5–4 y of age with a range from 4 mo to 7 y
3. Typically large angle of 25–40°
4. Concomitant
5. Normal correspondence
6. Seldom have significant amblyopia
7. Refractive type:
   Normal AC/A
   Hyperopia between 2.00–7.00 D, with mean of 4.50 D
8. Nonrefractive type:
   High AC/A ratio (>6:1)
   Hyperopia between 0.50–4.50 D, with mean of 2.00 D
9. Can have a combination of refractive and nonrefractive components

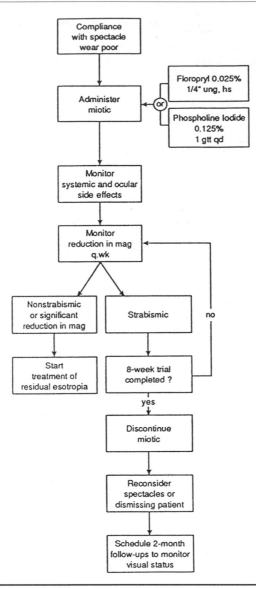

FIGURE 5.9. Accommodative esotropia treatment strategy using miotic agents.

OPHTHALMIC LUBRICANTS

Jill C. Autry

Ophthalmic lubricants represent the cornerstone of the management of ocular surface disease (OSD). New formulations of these all-important products have recognized the importance of limiting preservative toxicity while enhancing epithelial cell growth. Tables 5.26 to 5.30 list the most common products.

TABLE 5.26 Artificial Tear Solutions

Trade Name	Manufacturer	Major Components	Preservative
Adsorbotear	Alcon	Hydroxyethylcellulose, povidone	Thimerosal, EDTA
Akwa Tears	Akorn	Polyvinyl alcohol	Benzalkonium chloride, EDTA
Artificial Tears Solution	Rugby	Polyvinyl alcohol	Chlorobutanol, EDTA
Bion Tears	Alcon	Dextran 70 0.1%	None
Celluvisc	Allergan	Hydroxypropyl methylcellulose 2910 0.3%	None
Hypotears	Iolab	Carboxymethylcellulose	Benzalkonium chloride, EDTA
I-Liqui Tears	Americal	Polyvinyl alcohol, PEG-8000, dextrose	Benzalkonium chloride, EDTA
Isopto Alkaline	Alcon	Hydroxyethylcellulose, polyvinyl alcohol	Benzalkonium chloride
Isopto Plain	Alcon	Hydroxypropyl methylcellulose 1%	Benzalkonium chloride
Isopto Tears	Alcon	Hydroxypropyl methylcellulose 0.5%	Benzalkonium chloride
Just Tears	Blairex	Hydroxypropyl methylcellulose 0.5%	Benzalkonium chloride
Lacril	Allergan	Hydroxypropyl methylcellulose	Chlorobutanol
Liquifilm Forte	Allergan	Hydroxypropyl methylcellulose, gelatin A, polysorbate 80	Thimerosal, EDTA
Liquifilm Tears	Allergen	Polyvinyl alcohol 3%	Chlorobutanol
Moisture Drops	Bausch & Lomb	Polyvinyl alcohol 1.4%	Benzalkonium chloride, EDTA
Murine	Ross	Hydroxypropyl methylcellulose, dextran 40	Benzalkonium chloride, EDTA
Murocel	Bausch & Lomb	Polyvinyl alcohol, povidone, dextrose	Methylparaben, propylparaben
Muro Tears	Bausch & Lomb	Methylcellulose	Benzalkonium chloride, EDTA
Neo-Tears	Soia/Barnes-Hind	Hydroxypropyl methylcellulose, dextran 40	Benzalkonium chloride, EDTA
Refresh	Allergan	Polyvinyl alcohol, hydroxyethylcellulose	Purite
Refresh Plus	Allergan	Carboxymethylcellulose 0.5%	None
Refresh Liquigel	Allergan	Carboxymethylcellulose 0.5%	Purite
Refresh Endura	Allergan	Carboxymethylcellulose 1.0%	None
Systane	Alcon	Glycerin 1%, Polysorbate 80 1% Polyethylene glycol 400 0.4% Propylene glycol 0.3%	Polyquaternium-1
TearGard	Medtech	Hydroxyethylcellulose	EDTA
Tearisol	Iolab	Hydroxypropyl methylcellulose	Benzalkonium chloride, EDTA
Tears Naturale	Alcon	Hydroxypropyl methylcellulose, dextran	Benzalkonium chloride, EDTA
Tears Naturale II	Alcon	Hydroxypropyl methylcellulose, dextran	Benzalkonium chloride, EDTA
Tears Plus	Allergan	Polyvinyl alcohol, povidone	Chlorobutanol
Tears Renewed	Akorn	Hydroxypropyl methylcellulose, dextran 70	Benzalkonium chloride, EDTA
TheraTears PF	Advanced Vision Research	Carboxymethylcellulose 0.25%	None
Theratears liquid gel	Advanced Vision Research	Carboxymethylcellulose 1%	None
Ultra Tears	Alcon	Hydroxypropyl methylcellulose	Benzalkonium chloride

EDTA = ethylenediaminetetraacetic acid.

▶ **TABLE 5.27** Lubricating Ointments

Trade Name	Manufacturer	Major Components	Preservative
Akwa Tears	Akorn	White petrolatum, mineral oil, lanolin	None
Dey-Lube	Dey	White petrolatum	None
Duolube	Bausch & Lomb	White petrolatum, mineral oil	None
Duratears Naturale	Alcon	White petrolatum, mineral oil, lanolin	Methylparaben, propylparaben
Hypotears Ointment	Iolab	White petrolatum, mineral oil	None
Lacri-Lube NP	Allergan	White petrolatum, mineral oil, lanolin	None
Lacri-Lube S.O.P.	Allergan	White petrolatum, mineral oil, lanolin	Chlorobutanol
Refresh PM	Allergan	White petrolatum, mineral oil, lanolin	None

▶ TABLE 5.28 Dry Eye Questionnaire

1. Have you ever had drops prescribed or other treatment for dry eyes?
   A. Yes
   B. No
2. Do you ever experience any of the following eye symptoms?
   A. Soreness
   B. Scratchiness
   C. Dryness
   D. Grittiness
   E. Burning
3. How often do you have these symptoms?
   A. Never
   B. Sometimes
   C. Often
   D. Constantly
4. Do you regard your eyes as being unusually sensitive to smoke, smog, air conditioning, central heating?
   A. Yes
   B. No
5. Do you take:
   A. Antihistamines
   B. Diuretics (fluid tablets)
   C. Sleeping tablets
   D. Tranquilizers
   E. Stomach medicines
   F. High blood pressure medicines
6. Do you have arthritis?
   A. Yes
   B. No
7. Are your joints— especially fingers—sore or swollen in the morning?
   A. Yes
   B. No
8. Do you have dryness of the nose or mouth, or a persistent dry cough?
   A. Yes
   B. No
9. Do you have any thyroid abnormality?
   A. Yes
   B. No
10. Do you ever awaken with eye irritation or excessive dried mucus in the corners of your eyes?
    A. Yes
    B. No

(From McMonnies CW, Ho A. Patient history in screening for dry eye conditions. *J Am Optom Assoc* 1987; 58:296.)

▶ **TABLE 5.29 Pharmaceutical Agents That Can Affect Tear Quality**

Antibiotics	Antihistamines
Tetracycline	Allergy medications
Antihypertensives	Sinus medications
Methyldopate hydrochloride	Sleep medications
Reserpine	Diet medications
MAO inhibitors	Belladona alkaloids
Botulinum toxin	Bellergal
Dermatologicals	Donnatal
Isotretinoin	Pro-Banthine
Psychotomimetics	Diuretics
Choridazepoxide	Chlorothiazides
Diazepam	Furosemide
Amitriptyline	Hydrochlorothiazide
Thioridazine	Preserved topical ocular medications
Topical β-blockers	Long-term antiperspirants

▶ **TABLE 5.30 Diagnostic Tests for Dry Eyes**

Evaluation of tear meniscus	Schirmer tear test
Evaluation for corneal filaments	Rose bengal staining
Tear break-up time	Evaluation of tear protein
Evaluation of tear osmolarity	levels–lactoferrin, lysozyme
Cotton thread tear test	Conjunctival impression cytology
Evaluation for debris in tear film	

HYPEROSMOTIC AGENTS
Jill C. Autry

See Tables 5.31 and 5.32.

▶ **TABLE 5.31 Topical Hyperosmotic Agents**

Trade Name	Formulation	How Supplied	Preservative
Adsorbonac Opthalmic (Alcon)	2% or 5% NaCl solution	15 mL	Thimerosal
Muro-128 Opthalmic (Bausch & Lomb)	2% or 5% NaCl solution with methylcellulose	15, 30 mL	Methylparaben Propylparaben
AK-NaCl (Akorn)	5% NaCl ointment	3.5 g	
Muro-128 Opthalmic (Bausch & Lomb)			
Glucose-40 Opthalmic (Cooper Vision)	40% ointment in petrolatum and lanolin	3.5 g	

▶ TABLE 5.32 Systemic Hyperosmotic Agents

Drug	Formulation	Dosage
Glycerin	50% solution	1–2 g/kg p.o.
Isosorbide	45% solution	1–3 g/kg p.o.
Mannitol	5, 10, 15, 20 25% injectable	1.5–2 g/kg as 20% solution

ANTI-ALLERGY MEDICATIONS
Jill C. Autry

Allergic eye disease is one of the most common problems facing the primary care eye clinician. The disorder can involve several types of reactions ranging from mild itching to significant inflammation with tissue damage. This section contains information regarding the various medications used to manage allergic eye disease (Tables 5.33 to 5.40).

▶ TABLE 5.33 Decongestants*

Drug	Dosage Form	Comment
TOPICALS		
Phenylephrine	0.12% OTC solution 2.5% RX solution	All decongestant agents are contraindicated in narrow angle glaucoma, unstable systemic hypertension, and individuals using MAO inhibitors. Overuse can produce rebound hyperemia
Naphazoline	0.0125–0.03% OTC solution 0.1% RX solution	Imidazole derivative
Oxymetazolone	0.025% OTC solution	Longest acting of the group
Tetrahydrozoline	0.05% OTC solution	
ORALS		
Pseudoephedrine	30- and 60-mg oral tablets pediatric solution	Avoid in heart disease and hypertension

*Action: Decongestants reduce hyperemia and edema via vasoconstriction. All are adrenergic agonists with direct vasoconstrictive activity.

▶ **TABLE 5.34 Antihistamine Indications and Drug Selection**

Indication	Appropriate Drug
Allergic rhinitis	All except phenothiazines
Allergic dermatitis/urticaria	Diphenhydramine
	Phenothiazine
	Astemizole
	Cetirizine
Type I hypersensitivity reaction	Any antihistamine with epinephrine and steroids
Motion sickness/nausea and vomiting	Diphenyhydramine
	Promethazine

▶ **TABLE 5.35 Topical Antihistamines***

Drug	Dosage Form	Comment
Pheniramine	0.3% solution	Only available with naphazoline
Antazoline	0.5% solution	Only available with naphazoline
Levocabastine	0.05% RX solution	Only antihistamine available without decongestant

*Action: Inhibit the immediate hypersensitivity reaction associated with the release of histamine by blocking H-1 receptors.

▶ **TABLE 5.36** Topical Anti-Allergy Preparations

Rx	Manufacturer	Decongestant	Antihistamine	Other
OTC				
Optised	Various	P—0.12%		ZS 0.25%
Phenylzin	Cooper	P—0.12%		ZS 0.25%
Zincfrin	Alcon	P—0.12%		ZS 0.25%
Prefrin	Allergan	P—0.12%		AP 0.1%
Relief	Allergan	P—0.12%		Ap 0.1%
VasoclearA	Iolab	N—0.02%		ZS 0.25%
Visine AC	Leeming	T—0.05%		ZS 0.25%
Prefrin-A	Allergan	P—0.12%	Pyril 0.1%	AP 0.1%
AK-Vernacon	Akorn	P—0.125%	Phen 0.5%	
AK-Con-A	Akorn	N—0.025%	Phen 0.3%	
Naphcon-A	Alcon	N—0.025%	Phen 0.3%	
Opcon-A	Bausch & Lomb	N—0.025%	Phen 0.3%	
Albalon-A	Ciba	N—0.05%	Antaz 0.5%	
Vasocon-A	Ciba	N—0.05%	Antaz 0.5%	
RX				
Livostin	Ciba		Levocabastine 0.05%	
Alomide	Alcon			Lodoxamide 0.1%
Crolom	Bausch & Lomb			Cromolyn Na 4%
Acular	Allergan			Ketorolac 0.5%
Alocril	Allergan			Nedocromil 2 %
Patanol	Alcon		Olopatadine 0.1%	
Emadine	Alcon		Emedastine 0.05%	
Zaditor	Novartis		Ketotifen Fumarate 0.025%	
Alamast	Santen			Pemirolast K 0.1%
Optivar	Bausch & Lomb		Azelastine 0.05%	
Elestat	Inspine		Epinastine 0.05%	

P = Phenylephrine; Pyril = Pyrilamine maleate; N = Naphazoline; Phen = Phentiramine; ZS = Zinc sulphate; Anyaz = Antazoline; T = Tetrahydozoline; AP = Antipyrine.

▶ **TABLE 5.37** Systemic Antihistamines*

Drug	Sedative Effects	Antihistamine Activity	Anticholinergic Activity
Brompheniramine	Low	High	Moderate
Cetirizine	Low	High	Low
Chlorpheniramine	Low	Moderate	Moderate
Clemastine	Moderate	Moderate	High
Dexchlorpheniramine	Low	High	Moderate
Diphenhydramine	High	Moderate	High
Loratadine	Low	High	Low
Promethazine	High	High	High
Pyrilamine	Low	Moderate	Low
Tripelennamine	Moderate	Moderate	Low
Triprolidine	Low	High	Moderate

*Sedating antihistamines have greater CNS penetration and increased anticholinergic side effects, i.e., dryness and drowsiness. Nonsedating antihistamines have reduced CNS penetration and fewer anticholinergic side effects.

▌ TABLE 5.38 Oral Antihistamine Dosages

Drug	Dose (mg)	Dose Interval (h)	Max. Daily Dose (mg)
Brompheneramine	4	4–6	24
Cetirizine	10	24	10
Chlorpheniramine	4	4–6	24
Clemastine	1	12	8
Dexchlorpheniramine	2	4–6	12
Diphenhydramine	25–50	6–8	400
Loratadine	10	24	10
Promethazine	12.5–25	6–24	100
Pyrilamine	25–50	6–8	200
Tripelennamine	25–50	4–6	300
Triprolidine	2.5	4–6	10

▌ TABLE 5.39 Mast-Cell Inhibitors*

Drug	Dosage Form	Comments
Lodoxamide tromethamine	0.1% RX suspension	Most potent topical mast-cell inhibitor
Cromolyn sodium	4% solution	Effective in VKC, GPC, and AKC
Nedocromil	2% solution	Stops itching fast
Pemirolast potassium	0.1% solution	

*Action: Inhibit type I immediate hypersensitivity reactions by inhibiting mast-cell degranulation. *Note:* No antihistaminic activity. They are most effective when used regularly as a prophylactic agent.

▌ TABLE 5.40 Nonsteroidal Anti-inflammatory Agents (NSAIDs)*

Drug	Dosage Form	Comment
Ketorolac tromethamine	0.5%	Only NSAID approved for seasonal allergy
Ketorolac tromethamine	0.4%	(As Acularls)

*Action: Inhibit the synthesis of prostaglandins by blocking the enzyme cyclooxygenase.

ANTI-INFECTIVE AGENTS
Jill C. Autry

See Tables 5.41 to 5.51.

▶ **TABLE 5.41** The Aminoglycosides*

Drug	Dosage Form	Comment
Neomycin	Solution and ointment and corticosteroid	Only in combination form; greatest potential for sensitivity RX of all in group
Gentamicin	Solution and ointment and corticosteroid	Relatively high corneal toxicity
Tobramycin	Solution and ointment and corticosteroid	Good antipseudomonal activity
Amikacin	No ophthalmic	Excellent for treatment of resistant *P. aeruginosa* strains; must be extemporaneously prepared in a 6.7-mg/cc solution

*Action: Inhibition of protein synthesis; bactericidal.

▶ **TABLE 5.42** The Macrolides*

Drug	Dosage Form	Comment
Erythromycin	Ophthalmic ointment; oral tablets and pediatric suspension	Classic alternative for penicillin-sensitive patients; marked GI upset; med. spectrum
Clarithromycin	Only systemic dosage forms; tablets and pediatric suspension	Long half-life allows twice daily dosing; excellent for *Hemophilus*
Azithromycin	Only systemic dosage forms; tablets and pediatric suspension	Long half-life allows daily dosing; drug of choice for chlamydia in all age groups

*Action: Inhibition of protein synthesis; bacteriostatic and bactericidal activity

▶ **TABLE 5.43** The Tetracyclines*†

Drug	Dosage Form	Comments
Tetracycline	Ophthalmic suspension and ointment; oral capsules and syrup	Effective oral treatment for marginal *Staphylococcal blepharitis;* alternative treatment for chlamydia
Doxycycline	Oral dosage form only	Long half-life allows once or twice daily dosing; OK to take with food; tetracycline of choice
Minocycline	Oral dosage form only	Once to twice daily Gram (+) and Gram (−) coverage

*Action: Inhibition of protein synthesis; bacteriostatic.
†WARNING: All tetracyclines are contraindicated in children and pregnant women. Avoid dairy products and antacids with tetracycline. Tetracyclines can produce photosensitivity.

▶ **TABLE 5.44 The Sulfonamides***

Drug	Dosage Form	Comment
Sulfacetamide	Ophthalmic solution and ointment and corticosteroid	Marked *S. aureus* resistance
Sulfasoxazole	Opthalmic solution	Same as above; less sting upon instillation than sulfacetamide
Sulfamethoxazole and trimethoprim TMP-SMZ	Oral tablets and suspension	Synergistic combination effectively inhibits folic acid; very effective in treating toxoplasmosis; alternative treatment for chlamydia; avoid in pregnant women and sulfonamide-sensitive patients

*Action: Inhibition of bacterial folic acid synthesis by inhibiting the enzymatic conversion of para-aminobenzoic acid (PABA) to dihydrofolic acid; bacteriostatic.

▶ **TABLE 5.45 The Fluoroquinolones***

Drug	Dosage Form	Comment
Ciprofloxacin	Ophthalmic solution; oral tablets	Approved for monotherapy of bacterial keratitis; increasing bacterial resistance; incidence of corneal precipitates
Ofloxacin	Ophthalmic solution; oral tablets	No corneal precipitates; approved for monotherapy of bacterial keratitis
Norfloxacin	Ophthalmic solution; oral tablets	Not approved for bacterial keratitis; useful for bacterial conjuctivitis
Moxifloxacin	Ophthalmic solution; oral tablets	Improved Gram (−) and Gram (+) coverage
Gatifloxacin	Ophthalmic solution; oral tablets	Improved Gram (−) and Gram (+) coverage
Leuofloxacin	Ophthalmic solution	Purified Leuoisomen of Ofloxacin-lower mic-90 than Ofloxacin

*Action: Inhibit bacterial reproduction by inhibiting DNA gyrase; bactericidal.

▶ **TABLE 5.46 The Penicillins***†

Drug	Dosage Form	Comments
Ampicillin	Oral tablets, suspension, and injection	First broad-spectrum, semisynthetic penicillin; not effective against β-lactamase–producing bacteria
Amoxicillin	Oral tablets and suspension	Pro-drug of ampicillin, therefore, less GI upset, better absorption and tid vs qid dosing
Dicloxacillin	Oral capsules and suspension	Excellent resistance to β-lactamase
Amoxicillin/potassium clavulanate	Oral tablets and suspension	Excellent resistance to β-lactamase, but much more expensive than dicloxacillin

*Action: Inhibit cell-wall synthesis; bactericidal.
†WARNING: Approximately 3% of the population (1–10%) reports penicillin sensitivity. A careful history to evaluate for penicillin sensitivity is absolutely necessary prior to their use. Non-penicillinase *Staphylococcus* and *Hemophilus sp.* are now the exception. When prescribing penicillins for eye infections commonly caused by these microbes, one should assume that they are β-lactamase–producing strains and select the drug accordingly.

▶ **TABLE 5.47 The Cephalosporins***

Drug	Dosage Form	Comments
FIRST GENERATION		
Cephalexin	Oral capsules and suspension	Inexpensive alternative in penicillin-sensitive patients
Cefazolin	Powder for injection	Used to formulate fortified topical antibitotic to treat bacterial keratitis
SECOND GENERATION		
Cefaclor	Oral tablets and suspension	Excellent action against *Hemophilus influenzae;*
Cefuroxime	Oral and IV	Same as above

Note: Approximately 3–15% of the population that reports penicillin sensitivity will also exhibit sensitivity to the cephalosporins.
First-generation cephalosporins show excellent activity against β-lactamase–producing Gram (+) microbes, but limited Gram (−) activity.
Second-generation cephalosporins are quite useful in managing *Hemophilus influenzae*, which is particularly common in children. They also have the advantage of twice-daily dosing. A simple way to remember the spectrum of activity of the second-generation cephalosporin agents is by the pneumonic HENPEK:
H: *Hemophilus*
E: *Enterococci*
N: *Neisseria*
P: *Proteus*
E: *E. Coli*
K: *Klebsiella*
*Action: Inhibit cell-wall synthesis; greater resistance to β-lactamase than some of the penicillins.

▶ **TABLE 5.48 Chloramphenicol*†**

Drug	Dosage Form	Comment
Chloramphenicol	Ophthalmic solution and ointment; oral capsule and suspension	High lipid solubility; excellent corneal penetration; low corneal toxicity; crosses blood-brain barrier useful in meningitis

*Action: Inhibition of protein synthesis; bacteriostatic.
†WARNING: Chloramphenicol can produce dose-related CNS toxicity in children or adults with reduced hepatic microsomal activity.
Both topical and systemic chloramphenicol can produce aplastic anemia. This is a potentially fatal, nondose-related reaction.

▶ **TABLE 5.49 Bacitracin***

Drug	Dosage Form	Comments
Bacitracin	Ophthalmic ointment Powder for injection	Useful for Gram (+) species Can be prepared as fortified solution for treatment of bacterial keratitis

*Action: Inhibition of cell-wall synthesis; bactericidal.
Bacitracin is used in combination with a variety of other topical ophthalmic agents. It is primarily used in these products to enhance their ability to kill Gram (+) (staphylococcal and streptococcal sp.). Products that contain bacitracin include: Polysporin ophthalmic ointment; Polytrim ophthalmic solution; Neosporin ophthalmic ointment.

▶ **TABLE 5.50 Polymyxin B***

Drug	Dosage Form	Comments
Polymyxin B	Combined with other agents in a variety of ophthalmic products	Very effective against Gram (−) bacteria, particularly *P. aeruginosa*

*Action: Cell-wall inhibitor; bactericidal.
Polymyxin B is used in combination with other antibacterial agents to enhance their spectrum of activity. It is particularly useful against Gram (−) organisms, in particular *P. aeruginosa*. Polymyxin B combination products include: Polysporin ophthalmic ointment; Terramycin with polymyxin B ophthalmic ointment; Neosporin ophthalmic solution; Neosporin ophthalmic ointment.

▶ **TABLE 5.51 Vancomycin***

Drug	Dosage Form	Comments
Vancomycin	No ophthalmic dosage form; oral capsules and powder for injection	Major ophthalmic use is as topical prepared from powder to manage resistant *Staphylococcus* sp.; oral drug of choice to manage *C. dificile* infection

*Action: Inhibits cell-wall synthesis, increases cell-wall permeability, and alters RNA synthesis.

ANTIVIRAL AGENTS

These pharmaceutical agents are used to treat primarily herpetic eye disease, with many of the new systemic agents directed toward the management of the HIV-infected patient (Table 5.52).

▶ **TABLE 5.52 Approved Antiviral Agents**

Drug	Dosage	Comment
TOPICAL AGENTS		
Idoxuridine	0.1% Ophthalmic solution	Topical treatment of h. simplex
	0.5% Ophthalmic ointment	Poor corneal penetration
Vidarabine	3.0% Ophthalmic ointment	Only available as ointment
Trifluridine	1.0% Ophthalmic solution	Use 5–8 × daily. Drug of choice for h. simplex; must be refrigerated
ORAL AGENTS		
Acyclovir	200-, 400-, 800-mg tablets	H. simplex 800–1000 mg/d
	200 mg/5 cc suspension	H. zoster 400–800 mg 5 ×/d
Famciclovir	500-mg tablets	H. zoster 500 mg tid
Valciclovir	500-mg tablets	H. zoster 500 mg bid
Ganciclovir	250-mg capsules	CMV retinitis
INJECTABLES		
Ganciclovir	500-mg powder for injection	CMV retinitis
		May produce severe granulocytopenia
Ganciclovir	Implant	Surgically implanted intravitreal release for CMV retinitis
Foscarnet sodium	24 mg/cc in 250, 500 cc	CMV retinitis
		May produce severe nephrotoxicity

MANAGEMENT OF COMMON BACTERIAL EYE DISORDERS: A QUICK REFERENCE
Jill C. Autry

See Figure 5.10 and Tables 5.53 to 5.56.

Hyperacute conjunctivitis (gonococcal ophthalmia) is a highly contagious, sight-threatening condition. Tables 5.57 and 5.58 list the appropriate antibiotic therapy for this emergent ocular disorder.

PATIENT INSTRUCTIONS

Blepharitis is a complex disorder that requires complete patient cooperation in order to manage the disease process. It can take weeks, even months, to establish control of the condition. On occasion, lifetime treatment may be necessary.

The following treatment program has been designed specifically for you. If you have any questions concerning the medications or procedures, please contact our office.

PROCEDURES	HOW OFTEN	CONTINUE
warm compresses		
lid massage		
lid scrubs		
saline rinses		
medications		

Please return for a progress evaluation in __3 weeks___ .

FIGURE 5.10. Sample instruction sheet for staphylococcal blepharitis.

▌**TABLE 5.53 Treatment Protocol for Staphylococcal Blepharitis**

	Mild	*Moderate*	*Severe*
Warm compresses	bid × 7 d	qid × 7 d	q2h × 2 d
		bid × 7 d	qid × 10 d
Lid scrubs	bid × 7 d	bid × 7–14 d	bid × 14 d
	qd × 7 d	qid × 7–14 d	qid × 7–14 d
Saline rinses		bid × 7–14 d	bid × 14 d
Antibiotic agents			
Drops		Ofloxacin qid × 7 d	Ofloxacin qid × 7 d
Ointment	Polysporin hs × 7 d	Polysporin hs × 14 d	Polysporin hs × 14 d
Oral			Dicloxacillin Keflex 1 g/d × 5 d; then 500 mg/d × 5 d
Anti-inflammatory agents*	Optional[†]	Prednisolone 1%[†] qid × 7–14 d	Prednisolone 1%[‡] qid × 7–14 d

*May use combination drops (especially Pred G).
[†]Withhold if there is corneal involvement.
[‡]Withhold for the first 48 hours or if there is corneal involvement.

▶ **TABLE 5.54** Characteristics of Antibiotics Used to Manage Lid Disease

Antibiotic	Commonly Available Products	Mode of Delivery	Surface Toxicity	Allergic Reactions	Sensitivity	Resistance
Bacitracin	Bacitracin Polysporin Neosporin	Ung	Low	Seldom	Gram (+)	Gram (−)
Polymyxin	Polysporin Neosporin Statrol	Ung, gtt	Low	Seldom	Gram (−)	Gram (+)
Erythromycin	Ilotycin	Ung	Rare	Seldom	Gram (+)	Gram (−)
Aminoglycoside	Gentamicin Tobrex	Ung, gtt Oral	High	Moderate	Gram (+) Gram (−)	Streptococcus
Sulfa	Various	Ung, gtt	Low	Moderate	Some Gram (+) Gram (−)	Many Gram (+) Gram (−)
Penicillin	Ampicillin Amoxicillin Dicloxacillin	Oral, IV	N/A	Moderate	Streptococcus Hemophilus	Pseudomonas
Cephalosporin	Keflex	Oral	N/A	Low	Staphylococcus Streptococcus Hemophilus	Pseudomonas
Diaminopyrimidine	Trimethoprim	Gtt	Low	Low	Gram (+)	Gram (−)
Tetracycline	Tetracycline Doxycycline	Ung, gtt	Low	Moderate	Variable	Variable

▶ **TABLE 5.55** Initial Therapy of Bacterial Corneal Ulcer

Route of Delivery	Drug	
	First Choice	Alternative
Nonfortified topical	Gatifloxacin 3.5 mg/cc Polytrim (polymyxin B and trimethoprim)	Moxifloxacin 3 mg/cc
Fortified topical	Cefazolin 33–50 mg/cc Tobramycin 9.0–13.5 mg/cc	Bacitracin 9600 U/cc Gentamycin 14 mg/cc
Subconjunctival injection	Cefazolin 100 mg (0.75 cc) Tobramycin 40 mg (1.0 cc)	Methacillin 100 mg (0.75 cc) Gentamycin 20 mg (1.0 cc)

Note: Predosing patient with 5 drops of topical antibiotic in 5 min (1 drop per min) can greatly increase tissue levels of antibiotic. Fluoroquinolones should then be administered every 15 min for the first 4 h, then hourly thereafter.

TABLE 5.56 Preparation and Final Concentration of Fortified Topical Antibiotic Solutions

	Peni-cillin G	Carben-cillin	Oxa-cillin	Cephal-oridine	Genta-micin	Tobramycin	Amikacin	Neomycin	Vanco-mycin	Bacit-racin	Ticar-cillin
Physical state of antibiotic	Powder	Powder	Powder	Powder	Liquid	Liquid	Liquid	Powder	Powder	Powder	Powder
Amount in commercial antibiotic vial	5 million U	1 gm	1 gm	500 mg	80 mg; 40 mg/mL	80 mg; 40 mg/mL	200 mg; 100 mg/mL	500 mg	1 gm	50,000* U	1 gm
Volume of diluent added to commercial antibiotic	5 mL artificial tears	9.5 mL water	7 mL artificial tears	2 mL saline	—	—	—	2 mL artificial tears	10 mL water	3 mL artificial tears	10 mL water
Volume (mL) artificial tears discarded	—	—	—	2 mL	—	—	2 mL	—	—	—	—
Volume of parenteral antibiotic added to artificial tear bottle	5 mL	1 mL†	7.2 mL	2.4 mL	2 mL‡	4 mL	2 mL	2 mL	10.2 mL	9.6 mL	1 mL
Final therapeutic concentration of antibiotic in tear bottle	333,000 U/mL	6.2 mg/mL	66 mg/mL	32 mg/mL	14 mg/mL	1 mg/mL	6.7 mg/mL	33 mg/mL	31 mg/mL	9600 U/mL	6.3 mg/mL

*3 mL of artificial tears are added to each of three vials.
†1 mL of the 9.5-mL solution is added to 15 mL of artificial tears.
‡2 mL of parenteral gentamicin is added to 5 mL of commercial gentamicin ophthalmic solution (0.3%).
(From Baum J., Initial therapy of suspected microbial corneal ulcers. I. Broad antibiotic therapy based on prevalence of organisms. *Surv Ophthalmol* 1979; 24:102–103.)

▶ **TABLE 5.57 Treatment of Adult Gonococcal Ophthalmia**

Conjunctivitis
  Ceftriaxone 1.0 g IM (one dose)
  In penicillin-allergic patients, spectinomycin 2.0 g IM (one dose)
Keratoconjunctivitis
  Ceftriaxone 1.0 g IV every 12 h for 3 d
  In penicillin-allergic patients, spectinomycin 2.0 g IM every 12 h for 2 d
Concurrent treatment with
  Topical saline lavage and topical erythromycin ointment or gentamicin ointment or bacitracin
    ointment 4 times daily
Treatment for *Chlamydia trachomatis* infection with
  Tetracycline hydrochloride 500 mg by mouth 4 times daily for 14 d
                                   OR
  Doxycycline 100 mg by mouth twice daily for 14 d
                                   OR
  For patients in whom tetracycline is contraindicated, erythromycin base or stearate 500 mg by mouth
    4 times daily for 14 d

(From Ullman S, Roussel TJ, Forster RK. Gonococcal keratoconjunctivitis. *Surv Ophthalmol* 1987; 32:199.)

▶ **TABLE 5.58 Treatment of Neonatal Gonococcal Ophthalmia**

Conjunctivitis
  Ceftriaxone 50 mg/kg IM (one dose)
  In penicillin-allergic neonates, gentamicin 2 to 2.5 mg/kg IV every 8 h for 3 d
Keratoconjunctivitis
  Ceftriaxone 24–40 mg/kg IV every 12 h doses for 3 d
  In penicillin-allergic neonates, gentamicin 2 to 2.5 mg/kg IV every 8 h for 3 d
Concurrent treatment with
  Topical saline lavage and topical erythromycin ointment or gentamicin ointment or bacitracin ointment
    4 times daily
Treatment for *Chlamydia trachomatis* infection with
  Oral erythromycin syrup 50 mg/kg/day in 4 divided doses for 14 d

(From Ullman S, Roussel TJ, Forster RK. Gonococcal keratoconjunctivitis. *Surv Ophthalmol* 1987; 32:199.)

GLAUCOMA AGENTS
Jill C. Autry

This supplement has been designed to provide the clinician with a quick reference to the most commonly used glaucoma medications (Table 5.59). All pertinent pharmacologic information has been included with an emphasis on adverse effects. One section deals with risk of use during pregnancy or nursing. The following is a synopsis of important principles of glaucoma therapy.

▶ **TABLE 5.59 Quick Reference for Most Commonly Used Glaucoma Medications**

Active Ingredients	Trade Name	Concentration	How Supplied	Administration and Dosage
CLONIDINE DERIVATIVES				
Apraclonidine hydrochloride				
Ophthalmic solution	Iopidine (Alcon)	0.5%	5 mL	Instill 1 or 2 drops in the affected eye(s) 3 times daily.
Brimonidine Tartrate Opthalmic solution	Alphagan	0.2%	5, 10 mL	Instill 1 or 2 drops in the affected eye(s) 2–3 times daily.
Brimonidine Tartrate with Purite	Alphagan P	0.15%	5, 10, 15 mL	Less incidence of allergy
MIOTICS—CHOLINERGIC AGENTS				
Carbachol				
Ophthalmic solution	Isopto Carbachol (Alcon)	0.75% 1.5% 2.25% 3%	15 mL 15, 30 mL 15 mL 15, 30 mL	2 drops topically in the eye(s) up to 3 times daily.
Ophthalmic solution	Miostat Intraocular (Alcon)	0.01%	1.5 mL	Instill no more than 0.5 mL into the anterior chamber.
Pilocarpine Hydrochloride				
Ophthalmic solution	Adsorbocarpine (Alcon)	1% 2% 4%	15 mL 15 mL 15 mL	1 or 2 drops topically in the eye(s) up to 3 or 4 times daily. Under selected conditions, more frequent instillations may be indicated. Individuals with heavily pigmented irides may require higher strengths. During acute phases, the miotic must be instilled into the unaffected eye to prevent an attack of angleclosure glaucoma.
Ophthalmic solution	Akarpine (Alcon)	1% 2% 4%	15 mL 15 mL 15 mL	
Ophthalmic solution	Isopto Carpine (Alcon)	0.25% 0.5% 1%	15 mL 15, 30 mL 15, 30 mL	

Dosage form	Product (manufacturer)	Strength	Size	Notes
		2%	15, 30 mL	
		3%	15, 30 mL	
		4%	15, 30 mL	
		5%	15 mL	
		6%	15, 30 mL	
		8%	15 mL	
		10%	15 mL	
Ocular therapeutic system	Ocusert-Pilo (ALZA)	P.20	5 mg	Ocular therapeutic system applied once a week.
		P.40	11 mg	
Ophthalmic solution	Filostat (Bausch & Lomb)	0.5%	15 mL	
		1%	15 mL	
		2%	15 mL	
		3%	15 mL	
		4%	15 mL	
		6%	15 mL	
Ophthalmic gel	Pilopine HS Gel (Alcon)	4%	3.5 g	
Ophthalmic solution	Piloptic (Optopics)	0.5%	15 mL	May be instilled up to 6 times daily.
		1%	15 mL	
		2%	15 mL	
		3%	15 mL	
		4%	15 mL	
		6%	15 mL	
Ophthalmic solution	Pilocar (Ciba Vision) (Ophthalmics)	0.5%	15, 2 × 15 mL	1 or 2 drops topically in the eye(s) up to 3 or 4 times daily. Under selected conditions, more frequent instillations may be indicated. Individuals with heavily pigmented irides may require higher strengths. During acute phases, the miotic must be instilled into the unaffected eye to prevent an attack of angleclosure glaucoma.
		1%	1, 15, 2 × 15 mL	
		2%	1, 15, 2 × 15 mL	
		3%	15, 2 × 15 mL	
		4%	1, 15, 2 × 15 mL	
		6%	15, 2 × 15 mL	

(continued)

TABLE 5-59 Quick Reference for Most Commonly Used Glaucoma Medications (Continued)

Active Ingredients	Trade Name	Concentration	How Supplied	Administration and Dosage
Pilocarpine Nitrate				
Ophthalmic solution	Pilagan (Allergan)	1% 2% 4%	15 mL 15 mL 15 mL	1 to 2 drops 2 to 4 times daily.
Physostigmine Salicylate				
Ophthalmic solution	Eserine salicylate (Alcon)	0.5%	2 mL	Instill 2 drops into the eye(s) up to 4 times daily.
	Isopto-Eserine (Alcon)	0.25%	15 mL	
Physostigmine Sulfate				
Ophthalmic ointment	Available generically	0.25%	3.5 g	Apply a small quantity to lower fornix, up to 3 times daily.
Demecarium-bromide				
Ophthalmic solution	Humorsol (Merck & Co.)	0.125% 0.25%	5 mL 5 mL	Initially place 1 or 2 drops into the eye. Usual dose—1 or 2 drops twice a week to 1 to 2 drops twice a day. The 0.125% strength used twice daily usually results in smooth control of the physiologic diurnal variation in IOP.
Echothiophate Iodide				
Ophthalmic powder	Phospholine Iodide (Wyeth-Ayerst)	0.03% 0.06% 0.125% 0.25%	1.5 mg 3 mg 6.25 mg 12.5 mg	Early chronic simple glaucoma, advanced chronic simple glaucoma, and glaucoma secondary to cataract surgery—instill a 0.03% solution just before retiring and in the morning.
Isoflurophate				
Ophthalmic ointment	Floropryl (Merck & Co.)	0.025%	3.5 g	0.25-in strip in eye every 8–72 h.

SYMPATHOMIMETICS

Dipivefrin Hydrochloride

Ophthalmic solution	Propine (Allergan)	0.1%	5, 10, 15 mL	1 drop in the eye(s) every 12 h.

Epinephrine Borate

Ophthalmic solution	Epinal (Alcon)	0.5% 1%	7.5 mL 7.5 mL	1 drop in the affected eye(s) once or twice daily.
Ophthalmic solution	Eppy/N (Barnes-Hind)	0.5% 1% 2%	7.5 mL 7.5 mL 7.5 mL	

Epinephrine Hydrochloride

Ophthalmic solution	Epifrin (Allergan)	0.5% 1% 2%	15 mL 15 mL 15 mL	1 drop in the affected eye(s) once or twice daily.
Ophthalmic solution	Glaucon (Alcon)	1% 2%	10 mL 10 mL	

ADRENERGIC BLOCKING AGENTS

Betaxolol Hydrochloride

Ophthalmic suspension	Betoptic S (Alcon)	0.25%	2.5, 5, 10, 15 mL	1 to 2 drops in the affected eye(s) twice daily.
Ophthalmic solution	Betoptic (Alcon)	0.5%	2.5, 5, 10, 15 mL	

Carteolol Hydrochloride

Ophthalmic solution	Ocupress (Otsuka America)	1%	5, 10 mL	1 drop in the affected eye(s) twice a day.

Levobunolol Hydrochloride

Ophthalmic solution	Betagan (Allergan)	0.25% 0.5%	5, 10 mL 2, 5, 10, 15 mL	1 or 2 drops in the affected eye(s) once a day.
Ophthalmic solution	A K Beta (Akorn)	0.25% 0.5%	5, 10 mL 5, 10, 15 mL	

Metipranolol Hydrochloride

Ophthalmic solution	OptiPranolol (Bausch & Lomb)	0.3%	5, 10 mL	1 drop in the affected eye(s) twice a day.

(continued)

155

TABLE 5-59 Quick Reference for Most Commonly Used Glaucoma Medications (Continued)

Active Ingredients	Trade Name	Concentration	How Supplied	Administration and Dosage
Timolol Maleate				
Ophthalmic solution	Timoptic (Merck & Co.)	0.25% 0.5%	2.5, 5, 10, 15 mL 2.5, 5, 10, 15 mL	1 drop in the affected eye(s) twice a day. May be changed to 1 drop a day if IOP is maintained at satisfactory levels.
	Istalol (Ista)	0.5%	5 mL	
Preservative-free	Timoptic (Merck & Co.)	0.25% 0.5%	0.45 mL 0.45 mL	
Ophthalmic gel	Timoptic-XE (Merck & Co.)	0.25% 0.5%	2.5, 5 mL 2.5, 5 mL	
Timolol Hemi-Hydrate				
	Betimol (Ciba Vision Ophthalmics)	0.25% 0.5%	2.5, 5, 10, 15 mL 2.5, 5, 10, 15 mL	1 drop in the affected eye(s) twice a day. May be changed to 1 drop a day if IOP is maintained at satisfactory levels.
HYPEROSMOTIC AGENTS				
Glycerin				
Oral osmotic agent	Osmoglyn (Alcon)	50%	220 mL (Discon)	2–3 mL/kg body weight given 1–1.5 h before surgery.
Isosorbide				
Ophthalmic solution	Ismotic (Alcon)	45% w/v	220 mL (Discon)	1.5 g/kg body weight. Use 2 to 4 times a day.
Mannitol				
Solutions	Mannitol (Abbott)	5% 15%	1000 mL 150, 500 mL	Adult dose ranges from 50–200 g/24 h. Administer to maintain a urine flow rate of 30–50 mL/h. 1.5–2 g/kg given as a 15%–20% solution may be given over a period as short as 30 min.
	Osmitrol (Travenol)	5% 10% 15% 20%	1000 mL 500, 1000 mL 500 mL 250, 500 mL	
	Available generically	10% 20% 25%	1000 mL 250, 500 mL 50-mL vials and syringes	

CARBONIC ANHYDRASE INHIBITORS

Acetazolamide				
Tablets	Diamox (Lederle)	125 mg 250 mg	100s, 1000s UD 100s	250 mg to 1 g/day, in divided doses for amounts over 250 mg.
Powder for injection	Diamox (Lederle)	500 mg	Vial	
Capsules	Diamox Sequels (Lederle)	500 mg	30s, 100s	1 capsule 2 times a day.
	Available generically	125 mg 250 mg	50s, 100s, 250s, 500s 1000s, UD 100s	
Dichlorphenamide				
Tablets	Daranide (Merck & Co.)	50 mg	100s	100–200 mg initially, followed by 100 mg every 12 h until the desired response is obtained.
Methazolamide				
Tablets	Neptazane (Lederle)	25 mg 50 mg	100s 100s	50–100 mg, 2 to 3 times daily.
	GlaucTabs (Akorn)	25 mg 50 mg	100s 100s	
	MZM (Ciba Vision Ophthalmics)	25 mg 50 mg	100s 100s	
Dorzolamide Hydrochloride				
Ophthalmic solution	Trusopt (MSD)	2%	5 mL	Instill 1 drop in affected eye(s) 3 times daily.
Brinzolamide	Azopt (Alcon)	1.0%	5, 10 mL	
PILOCARPINE COMBINATIONS			2.5, 5, 10, 15 mL	
Pilocarpine and Epinephrine Bitartrate				
Ophthalmic solution	E-Pilo-1 (Ciba Vision Ophthalmics)	1% pilocarpine HCl, 1% epinephrine bitartrate	10 mL	Instill 1 or 2 drops in the eye(s) 1 to 4 times daily. Individuals with heavily pigmented irides may require larger doses.

(continued)

▶ TABLE 5.59 Quick Reference for Most Commonly Used Glaucoma Medications (Continued)

Active Ingredients	Trade Name	Concentration	How Supplied	Administration and Dosage
Ophthalmic solution	E-Pilo-2 (Ciba Vision Ophthalmics)	2% pilocarpine HCl, 1% epinephrine bitartrate	10 mL	
Ophthalmic solution	E-Pilo-4 (Ciba Vision Ophthalmics)	4% pilocarpine HCl, 1% epinephrine bitartrate	10 mL	
Ophthalmic solution	E-Pilo-6 (Ciba Vision Ophthalmics)	6% pilocarpine HCl, 1% epinephrine bitartrate	10 mL	
Ophthalmic solution	P_1E_1 (Alcon)	1% pilocarpine HCl, 1% epinephrine bitartrate	15 mL	
Ophthalmic solution	P_2E_1 (Alcon)	2% pilocarpine HCl, 1% epinephrine bitartrate	15 mL	
Ophthalmic solution	P_3E_1 (Alcon)	3% pilocarpine HCl, 1% epinephrine bitartrate	15 mL	
Ophthalmic solution	P_4E_1 (Alcon)	4% pilocarpine HCl, 1% epinephrine bitartrate	15 mL	
Ophthalmic solution	P_6E_1 (Alcon)	6% pilocarpine HCl, 1% epinephrine bitartrate	15 mL	
Pilocarpine and Physostigmine				
Ophthalmic solution	Isopto P-ES (Alcon)	2% pilocarpine HCl, 0.25% physostigmine salicylate	15 mL	Instill 1 or 2 drops in the affected eye(s) up to 4 times daily.
PROSTAGLANDINS				
Latanoprost				
Ophthalmic solution	Xalatan	0.005%	2.5 mL	Instill 1 drop at bedtime.
Bimatoprost				
Ophthalmic solution	Lumigan (Allergan)	0.03%	2.5, 5 mL	Instill 1 drop at bedtime.
Travaprost				
Ophthalmic solution	Travatan (Alcon)	0.004%	2.5 mL	Instill 1 drop at bedtime.

PRINCIPLES OF GLAUCOMA MANAGEMENT

1. Do not continue to add second and third medications unless it has been firmly established that prior therapy is not effective. There are many patients on two or three medications who could be equally cared for with one effective medication.
2. Rule out any contraindications, such as chronic obstructive pulmonary disease or significant heart disease, prior to initiating β-blocker therapy.
3. All β-blockers (including β-1 selective agents) are contraindicated in patients with cardiac disease (particularly heart block).
4. Record baseline pulse rate and monitor blood pressure prior to initiating β-blocker therapy.
5. When contemplating therapy with an agent having two concentrations (0.25% or 0.5%), initiate therapy with the lower concentration.
6. Always conduct a monocular therapeutic trial to establish efficacy if at all possible.
7. Always try once daily dosing in the morning with β-blocker therapy to determine effectiveness of single-dose daily therapy.
8. Using sound clinical judgment, set a target goal of intraocular pressure reduction, and direct your energies methodically toward that goal.
9. Recheck the patient in approximately 3 weeks to determine efficacy of therapy. Dipivefrin therapy is the exception to this rule. It may take up to 3 months to reach its maximum efficacy.
10. Approximately 10% of patients do not respond to β-blocker therapy.
11. When a second agent is indicated, the drugs of choice are, in the following order: dorzolamide, apraclonidine, dipivefrin, and pilocarpine.
12. Dorzolamide or dipivefrin are excellent agents for asthmatics.
13. Dorzolamide should be started two times a day initially; go to three times a day only if clinically indicated. (See Tables 5.60 and 5.61.)
14. With all topical ophthalmic therapy, have patients gently close their eyelids for at least 30 seconds following instillation.
15. When initiating pilocarpine therapy, start with a 0.5% sample and gradually increase to the concentration necessary to control intraocular pressure. The most common final concentrations are 2% and 4%. There is rarely a reason to exceed the 4% concentration.
16. Once intraocular pressure control has been established, routinely follow up every 3 to 6 months; however, this schedule depends on the patient's response to medication and the stability of the disease.
17. At least two baseline visual fields should be obtained during the first 3 to 6 months of evaluation or therapy, and repeat field testing should be done annually for most patients.
18. If glaucoma is suspected, gonioscopy should be performed.
19. There are many patients using glaucoma medications who do not have glaucoma, nor any significant risk factors. Keep this in mind when you "inherit" a new patient on glaucoma therapy. Always thoroughly reassess the patient to confirm the diagnosis and need for continued therapy. If possible, consider alternative treatment that may minimize adverse effects and maximize efficacy.

▌ **TABLE 5.60** Guidelines for NSAIDS Dosages

NSAID	Brand Name	Usual Adult Dose	Usual Pediatric Dose
Acetaminophen		650–975 mg q 4 h	10–15 mg/kg q 4 h
Aspirin		650–975 mg q 4 h	10–15 mg/kg q 4 h (contraindicated in fever or viral illness)
Choline magnesium trisalicylate	Trilisate	1000–1500 mg bid	25 mg/kg bid
Diflunisal	Dolobid	1000 mg initially, then 500 mg q 12 h	
Etodolac	Lodine	200–400 mg q 6–8 h	
Fenoprofen calcium	Naflon	200 mg q 4–6 h	
Ibuprofen	Motrin, others	400 mg q 4–6 h	10 mg/kg q 6–8 h
Ketoprofen	Orudis	25–75 mg q 6–8 h	
Magnesium salicylate		650 mg q 4 h	
Meclofenamate Na	Meclomen	50 mg q 4–6 h	
Mefenamic acid	Ponstel	250 mg q 6 h	
Naproxen	Naprosyn	500 mg initially, then 250 mg q 6–8 h	5 mg/kg q 12 h
Naproxen Na	Anaprox	550 mg initially, then 275 mg q 6–8 h	
Salsalate	Disalcid	500 mg q 4 h	
Sodium salicylate		325–650 mg q 3–4 h	
Ketorolac	Toradol	30 or 60 mg IM initially, then 15 or 30 mg IM q 6 h Oral dose following IM dose: 10 mg q 6–8 h	
Nabumetone	Relafen	1 g q night	

(Adapted from: Acute Pain Management Guideline Panel: Acute pain management. Operative or medical procedures and trauma (AHCPR Pub. No. 92-0032). Agency for Health Care Policy and Research, U.S. Department of Health and Human Services, 1992.)

▶ **TABLE 5.61** Guidelines for Adult Narcotic Analgesic Dosages

Opioid Agonist	Brand Name	Starting Oral Dose Adult >50 kg wt (Child and Adult <50 kg wt)	Starting Parenteral Dose Adult >50 kg wt (Child Adult <50 kg wt)
Morphine		30 mg q 3–4 h (0.3 mg/kg q 3–4 h)	10 mg q 3–4 h (0.1 mg/kg q 3–4 h)
Codeine		60 mg q 3–4 h (1 mg/kg q 3–4 h)	60 mg q 3–4 h (IM, SC) (Not recommended)
Hydromorphone	Dilaudid	6 mg q 3–4 h (0.06 mg/kg q 3–4 h)	1.5 mg q 3–4 h (0.015 mg/kg q 3–4 h)
Hydrocodone	in Vicodin, others	10 mg q 3–4 h (0.2 mg/kg q 3–4 h)	Not available (Not available)
Levorphanol	Levo-Dromoran	4 mg q 6–8 h (0.04 mg/kg q 6–8 h)	2 mg q 6–8 h (0.02 mg/kg q 6–8 h)
Meperidine	Demorol	Not recommended (Not recommended)	100 mg q 3 h (0.75 mg/kg q 2–3 h)
Methadone	Dolophine	20 mg q 6–8 h (0.2 mg/kg q 6–8 h)	10 mg q 6–8 h (0.1 mg/kg q 6–8 h)
Oxycodone	in Percocet, Percodan, Tylox	10 mg q 3–4 h (0.2 mg/kg q 3–4 h)	Not available (Not available)
Oxymorphone	Numorphan	Not available (Not recommended)	1 mg q 3–4 h (Not recommended)
OPIOID AGONIST—ANTAGONIST AND PARTIAL AGONIST			
Buprenorphine	Buprenex		0.4 mg q 6–8 h (0.004 mg/kg q 6–8 h)
Butorphanol	Stadol	Not available (Not available)	2 mg q 3–4 h (Not recommended)
Nalbuphine	Nubain		10 mg q 3–4 h (0.1 mg/kg q 3–4 h)
Pentazocine	Talwin	50 mg q 4–6 h (Not recommended)	Not recommended (Not recommended)

(Adapted from Acute Pain Management Guideline Panel. Acute pain management. Operative or medical procedures and trauma (AHCPR Pub. No. 92-0032). Agency for Health Care Policy and Research, U.S. Department of Health and Human Services, 1992.)

ANALGESIC AGENTS
Jill C. Autry

PRINCIPLES OF PAIN MANAGEMENT

1. Appreciate the patient's report of pain, and intervene before the pain worsens.
2. Place the symptoms of pain within the total evaluation of the patient. Look beyond the eye injury itself when indicated.
3. Always make an accurate diagnosis of the underlying disease process. Do not mask the disease with pain relievers.
4. Obtain a thorough medical and drug history to avoid drug-drug and drug-patient adverse reactions. (See Table 5.62.)
5. Use an effective drug and dose appropriate for the patient's pain. Opioids should not be used indiscriminately. They also should not be withheld if nonopioids prove ineffective.
6. Adjust therapeutic pain relief measures on the basis of patient response.
7. Analgesic therapy should be provided on a 24-hour schedule. Duration of effect depends on the drug and its route of administration.
8. All analgesics have potential side effects. Monitor for nausea, sedation, itching, or constipation. Adjust dosage as needed to minimize side effects. Refer to internist when necessary.
9. Consider cost and use over-the-counter (OTC) drugs when possible. Always prescribe generic equivalents when available.

▶ **TABLE 5.62** Narcotic Agonist Comparative Pharmacology

Drug	Analgesic	Anti-tussive	Constipation	Respiratory Depression	Sedation	Emesis	Physical Dependence
PHENANTHRENES							
Codeine	+	++-	+	+	+	+	+
Hydrocodone	+	++-	nd	+	nd	nd	+
Hydromorphone	++	+++	+	++	+	+	++
Levorphanol	++	-+	++	++	++	+	++
Morphine	++	+++	++	++	++	++	++
Oxycodone	++	+++	++	++	++	++	++
Oxymorphone	++	-	++	+++	nd	+++	+++
PHENYLPIPERIDINES							
Alfentanil	++	nd	nd	nd	nd	nd	nd
Fentanyl	++	nd	nd	+	nd	+	nd
Meperidine	++	+	+	++	+	nd	++
Sufentanil	+++	nd	nd	nd	nd	nd	nd
DIPHENYLHEPTANES							
Methadone	+-	++	++	++	+	+	+
Propoxyphene	+	nd	nd	+	+	+	+

nd = No data available.

NUTRITIONAL AGENTS
Jill C. Autry

The use of nutritional agents in the management of ocular disease, albeit controversial, may be of benefit in the prevention of cataracts and the treatment of age-related macular degeneration (ARMD) and dry eye syndrome.

In general, the compounds that have attracted the most interest are the vitamin/mineral combinations that exhibit antioxidant activity. They are listed in Table 5.63.

▶ TABLE 5.63 Currently Available Over-the-Counter Ocular Vitamin/Mineral
Supplements

Tablet Information	Icaps Plus	Ocuvite	Ocusoft VMS	Nutrivision	US RDA
Zinc	30 mg (zinc acetate)	40 mg (zinc oxide)	40 mg (zinc oxide)	20 mg (zinc gluconate) 10 mg (zinc picolinate)	15 mg
Copper	1.5 mg	2 mg	2 mg	1.5 mg	2 mg
Selenium	60 mcg	40 mcg	40 mcg	50 mcg	not established
Manganese	5 mg	—	—	—	not established
Chromium	—	—	—	25 mcg	not established
Vit A (beta carotene)	6000 IU	5000 IU	5000 IU	5000 IU	5000 IU
Vit B-2 (riboflavin)	20 mg	—	—	—	1.7 mg
Vit C (ascorbic acid)	200 mg	60 mg	60 mg	300 mg	60 mg
Vit E (α-tocopherol)	60 IU	30 IU	30 IU	100 IU	30 IU
Daily dose	1–2 tablets w/meal	1–2 tablets	1–2 tablets w/meal	1–2 tablets w/meal	
Source	La Haye	Storz-Lederle	Ocusoft	Bronson	
Telephone no.	1-800-344-2020	1-800-325-9929	1-800-233-5469	1-800-235-3200	
Notes	new formula 12/91		new name 3/92		

Chapter 6

Bacterial Infectious Diseases

BACTERIAL BLEPHARITIS

Marcus Piccolo

ICD—9: 373.01 - Blepharitis, ulcerative
ICD—9: 372.21 - Blepharitis, angular

THE DISEASE

Pathophysiology

Blepharitis occurs when there is colonization and infection of the lid margin, lid glands, or cilia follicle by bacterial pathogens. The liberation of bacterial enzymes and exotoxins may result in inflammation and potential morphological changes to the lid, cilia, conjunctiva, and cornea. Inflammatory changes of the external adnexa and alteration of the sebaceous secretions may also produce various ocular surface disorders (OSD).

Etiology

The most common pathogens responsible for bacterial blepharitis are *Staphylococcus aureus, Staphylococcus epidermidis, P. acnes,* and *Moraxella spp.* Other causes of infectious blepharitis should be excluded (i.e., herpes simplex, herpes zoster, *Candida spp.* vaccinia, and molluscum).

The Patient

Clinical Symptoms

Chronic itching, redness, burning, tearing, foreign body sensation, and lash crusting with intermittent exacerbations are common features. Symptoms are typically worse in the morning. Patients may also complain of dryness of the eyes.

Clinical Signs

- Lids: Thickened, irregular lid margins with telangectasias are common features. Infection of the base of the cilia leads to deposition of fibrin, which eventually hardens and separates from the lid as a disc upon growth of the cilia. What results is the classic collerette pierced by a cilia. Collerettes are the hallmark of staphylococcal blepharitis and should be differentiated from the scaly, grayish sleeve that is associated with *Demodex* infestation. In addition, fine flakes of keratinized epithelium may surround the base of the lashes. Deeper infection within the cilia follicle may result in poliosis (white lashes), madarosis (missing lashes), and trichiasis (misdirected lashes). Other findings may include ulcerated lid margins, meibomitis, hordeola, chalazia, and/or preseptal cellulitis.

- Corneal and Conjunctiva: Chronic inflammation of the lids may result in a papillary conjunctivitis, with occasional exacerbations. Exotoxins produced by *Staphylococcal* organisms are typically implicated in a toxic conjunctivitis, as well as the development of inflammatory infiltrates of the cornea. Fine punctate keratopathy may be present in the inferior portions of the cornea. Subepithelial infiltrates are usually found adjacent to the limbus most prominently superiorly and inferiorly and where the lid crosses the limbus (11, 2, 4 and 8 o'clock). An infiltrate may necrose, resulting in a sterile ulcer. If the corneal involvement is chronic or recurrent, visually significant vascularization and scarring may occur. In addition, phlyctenules may form, which are immunologic reactions to bacterial exotoxins. Phlyctenules are typically raised lesions consisting of lymphocytes. They may be found on the cornea or conjunctiva, but are most frequently seen in the limbal area. Phlyctenules may ulcerate with neutrophils appearing as necrosis occurs. (See section on Phlyctenulosis.)

Demographics

Bacterial blepharitis may occur in all ages, including children. Bilaterality is the rule, although unilateral involvement may rarely occur. Women are more frequently affected than men.

Significant History

Dry eyes and tear deficiencies may be contributing factors. Other conditions found in association with bacterial blepharitis include acne vulgaris, ocular rosacea, seborrheic blepharitis, eczema, impetigo, and other infectious skin diseases.

Ancillary Tests

The diagnosis of bacterial blepharitis is usually based on clinical findings; however, cultures of the conjunctival cul de sac and lid margins should be performed and plated on chocolate and blood agar in patients who do not respond to empiric therapy.

Technique: a calcium alginate swab, moistened with a liquid media such as thioglycolate broth, should be gently drawn through the upper and lower cul de sacs (total contact time should be ~5 seconds) and then applied to both blood and chocolate agar. A new swab should be used to wipe the inferior and superior lid margins and then applied to the same plates. The procedure should be repeated for the opposite eye using fresh swabs (Figure 6.1).

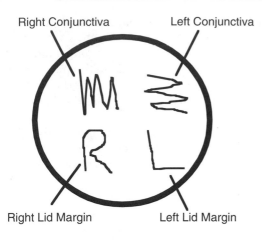

Right Conjunctiva   Left Conjunctiva

Right Lid Margin   Left Lid Margin

FIGURE 6.1. *S. epidermidis* is commonly found on normal patients, although heavy growth is more significant. Any growth of *S. aureus* maybe significant, but is isolated in over 50% of patients. Sensitivity testing should be performed in cases resistant to emperic treatment.

The Treatment

Topical

Warm compresses followed by a commercial lid scrub preparation (diluted baby shampoo may be substituted, but may be more irritating to the eye) are the mainstay of therapy. Lid scrubs may be required several times per day depending on the severity of the disease and then tapered to a maintenance schedule as the condition improves. Warm compresses and lid scrubs decrease the bioload on the lids, as well as stimulate the flow of the meibomian glands.

Topical bacitracin or erythromycin ointment applied to the lids and lashes qhs × 3–4 weeks then tapered to a maintenance dose. Alternation of antibiotics may reduce the tendency of developing resistant organisms.

Topical steroid/antibiotic drops may be helpful for bulbar conjunctival and corneal involvement: Maxitrol drops (neomycin/polymyxin B/dexamethasone) 1 gtt qid × 7–10 d.

Unresponsive patients may be carriers and require culturing of the nasopharynx and ear canal and skin, as well as systemic antibiotic therapy.

Systemic

Systemic antibiotics are not used in this condition for their antibiotic properties, but rather to stabilize meibomian gland secretions by reducing inflammation and by inhibiting bacterial enzymes. Suggested regimens include:

- Tetracycline (do not use in pregnant women or children under age 8), 250 mg qid p.o. × 2–4 mo
- Erythromycin, 250 mg qid p.o. × 2–4 mo
- Doxycycline or minocycline, 100 mg bid p.o. × 1 mo, then tapered and used for several additional months
- If a penicillinase resistant antibiotic is necessary, consider cloxacillin:
  >20 kg—250 mg q6h p.o. × 10 d. or
  <20 kg—50 mg/kg/day in equally divided doses q6h p.o. × 10 d

In general, blepharitis is a chronic condition, and treatment is aimed at control rather than cure. It is likely that some form of maintenance therapy, such as daily lid hygiene, will be required lifelong.

BACTERIAL CONJUNCTIVITIS
Marcus Piccolo

ICD—9: 372.0 - Conjunctivitis, acute, unspecified
ICD—9: 372.11 - Conjunctivitis, chronic, simple
ICD—9: 098.49 - Gonococcal, eye infection, other
ICD—9: 098.4 - Conjunctivitis, gonococcal, neonatorum
ICD—9: 372.04 - Conjunctivitis, membranous

THE DISEASE
Pathophysiology

Bacterial conjunctivitis results from infection of the conjunctival tissue with bacterial pathogens. The resultant inflammatory process may present with a wide range of severity and of clinical appearances.

Etiology

Bacterial conjunctivitis results when a bacterial innoculation overcomes the natural defense mechanisms of the conjunctiva. The pathogens may be normal flora of the conjunctiva or lids or may be the result of innoculation from an adjacent infection (silent dacryocystitis), hand-to-eye contact, or airborne respiratory droplets. The defense mechanisms of the conjunctiva include the mechanical actions of the lids and tears, enzymes such as lysozyme, lactoferin and B-lysin present in the tears, immunoglobulins (IgA and IgG) present in the tears, conjunctival associated lymphoid tissue, and an intact epithelial barrier.

Bacterial conjunctivitis can be classified as hyperacute, acute, pseudomembranous/membranous and chronic (Table 6.1).

▌ **TABLE 6.1 Common Conjunctival Bacterial Pathogens in Adults**

Hyperacute	Acute	Membranous	Chronic
Neisseria gonorrhea	Streptococcus pneumoniae	*Neisseria* spp	*Staphylococcus aureus*
Neisseria meningitides	*Haemophilus aegyptius*	Corynebacterium diphtheriae	Moraxella lacunata
	Haemophilus influenzae	*Streptococcus pyogenes*	
	Staphylococcus spp	*S. aureus*	

The Patient

Clinical Symptoms

Hyperacute Conjunctivitis

- Onset is usually within 12 hours of exposure and is rapidly progressive.
- The patient reports irritation, redness, and copius purulent discharge. The eye lids may be adherent upon awakening. Infection may start in one eye and migrate to the other eye because of hand-to-eye contact or fomites.
- Visual acuity is unaffected if the cornea is not involved and if the discharge can be irrigated from the corneal surface.

Acute Conjunctivitis

- Redness, irritation, grittiness, and mucopurulent discharge are common symptoms.
- Visual acuity is typically unaffected.
- The infection usually starts unilateral but often spreads to the fellow eye within a few days.

Membranous Conjunctivitis (Same as acute conjunctivitis.)

Chronic Conjunctivitis

- Symptoms include mild, chronic redness and irritation of the conjunctiva and lids especially in the fornices.
- Visual acuity is usually unaffected.
- Discharge may be mucoid or watery.

Clinical Signs

Hyperacute Conjunctivitis

- Classic presentation is a severely injected, chemotic conjunctiva with copious purulent discharge.
- PA nodes are commonly enlarged and tender to palpation.
- Corneal involvement may occur; resulting in SPK or frank corneal ulceration (*Neisseria* may invade an intact cornea). Peripheral ring infiltrates may be seen with gonococcus resulting in corneal perforation if left untreated.
- Conjunctival pseudo membranes may be evident.
- *Neisseria* meningitides may gain access to the central nervous system through infection of the conjunctiva via hematogenous spread, resulting in infectious meningitis. Other concomitant infections may involve the genitourinary tract and/or the pharynx if *N. gonorrhoeae* is responsible for the underlying infection.
- Other potential ocular and systemic complications of gonococcal conjunctivitis include: iritis, lid abscess, dacryoadenitis, and septicemia.

Acute Conjunctivitis

- The typical presentation is a mild to moderate bulbar and tarsal conjunctival injection with canthal involvement.
- There is usually minimal eyelid involvement and no PA lymphadenopathy, except in very severe cases.
- A papillary conjunctival tissue reaction is common.
- Pseudomembranes or small subconjuctival hemorrhages may exist (Streptococcus).

- Mucopurulent discharge may be mild to moderate and may seal the eyelids upon awakening.
- The cornea is usually uninvolved.

Membranous Conjunctivitis

- This disorder has the same clinical presentation as acute conjunctivitis, with the addition of pseudomembranes or membranes and markedly swollen lids.
- Pseudomembranes (fibrinous exudate that lies on the conjunctival surface without deep attachments and can be removed without significant bleeding) in bacterial conjunctivitis are most commonly caused by *Neisseria* or *Streptococcus pyogenes*; true membranes (fibrin strands project into the conjunctiva between epithelial cells, thus removal causes bleeding) are most often caused by Corynebacterium diphtheriae.
- Pain is a prominent feature of membranous conjunctivitis.
- Any severe bacterial conjunctivitis can cause a pseudomembrane.
- Membranous conjunctivitis may be associated with corneal ulceration and/or permanent loss of goblet cells, which could result in ocular surface disorders and chronic dry eye.

Chronic Conjunctivitis

- Staphylococcus

  The lids may show signs of crusting and formation of collerettes with associated madarosis and trichiasis. In addition, the skin of the lids may show an eczematous-type reaction. The bulbar conjunctiva may be mildly to moderately injected with or without the presence of phlyctenules. The palpebral conjunctiva usually demonstrates a papillary reaction. The cornea may be involved with inferior punctate keratitis, marginal infiltrates, or micropannus as a result of the presence of bacterial exotoxins. (See Bacterial Blepharitis.)

- Moraxella

  Moraxella may cause mild to moderate papillary conjunctivitis without corneal involvement. May result in angular blepharoconjunctivitis (Staph has also been implicated as a common cause in this presentation). On occasion, Moraxella may cause a chronic follicular conjunctivitis with corneal involvement, including punctate keratitis, subepithelial infiltrates, and preauricular lymphadenopathy. This latter presentation could be confused with adenovirus or chlamydial infections.

Demographics

Hyperacute Conjunctivitis

Hyperacute conjunctivitis can occur in men or women. It is usually associated with venereal disease (Gonococcus). Hyperacute conjunctivitis may be implicated in ophthalmia neonatorum.

Acute Conjunctivitis

Acute conjunctivitis is usually self-limiting in 1 to 3 weeks. It is a common cause of "pink eye" in the United States. Pneumococcus is the predominate etiology in the northern

United States, while *Haemophilus aegyptius* (Koch-Weeks bacillus) is the leading cause in the southern United States.

Haemophilus influenzae must be excluded in any conjunctivitis in young patients, as the ability to make appropriate antibodies for H. influenzae does not exist in children age 5 and under. However, the H. influenzae type B vaccine has greatly reduced the incidence of this disease.

Membranous Conjunctivitis
Rarely caused by C. diphtheriae because of immunizations in the United States.

Chronic Conjunctivitis
Chronic conjunctivitis may occur in men, women or children and may be the sequelae of an acute infection that received inadequate or inappropriate treatment.

Significant History

Hyperacute Conjunctivitis
History of urethritis or other urogenital involvement may be present. A history of a new sexual partner or of promiscuity is significant. The patient may have other venereal diseases as well.

Acute Conjunctivitis
The patient may have a history of an upper respiratory infection or contact with someone with a conjunctivitis or an upper respiratory infection. Children at daycare facilities may be more likely to come in contact with pathogens.

Membranous Conjunctivitis
C. diphtheria conjunctivitis may be associated with a history of respiratory involvement including airway obstruction with a pharyngeal membrane; exotoxins from C. diphtheriae may result in paralysis of accommodation and extraocular muscles as well as cardiac toxicity and liver necrosis.

S. pyogenes may be associated with chronic low-grade dacryocystitis, which erupts into an acute conjunctivitis.

Chronic Conjunctivitis
Chronic conjunctivitis is often associated with blepharitis or past episodes of acute bacterial infection.

Ancillary Tests

In general, the diagnosis of a nonsevere conjunctivitis is made clinically. However, cases of severe bacterial infections mandate further investigation.

Hyperacute Conjunctivitis
- Cytology
   PMN response with intracellular bacteria.

- Gram Stain
    Gram-negative intracellular, diplococci, with many PMNs – *Neisseria*.
    Gram-negative coccobacilli – H. influenzae.
- Cultures
    Purulent discharge should be streaked on blood and chocolate agar and incubated at 37° in 10% CO_2 or on a Thayer-Martin plate. Antibiotic sensitivities should also be performed.

    Note: Imaging may be indicated in cases of orbital abscess or advanced cellulitis.

Acute Conjunctivitis

- Cytology
    PMN response.
- Gram Stain
    Presence of bacteria. The clinician should note the morphology of the organism (rod, club, or cocci) as well as other characteristic features of the organism (e.g., clusters, chains, etc.).
- Cultures
    Cultures are necessary in persistent infections that do not respond to emperic treatment, and should include plating on blood and chocolate agar as well as thioglycolate broth. Antibiotic sensitivities should also be requested.

Membranous Conjunctivitis

- Cytology
    PMN response.
- Gram Stain
    Gram-positive cocci arranged in chains (*S. pyogenes*).
    Gram-positive pleomorphic rods that appear drumstick-shaped (*C. diphtheriae*).
    Gram-negative diplococci (*Neisseria*).
- Cultures
    Beta-hemolysis on blood agar (*S. pyogenes*).
    Loffler's blood serum (*C. diphtheria*).

Chronic Conjunctivitis

- Cytology
    PMN response.
- Gram Stain
    Gram-positive cocci in clusters (*Staphylococcus*).
    Gram-negative bacillus usually arranged in pairs (Moraxella).
- Cultures
    Staphylococcus: Blood agar with coagulase test and mannitol fermentation to differentiate *S. aureus* from *S. epidermidis*; sensitivities should be performed because of propensity toward resistance.
    Moraxella: Enriched media such as Loffler's medium.

The Treatment

Hyperacute Conjunctivitis

- Systemic treatment is mandatory in this condition; topical treatment is only adjunctive.
- Hospitalization is not uncommon, especially if keratitis exists.
- The patient and the sexual partners must be promptly referred for venereal aspects of *N. gonorrhea* (and coinfection with other STDs such as HIV, syphilis, chlamydia, etc.) to avoid significant morbidity.
  1. Topical Therapy
     Warm saline rinses qid until the discharge has resolved.
     Erythromycin, tobramycin, or bacitracin ung qid.
     Fluoroquinolones (ciprofloxacin, levofloxacin, ofloxacin, moxifloxacin, or gatifloxacin) q2h × 4–7 days.
  2. Systemic Therapy
     No keratitis present
         ceftriaxone 1g IM in a single dose.
     Keratitis present
         ceftriaxone 1 g IV q12h to 24h × 3 days or until symptoms subside and there is an appropriate clinical response.
     Treatment for a concomitant chlamydial infection includes erythromycin, tetracycline, or sulfacetamide ointment 2–3 ×/d plus:
         tetracycline 250—500 mg qid p.o. × 2–3 weeks, or
         doxycycline 100 mg bid p.o. × 2–3 weeks, or
         erythromycin 250–500 mg qid p.o. × 2–3 weeks, or
         azithromycin 1 g p.o. (single dose) preferred treatment.

Acute Conjunctivitis (Table 6.2)

Nonsevere cases of acute conjunctivitis generally subside in 1 to 2 weeks; however, topical antibiotics may accelerate resolution of the infection and reduce the risk of transmission.

Polytrim (trimethoprim/polymyxin B) 1 gtt qid × 7–10d, or
Ocuflox (ofloxacin) 1 gtt qid × 7–10d, or
Tobrex (tobramycin) 1 gtt qid × 7–10d, or
Ilotycin (erythromycin ophthalmic) ung bid × 7–10d, or
Vigamox (moxifloxacin) 1 gtt tid × 4–7 d, or
Zymar (gatifloxacin) 1 gtt q2h while awake × 2d, then 1 gtt qid days 3–7

Membranous Conjunctivitis

After installation of a topical anesthetic, remove the membranes with forceps. Removal can be difficult and causes bleeding.

- C. diphtheriae
    C. diphtheriae antitoxin 10,000–100,000 units parenterally
    Topical penicillin
- *S. pyogenes*

▶ **TABLE 6.2** **Acute Conjunctivitis Differential Diagnosis**

	Adenoviral	*Chlamydial*	*Bacterial*
Incubation	3–5 days	6–12 days	1–3 days
Onset	Rapid	Slower	Rapid
	1–3 days	3–7 days	1–3 days
Age	Any age	Sexual age	Any age
Exposure	Pink eye	Sexual contact	Pink eye
Discharge	Watery	Either	Mucopurulent
Membranous	Adeno 8 most common	Newborn only	Strep most common
Keratitis	Usually central	Usually superior	None
Infiltrates	Subepithelial	Subepithelial	None
Pannus	None	Superior micropannus	None
Duration	2–4 weeks	4–14 months	1–2 weeks
Leukocytes	Mononuclear	PMN	PMN
Inclusions	None	Difficult to find in adult IC, common in newborn IC	None
PA node	Yes	Yes	No—only in GC
Response	Follicular	Follicular	Papillary

From: JD Lanier

Topical: bacitracin or erythromycin ung bid-qid

Systemic: cephalexin or erythromycin 250mg q6h p.o. × 7d

Note: Topical steroids are often helpful in reducing inflammation and preserving the conjunctiva architecture.

Chronic Conjunctivitis

■ Topical:

Lid hygiene with a commercial lid scrub preparation (diluted baby shampoo may be substituted, but may be more irritating to the eye).

Topical bacitracin or erythromycin ointment applied to the lids and lashes hs × 3–4 weeks then tapered to a maintenance dose.

Topical steroid/antibiotic gtts may be helpful for bulbar conjunctival and corneal involvement: Maxitrol drops (neomycin/polymyxin B/dexamethasone), or Tobradex (tobramycin/dexamethasone) 1 gtt tid × 7–10 d.

Unresponsive patients may be carriers and require culturing of the nasopharynx, ear canal, and skin, as well as systemic therapy.

■ Systemic:

Tetracycline (do not use tetracycline in pregnant women or children under age 8) or erythromycin 250 mg qid p.o. × 2–4 mo or

Doxycycline or minocycline 100 mg bid p.o. × 1 mo, then tapered and used for several additional months or

If penicillinase resistant antibiotic is necessary, consider cloxacillin:

>20 kg—250 mg q6h p.o. × 10 d or

< 20 kg—50 mg/kg/day in equally divided doses q6h p.o. × 10d

PHLYCTENULOSIS
Marcus Piccolo

ICD—9: 370.31

THE DISEASE

Pathophysiology

Phlyctenulosis is an immune reaction of the conjunctiva, limbus, or cornea, most commonly initiated by bacterial proteins that are recognized as antigenic. The immune reaction is classified as a Type IV delayed hypersensitivity response resulting in a raised nodule and localized perivascular inflammation. The nodule may necrose and ulcerate, further amplifying the resultant inflammatory response. Although the antigen is usually bacterial protein, other pathogens have also been responsible for initiating a phlyctenular response, including virus, fungus, chlamydia, and nematodes.

Etiology

The etiology of phlyctenulosis is the result of systemic or local infection by a pathogen that acts as an antigen in the eye. The organisms most likely to cause a phlyctenular response are tubercle bacillus and *Staphylococcus spp*. Classically, systemic tuberculosis was implicated as the primary cause. More recently, hypersensitivity to *Staphylococcus spp*, associated with bacterial blepharitis, has been a more common presentation. Other less common pathogens include *Coccidioides immitis*, *Candida albicans*, *Chlamydia spp*, *Haemophilus aegyptius*, herpes simplex virus, and various nematodes.

The Patient

Clinical Symptoms
Patients presenting with phlyctenulosis often experience discomfort or pain (especially if the phlyctenule is limbal or corneal), photophobia, tearing, and irritation.

Clinical Signs
Phlyctenulosis typically causes a red irritated eye. The phlyctenule itself is a small (1–3 mm) elevated nodule. The nodule is usually yellow, grey, or white in color and can be found on the bulbar conjunctiva, at the limbus (the most common location), or on the cornea. The lesion is frequently inflamed and surrounded by dilated vessels. On rare occasion, a phlyctenule can be found on the tarsal conjunctiva. Limbal phlyctenules typically take on a more triangular shape with the apex toward the cornea. It is common for the nodule to ulcerate, in which case it will stain with fluorescein. In most cases the nodule will appear, necrose, and then subside within 14 days. However, it is possible for the phlyctenule to persist and to recur. Phlyctenules on the conjunctiva typically do not scar; however, limbal and especially corneal phlyctenules often

result in scarring. A peripheral corneal phlyctenule may advance onto the cornea. In so doing, a leash of vessels will trail behind the nodule creating a superficial fibrous vascular bundle with an underlying infiltrate. This fibrovascular response has the potential to cause significant visual impairment and may ultimately require a corneal graft. Past episodes of limbal phlyctenules may be visible by identifying triangle shaped scars at the limbus.

Demographics

Phlyctenulosis most commonly affects children and young adults, with a slight predilection for females. Populations that have a higher prevalence of tuberculosis (TB) may be more at risk. This systemic factor is greater in many third world countries where TB is endemic, as well as some locations within the United States that are inhabited by large third world populations. Although TB has historically been a prominent cause of phlyctenulosis, most authorities agree that the major cause of phlyctenulosis in the United States is secondary to Staphylococcal blepharitis.

Significant History

A history of chronic lid infection/inflammation is significant for the presence of bacterial blepharitis and should be investigated as an etiology for phlyctenulosis.

A history of chronic cough or being in close contact with others that may have TB is important.

Ancillary Tests

Laboratory studies should focus on known etiologies. Included should be a PPD skin test for TB and potentially tests to rule out a chlamydial infection.

In recalcitrant cases, cultures (and sensitivities) of the lids and lashes may prove beneficial.

The Treatment

Treatment may take two directions. First, underlying infective diseases must be controlled. In the case of TB or chlamydia, appropriate systemic therapy must be initiated. Bacterial blepharitis, if present, should be addressed with lid hygiene and the appropriate topical antibiotics. Both bacterial blepharitis and chlamydial infections are discussed elsewhere in this text.

The specific therapy for phlyctenulosis is topical steroid therapy. A course of topical steroids will quickly cause the nodule and symptoms to abate, usually within 5 to 7 days.

Prednisolone acetate 1% qid × 5–10 days will in most cases be sufficient to relieve symptoms and signs. Concomitant use of topical antibiotics is appropriate while steroid drops are used. A combination drug such as Tobradex (tobramycin/dexamethasone) could also be used qid × 5–10 days.

Recurrences are not uncommon and should be treated aggressively, especially when corneal involvement is present.

BACTERIAL KERATITIS

BACTERIAL INFECTIOUS CORNEAL INFILTRATES AND BACTERIAL CORNEAL ULCERS

Nicky R. Holdeman

ICD—9: 370.01 - Bacterial infectious corneal infiltrates
ICD—9: 370.03 - Bacterial corneal ulcers

THE DISEASE

Pathophysiology

Bacterial keratitis is a potentially sight threatening infection of the cornea. A wide range of pathogens have been implicated; however, the lid margins provide a common source of bacteria that may, under the right conditions, invade the cornea. The severity of the condition and the complications incurred depend on the infectious agent, the production of toxins and enzymes by the organism, and the inflammatory response of the host. Vision compromise may occur by corneal scarring, by the development of glaucoma and cataracts, or by loss of the eye following corneal perforation.

Etiology

Bacterial infections of the cornea may be produced by a number of microorganisms. While regional variations within the United States may exist, the most common pathogens cultured from clinical cases of keratitis include *S. aureas, S. epidermidis, Streptococcus viridans, Streptococcus pneumoniae, Pseudomonas aeruginosa,* and species of *Moraxella, P. acnes, Klebsiella, Proteus, Serratia, Hemophilus,* and *Neisseria.*

Up to 70% of contact lens–related microbial keratitis is because of *Pseudomonas aeruginosa* and about half the reported cases of post-LASIK infections are secondary to atypical mycobacteria, such as *M. chelonae.*

The Patient

Clinical Symptoms

- Conjunctival injection
- Pain or foreign body sensation
- Decreased visual acuity
- Swelling of the lids
- Photophobia
- Discharge

Clinical Signs

An infectious keratitis is often accompanied by:

- lid and conjunctival edema and hyperemia
- purulent or mucopurulent discharge

- anterior chamber inflammation (with or without hypopyon)
- papillary conjunctival response

A bacterial corneal ulcer is present when an infectious infiltrate is associated with a loss of epithelial or stromal tissue.

- The ulcerated defect may have well demarcated borders with an ill-defined dense, grey stromal infiltrate, and underlying endothelial plaque.
- WBC infiltration and edema may extend well beyond the epithelial defect.

An infectious infiltrate typically has the following features:

- Overlying epithelial defect that stains with sodium fluorescein
- Anterior to midstromal location
- Diffuse appearance with poorly defined borders
- No clear zone between the infiltrate and the limbus
- >2 mm in diameter
- Pain

The patient should be quickly assessed as to whether the keratitis is potentially sight threatening. Bacterial ulcers may progress to corneal perforation within 24 hours if not properly identified and treated. Any of the following characteristics is highly suggestive of a serious infection:

- AC response of 2+ or more (>10 cells/1 mm beam)
- Infiltrate is >2 mm in size
- Infiltrate is <3 mm from the visual axis
- The condition is worse (signs and symptoms have not improved) after 24 hours of empiric therapy

Note: Several features have been identified in which a microbial keratitis often leads to a poorer prognosis or results in a higher incidence of penetrating keratoplasty. These risk factors may serve as indicators for primary treatment failures and identify patients who may require intensive, tertiary care:

- >60 years of age
- Central location or limbal involvement of the ulcer
- Past ocular surgery, including LASIK
- Poor visual acuity at presentation
- Large ulcer (>5 mm), thinning, and/or hypopyon
- Previous treatment with a topical steroid
- Delay in treatment or delay in referral (>7 days) to a corneal specialist

The patient should also be examined and monitored for secondary manifestations of inflammation, including:

- Synechiae formation
- Elevated IOP
- Cataracts
- Progressive corneal thinning/perforation
- Scarring

Demographics

Approximately 30,000 cases of bacterial keratitis occur annually in the United States.

Bacterial keratitis may affect anyone at any age, but is more often associated with mechanical/chemical corneal trauma or soft contact lens wear.

The incidence of infection is also higher in patients with other risk factors such as:

- Neuroparalytic keratopathy
- Keratitis sicca
- Blepharitis
- Defective immune system (local or systemic)
- Alcohol abuse
- Vitamin deficiency
- Epithelial compromise
- Certain systemic diseases (e.g., diabetes mellitus, rheumatoid arthritis, atopic dermatitis)

Significant History (see risk factors cited earlier)

- Soft contact lens use (especially extended wear)
- Immunosuppression (acquired or iatrogenic)
- Malnutrition
- Bell's palsy
- Topical steroid use
- Epithelial defects (trauma, erosions, dystrophies)
- Recent exposure to hospital environment (inpatient, nurse, employee, etc.)
- Past ocular surgery (suture abscess, bleb infection)

Ancillary Tests

Microbiologic studies (stains and cultures) of the lids, the conjunctiva, and especially the cornea are essential any time a sight-threatening infection of the cornea is suspected. A small proportion, yet clinically significant number of eyes with bacterial ulcerative keratitis, does not respond to empirically selected therapy. Culturing and sensitivity testing at the time of presentation will facilitate appropriate modification of treatment.

Stains (Routine)

- Gram stain—demonstrates bacteria and yeasts.
- Giemsa stain—demonstrates fungal and viral elements.

Note: Stains analyzed by a general microbiology lab will often have less diagnostic value than when interpreted by an experienced ophthalmic microbiology technician. Slides fixed by immersing in methanol can be used for special stains if required at a later time.

Microbiologic Media (Routine)

- Blood agar—supports most aerobic bacteria and fungal organisms; will not support *Haemophilus;* poorly grows *Neisseria.*

- Chocolate agar—supports most bacteria, including *Haemophilus* and *Neisseria;* does not provide information on alpha or beta-hemolysis.
- Sabouraud's agar (without cyclohexamide)—supports fungal pathogens while inhibiting bacterial growth.
- Thioglycolate broth—used to isolate anaerobic bacteria and to saturate swabs prior to plating blood and chocolate agar.

In contact lens associated ulcers (CLAUs), the patients' lenses, solutions, and case should also be cultured, especially if the corneal cultures reveal no growth and the patient is not improving.

Note: One can expect a positive corneal culture to be obtained in approximately 50% of cases. Percentages may be increased by using nonpreserved topical anesthetics and proper culture techniques in patients with an adequate inoculum.

Corneal biopsy may be indicated when conventional cultures have not identified an organism and the infection has not responded to broad spectrum antibiotics.

The Treatment

The basic principles in the treatment of bacterial keratitis is to rapidly eradicate the affected tissue of replicating microorganisms, to limit the structural damage caused by the infectious process, and to taper therapy appropriately in order not to impede healing.

The cornea is best treated by frequent application of bacteriacidal concentrations of topical antibiotics in conjunction with ancillary therapy. Patients should be followed on a daily basis until clinical improvement has been demonstrated.

Treatment of infectious infiltrates and infectious ulcers typically involves:

- Cycloplegics (5% homatropine, 1% atropine, or 0.25% scopolamine) bid-tid depending on the level of inflammation
- Topical antibiotics—antibiotic selection should be based on the organisms demonstrated by the Gram and Giemsa stains, severity of the infection, risk factors, and clinical impression. In cases of serious keratitis, it is best to treat with multiple broad-spectrum antibiotics until the organism and sensitivity patterns are identified by culture. Depending on severity, treatment may involve fortified and/or commercially prepared antibiotics.
  1. Fortified antibiotics—For sight-threatening infections, many external disease specialists advocate the use of tobramycin or gentamycin (9.1 mg/mL or 14 mg/mL) q30–60 minutes on the hour alternating with cefazolin (50 mg/mL) q30–60 minutes on the half hour, tapering with clinical response. This combination is a common and well evaluated regimen. However, there have been reports of increasing resistance to the aminoglycosides and to cefazolin. Retrospective studies have suggested the use of fortified vancomycin (25–50 mg/mL) alternating with ceftazidime (50 mg/mL). This latter combination typically covers methicillin resistant *S. aureus* (MRSA) and difficult gram-negative bacteria, but the use of vancomycin and ceftazidime is limited because of the expense of these drugs and severe stinging on instillation. Consequently, the aminoglycosides and cefazolin are still considered by some as the mainstay of fortified antibiotic therapy in sight-threatening infections (see Table 6.3). Unfortunately,

> **TABLE 6.3 Formulation of Fortified Antibiotics**

Tobramycin, 9.1 mg/mL
Add 2 cc of parenteral tobramycin (20 mg/mL) to 5 cc of commercial ophthalmic tobramycin solution (3 mg/mL). This concentration has good potency and may be less toxic than higher concentrations.

Tobramycin, 10 mg/mL
Add 1 cc of parenteral tobramycin (40 mg/mL) to 5 cc of commercial ophthalmic tobramycin solution (0.3%).

Tobramycin or (gentamycin) 14 mg/mL
Add 2.0 mL of parenteral tobramycin or gentamycin (40 mg/mL) to 5.0 mL of commercial ophthalmic solution (0.3%).

Cefazolin 50 mg/mL
A. Reconstitute cefazolin dry powder (500 mg) with 2.5 mL sterile water (without preservative). Add 1.0 mL of this solution to 3.0 mL of artificial tears.
B. Add sterile water (without preservative) to cefazolin dry powder (500 mg) to form 10 mL of solution.

Vancomycin 33 mg/mL
Reconstitute a 500-mg vial of parenteral vancomycin with 10 mL of sterile water (without preservative). 10.2 mL of this solution is then added to 6 mL of artificial tears.

Vancomycin 50 mg/mL and 25 mg/mL
Reconstitute a 500-mg vial of parenteral vancomycin with 10 mL of sterile water (without preservative) or artificial tears for a final concentration of 50 mg/mL. For a 25 mg/mL-concentration, take 5 mL of the 50 mg/mL-solution and add another 5 cc of sterile water or artificial tears.

Bacitracin 10,000 U/mL
Add 5 mL of sterile water (without preservative) or artificial tears to 50,000 units of dry bacitracin powder.

Ceftazidime 50 mg/mL
Reconstitute a 500-mg vial of parenteral ceftazidime with 10 mL of sterile water (without preservative) or artificial tears.

Note: Fortified antibiotics should be refrigerated and shaken before each use. In general, they are good for 4–7 days after reconstitution.

fortified antibiotics are not readily available, are slower acting, have variable corneal penetration, require refrigeration, and are more toxic to the cornea when compared to the newer fluoroquinolones.

2. Commercial antibiotics—Currently, ciprofloxacin (Ciloxan), ofloxacin (Ocuflox), and levofloxacin (Quixin and Iquix) have FDA approval for monotherapy treatment of bacterial keratitis. However, it is abundantly evident that there has been increasing development of bacterial resistance to these fluoroquinolones (FQs) since their introduction.

Two "next generation" FQs are available for topical use and both target DNA gyrase and topoisomerase IV; they are gatifloxacin (Zymar) and moxifloxacin (Vigamox). These new FQs are bactericidal, rapid acting, highly soluble, broad spectrum with low toxicity, and are commercially available.

Note: Gatifloxacin (Zymar) may induce less damage to the corneal epithelium than other antibiotic solutions, especially in patients with dry eye. Gatifloxacin also appears to be less inhibitory to the processes involved in ocular surface healing than moxifloxacin. Because moxifloxacin does not contain a preservative, the disruption to the epithelium may be a result of the inherent qualities of the molecule.

Both of the new FQs maintain the excellent coverage of gram-negative bacteria, just as the earlier agents did. In addition, they clearly offer increased effectiveness against older FQ-resistant gram-positive bacteria such as S. *epidermidis*, S. *aureus*, and S. *pneumoniae* and markedly better coverage of atypical mycobacteria, the most common infection seen after LASIK. Thus far, in-vitro susceptibility studies show that Zymar appears to be slightly more effective than Vigamox against gram-negative bacteria while Vigamox seems slightly more effective against gram-positive organisms than Zymar. Only time will tell which drugs perform better in clinical settings, but no single antibiotic will ever have complete coverage.

Note: Both Zymar and Vigamox appear equally effective against M. *fortuitum* and M. *gastri*; however, M. *absessus* has shown resistance to all topical FQs. In cases of late-onset, post-LASIK infections suspected to be caused by atypical nontuberculous mycobacteria, one should obtain cultures and begin aggressive treatment with a topical new generation fluoroquinolone (gatifloxacin or moxifloxacin) and a topical macrolide (clarithromycin or azithromycin) until cultures and sensitivities are available. This combination of drugs appears effective against M. *fortuitum* and M. *chelonae*, the two most common pathogens of post-LASIK, mycobacterial, intralamellar corneal infections.

Clinicians should also be aware that in-vitro susceptibility studies have shown that *Pseudomonas* strains that were resistant to ciprofloxacin (ciprofloxacin-resistant *Pseudomonas aeruginosa* CRPA) and ofloxacin were also resistant to the newer FQs. Up to 70% of contact lens—related cases of microbial keratitis is because of P. *aeruginosa*, thus clinicians should recognize this resistance. Animal models suggest that CRPA keratitis might best be treated with a combination of fortified tobramycin and 0.6% ticarcillin.

Community strains of MRSA are affecting athletes, prisoners, and small children in growing numbers across the United States. These community strains appear to be highly transmissible and commonly take the form of a skin abscess. MRSA now makes up a significant number of all diagnosed staph infections and could potentially involve the eye.

While bacterial resistance will continue (despite the need for multiple genetic mutations), and newer antibiotics will be introduced, the current recommendations for potentially sight-threatening infections include:*

Vigamox (moxifloxicin) 0.5% q30–60 minutes on the hour alternating with fortified tobramycin 10 mg/mL q30–60 minutes on the half hour. Antibiotic modification and tapering should be based on the results of the culture and sensitivities and clinical response respectively. When cultures show stronger sensitivity to one of the two medications, the other one should be discontinued. If an unsuspected organism should be identified, such as a CRPA or MRSA, medications should be altered to maximize therapy.

Oral pain medication may be prescribed depending on the level of discomfort and the patients overall medical condition.

---

*Suggested web site for updates on ocular antimicrobial therapy: http://eyemicrobiology.upmc.com.

Most small, peripheral, community-acquired corneal ulcers with little thinning and/or inflammation (i.e., potentially nonsight-threatening infections) can usually be treated with a single flouroquinolone such as levofloxacin, gatifloxacin, or moxifloxacin. Drug penetration into the cornea is increased by frequent instillations (i.e., q1 hour during the day following a loading dose of 1 qtt every 15 minutes for 2 hours; use 1 qtt every 2–3 hours during the night for the first 24–48 hours) and the typical presence of an epithelial defect, which often results in antibiotic levels in excess of the MIC as determined by in-vitro antibiotic susceptibility testing.

- Adjunctive therapy—Several other modes of therapy have been employed in the treatment of corneal ulcers (e.g., collagenase inhibitors [topical acetylcystine, oral tetracycline], cyanoacrylate adhesives, antibiotic soaked collagen shields and amniotic membrane transplants). Future delivery systems may include contact lenses made with particle-laden hydrogels that release therapeutic levels of drugs for extended periods.
- Topical steroids—The use of steroids is controversial. Suppression of the inflammatory response may lessen the structural damage caused by the inflammatory process but may make the infectious process more difficult to control. While clinical studies have not shown a significant effect of topical corticosteroid therapy on the outcome of bacterial keratitis, the use of steroids (e.g., prednisolone acetate 1%) may be appropriate in certain cases if the following criteria have been fulfilled:
  1. the organism has been identified by culture
  2. lab sensitivities have been reported
  3. concurrent use of a microbicidal antibiotics
  4. demonstrated clinical improvement for 48 to 72 hours
  5. eliminated epithelial herpes simplex or fungal infection as an etiology
  6. no threat of corneal perforation.

While most patients can be successfully managed on an outpatient basis with aggressive topical treatment and frequent follow-up, occasionally subconjunctival antibiotics and/or hospital admission may be required (Table 6.4).

▌ **TABLE 6.4 Comparison of Topical Fluoroquinolones**

Brand Name	Ciloxan	Ocuflox	Zymar	Vigamox	Quixin*
Active ingredient	Ciprofloxacin	Ofloxacin	Gatifloxacin	Moxifloxacin	Levofloxacin
Preservative	BAC .006%	BAC .005%	BAC .005%	None	BAC .005%
Formulated concentration (mg/mL)	3.0	3.0	3.0	5.0	5.0
pH	4.5	6.4	6.0	6.8	6.5
Aqueous solubility at pH 7 (mg/mL)	0.09	3.23	Not reported	Not reported	35.8
Approved age group	>1 year	>1 year	>1 year	>1 year	>1 year
Pregnancy category	C	C	C	C	C
How supplied	2.0 & 5.0 mL	5.0 & 10.0 mL	2.5 & 5.0 mL	3 mL	2.5 & 5.0 mL

*Levofloxacin 1.5% (Iquix) has been approved by the FDA as a self-preserved formulation.
September 2004

ADULT INCLUSION CONJUNCTIVITIS (AIC)
Marcus Piccolo

ICD—9: 077.98

THE DISEASE
Pathophysiology

AIC is a sexually transmitted disease that can produce an acute to subacute inflammation of the conjunctiva and cornea that will often progress to a more chronic follicular conjunctivitis. The inferior conjunctiva is the primary area of involvement, and significant visual loss is uncommon. However, *Chlamydia trachomatis* has the ability to cause recurrent or persistent infections that often lead to greater tissue damage than the initial infection.

The incubation period is 4 to 14 days after exposure to the organism.

Etiology
- AIC is caused by infection with *C. trachomatis*, an obligate intracellular organism, serotypes D–K.
- Transmission is via sexual contact or by hand–eye autoinoculation with infected genital or urinary secretions.
- Humans are the only reservoir of *C. trachomatis.*

The Patient

Clinical Symptoms
- Symptoms may be acute or subacute in onset and include ocular irritation, discharge, discomfort, redness, and mild photophobia.
- AIC often has a chronic presentation lasting 4 to 14 months if not treated.
- It is possible that the patient (especially men) may be systemically asymptomatic, but if present, may include symptoms associated with urethritis, epididymitis, salpingitis, endometritis, cervicitis, or pelvic inflammatory disease (PID).

Clinical Signs
- Mild to moderate mucopurulent discharge
- Conjunctival appearance:
  1. Follicular conjunctival reaction greater on inferior tarsus
  2. Hyperemia and chemosis
  3. Scarring is minimal to nonexistent
  4. No membranes in adults
- Corneal appearance:
  1. Superior micropannus (<2 mm)
  2. Mild SPK to course SPK
  3. Small subepithelial infiltrates are occasionally seen and may scar

- Preauricular lymphadenopathy, palpable and sometimes tender; which may be visible upon gross inspection

Demographics
- *C. trachomatis* is the leading cause of STDs; an estimated 460,000 cases are contracted annually in the United States.
- AIC may occur in males or females and is most common in sexually active young adults.
- Racial and ethnic distributions are equal.

Significant History
- AIC may cause urethritis in men and cervicitis or vaginitis in women.
- Other venereal diseases may be present, such as syphilis, gonorrhoeae, HIV, herpes, and so on.
- Otitis media occurs in 15% of cases.
- AIC may rarely be associated with swimming pools with inadequate chlorine.
- A history of new or multiple sexual partners or previous treatment for a sexually transmitted disease is significant.

Ancillary Tests
- Cytology
    Initial PMN response in acute phase.
    50/50 PMN to lymphocyte response in chronic phase.
    Basophilic, intracytoplasmic, epithelial inclusions with Giemsa staining.
- IFA (Immunofluorescent antibody testing)
    Stained conjunctival scrapings and serum titers (Microtrak testing is >90% sensitive and provides a rapid diagnostic method). Topical NaFl can interfere with this test.
- Polymerase chain reaction (PCR) and DNA probe is highly sensitive and specific for analysis of cervical and urine samples.
- Other STD testing as deemed appropriate.

The Treatment
- Systemic Antibiotics
    tetracyline 500 mg tid p.o. × 1–2 weeks (not to be used in pregnant women) or
    doxycycline 100 mg bid p.o. × 1–2 weeks or
    erythromycin 250–500 mg qid p.o. × 1–2 weeks or
    azithromycin 1 g p.o. (single dose)—preferred treatment
- No topical antibiotics are necessary, but topical antibiotics will suppress the ocular manifestations.
- A referral for venereal aspects of disease and to exclude other STDs is required for the patient and their sexual partners.
- If sexual partners are not treated, reinfection may occur.
- Untreated infections in women may lead to PID, sterility, or ectopic pregnancy.

TRACHOMA
Marcus Piccolo

ICD—9: 076.9

THE DISEASE

Pathophysiology

Trachoma causes inflammation and scarring of the conjunctiva and cornea secondary to infection with *C. trachomatis*. The condition is often related to poor hygienic conditions, with transmission through contact of infected ocular secretions, respiratory droplets, or fecal contamination.

Presentation is typically 5 to 6 days after inoculation.

Etiology

- Infection occurs from serotypes A, B, Ba, and C of *C. trachomatis*.
- The common fly often serves as a vector.
- The chief reservoir is contaminated children with active disease.

The Patient

Clinical Symptoms

- Trachoma is characterized by an acute inflammation of the eye in the first decade of life with slow progression and then resolution in the second decade of life.
- Pain, mucopurulent discharge, and photophobia are typically present during acute phases.
- A secondary bacterial conjunctivitis is not uncommon.

Clinical Signs

- MacCallan Classification
  Stage I: Immature follicles on the upper palpebral conjunctiva with no scarring.
  Stage II: Mature follicles on the upper palpebral conjunctiva with no scarring. Papillary hypertrophy may be present.
  Stage III: Necrotic follicles and linear scarring of the upper tarsal conjunctiva (Arlt's lines).
  Stage IV: Inactive trachoma—no follicles, no active infiltrates, but often extensive conjunctival scarring.
- A more severe follicular response is noted in the superior tarsus versus the inferior tarsus.
- Limbal follicles, when resolved, leave well demarcated depressions called "Herbert's pits."
- Corneal findings include: epithelial keratitis, peripheral and central infiltrates, and superficial fibrovascular pannus (usually >2 mm), all of which occur predominantly superiorly.

- Late complications of trachoma include lid scarring, corneal scarring, trichiasis, and tear deficiencies.

Demographics
- The acute phase usually occurs in children, with no predilection for race or sex.
- Cicatrizing trachoma is 2 to 3 times more common in women than men.
- Trachoma is considered a disease of the underprivileged and is common in third world countries; however, trachoma is rare in the United States.
- Reinfection is common.
- Trachoma is the leading cause of preventable blindness in the world.

Significant History
- A history of acute and chronic ocular inflammation is significant, as is exposure to hyperendemic (third world) areas, such as the Gurage Zone in Ethiopia.
- Past infection confers no immunity to recurrent disease.

Ancillary Tests

The trachoma organism cannot be identified in every active case. Polymerase chain reaction (PCR) and ligase chain reaction (LCR) tests, which employ DNA amplification, have the highest sensitivity and specificity. Other tests include:

- Cytology: Basophilic, cytoplasmic epithelial inclusions (rare)
    PMNs—Acute phase
    PMNs and mononuclear cells—Chronic phase
  - Giemsa staining is less sensitive in detecting the organism compared to PCR or LCR.
  - IFA testing identifies antibodies to certain serotypes of *C. trachomatis* antigens. This test is rarely useful for individual cases but is sometimes used for epidemiologic studies.

The Treatment
- Treatment involves both topical and systemic therapies. Practitioners should select one ointment and one oral agent.
- Topical:
    Tetracycline ung, erythromycin ung or sulfacetamide ung bid to qid for 3–6 weeks
- Systemic (adult dosage):
    Azithromycin 1 g p.o. (single dose)—preferred form of treatment or
    Tetracycline 250–500 mg qid p.o. × 3–6 weeks or
    Doxycycline 100 mg bid p.o. × 3–6 weeks or
    Erythromycin 250–500 mg qid p.o. × 3–6 weeks or
    Ofloxacin 300 mg qid p.o. × 3–6 weeks
- Improved hygiene:
    Improved cleanliness of young patients is mandatory in lowering the prevalence of active trachoma. Reducing the densities of eye-seeking flies is also effective in preventing this devastating disease.

- Mass antibiotic administration:
  It appears that biannual mass azithromycin administration could eliminate chlamydia from hyperendemic areas.

PRESEPTAL CELLULITIS/ORBITAL CELLULITIS
Nicky R. Holdeman

ICD—9: 373.13 - Preseptal cellulitis
ICD—9: 376.01 - Orbital cellulitis

THE DISEASE

Pathophysiology

Infections of the orbit and periorbital tissues are an important group of diseases, not only because of the frequency of presentation, but also because these conditions can be potentially life threatening.

Preseptal cellulitis is a diffuse, deep infection of the eyelid tissues localized anterior to the orbital septum. (The orbital septum is a fibrous connective tissue that extends vertically from the periosteum of the orbital rim to the levator aponeurosis of the upper lid and to the tarsal plate of the lower lid.) Preseptal cellulitis may occur by itself or may progress to involve the orbit.

Orbital cellulitis is an infection of the soft tissue within the orbit, posterior to the orbital septum characterized by infiltration of the orbital tissues by microbial organisms, inflammatory cells, and edema. Orbital infections are commonly associated with sinusitis, as sinuses form the walls of the orbit thus predisposing the orbit to extension of infections originating from the sinuses.

Etiology

Preseptal cellulitis is typically a unilateral condition that may be caused by several entities; conditions include:

- Eyelid trauma: Most common organisms are *S. aureus* or *S. pyogenes*. Anaerobes and polymicrobial infections are less common.
- Extraocular skin infections: May be seen with impetigo (because of *S. aureus* or *S. pyogenes* group A); erysipelas (because of *S. pyogenes* group A); or viral associated skin rashes (HSV or HZV).
- Spread of infection from the upper respiratory tract or middle ear: Most common offending pathogens are *H. influenzae* and *S. pneumoniae*. However, the incidence of *Haemophilus*—associated bacteremia in patients with preseptal cellulitis—has decreased dramatically over the past several years as a result of the introduction of H. influenzae type B vaccine in 1985.

The differential diagnosis of preseptal cellulitis includes orbital cellulitis, cavernous sinus thrombosis, dacryocystis, dacryoadenitis, hordeolum, viral conjunctivitis with lid swelling, angioneurotic edema, and allergic eyelid swelling.

Note: Preseptal cellulitis, with or without orbital involvement, may cause noninfectious, contralateral eyelid edema.

Orbital cellulitis is characterized by a unilateral infection of rapid onset and may originate from a number of sites. Common routes of infection include:

- Sinusitis, particularly ethmoidal disease in adults and maxillary disease in children. The most common organisms associated with sinusitis are *S. pneumoniae*, *S. pyogenes*, *S. aureus*, and *H. influenzae* (especially in children). Anaerobes are less common. Sinusitis accounts for ~58% of cases.
- Surrounding (periorbital) structures such as the face, lacrimal sac, teeth, and globe. Periorbital infections are responsible for ~28% of cases.
- Trauma to the eye or periocular tissues. Trauma and foreign bodies are involved in ~11% of cases.
- Hematogenous spread during a systemic infection (bacteremia). This source of infection is the primary etiology in ~4% of cases.
- Direct inoculation from surgery. There is a potential, yet low incidence of infection with proper sterile technique. Orbital surgery, especially placement of an orbital implant, carries increased risk.

Post-traumatic and postsurgical orbital cellulitis is seen after violation of the orbital septum. The most common organism is *S. aureus*, although anaerobic and polymicrobial infections are possible. Gram-negative rods can be seen with orbital foreign bodies.

Fungal infections are rare and are primarily seen in diabetic ketoacidosis and immunocompromised patients, such as HIV-positive individuals and those on steroids or other immunosuppressive agents.

The differential diagnosis of orbital cellulitis includes cavernous sinus thrombosis, orbital pseudotumor, orbital myositis, dysthyroid ophthalmopathy, rhabdomyosarcoma, retinoblastoma, metastatic carcinoma, infiltrative disorders (leukemia, lymphoma), Wegener's granulomatosis, sarcoidosis, or a retained foreign body.

Note: Bilateral involvement or decreased sensation of V_1 suggests life-threatening cavernous sinus disease.

The Patient

Symptoms and signs will depend on the underlying etiology. Typical findings in preseptal cellulitis include the following.

Clinical Symptoms
- Unilateral, swollen, red eyelid
- Tenderness

Clinical Signs
- The patient is generally well, although a mild fever may be present.
- Eyelid edema (possibly with ptosis).
- Skin tenderness, erythema, and warmth.
- Conjunctival chemosis may be present.
- Foul-smelling discharge, crepitus, or necrosis may indicate an anaerobic organism.

▶ **TABLE 6.5** Bacterial Preseptal Cellulitis Versus Orbital Cellulitis

Clinical Finding	Preseptal Cellulitis	Orbital Cellulitis
Visual acuity	Normal	May be reduced
Pain or eye movement	Absent	Present
Orbital pain	Absent	Present
Proptosis	Absent	Present
Chemosis	Rare or mild	Common
Pupillary reaction	Normal	May be abnormal
Motility	Normal	Decreased
Corneal sensation	Normal	May be reduced
Ophthalmoscopy	Normal	May be abnormal
Fever/malaise	Mild	Often severe
White blood count	Normal to elevated	Increased
Intraocular pressure	Usually normal	May be increased
CNS involvement	Absent	May be present

- Hemophilus infection is typically nonpurulent, with a bluish-purple (violaceous) discoloration of the lid.
- Erysipelas usually manifests as a sharply demarcated, bright red, elevated plaque.
- Impetigo is suggested by a thick golden or honey-colored crust.
- HSV, HZV, and VZV have a characteristic vesicular skin rash.

Important negative findings include no proptosis, the globe is quiet and white, vision is normal, and there is no ocular muscle restriction or pain with movement (see Table 6.5). However, these infections can progress quickly, especially in children, to involve the orbital structures or even meninges.

Postseptal infections have been categorized into subsets of orbital involvement: orbital cellulitis, subperiosteal abscess, orbital abscess, and cavernous sinus thrombosis. Consequently, potential findings seen with retroseptal involvement may include the following.

Clinical Symptoms
- Lid swelling, tenderness, and redness
- Decreased vision
- Pain on eye movement
- Diplopia
- Headache
- Conjunctival redness and swelling
- Symptoms of sinusitis (rhinorrhea, sinus pressure)

Clinical Signs
- Systemically unwell, febrile patient
- Periorbital edema, erythema, and pain (signs of preseptal cellulitis)
- Reduced visual acuity; reduced color vision
- Relative afferent pupillary defect (RAPD)

- Restriction of ocular motility
- Proptosis with resistance to retropulsion
- Ptosis
- Conjunctival hyperemia and chemosis
- Globe involvement (episcleritis or scleritis)
- Increased intraocular pressure
- Decrease in corneal sensation (neurotrophic keratitis)
- Acutely tender over the inflamed sinus
- Congestion of retinal veins; CRAO
- Chorioretinal stria
- Optic neuropathy
- Nausea and vomiting
- Cavernous sinus thrombosis
- Decreased consciousness
- Intracranial abscess and meningitis
- Death

Demographics

Preseptal cellulitis may occur in any age group but is much more common in childhood. Eighty-five percent of patients are younger than 20 years old and 56% are younger than 5 years of age.

Preseptal cellulitis is most prevalent during the summer in warm, humid climates. True orbital infections are rare in children less than 5 years of age but are potentially lethal in all age groups.

Twelve percent to 25% of patients with H. influenzae infection and positive blood cultures develop meningitis.

Significant History

- Is there a history of sinusitis, trauma, surgery, or dental infection?
- Is the patient immunocompromised, alcoholic, or diabetic?
- Has there been a recent hordeolum, dacrocystitis, or orbital floor fracture?
- Is there a history of a recent ear, nose, throat, or systemic infection?
- Does the patient have a stiff neck or mental status changes?

Ancillary Tests

In cases involving preseptal or orbital cellulitis, the ocular and systemic examination should be as prompt and as comprehensive as possible. Testing should include:

- Vital signs (especially temperature)
- Best corrected visual acuities
- Color vision testing or red desaturation testing
- Checking for afferent pupillary defect
- Evaluation of the ocular adnexae and regional lymph nodes
- Ocular motility restrictions or pain with eye movement
- Exophthalmometry for proptosis

- Visual fields
- Checking for decreased corneal sensation and decreased periorbital skin sensation (especially V_1 and V_2)
- Palpating the lids for hordeolum and percuss the sinuses to elicit pain secondary to sinusitis
- Checking mental status, neck flexibility or rigidity
- Biomicroscopy of the anterior segment; apply pressure to the nasolacrimal system, observing for discharge
- Tonometry
- Ophthalmoscopy

If the patient's history and physical exam are suggestive of orbital involvement, the patient should have additional testing.

- CBC with differential should be obtained in all cases in which systemic symptoms of fever, chills, or malaise are present.
- Blood cultures (positive in ~23% of patients with orbital cellulitis).
- Explore and debride wound if present and obtain Gram stain and cultures of drainage.
- CT scan, with contrast, of the orbits, sinuses, and brain. Include axial and coronal thin cuts (2 mm or less) to look for abscess formation, foreign bodies, and/or sinusitis. An abscess enhances with contrast.
- MRI is the imaging modality of choice for suspected cases of cavernous sinus thrombosis.
- ENT consultation is recommended in cases likely related to sinusitis Aspiration of sinus material for culture may be helpful and nasal decongestion should be initiated to promote drainage of any affected sinus.
- Pediatric consultation is suggested if the patient is a child.
- Neurology consultation and lumbar puncture is recommended if meningitis or intracranial pathology is suspected.

Note: Culture of discharge from the nasal mucosa, nasopharynx, and conjunctiva rarely yield the causative agent, but may sometimes be useful. However, aspiration of fluid from the orbit is contraindicated.

The Treatment

Rapid diagnosis and medical intervention are the mainstay of treatment.

Therapy will vary depending on the age of the patient, the overall clinical presentation, the site of origin, the site and extent of involvement, and the suspected organism. A multidisciplinary approach to management may be needed and can include ophthalmologists, otolaryngologists, infectious disease specialists, radiologists, pediatricians, neurologists, and even neurosurgeons.

Preseptal Cellulitis

Immunocompetent adults with mild cases of preseptal cellulitis who are systemically well and reliable can often be managed on an outpatient basis. Conversely, children under age 5 or any patient with a severe infection are best hospitalized for initial treatment.

Local therapy includes the application of warm, moist compresses qid and a topical broad spectrum antibiotic ointment (i.e., Polysporin, erythromycin) qid if a secondary conjunctivitis is present.

In mild, uncomplicated cases, systemic therapy consists of oral antibiotics effective against likely strains of staphylococci and streptococci.

- Amoxicillin/clavulanic acid (Augmentin) 250–500 mg p.o. tid or 875 mg p.o. bid
- Dicloxacillin (Dynapen) 250 mg p.o. q6 hours
- Cefaclor (Ceclor) 250–500 mg p.o. tid

If the patient is allergic to penicillin:

- Trimethoprin/sulfamethoxazole (Bactrim) one double strength tablet p.o. bid
- Azithromycin (Zithromax) 500 mg p.o. as a single dose on day 1, then 250 mg p.o. q day
- Levofloxacin (Levaquin) 500 mg p.o. q day

Select one agent with daily follow-up and treat for 7 to 10 days. If there is no improvement (or worsening) after two days of oral antibiotics, CT scanning and IV antibiotics are in order.

For moderate to severe disease, or if confronted with a toxic appearing patient, an immunocompromised patient, or a child younger than 5 years of age, or if there is concern regarding reliability, hospitalize the patient.

Initiate IV antibiotics such as ceftriaxone and vancomycin. Chloramphenicol should be considered if anaerobic organisms or H. influenzae is suspected.

Tetetanus vaccine, if indicated, in cases of traumatic etiology.

Exploration and debridement of a flocculent mass or an abscess.

Orbital Cellulitis

If orbital cellulitis is suspected in any age group, it should be considered an urgent situation with prompt hospitalization. Intravenous antibiotics must be started as soon as possible. Choice of antibiotics depends on the pathogen and the age of the patient. Recommendations vary but may include:

- Ceftriaxone and vancomycin
- Ceftazidime and clindamycin
- Cloxacillin or nafcillin in combination with chloramphenicol
- Cefuroxine (plus gentamycin or tobramycin if a foreign body were present)
- Ampicillin/sulbactam (Unasyn)

Changes in therapy are contingent on clinical response, blood cultures, or direct culture of an abscess. If a definitive organism is isolated, the antibiotic therapy may be adjusted for the specific pathogen.

Clinical signs (i.e., vital signs, CBC, ophthalmic examination), should start improving 24 to 48 hours after initiation of antibiotic therapy. Complete regression of the exophthalmos may take 2 weeks.

Once definitive improvement is seen, the patient may be converted to oral antibiotics to complete a total 2 week course of antibiotics.

Failure to improve with IV antibiotics may suggest an alternative diagnosis (see differential diagnosis cited earlier) or a resistant organism. Mucormycosis should be considered in all diabetics, alcoholics, and immunocompromised patients. The mortality rate is high.

PARINAUD'S OCULOGLANDULAR CONJUNCTIVITIS (POC)

Marcus Piccolo

ICD—9: 372.30

THE DISEASE

Pathophysiology

POC is an infection and subsequent development of a granulomatous inflammatory conjunctivitis, associated with pronounced preauricular lymphadenopathy. Infection of the conjunctiva is usually because of direct inoculation with cat saliva after being bitten or scratched by a cat. The offending organisms are found in cat saliva 100% of the time and in human saliva to a much lesser extent. Fleas may transmit the disease from one cat to another.

The pathogen causes a granulomatous tissue reaction of the palpebral conjunctiva and can be found in the vessel walls of small capillaries and as inclusions in macrophages. The vessel infiltration can result in occlusion of the vessel's lumen resulting in focal areas of necrosis.

Etiology

POC is caused primarily by *Bartonella henselae*, *Bartonella quintana*, or *Afipia felis*, pathogens responsible for cat scratch disease. Other infectious agents are responsible for causing a similar syndrome (i.e., Parinaud's oculoglandular syndrome). These pathogens and conditions include *Francisella tularensis* (tularemia), *Mycobacterium tuberculosis* (tuberculosis), *Sporothrix schenckii* (sporotrichosis), *Treponema pallidum* (syphilis), and others such as chlamydia, sarcoid, rickettsiae, virus, and fungi. This review will concentrate on Parinaud's oculoglandular conjunctivitis associated with cat scratch disease.

The Patient

Clinical Symptoms
POC usually presents as a unilateral red eye. The patient may experience ocular irritation, photophobia, fever, malaise, anorexia, painful regional lymphadenopathy, and headache. Symptoms begin about 2 weeks after inoculation.

Clinical Signs

Classic findings include diffuse injection of the bulbar conjunctiva, mild mucopurulent discharge, and on occasion a mild ptosis of the affected lid. The palpebral conjunctiva (and on rare occasion the bulbar conjunctiva) will show a follicular conjunctivitis with a focal granuloma, which may ulcerate. The granuloma may be single, large, and flat, or there may be multiple granulomas of the same description.

Regional lymphadenopathy may be noted, which is preceded by an inflamed papule or ulcer at the site of inoculation. Tender enlarged lymph nodes may be palpated in the preauricular, submandibular, or cervical regions.

Other ocular manifestations include retinal nodules, optic nerve head swelling, afferent pupillary defect, neuroretinitis with a macular star formation, various forms of uveitis, vessel occlusions, serous retinal detachments, and visual field defects.

Demographics

POC usually occurs in children and young adults. The disease is unilateral, and males are typically affected more than females. No racial predilection has been reported.

Significant History

Patients will frequently provide a history of being around cats or kittens, as *Bartonella* organisms live on cats and their fleas. Having a recent scratch or bite by a cat is significant; however, a scratch is not necessary for contracting the illness. The transmission of the pathogen may be directly from cat saliva or from coming in contact with cat saliva that may be present on a pillow, and so on.

Ancillary Tests

- Serology—Confirmation of disease is most commonly made by immunofluorescent antibody (IFA) testing, which is highly sensitive and specific.
- PCR testing—DNA amplification of a lymph node aspirate may be a useful diagnostic test.
- Biopsy—Conjunctival biopsy is rarely needed but may help establish the diagnosis and the removal of the granuloma may hasten the course of the disease. A positive biopsy will show mononuclear infiltration of the tissue and specifically infiltration of small vessel walls by lymphocytes and histiocytes. In addition, slender rod shaped pleomorphic bacteria may be visible.
- Skin test—A skin test for cat scratch fever is available (Hanger-Rose test) but is seldom used. Pus taken from active cases and diluted 1:5 and processed by heating at 60°C for 10 hours can be injected intradermally. A positive test consists of a central papule or area of erythema of 0.5–1.0 cm in size. A positive test may be present for those infected or those who have had the infection in the past.

The Treatment

Mild disease is generally benign and self-limiting and may not require active therapy. While antibiotics have not proven to be overly efficacious and visual recovery tends to occur spontaneously in patients with neuroretinitis, severe cases may improve more rapidly with treatment. Anecdotal reports indicate resolution of disease with a variety of anti-infective agents.

Treatment for aggressive disease has included several systemic antibiotics— azithromycin, doxycycline, or ciprofloxacin are most commonly suggested. Because comparative trials have not been conducted, firm recommendations cannot be made. Care should be given not to prescribe the tetracyclines for children under the age of 8 years.

Specific Regimens (adult dosage)
- Azithromycin 500 mg p.o. × 1, then 250 mg/d × 4 days—preferred treatment, or
- Doxycycline 100 mg bid p.o. × 14–21 days, or
- Ciprofloxacin 250 mg bid p.o. × 14–21 days, or
- Tetracycline 250 mg qid p.o. × 14–21 days

In addition to systemic drugs, topical erythromycin ointment may be used bid × 14 days as adjunctive therapy.

Excision of conjunctival granulomas may hasten resolution and can be curative.

Other causes of Parinaud's oculoglandular syndrome (e.g., tuberculosis, tularemia, etc.) should be treated on an etiology specific basis.

HORDEOLA/CHALAZIA/MEIBOMITIS (MEIBOMIANITIS)
Marcus Piccolo

ICD—9: 373.11- Hordeolum, externum (styc)
ICD—9: 373.12 - Hordeolum, internum
ICD—9: 373.2 - Chalazion
ICD—9: 373.12 - Meibomianitis

THE DISEASE
Pathophysiology
- Hordeola arise from an infection of either the sebaceous glands associated with the cilia (glands of Moll or Zeiss), resulting in an external hordeolum, or an infection of the meibomian glands, resulting in an internal hordeolum. Inflammation may result in swelling of the adjacent tissue with accompanying pain, especially in external hordeola. The infected gland may spontaneously point and drain a purulent material either to the skin side of the lid or internally into the conjunctival cul de sac.
- Chalazia are the result of a sterile lipo-granulomatous inflammation of the meibomian glands. They may appear singly or in multiples. The presence of the granuloma creates a nontender, sometimes reddened, palpable lesion within the lid.
- Meibomitis represents a more generalized inflammation and dysfunction of the meibomian glands. This condition results in stagnation and inability of the lipid content of the gland to properly excrete. This dysfunction may result in a breakdown of

glandular lipids into free fatty acids and on occasion, obliteration of output ducts, or the capping of the gland orifice with abnormal, waxy, meibomian plugs (inspissated meibomian glands). The normally clear meibomian lipids may degrade into a turbid secretion or a 'toothpaste like' product. These abnormal meibomian secretions may result in a frothing of the tears on the eye lid margins and result in tear film abnormalities, culminating in a dry eye syndrome.

Etiology

- Hordeola are caused by a bacterial infection of either the glands of the anterior lid margin (Moll or Zeiss) or the internal meibomian glands. The most likely bacteria to cause this condition are staphylococcal organisms, in particular *S. aureus* or *S. epidermidis*. The condition is often found in the presence of bacterial blepharitis.
- Chalazia may have more than one etiology or origin. In some cases, chalazia may result from a resolved hordeolum, where the infection is no longer present but the lipases produced by the offending organism cause a change in character of the meibomian content, with an ensuing granuloma formation. Another potential etiology may be secondary to meibomian dysfunction, resulting in an accumulation of lipid, with breakdown and extrusion of the meibomian product within the gland. The dysfunctional gland may then stimulate the formation of a chalazia. In either case, a sterile granuloma is formed within the meibomian gland.
- Meibomitis, or meibomian dysfunction, may be the result of breakdown and stagnation of the lipid content of the meibomian gland without the formation of a granuloma. The presence of seborrheic or bacterial blepharitis may be contributing factors. In addition, conditions that affect other sebaceous glands of the face have a tendency to affect the meibomian glands, resulting in meibomian dysfunction. It is common that meibomitis is associated with acne rosacea and/or seborrheic dermatitis.

The Patient

Clinical Symptoms

- The hallmark symptom for hordeola is focal pain of the lid or lid margin. Discomfort is likely more acute in external presentations; however, internal hordeola may still be quite uncomfortable. Mild blurring of vision may be present if the lid is swollen to the extent that the eye is only partially open or if the lesion is draining into the cul de sac producing a purulent discharge.
- Chalazia are typically symptom free; however, they may present a cosmetic concern. In rare instances, chalazia that have existed for some time may induce an irregular corneal astigmatism, which could impact the patient's vision. The lesion is typically nontender to palpation.
- Symptoms of meibomitis are typically those associated with a poor tear film and consist of burning, irritation, and foreign body sensation.

Clinical Signs

- The signs of hordeola are swelling of the lid and the presence of an elevated nodule of the lid margin, in an external hordeolum, or proximal to the external lid margin, in an internal hordeolum. The lid may be edematous to the extent that it may be difficult to localize the lesion by gross inspection. In this case, palpating the lid or lid margin should yield an area of localized tenderness, which is readily identifiable. The conjunctiva is usually quiet, but spontaneous drainage of the lesion may result in mild injection of the conjunctiva and a papillary response in some cases. External hordeola may show a white head at the orifice of the gland, which may spontaneously drain. An internal hordeolum may point and drain to either the skin or conjunctival surface. Although these lesions are frequently found singly, it is possible for them to appear as multiples. In rare cases, they may appear in the conjugate glands of both the upper and lower lids creating what is known as "kissing lesions," representing the contact points where the upper and lower lids touch during eye closure. Infection or inflammation which extends beyond the glands may result in a preseptal cellulitis.

- Chalazia appear as a nontender growth within the lid. These lesions may be single or multiple and are sometimes referred to as a "crop" when in multiples. The remainder of the eye and adnexa is typically quiet with no inflammation of the conjunctiva or adjacent lid. Recurrences, or chronic chalazia in the same position should be suspect for sebaceous gland carcinoma. In addition, atypical basal cell carcinoma and/or squamous cell carcinoma may masquerade as a chalazion.
- Meibomitis is identified by the presence of nonfunctional or blocked meibomian glands or by the presence of an inadequate tear film. Tear insufficiency is evidenced by a rapid tear break-up time, as well as the potential of a frothy foam along the lid margins. The orifices of the meibomian glands may be capped by waxy plugs and may appear pouting or erythematous. The conjunctiva is usually quiet unless the tear film is significantly inadequate, resulting in irritation and injection.

Demographics

- Hordeola may occur in any race, either gender, or at any age. The presence of predisposing conditions such as bacterial blepharitis is common.
- Chalazia occur regardless of race, gender, or age. The presence of acne rosacea, previous hordeolum, bacterial or seborrheic blepharitis, meibomitis, or any form of meibomian gland dysfunction may be significant.
- Meibomian gland dysfunction may occur in any race, gender, or age. There is, however, a strong association with acne rosacea and chronic forms of blepharitis.

Significant History

- In hordeola, the presence of bacterial blepharitis or poor hygiene is important.
- In chalazia, previous episodes of hordeolum, as well as, chronic blepharitis, acne rosacea, and seborrheic dermatitis are significant.
- In meibomitis, a history of acne rosacea, seborrhea, or bacterial blepharitis is noteworthy.

Ancillary Tests

Hordeola, Chalazia, and Meibomitis—Typically no laboratory tests are necessary and the diagnosis is made on a clinical basis. However, cultures and sensitivities of the lids and/or lesions are sometimes helpful.

Atypical or recurrent chalazia in the same location should be excised and sent for pathological analysis.

The Treatment

Hordeola

The treatment for hordeolum may take several forms. Initial therapy consists of frequent, warm, moist compresses applied directly to the lid followed by a light massage and application of bacitracin or erythromycin ointment to the lesion. In an internal hordeolum, ointment may be applied to the cul de sac to prophylax for spontaneous rupture. If resolution does not occur within 2 to 3 days, or if the presence of preseptal cellulitis is noted, a systemic antibiotic may be appropriate.

Specific therapies include:

- Warm compresses qid for 15 minutes until resolution, and
- Erythromycin ung bid × 1–2 weeks, and/or
- Dicloxacillin 250 mg q6h p.o. × 1–2 weeks, or
- Cephalexin 250–500 mg q6h p.o., × 1–2 weeks, or
- Augmentin 250 mg q8h p.o. × 1–2 weeks

On occasion, incision and drainage may be useful for a hordeolum. If surgery is performed, it could be accomplished by vertical incision through the conjunctiva or a horizontal incision through the skin. In either case, the lesion should be allowed to drain without compression to express the residual material. When drainage occurs, especially into the cul de sac, a topical antibiotic should be used for prophylaxis.

Chalazia

Management of chalazia consists of several options. The most benign therapy consists of the application of warm compresses. This therapy, over a period of weeks, may significantly reduce the size of a chalazia or may result in total resolution. The use of oral tetracycline may be helpful, particularly in cases preceded by a hordeola. Tetracycline has the ability to stabilize the free fatty acids that are formed by the breakdown of meibomian lipids, ultimately altering the stimulus to granuloma formation.

Intralesional injection of the chalazia with steroids may be useful in accelerating the resolution of the lesion. Intralesional injections should be performed with caution in persons of color, as permanent depigmentation of the skin may occur.

Surgical incision and curettage is the definitive management for persistent or large lesions. This procedure involves injection of a local anesthetic, stabilization of the lesion with a chalazion clamp, and a vertical incision through the tarsal conjunctiva with removal of the granuloma and the contents of the gland. Postsurgical management consists of application of erythromycin ointment to the wound.

Specific therapies include:

- Warm compresses qid for 15 minutes until resolution, and
- Tetracycline (contraindicated in children under 8 and in pregnant women) 250 mg qid p.o. × 3–4 weeks, or
- Doxycycline or minocycline 50–100 mg bid p.o. × 3–4 weeks

- Intralesional injection of 0.2–1.0 mL of triamcinolone, 40 mg/mL, using a 26-gauge needle
- Incision and curettage

Meibomitis

Warm compresses and lid scrubs with diluted baby shampoo are the mainstays of therapy. In recalcitrant cases, gentle message of the meibomian glands immediately following the compresses and scrubs may be beneficial. A week of warm compresses and lid scrubs may aid in removing debris from around the gland orifices and the warm, moist, heat may help liquefy the contents of the gland. In the office, under topical anesthetic, squeezing and rolling a cotton tipped applicator on the conjunctival side of the lid while maintaining digital pressure over the skin surface of the lid will often result in expression of the gland content. The content of the gland may be quite turbid containing some solids, or it may be very viscous resembling toothpaste in consistency. Long-term use of warm compresses and lid scrubs may help to prevent recurrences.

Oral tetracycline may reduce inflammation and may decrease the conversion of glandular lipids to free fatty acids, thus reducing the dysfunction of the glands.

Specific therapies include:

- Tetracycline 250 mg qid p.o. × 3-4 weeks, or
- Doxycycline or minocycline 50–100 mg bid p.o. × 3–4 weeks

Decreasing the doxycycline or minocycline to once a day over a period of months may help to control the condition.

Chapter 7

Viral Infectious Diseases

ADENOVIRUS/EPIDEMIC KERATOCONJUNCTIVITIS (EKC)
Marcus Piccolo

ICD—9: 077.1 - Epidemic keratoconjunctivitis
ICD—9: 077.3 - Adenoviral keratoconjunctivitis

THE DISEASE
Pathophysiology

EKC causes infection and subsequent inflammatory responses in the conjunctiva and cornea to various serotypes of adenovirus.

Etiology

EKC is most commonly caused by adenovirus 8 and less frequently by adenovirus 19, but multiple serotypes are capable of producing a similar clinical presentation. The incubation period is typically 5 to 10 days following inoculation of the conjunctiva.

The Patient

Clinical Symptoms
The patient experiences marked foreign body sensation, photophobia, burning, and profuse tearing. Tenderness of the ipsilateral preauricular lymph node is often present. Visual acuity is usually not affected in the early stages of the disease; however, acuity may decrease if and when the cornea becomes involved.

Clinical Signs
- Conjunctiva—Acute onset of redness and edema of the lids, plica, caruncle, and conjunctiva over a 24- to 48-hour period. Approximately 5 days after initial onset, follicles develop on the palpebral conjunctiva, occurring more noticeably inferiorly. Pseudomembranes may be present that can make visualization of the follicles difficult. On occasion, a papillary conjunctivitis or subconjunctival hemorrhages may obscure the follicles as well. Initial presentation is usually unilateral with the second eye becoming less severely involved after 5 to 10 days. The conjunctival findings are usually self-limiting in 2 to 4 weeks.

■ Cornea—A diffuse superficial keratitis may occur 2 to 3 days after the onset of symptoms. Seven to 10 days later, a grayish, focal, punctate, epithelial infiltrate occurs that may stain with fluorescein. Approximately 15 days after initial onset, gray subepithelial opacities begin to occur under the epithelial lesions. In time, these lesions resolve, leaving the characteristic subepithelial infiltrates. The subepithelial infiltrates may persist for weeks to months.

In severe cases, epithelial sloughing and/or an accompanying iritis may occur.

The course of the disease is usually of about 1 month's duration. The patient is considered infectious for 2 weeks after initial onset.

Demographics

EKC usually occurs in young adults, ages 20 to 40 years, but children and the aged may also become infected. The virus can survive on nonporous surfaces (i.e., tonometer tips, countertops, magazine covers) for up to 34 days. It was initially named "shipyard disease" because of its epidemic occurrence within populations living in close proximity (first described in shipyards and military compounds). Adenovirus is commonly spread by hand-to-eye contact or from contaminated ophthalmic instruments that come into contact with the eye. Because of the contagious nature of this disease, a 2-week quarantine should be imposed on infected health-care workers or other personnel who have contact with the public. Care should be taken to avoid spread of the disease via vectors such as tissues, towels, or pillows. Frequent hand washing is mandatory.

Significant History

A history of association with other individuals with acute onset of red eyes is significant. Associated systemic findings such as an upper respiratory tract infection or fever are less common with EKC than with other viral eye diseases.

Ancillary Tests

Laboratory confirmation of adenovirus can be made via a number of methods, including immunofluorescent techniques, immunoperoxidase techniques, serum titers to virus antibodies, and direct inoculation to animal and human cell cultures. These techniques are infrequently needed and are seldom used clinically.

Cytology
Giemsa staining typically yields lymphocytes in the absence of a pseudo or true membrane. If a membrane is present, PMNs may predominate. Eosinophilic intranuclear inclusion bodies may be present early with basophilic intranuclear inclusion bodies appearing late.

The Treatment

Treatment is aimed at prevention and support. Patients should be advised that their condition may worsen before it improves.

Cool compresses and artificial tears may help in alleviating symptoms as may the application of topical vasoconstrictors (i.e., naphozaline drops 4 to 6 times per day). Topical antiviral agents are not effective or useful for EKC. The use of corticosteroid drops is controversial. It may be appropriate to use medium-potency (FML Forte, Flarex) or high-potency (prednisolone acetate 1%) corticosteroid drops to quiet the initial inflammatory response during the first 2 weeks, and then rapidly tapered. Rarely, steroid therapy may be reinstituted at a later date for treatment of severe subepithelial opacification (prolonged or severe symptoms, significant visual loss), but steroid use may also prolong the duration of the disease. In addition, steroids can produce unwanted side effects (i.e., corneal immunosuppression, IOP elevations, and cataracts) and tapering is often difficult.

Topical antibiotics (erythromycin ointment) may be employed to prevent a secondary bacterial infection.

PHARYNGEAL CONJUNCTIVAL FEVER (PCF)
Marcus Piccolo

ICD—9: 077.2

THE DISEASE
Pathophysiology

PFC is an infection and subsequent inflammatory response in the conjunctiva and cornea to several serotypes of adenovirus. The disease usually presents unilaterally but the fellow eye is ultimately involved in ~50% of cases.

Etiology

PCF is most commonly caused by adenoviruses 3, 4, and 7, and less commonly by adenoviruses 1, 2, 5, 6, and 14. However, all 37 serotypes of adenovirus are capable of producing PCF in rare instances.

The Patient

Clinical Symptoms
Acute presentation of a unilateral red eye with associated pharyngitis and fever is the hallmark of PFC. Foreign body sensation, photophobia, and a watery or scant mucoid discharge may occur. In addition, the patient may experience malaise, myalgia, headache, abdominal discomfort, or diarrhea. The disease typically manifests 5 to 7 days after inoculation. Visual acuity is usually unaffected unless the cornea is significantly involved.

Clinical Signs
- Lids, Conjunctiva, and Adnexa—The tarsal conjunctiva demonstrates a follicular reaction more evident inferiorly. The bulbar conjunctiva becomes inflamed and chemotic

and may demonstrate some hemorrhagic changes. Conjunctival membranes and pseudomembranes can occasionally occur and the superior and inferior lids are usually edematous. A small ipsilateral nontender preauricular lymph node is typically palpable. Less frequently, a nontender cervical lymph node is noted.

- Cornea—The cornea occasionally shows a superficial punctate keratitis early in the disease. Six to 8 days after the initial symptoms, a focal epithelial keratitis may occur. This focal keratitis may lead to subepithelial infiltrates, which manifest 1 to 2 weeks after the onset of the conjunctivitis. The infiltrates are typically smaller and less severe than the classic infiltrates associated with an adenoviral epidemic keratoconjunctivitis (EKC). In general the cornea has a less severe presentation in PCF as compared to EKC.

The infection is self-limiting with complete resolution without sequelae in 3–4 weeks. The virus can be found in ocular tissue for up to 2 weeks after onset. However, the virus can be isolated in the feces for up to 30 days.

Demographics

Although any age can be affected, PCF tends to occur more frequently in children and may become epidemic in schools as a result of the highly contagious nature of the virus. For this reason, infected children should be quarantined for at least 2 weeks.

Transmission often occurs via droplets or it may be water borne via swimming pools. Chlorination of pools does not significantly inhibit the virus. Fecal contamination of swimming pools may be responsible for outbreaks.

Intrafamilial transmission is not uncommon.

Significant History

Association with children or other individuals with an acute onset of red eyes is significant. History of swimming in contaminated pools could be important.

Ancillary Tests

Confirmation of adenovirus can be made via a number of methods, including immunofluorescent techniques, immunoperoxidase techniques, serum titers to virus antibodies, and direct inoculation to animal and human cell cultures. These techniques are seldom required and infrequently used.

Cytology

Giemsa staining typically yields lymphocytes in the absence of a pseudo- or true membrane. If a membrane is present, PMNs may predominate. Eosinophilic intranuclear inclusion bodies may be present early with basophilic intranuclear inclusion bodies appearing late.

The Treatment

Treatment of PCF relies on supportive measures and isolation of affected individuals. Cool compresses, artificial tears, and vasoconstrictors (naphozaline drops 4 to 6 times per day) may be of some value. The disease is self-limiting in approximately 21 days with no ocular sequelae; therefore, drugs such as corticosteroids are not necessary and may in themselves pose more of an ocular risk.

Prevention of disease relies on prompt diagnosis, quarantine of affected individuals, and frequent hand washing. In addition, use of separate hand towels, pillows, eating utensils, and washcloths is important.

ACUTE HEMORRHAGIC CONJUNCTIVITIS (AHC)
Marcus Piccolo

ICD—9: 077.4

THE DISEASE
Pathophysiology

AHC is a viral infection and subsequent inflammation of the conjunctiva, cornea, and lids. The acute and rapid inflammatory response causes petechial or subconjunctival hemorrhages giving the descriptive name to the disease. In addition to conjunctival secretions, transmission of the virus by respiratory and oral routes accounts for the rapid and extensive spread of the disease during an outbreak.

Etiology

AHC is caused by inoculation of the conjunctiva with enterovirus 70 (EV-70) or coxsackie virus A24 (CA-24). The infection is most commonly the result of hand-to-eye contamination or contact with fomites. The disease is extremely contagious and has occurred in epidemic or pandemic proportions in dense population centers. Epidemics of AHC have been documented since 1969 when it was first seen in Ghana and given the name "Apollo II" conjunctivitis (this was during the U.S. Apollo space missions). It was later more descriptively named acute hemorrhagic conjunctivitis. The incubation period for AHC is very short, consisting of 1 to 2 days with a rapid onset of signs and symptoms. Resolution usually occurs within 7 to 14 days after onset.

The Patient

Clinical Symptoms
Symptoms of AHC include sudden onset of an unilateral conjunctivitis, which rapidly becomes bilateral. The patient will likely experience epiphora, photophobia, lid swelling, itching, ocular irritation, and/or periorbital pain. Systemically the patient may experience flulike symptoms of myalgia, malaise, headache, and pharyngitis.

Clinical Signs
Patients characteristically show a follicular reaction of the inferior conjunctiva. Although this disease is typically bilateral, one eye is usually more involved than the other. The patient will show eyelid edema, conjunctival chemosis, and a profuse mucoid

discharge. Small, palpable, nontender preauricular lymphadenopathy is often noted. The "hallmark" sign is the presence of subconjunctival hemorrhages. The hemorrhages may be petechial or diffuse, but are more commonly confluent, especially late in the presentation. Early in the disease, hemorrhages under the superior bulbar conjunctiva may show a pattern of concentric semilunar patterns following the arch of the limbus. Hemorrhage may also be present in the upper palpebral conjunctiva. Some patients may have a unilateral or bilateral ecchymosis.

The cornea may show a fine punctuate epithelial keratitis with mild subepithelial infiltrate similar to an adenoviral infection.

Rarely the patient may experience paralysis of the lower extremities (Guillain-Barre syndrome), as well as a transient Bell's palsy.

Demographics

AHC affects men and women equally and all age groups are susceptible. The disease tends to be epidemic and has a predilection for populations that are living in very close quarters without proper hygiene.

Significant History

An association with others that have a similar ocular presentation is significant because of the very contagious nature of AHC.

Ancillary Tests

Diagnosis is usually made on a clinical basis; however, viral isolation is most likely during the first week of the infection.

Conjunctival scrapings will likely yield the presence of lymphocytes in the smear.

The Treatment

Treatment for AHC is largely supportive since the disease is self-limiting with very rare ocular sequelae. The use of analgesics, ocular astringents, cool compresses, and lubricants may make the patient more comfortable during the acute phases of the disease.

Since the disease is highly contagious, the patient should be quarantined for 7 to 10 days following the onset of symptoms.

Topical corticosteroids have not demonstrated a significant advantage because of the typically short course of the disease. In addition, steroids may predispose the patient to a corneal superinfection, thus increasing the risk of microbial keratitis.

Patients should be educated on proper hygiene including using their own hand towels, face towels, and pillowcases. The patient should limit touching of his or her eyes and hand washing should be performed frequently.

On occasion, secondary bacterial infections may arise. The presence of a purulent discharge may signal a secondary bacterial infection. These infections should be treated with appropriate antibiotics; however, the use of antibiotics without the development of a secondary bacterial infection is not necessary.

HERPES SIMPLEX VIRUS: OCULAR MANIFESTATIONS

Nicky R. Holdeman

ICD—9: 054.40

THE DISEASE

Pathophysiology

HSV is a ubiquitous DNA virus that affects the majority of the population by the age of 5. While the primary infection may be mild or subclinical in nature, the virus may reactivate and ultimately involve various ocular structures. Potential manifestations include blepharitis, conjunctivitis, corneal epithelial disease, stromal disease, endotheliitis, trabeculitis, uveitis, retinitis, and/or metaherpetic ulceration. Active viral replication, pathogenicity of the virus, and host immune responses are major factors of recurrent ocular herpes.

Etiology

There are two types of HSV, HSV-1 and HSV-2. HSV-1 commonly causes labialis and ocular manifestations and is transferred by direct contact with cold sores, saliva, or fomites. HSV-2 is usually genital and is typically acquired by sexual contact or may be transferred to an infant during birth. The initial HSV-1 infection may involve the face, mouth, eye, or nose and is often obscure, with the virus becoming dormant in the trigeminal ganglion or remaining latent in the skin or cornea. HSV-2 is harbored in the sacral ganglion.

Note: It was once held that recurrent eruptions were triggered by physical or emotional stress, febrile illnesses, fatigue, trauma, exposure to ultra-violet rays, contact lens wear, surgery, steroids, menstruation, and/or certain foods. However, the association and significance of these factors has not been well documented.

The Patient

Clinical Symptoms

The principal symptoms are foreign body sensation, burning, stinging, skin rash, photophobia, pain, lacrimation, conjunctival hyperemia, and reduced acuity. HSV is often in the differential diagnosis of any inflammatory eye disease of the anterior segment that has an unclear etiology.

Unilateral disease is present in >90% of the patients, thus, bilateral HSV disease should increase suspicion of systemic immune depression.

Clinical Signs

Physical findings will vary depending on the structures involved. Each of the following conditions can potentially occur (see Table 7.1).

▶ **TABLE 7.1** Ocular Manifestations of Herpes Simplex Virus

Viral Disease
- Dermatitis
- Blepharitis
- Conjunctivitis
- Corneal epithelial disease
  - punctate keratitis
  - dendritic keratitis
  - geographic (ameboid) keratitis
- Corneal stromal disease
  - necrotizing interstitial keratitis
  - disciform keratitis
  - immune rings
  - limbal vasculitis
- Endothelitis
- Trabeculitis (peripheral endothelitis)
- Iridocyclitis
- Retinitis

Nonviral Disease (postinfectious)
- Indolent ulceration of the cornea
- Metaherpetic (trophic) ulceration of the cornea
- Altered stromal structure
- Irreversible damage to the trabecular meshwork

- Dermatitis/blepharitis—Clear lid vesicles, atop an erythematous base, may appear on the upper or lower lids or on the lid margin. May be present in primary or recurrent disease, but recurrent episodes are more commonly associated with other eye findings than the primary infection. Lid swelling is usually present, but visual acuity is unaffected.
- Conjunctivitis—Typically produces diffuse conjunctival injection, watery discharge, follicles, and tender preauricular lymph node enlargement. Pseudomembranes may be seen in more severe infections and could lead to conjunctival scarring, loss of goblet cells, and a permanent dry eye condition. May occur in primary disease or in recurrent infections, with or without eyelid vesicles or epithelial keratitis.
- Corneal epithelial infections—Caused by live HSV replication. May manifest as a superficial punctate keratitis, a classic dendritic keratitis, or geographic ulceration. Corneal sensitivity is often reduced in the involved eye.

  About 11% of patients with an epithelial ulceration will ultimately develop stromal disease.
- Corneal stromal disease—Three forms of stromal disease may be caused by HSV. Stromal keratitis is less common but a more sight-threatening form of herpetic disease.
  1. Necrotizing interstitial keratitis—Deep inflammation throughout the cornea, often associated with uveitis, synechia, elevated IOP, thinning, and neovascularization.

In severe cases with dense infiltrates, there may be necrosis, melting, and hypopyon, mimicking the appearance of a bacterial keratitis. Immune response; antigen-antibody-complement mediated. The role of active virus in this disease is ill defined, but live viruses have been found within corneal tissue.

2. Disciform keratitis—Focal disc of stromal edema typically without necrosis or corneal neovascularization, usually associated with an intact epithelium. However, severe cases may show diffuse edema, folds in Descemet's membrane, KPs, neovascularization, iritis, and necrotic thinning of the stroma. Probably a cell mediated (lymphocyte), delayed hypersensitivity response but may involve active viral disease of the corneal endothelium.

3. Altered stromal structure (i.e., old disciform scar)—Repeated bouts of stromal inflammation may result in endothelial dysfunction resulting in a permanently vascularized, scarred, and/or edematous cornea.

- Endotheliitis—Rarely, keratouveitis may result in endothelial cell swelling, pleomorphism, and decompensation with secondary stromal edema. Endothelial cell damage is believed to be an immune reaction.

- Trabeculitis—Inflammation, edema, and obstruction of the trabecular meshwork may result in transient or permanent glaucoma. Inflammation may occur with or without active corneal disease.

- Uveitis—A nongranulomatous iridocyclitis is usually associated with corneal disease but can occur as an isolated finding. This condition is felt to result from an immune inflammatory reaction but may also have a live virus component.

- Metaherpetic keratopathy—Occasionally, repeated bouts of herpetic keratitis will cause structural damage to the basement membrane, resulting in a sterile ulceration of the cornea. Persistence of trophic ulceration may lead to stromal melting and subsequent perforation. Etiologic factors include drug toxicity, corneal hypoesthesia, and decreased tear formation.

Demographics

About 90% of the U.S. population has been infected with HSV, but <20% will manifest cutaneous or ocular disease.

Nearly 500,000 people in the United States have experienced a HSV-related ocular disease. There are 20,000 new cases of ocular HSV and 28,000 reactivations of ocular HSV per year in the United States. HSV is the most common infectious cause of corneal blindness in the Western hemisphere and a leading cause for corneal transplantation.

HSV infections can affect males and females at any age although the initial infection is often subclinical. Incidence may be higher in males than females over the age of 40.

Transmission of the virus occurs by direct contact with infected lesions, by salivary droplets, by fomites, and by healthy, asymptomatic carriers.

Possible increased incidence in fall and winter months.

Incubation period, between contact and disease, is 3 to 9 days.

Roughly 24–30% of patients with ocular disease will experience a recurrence within 2 to 5 years after the first episode.

Significant History

- Recent exposure to a known source of infection?
- Previous episodes of HSV disease?
- Rashes involving the mouth, lips, nose, or genitalia?
- Immune deficiency?
- Recent use of topical or systemic steroids?
- History or presence of atopic skin disease?
- Proposed stimuli of reactivations include physical or mental stress, heat, illness, UV light exposure, fever, trauma, and menstruation. Topical prostaglandins may be another potential trigger factor.

Ancillary Tests

Most cases (>90%) of HSV disease can be diagnosed by the patient's history, symptoms, and physical findings. If the diagnosis is questionable or confirmation is required, several laboratory tests may prove useful.

- Tzanck cell tests or Giemsa stains reveal the large, multinucleated epithelial giant cells of scrapings from a skin lesion or corneal ulcer.
- Viral cultures from the cornea, conjunctiva, or skin obtained within several days of onset, and prior to antiviral therapy, have a high sensitivity in identifying the organism. Results can take several weeks, but provide a definitive diagnosis.
- Enzyme immunoassay (EIA) tests can be performed in the office (Herpchek; Kodak SureCell). These tests have relatively good sensitivity and specificity to detect HSV antigens.
- Polymerase chain reaction (PCR) from an anterior chamber tap may detect viral DNA in cases of herpetic keratouveitis.
- The Captia test (Trinity Biotech) is a blood test to detect antibodies to the herpes simplex virus. Unlike other tests, it can reportedly differentiate between HSV-1 and HSV-2.

Note: Pseudodendrites can result from ocular surface disease, healing abrasions, and ABMD. Herpes zoster, Epstein-Barr virus, adenovirus, and acanthamoeba can also resemble HSV at certain stages of the disease.

The Treatment

Treatment will vary depending on the structures involved and whether live virus or immunologic factors (or both) account for the disease.

- Dermatitis/blepharitis—Currently there is a lack of clinical efficacy in the treatment of skin disease. There is no clear evidence that topical antiviral medication promotes healing or prevents corneal disease, thus virustatic agents are probably not required. Skin hygiene and warm, moist, sterile compresses tid, may help prevent secondary bacterial infections. Consider applying topical povidone-iodine on severe skin ulcers, avoiding the immediate periocular area.

If viral vesicles involve the lid margins, ophthalmic antiviral drops (e.g., trifluridine 1%) or ointment (e.g., vidarabine 3%) applied 3 to 5 times/d is advised. HSV skin infections usually heal within 10 days without scarring.

Note: Certain studies have implied that early administration of oral acyclovir, 400 mg p.o. 5 times/d for 5 days, may accelerate healing and reduce patient discomfort.

- Conjunctivitis—While the use of antiviral agents has not been clearly defined, most would advocate topical antiviral therapy with either drops (trifluridine 1%) or ointment (vidarabine 3%) 5 times/d to speed resolution and potentially reduce the risk of keratitis. Conjunctivitis usually resolves within 7 to 10 days.

  Monitor for corneal involvement, as epithelial keratitis develops in approximately one third of eyes.
- Corneal epithelial infections—Minimal wipe debridement of the infected epithelium with a damp, sterile, cotton-tipped applicator serves to remove the viral load and the viral antigens that may induce stromal keratitis.

  Trifluridine 1% solution q 2 hrs, up to, but not to exceed, 9 times/d or vidarabine 3% ointment 5 times/d until the epithelium heals, usually after 5 to 10 days.

  Topical antiviral agents should then be used qid for 3 to 5 days after complete epithelialization of the cornea, but not used for more than 21 days total. Epithelial lesions usually heal within 1 to 2 weeks, but antiviral use for more than 21 days can result in significant epithelial toxicity.

Note: Use of both topical antiviral agents may be advised in large geographic ulcers. Idoxuridine may also be used if an allergy develops to the other topical antiviral agents as cross-reactivity is rare. Watch for antiviral toxicity. If topical toxicity occurs, or in cases of severe or recalcitrant infections, oral acyclovir 200–400 mg 5 times/d or valacyclovir 500 mg p.o. bid for 10–14 days may be used and has been shown to achieve therapeutic concentrations in the tear film and aqueous humor. Oral antiviral agents may also be preferred in children, in patients with preexisting ocular surface disease, and in patients unable to use topical agents (i.e., severe arthritis of the hands).

It should be noted, however, that a short course of oral acyclovir does not reduce the risk of developing stromal keratitis or iridocyclitis in patients treated with topical antivirals:

Homatropine 5% or scopolamine 0.25% bid-tid for iritis.
Topical antibiotics (e.g., Polytrim) qid while active ulcers are present.

Note: Topical steroids are contraindicated in almost all conditions with active epithelial disease. If stromal disease occurs simultaneously with active epithelial infections, using steroids will make the situation worse.

- Necrotizing interstitial keratitis—If active corneal epithelial disease is present, treat as indicated previously. Dendritic or geographic ulcers indicate the presence of live virus. Cyclopegics PRN for iridocyclitis.

  If the disease is mild and is not threatening the visual axis, no treatment may be required. Best to avoid steroids in mild cases and if the patient has not previously been treated with steroids.

In cases of more severe inflammation, and/or a threat to the visual axis, topical steroids (minimal concentration and dosage needed to control inflammation, with a slow taper based on the level of disease severity and the rate of clinical improvement) and an oral antiviral agent, should be employed to reduce scarring and neovascularization (e.g., acyclovir 400 mg 5 times daily for 2–3 weeks, then 200–400 mg bid-tid for several additional weeks).

Artificial tears (e.g. Celluvisc) q 2 hrs to facilitate epithelial healing.

Follow the patient for bacterial or fungal superinfection.

- Disciform keratitis—Responds dramatically to topical steroids; however, rules for treatment are the same as HSV interstitial keratitis described previously. If steroids are used, treatment must generally be maintained for several months with concurrent, prophylactic antiviral agents (i.e., topical trifluridine or oral acyclovir).

Topical corticosteroids appear to shorten the duration of HSV stromal keratitis but does not offer a long-term difference in visual outcome or influence recurrence rates in most patients.

Postponing steroids for several days may delay resolution of disciform edema but again, does not appear to have long-term detrimental effects.

Some patients require chronic low dose steroids to maintain an uninflamed state. IOP should always be monitored regularly.

Note: Oral acyclovir is not helpful in the treatment of HSV disciform keratitis in patients receiving concomitant topical corticosteroids and trifluridine. However, in cases where pronounced keratouveitis or trabeculitis supervene, oral antiviral agents are often recommended.

- Altered stromal structure—Does not respond to steroids or other medical therapy. Depending on symptoms, the visual requirements of the patient, and condition of the fellow eye, treatment options include bandage soft contact lenses, conjunctival flap, and penetrating keratoplasty.
- Endotheliitis/trabeculitis/uveitis—Treatment for these conditions is nonspecific involving topical and/or oral medications. While topical antiviral agents will not penetrate in therapeutic titers, they should be used as a prophylactic cover when topical corticosteroids are given. Antiviral coverage can typically be discontinued when the steroids are tapered to once a day or less. The following drugs should be employed as needed to control the patient's condition:

Cycloplegics (e.g., homatropine 5%, atropine 1%, scopolamine 0.25%) bid-tid as required for cells and flare.

Topical steroids (e.g., prednisolone acetate 1%) q1–3 hrs to once per day depending on the severity of the condition.

Antiviral agents (e.g., trifluridine 1%) tid-qid for prophylaxis with topical steroids.

Beta-blockers (e.g., timolol maleate 0.5% bid) and/or topical or oral carbonic anhydrase inhibitors (e.g., acetazolamide 250 mg p.o. bid-qid) for secondary glaucoma. Topical prostaglandins should be avoided as they may increase recurrences in some patients.

Oral acyclovir, 200–400 mg p.o. 5 times/day for 4–6 weeks, may be beneficial for patients not responding to 7 days of topical antiviral therapy.

Oral steroids (e.g., prednisone 20–40 mg p.o. bid for 7–14 days, then tapered over 10 days) may be given if corneal ulceration or melting contraindicates the use of topical steroids.

Note: Argon laser trabeculoplasty is not indicated in HSV trabeculitis and may increase scarring.

It should also be noted that the long-term administration of oral acyclovir (400 mg p.o. bid for 1 year), in patients with any form of ocular HSV disease, reduces the risk of the development of recurrent HSV disease by 40%. This regimen would appear to be particularly important in patients with a history of previous stromal disease as the reduction in risk for recurrent stromal disease is reduced by ~50%. Superficial forms of HSV such as blepharitis, conjunctivitis, and epithelial keratitis, are effectively treated with topical antiviral agents and the use of long-term oral acyclovir in these patients is questionable.

- Metaherpetic keratopathy—Treatment for these postinfectious lesions is aimed at protecting the damaged basement membrane of the cornea. Treatment involves the following: eliminating toxic agents (i.e., antiviral drugs, steroids, and all eye drops containing preservatives) and frequent application of unpreserved tears and ointments to promote corneal healing.

  Therapeutic or bandage soft contact lens may be considered for weeks to months to protect and lubricate the cornea. Artificial tears q2–3 hrs. and prophylactic antibiotic drops (e.g., Polytrim) bid should be used while the lens is in place.

  Cycloplegics, bid, prn, if an iritis is present.

  Mild steroids (e.g., prednisolone phosphate 0.125%) qd-qid may be warranted if major stromal edema is slowing the healing process. If corneal thinning is present, 1% medroxyprogesterone can be formulated and instilled 2 to 5 times daily, which will not interfere with collagen synthesis. Viroptic 1% bid-qid should be used concurrently, as a prophylaxis, if a steroid equivalent of 1% prednisolone bid or more is in use.

  Cyanoacrylate adhesives may be applied if active corneal melting with impending perforation develops.

  Conjunctival flap or keratoplasty may be required in some cases.

HERPES ZOSTER OPHTHALMICUS
Nicky R. Holdeman

ICD—9: 053.29

THE DISEASE

Pathophysiology

HZO is a multivariate disorder that may affect every structure of the eye. The classic presentation of HZO is seen when the first division of the trigeminal nerve (V_1) is affected by the varicella zoster virus (VZV). HZO is caused by the reactivation of the primary disease, varicella (or chicken pox), which usually occurs during childhood. Varicella gains access to the sensory ganglion where it enters a latent state. If the virus reactivates it can lead to substantial visual disability, and rarely, can be associated with fatal CNS complications. The basic mechanisms of the disease are direct viral tissue invasion and vasculitis, which can lead to ischemia, inflammation, and/or necrosis.

Etiology

The herpes viridae are a large group of linear double-stranded DNA viruses that are found throughout the world. Varicella (chicken pox) is principally a disease of childhood and often occurs in epidemics during the winter and spring. The virus is highly contagious and is spread through direct contact with respiratory secretions or skin lesions. Zoster (shingles) is the result of the reactivation of a latent varicella virus infection and is usually seen in adults. Following activation, the virus travels along a nerve (or nerves) to the skin, where it produces lesions over the area of skin supplied by the affected nerves. Children and other susceptible persons who are exposed to an adult with zoster may develop a typical case of chicken pox.

The Patient

Clinical Symptoms

The characteristic prodromal symptoms of acute HZO include 2 to 3 days of generalized malaise, fever, and headache, with the affected dermatome showing evidence of hyperesthesia, pain, burning, and/or itching. The patient may also report skin redness, edema, and a rash, which is first papular, then becoming vesicular within 12 to 24 hours. Rarely, a patient may manifest herpes zoster sine herpete (HZSH), which is zoster without an associated rash.

Without antiviral therapy, ocular complications will develop in 50–70% of patients with ophthalmic branch involvement. If that is the case, the patient may complain of conjunctival injection, eye pain, photophobia, and blurred vision.

Clinical Signs

HZO may manifest a variety of ocular findings; some have potentially sight-threatening complications. If the rash involves the nasociliary branch of V_1, characterized by vesicles on the tip of the nose (Hutchinson's sign), it may predict a greater risk of ocular involvement.

In addition to a midline respecting dermatitis, which can lead to permanent contraction scars of the lids, other ocular manifestations may include:

- Conjunctivitis—Conjunctival inflammation is common and may occur as watery hyperemia with petechial hemorrhages, follicles, regional adenopathy, and/or membranous inflammation.
- Episcleritis—Usually sectorial, flat, or nodular.
- Scleritis—May be diffuse or focal nodular; resolution may lead to scleral thinning and staphyloma.
- Keratitis—Occurs in ≈40–66% of patients with HZO and may precede the neuralgia or skin lesions. There can be a multitude of effects, ranging from SPK and pseudodendrites to neurotrophic keratopathy.

- Iridocyclitis—Occurs in up to 40% of patients with HZO. May appear independent of corneal involvement, and onset may be delayed for months after the disappearance of the rash. Findings in patients with anterior uveal involvement include diffuse, focal, or sector iris atrophy (because of occlusion of iris vessels), granulomatous KP, or anterior and posterior synechiae.
- Glaucoma—≈40% of patients show an elevated IOP, usually because of trabeculitis. Formation of synechia may result in long-term complications.

Less common manifestations of HZO include cataract formation, cranial nerve palsies (Ramsey-Hunt syndrome), retinitis (acute retinal necrosis [ARN] and progressive outer retinal necrosis [PORN]), CRVO, CRAO, optic neuritis, and multifocal choroiditis. In addition, postherpetic neuralgia (PHN) commonly follows HZO and can be the most distressing complication of the disease (see the next section).

Demographics

Over 90% of adults in the United States have serologic evidence of varicella zoster virus infection and are at risk for herpes zoster. It is estimated that herpes zoster may occur in as many as 850,000 people in the United States each year.

Caucasians appear to be four times more likely to be infected with zoster than are African Americans.

There appear to be two general risk factors for the disease: aging and a weakened immunity.

Children constitute only 7% of those with the ocular disease and the course of disease is shorter in children.

HZO is often the presenting sign in AIDS-related complex and AIDS.

Significant History

While the majority of cases occur in healthy, older adults, there is an increasing number of patients who have acquired or iatrogenic immunosuppression. The patient should be questioned regarding malignancies and immunosuppressive therapies.

Other predisposing factors include tuberculosis, malaria, syphilis, and physical or emotional trauma.

Ancillary Tests

The diagnosis of HZO is almost always made on the basis of the clinical picture. However, the virus can be detected by methods based on the polymerase chain reaction (PCR), which may prove useful in unusual presentations such as younger patients and those with absence of skin lesions. PCR is able to amplify small amounts of viral DNA in fluid and tissues and identify a specific DNA.

Viral culture is possible, but VZV is labile and relatively difficult to recover from swabs of cutaneous lesions.

Each patient should receive a complete medical/social history and comprehensive ocular examination.

Patients younger than 40 years, with no known cause of immunosuppression, should be referred for medical evaluation. One must consider HIV infection in young patients with zoster.

The Treatment

Since HZO may cause devastating complications, early and aggressive therapy should be instituted.

Oral antiviral agents are mandatory for patients presenting with HZO, in order to reduce the risk of serious ocular complications. These drugs are most efficacious if initiated within 48 to 72 hours of the rash, but some patients will benefit even when treatment is started after 3 days.

- Dermatitis

    Patients with zoster in an ophthalmic distribution should receive antiviral drugs for at least 7 days. Oral antiviral therapy reduces the frequency of ocular complications and have been shown to hasten healing of skin lesions, decrease virus shedding, and reduce the severity of acute pain. All three drugs are safe, efficacious, and well tolerated. (Dosage should be reduced in patients with renal insufficiency.)
    1. Acyclovir 800 mg p.o. 5 times per day, or
    2. Famciclovir 500 mg p.o. tid, or
    3. Valacyclovir 1000 mg p.o. tid

    Note: Valacyclovir is a pro-drug of acyclovir and produces serum acyclovir levels that are 3 to 5 times higher than those achieved with oral acyclovir therapy.

    1. Erythromycin or bacitracin ointment bid for 1 to 2 weeks for prophylaxis
    2. Warm compresses or Burow's solution (5% aluminum acetate) tid-qid to skin lesions

    The skin lesions often heal within 4 weeks, and the pain usually subsides as the skin lesions resolve. There is no role for topical antiviral drugs in the management of herpes zoster.
- Conjunctivitis

    Cool compresses; prophylactic erythromycin ointment bid.
- Episcleritis/Scleritis

    A mild episcleritis may not require treatment as it is often self-limiting.

    Nodular episcleritis or scleritis (which is more serious than episcleritis) can be treated with one of the following drugs when appropriate. Response to therapy may take 2 to 3 weeks:
    1. Indomethacin SR 75 mg p.o. bid
    2. Diflunisal 500 mg p.o. bid
    3. Naproxen 375–500 mg p.o. bid
    4. Ibuprofen 400–600 mg p.o. qid
    5. Piroxicam 20 mg p.o. qd
- In recalcitrant or severe cases of scleritis and in necrotizing scleritis, systemic steroids should be given. On occasion, peribulbar steroid injections or cytotoxic agents may be needed.

Note: Immunocompromised patients should not receive systemic steroids.

■ Keratitis

Pseudodendrites and SPK are often self-limiting and clear within a few days. Non-preserved artificial tears may be used q1–2 hours.

Disciform immune keratitis usually responds to topical steroids (prednisolone acetate 1% q1–6 hours), which should be slowly tapered. Some patients require minimal daily doses to prevent recurrence.

■ Iridocyclitis

1. Cycloplegic agents (homatropine 5% bid-tid; cyclopentolate 1–2% tid)
2. Topical steroids (prednisolone acetate 1%) q1–6 hours

■ Glaucoma

The treatment for glaucoma will vary depending on the etiology. Elevated IOPs may be caused by trabeculitis, trabecular meshwork debris, rubeosis with secondary angle closure, posterior synechia with pupillary block, PAS with angle closure, or secondary to steroids.

If inflammation is present, topical steroids may be utilized. Consider using the "soft" steroids such as rimexolone 1% or lotoprednol 0.5% and taper as clinically indicated.

Aqueous humor suppressants (timolol 0.5% bid, dorzolamide 2% tid, brinzolamide 1% tid, or methazolamide 50 mg p.o. bid or tid) may be employed if needed.

Topical antiglaucoma agents associated with uveal inflammation (prostaglandins, brimonidine, metipranolol) should be used with caution.

Note: If pain is of concern to the patient, oral analgesics may be required. Treatment usually includes extra-strength acetaminophen and 30–60 mg of codeine q4–6 hours as needed.

■ Post Herpetic Neuralgia (PHN), ICD—9:053.13

PHN, defined as pain persisting at least 1 month after the skin rash has healed, is one of the most feared complications in immunocompetent patients.

There is no universally accepted treatment for PHN, a condition that increases dramatically with age (>50% of patients over age 80). Management should involve the patients primary care physician as treatment is complex, often requiring a multifaceted approach. Consultation with a pain specialist is sometimes needed.

Suggested oral therapies have included:

1. Amitriptyline or nortriptyline (25–75 mg/d)
2. Carbamazapine (400–1200 mg/d)
3. Phenytoin (300–400 mg/d)
4. Gabapentin (300 mg tid)

Topical therapy may be useful for temporary relief from pain after the initial skin lesions have healed, but cannot be used around the eye.

1. Capsaicin 0.025% (3–4 times/d)
2. Lidocaine skin patch

Fortunately, the natural history of pain after an episode of herpes zoster is one of improvement, and even PHN of long duration may lessen with time.

VARICELLA
Marcus Piccolo

ICD—9: 052.7

THE DISEASE
Pathophysiology

Varicella is the primary infection from the varicella zoster virus, resulting in inflammatory as well as immunologic reactions. VZV is responsible for the systemic varicella infection (chicken pox) upon initial exposure to the virus, and for herpes zoster (shingles) upon reactivation of latent virus, which resides in the dorsal root ganglia of the spinal column. The primary varicella infection results in an exanthematous reaction of the skin (occasionally involving the conjunctiva or cornea), resulting in the formation of "pocks" containing live virus. The lesions are typically self-contained and tend to resolve over a period of 1 to 2 weeks. Secondary immunologic reactions to virus antibodies may result in stromal disciform disease of the cornea or phlyctenule-like disease on the conjunctiva.

Etiology

This condition results from inoculation of the varicella zoster virus, a human herpes virus 3, through inhalation of respiratory droplets or by direct contact with cutaneous lesions of infected individuals. The virus replicates in the lymph nodes and then gains access to the blood stream. Patients are infectious from 24 hours before appearance of the rash, until the final lesions have crusted.

The Patient

Systemic Symptoms
Primary systemic infection with VZV most frequently involves the respiratory tract, after a 10 to 21 day latency period. Prodromal symptoms of varicella often include fever, malaise, anorexia, and/or a mild headache, which is followed by skin involvement.

Systemic Signs
The rash undergoes progression from macule, papule, vesicle, to encrustation, and healing. The rash occurs in crops resulting in lesions of various states and appearance; the lids are sometimes involved. Resolution typically occurs without scarring in 1 to 2 weeks.

Ocular Symptoms
Ocular involvement results in a mild to moderate red eye with a watery discharge. The patient may experience a foreign body sensation or a decrease in vision if the cornea is significantly affected; however, the majority of cases do not demonstrate a reduction in acuity. Photophobia may be reported if an accompanying uveitis is present.

Ocular Signs

- Conjunctiva—Primary VZV infection of the eye results in an acute papillary conjunctivitis. The bulbar conjunctiva may demonstrate a raised, round, vesicular lesion ("pock"), which may be associated with subconjunctival hemorrhage. The pocks are typically located near the limbus or peripheral cornea. They usually occur during the systemic manifestation of the disease; however, they also may occur weeks to months after the systemic condition has resolved. Pocks are most likely reservoirs of live virus, whereas late-forming lesions may be sterile and the result of immunologic reactions to residual virus antigens. Ulceration of the pocks may occur prior to resolution.
- Cornea—Primary VZV infection of the cornea may cause a nonrecurring superficial punctate keratitis or dendritic keratitis. VZV corneal dendrites are typically finer and smaller, lack terminal end bulbs, and are more superficial in appearance as compared to the classic dendrites of herpes simplex virus (HSV). However, varicella dendrites may progress to amoeboid or geographic configurations. VZV dendrites have an elevated nonulcerated appearance and usually stain poorly with fluorescein. Immunologic reactions in the cornea may result in sterile disciform type lesions in the stroma. VZV disciform lesions are typically milder and resolve more rapidly as compared to HSV.

    A concurrent uveitis can occur and may be quite severe. Cataract, optic neuritis, retinitis, and ophthalmoplegia have all been reported.

    Corneal scarring and vascularization may result as a permanent sequellae of a VZV corneal infection.

Demographics

Primary infection with VZV is normally seen in childhood before the age of 9 but may appear in adolescence or early adulthood, especially in isolated, less populous areas of the world. The disease is highly contagious affecting 80–90% of exposed individuals

Significant History

A history of exposure to an individual with active chicken pox or active zoster should arouse suspicion. The abrupt onset of a skin rash with flulike symptoms is also important.

Ancillary Tests

While diagnosis of VZV is usually made on the basis of clinical findings, the following tests may be useful in isolated cases.

- Cultures—VZV can be retrieved from active vesicles as well as some mucus membranes. Cultures of VZV require inoculation of human tissue cultures.
- Serology—Serology to detect complement fixation or neutralizing antibodies can be performed. Seropositive reactions approach 100% by age 60.
- Ocular Cytology—Giemsa staining often reveals lymphocytes. The presence of ulcerated conjunctival pocks may result in the presence of PMNs in the smear, and multinucleated giant cells may also be noted. Papanicolaou-stained cytological

samples taken from the cornea, conjunctiva, or skin vesicles may reveal eosinophilic intranuclear inclusions (Lipschutz bodies).
- Smears can also be examined using direct immunofluorescent techniques.

The Treatment
- Systemic—Primary VZV is typically treated by supportive measures, using cool compresses, analgesics, antipyretics, antipruritics, and adequate hygiene of the cutaneous lesions. Aspirin should be avoided because of the reported risk of Reye's syndrome in children. Oral acyclovir may be indicated in severe cases, especially in older children and adults. Intravenous acyclovir or vidarabine may be required in immunocompromised individuals.
- Ocular—No topical antiviral agent has demonstrated efficacy for treatment of epithelial disease. Cool compresses and observation is often the treatment of choice as the lesions are usually self-limiting. Gentle, minimal wipe debridement or topical steroids may hasten resolution in some cases.

Topical antibiotics (erythromycin) should be used bid for ocular prophylaxis in patients with corneal epithelial disease and applied to the skin of patients with lesions involving the eyelids or periorbital area.

The use of corticosteroid drops may be indicated for stromal and disciform disease of the cornea secondary to VZV. Stromal disease may have a protracted course requiring careful and extended treatment.

Prednisolone acetate 0.12% (Pred mild) 1 drop tid to qid and tapered slowly over several weeks.

Associated uveitis may be treated with cycloplegics alone, although adjunct therapy with topical corticosteroids may be required.

Note: VZV vaccination is recommended for all children over 12 months of age who have not had chicken pox. While varicella vaccination is not 100% effective (~80% effective in preventing all disease), cases in vaccinated persons are usually milder, with fewer lesions and fewer constitutional symptoms. Also, patients who develop chicken pox despite being vaccinated (i.e., breakthrough varicella) are only about half as contagious as their unvaccinated counterparts, although contagiousness varies with the number of skin lesions.

MOLLUSCUM CONTAGIOSUM
Marcus Piccolo

ICD—9: 078.0

THE DISEASE
Pathophysiology

Molluscum contagiosum is a cutaneous or conjunctival viral infection that causes a raised, waxy, umbilicated lesion on the eyelids and face. Virus that is shed into the tear film may cause a toxic reaction on the cornea and conjunctiva resulting in a chronic follicular conjunctivitis and mild superior keratitis.

Etiology

This condition is caused by the Molluscum contagiosum virus, a double-stranded DNA poxvirus.

Inoculation occurs via contact, under moist conditions, with an infected individual or fomites, resulting in an infection of epidermal cells.

The Patient

Clinical Symptoms

Molluscum contagiosum results in a slow onset, chronic red eye with scant discharge. Minor irritation may be present; however, frank pain and photophobia are not commonly reported. Visual acuity is usually unaffected unless significant corneal involvement occurs.

Clinical Signs

- Lids—Infection may result in multiple or isolated, dome-shaped, elevated, noninflamed, waxy lesions with an umbilicated center, although flat, nonumbilicated lesions have also been observed. The lesions are typically painless, located near the lid margin, and may be hidden by the cilia. Nodular lesions range from 2 to 5 mm in size.
- Conjunctiva—Toxic reactions from viral products result in a chronic follicular conjunctivitis. Rarely, direct infection of the conjunctiva can occur resulting in lesions that appear as small white pimples on an erythematous base.
- Cornea—Toxic reactions to the virus can cause fine superior epithelial keratitis. Longstanding chronic presentations may result in a superior micro pannus, which along with the follicular conjunctivitis may mimic trachoma. Untreated, the condition can cause significant vascularization and scarring of the cornea resulting in loss of visual acuity.

  Infected individuals may have cutaneous lesions on other parts of their body besides their lids.

  Preauricular lymphadenopathy is usually not present.

Demographics

Molluscum contagiosum usually occurs in young adults and adolescents—there is no known racial or ethnic distribution. Venereal spread of the virus is not uncommon. The infection is usually self-limiting, although chronic over several months. If the individual is immunosuppressed, the lesions will not undergo spontaneous resolution.

Significant History

History of close contact with an infected individual is relevant. Sexual activity, promiscuity, or activities such as wrestling, may increase the risk of inoculation from infected individuals.

Patients who are immunocompromised (AIDS) may present with bilateral, recurrent, or disseminated disease.

Ancillary Tests

Diagnosis is based on clinical appearance, although identification and confirmation of the condition is sometimes necessary. Patients with recurrent or atypical lesions should be referred to exclude acquired immunodeficiency syndromes.

- Cytology—Lymphocytic reactions are observed with Giemsa staining.
- Biopsy—Biopsy of lesions reveals eosinophilic, cytoplasmic inclusion bodies (molluscum bodies) displacing the nuclei of infected epidermal cells.

The Treatment

No medical treatment or antiviral therapy exists for molluscum contagiosum. Spontaneous resolution is usually seen in 3 to 12 months in immunocompetent patients.

Treatment is by surgical excision, incision, cauterization, cryotherapy, or curettage of the central core of the lesion. All treatments seem equally effective if the central core is removed.

Exposure of the virus to the immune system via blood will typically result in a cure.

The conjunctivitis and keratitis typically resolve, assuming all the lesions were identified and appropriately treated.

THYGESON'S SUPERFICIAL PUNCTATE KERATITIS (TSPK)
Marcus Piccolo

ICD—9: 370.21

THE DISEASE
Pathophysiology

TSPK occurs because of a mild inflammation of the corneal epithelium, resulting in small, stellate, round, or linear opacities and a mild subepithelial infiltrate. These course lesions remain confined to the epithelium and tend to regress spontaneously.

Etiology

The etiology for TSPK is unknown, but viral etiologies are suspected. However, no confirmed virus has been identified. Varicella zoster virus was isolated in one patient but confirmation by other researchers has failed to replicate this finding, either by virus culture or by electron microscopy.

The Patient

Clinical Symptoms
The patient often complains of mild photophobia, burning, tearing, and foreign body sensation. A decrease in visual acuity may be present as a result of central corneal involvement.

Clinical Signs
Patients usually present with bilateral, discrete, granular, slightly elevated, corneal epithelial opacities. The lesions may be few to many in number and tend to be concentrated in the pupillary region. The superficial stroma rarely shows trace edema or a mild infiltrate directly under the epithelial lesions. The epithelial lesions may stain minimally with fluorescein. Although bilateral presentation is the rule, unilateral cases are not uncommon. The conjunctiva and lids are not involved, and other than the corneal findings, the eye appears quiet. The condition may wax and wane, but usually remains for years with spontaneous resolution.

Demographics

TSPK affects both men and women and typically manifests in the first to fourth decade of life.

Significant History

No particular history is associated with TSPK, except that the patient will not have had a recent conjunctivitis. While viral etiologies are suspected, the condition appears to be noncontagious as demonstrated by the likelihood that only one member of a family may be affected by the condition.

Ancillary Tests

There are presently no tests that are helpful in confirming TSPK; consequently, the diagnosis remains clinical in nature.

The Treatment

Treatment of TSPK is primarily aimed at controlling symptoms, and management is dependent on the severity at presentation. For patients with mild symptoms and signs, supportive therapy with artificial tears may be sufficient.

The use of bandage soft contact lenses has been effective at controlling symptoms in chronic cases.

If the condition is severe, the use of topical steroids may be indicated. If steroids are used, it is suggested that mild steroids be prescribed in dosages just ample to control symptoms. Steroid drops will usually result in resolution of the corneal lesions, but may ultimately prolong the course of the disease and may be difficult to taper. The possibility of adverse steroid effects such as glaucoma, increased risk of opportunistic infection, and cataracts are real concerns.

Some specialists have advocated the use topical 2% cyclosporine-A (CSA) as a substitute for steroid therapy. Topical cyclosporine is usually given tid, or up to 5 times per day to eliminate symptoms and to reverse corneal findings. Sustained therapy for up to 6 months may be necessary; however, there is little in the way of adverse effects.

Chapter 8

Fungal Infectious Diseases

FUNGAL KERATITIS
Nicky R. Holdeman

ICD—9: 370.05

THE DISEASE
Pathophysiology

Fungal keratitis results from invasion of the cornea by a fungal organism. While fungi are ubiquitous, they are responsible for less than 2% of corneal infections worldwide. Unfortunately however, because of the difficulty in diagnosing and treating these infections, they often result in devastating ocular consequences. The incidence of fungal keratitis has risen substantially in the last 20 to 30 years, probably because of the increased use of topical corticosteroids and broad spectrum antibiotics and better diagnostic techniques.

Etiology

Fungi do not invade the cornea easily and seem to require epithelial trauma, contact lens wear, or immunologic compromise for infection. The most common organism responsible for fungal keratitis on a worldwide basis is *Aspergillus*; however, keratomycosis is climate specific. In the southern United States, *Fusarium* is the most common cause of keratomycosis, whereas *Candida* and *Aspergillus* are isolated most frequently in the northern states. Up to 70 different fungi have been implicated as etiologic agents of fungal keratitis.

The Patient

The clinical presentation of keratomycosis may vary. The patient's immune status, duration of involvement, and prior treatment will modify the findings.
   Clinical symptoms include:

- Pain
- Conjunctival redness
- Light sensitivity
- Tearing/discharge
- Foreign body sensation

Clinical signs include:

- Conjunctival injection
- Epithelial defect (or less commonly an elevated epithelium)
- Gray or gray-white leukocytic stromal infiltrate often with irregular feathery borders or hyphate edge
- Anterior chamber reaction; possibly hypopyon with fibrinoid aqueous
- Dry, rough texture in the area of involved cornea
- Satellite lesions surrounding the primary infiltrate
- Endothelial plaque

Note: These findings may be useful in raising one's level of suspicion; however, fungal keratitis has no pathognomonic appearance.

Demographics

While keratomycosis may affect either sex, there seems to be a higher incidence in men, especially in farm workers and other outdoorsmen. In the southern United States, there is a bimodal distribution of occurrence with greater frequencies in the spring and late fall to early winter.

Incidence is estimated to be ≈1,500 cases/year in the United States.

Significant History

The history should cover the known risk factors associated with fungal keratitis. The following information should be obtained.

- Has the patient sustained corneal trauma, especially with organic material? (Infection usually occurs 36 to 48 hours after trauma, often slowly progressive.)
- Is the patient systemically or topically immunocompromised?
- Does the patient have any chronic systemic diseases, especially diabetes mellitus?
- Does the patient wear extended-wear contact lenses or a therapeutic bandage lens? (Fungal infection has been reported in contact lens wearers, but bacterial keratitis is more common in these patients.)
- Does the patient have a chronic preexisting ocular surface disorder that may compromise the epithelium (e.g., exposure keratitis, keratitis sicca, herpes simplex keratitis, prior keratoplasty, etc.) ?

Ancillary Tests

Diagnosing keratomycosis is often difficult. The primary obstacle in many cases is a failure to suspect a fungal etiology. It is therefore important for the clinician to perform a prompt and thorough laboratory investigation. One should complete the same culture procedure as previously described in the section on bacterial keratitis; however, several points should be emphasized.

1. Scraping the cornea with a sharpened Kimura spatula or a No. 15 scalpel blade is required to enhance the retrieval of fungal elements. The base and leading edge of

the infiltrate should be vigorously scraped then incubated on blood agar, thioglycolate broth, and Sabouraud's agar (without cyclohexamide) without breaking the surface of the media. (Cyclohexamide is an inhibitant of saprophytic fungi, which are considered contaminants elsewhere in the body, but can be potential pathogens of the cornea.)

Growth of fungi in culture is usually identifiable within 2 to 7 days, but cultures should be held for 3 weeks before discarding them as negative.

Occasionally, patients will have a mixed bacterial-fungal, herpetic-fungal, *Acanthamoeba*-fungal, or mixed-fungal keratitis.

If keratomycosis is the suspected diagnosis, yet the cultures are negative at 48 to 72 hours and the patient is not improving on antibacterial therapy, a corneal biopsy may be necessary to obtain diagnostic material. If biopsy fails to confirm keratomycosis and the ulcer is progressing, an anterior chamber paracentesis may be considered to analyze the hypopyon, but is rarely indicated.

2. Scrapings should also be used to make thin smears for both Gram and Giemsa stains. Gram stains may help to identify yeast forms of fungi (e.g., *Candida*) while Giemsa stain is more likely to define filamentous fungi (e.g., *Fusarium, Aspergillus, Cephalosporium*). Occasionally, specialized stains (i.e., potassium hydroxide with calcofluor white; acridine orange, etc.) and media (i.e., brain-heart infusion broth) are required to identify the more fastidious organisms.

   Note: Diagnosis requires laboratory confirmation and should never be made solely on the basis of the history or the appearance of the cornea. DNA amplification using polymerase chain reaction (PCR)–based assay is a promising method for rapid and sensitive diagnosis of fungal keratitis that may be more widely available in the future.

3. Sensitivities of isolated fungi to various antifungal agents can only be performed in a few specialized laboratories, such as the CDC in Atlanta. It is recommended, however, that isolated organisms not be discarded so that additional studies could be performed at one of these sites in the event the patient does not respond to therapy.

The Treatment

Typically, most infectious corneal infiltrates and ulcers are treated empirically with broad spectrum antibacterial therapy unless fungal elements are seen on smears or fungi are isolated on cultures. Medical therapy for keratomycosis is somewhat limited by FDA-approved topical antifungal agents and by the poor penetration into ocular tissues. If studies verify a fungal etiology, typical management often includes the following measures:

1. Currently, natamycin, 5% suspension (Natacyn), is the only commercially available, FDA-approved, antifungal agent for topical use. It is a polyene agent that is most effective against filamentous fungi such as *Fusarium*, but is also active against some yeast. A typical regimen would be one drop q1 to 2 hours for 1 to 4 days at which time it can usually be reduced to one drop 6 to 8 times daily depending on clinical response. Average duration of therapy runs 21 to 35 days, but several months of treatment may be required to assure the organism has been eliminated. While natamycin is well tolerated by the eye, refractory cases may require the addition of other

topical, sub-conjunctival, or systemic antifungal drugs (e.g., amphotericin B, flucyto-sine, itraconazole, fluconazole, econazole, voriconazole, miconazole, clotrimazole, or ketoconazole). Systemic antifungal agents are typically employed in patients with severe keratitis, scleritis, impending perforation, and endophthalmitis.

2. Epithelial debridement and debulkment of necrotic tissue often aids drug penetration.

3. Cycloplegics (e.g., scopolamine 0.25% tid) are used to prevent synechiae formation, reduce inflammation, and increase patient comfort.

4. Intraocular pressures should be monitored and secondary glaucoma controlled as needed. (See Glaucoma Section.)

5. Topical corticosteroids are contraindicated during early therapy of a fungal ulcer as they may exacerbate the infection and worsen the prognosis. Topical antifungal agents are typically fungistatic and efficacy may vary. After several weeks of effective antifungal therapy and documented clinical improvement, topical steroids are rarely, but judiciously employed to decrease corneal inflammation and scarring with the continued use of antifungal agents. However, most would agree that steroids are best avoided in a confirmed case of fungal keratitis.

Clinical signs of response to treatment are initially an arrest of progression, decreasing infiltrate size and opacity, blunting of the leading edge of the infiltrate, and resolution of a hypopyon.

Unfortunately, even with early, appropriate, and aggressive treatment, patients with fungal keratitis sometimes proceed to corneal perforation or develop keratoscleritis or endophthalmitis. Penetrating keratoplasties should be considered early in patients not responding to aggressive medical therapy to try and prevent these sight threatening complications. The excision should encompass the entire infiltrate plus 1 mm of clear cornea.

Note: Cyclosporine A has been shown to possess significant antifungal activity and can help prevent allograft rejection in patients incurring corneal transplant after mycotic infections.

Chapter 9

Other Infectious Diseases

ACANTHAMOEBA KERATITIS

Marcus Piccolo

ICD—9: 370.59

THE DISEASE

Pathophysiology

Acanthamoeba keratitis occurs following invasion of the cornea with the free-living protozoa *Acanthamoeba*. The inflammation is intensified by the release of proteolytic enzymes and stimulation of the immune system within the cornea. The organism is capable of existing in two forms: a free-living trophozoite form, which is mobile, proliferates, and feeds on bacteria and other unicellular organisms, and a cyst form, which develops in response to a hostile environment, such as drugs, chemicals (chlorine), temperature, or other adverse stimuli.

Etiology

Keratitis involves the exposure and subsequent infection of the cornea with *Acanthamoeba*. The most common species are *A. castellanii, A. polyphagia*, and *A. rhysodes*. A corneal epithelial break or bacterial coinfection may be necessary for *Acanthamoeba* infection, since the *Acanthamoeba* organism will initially self sustain by ingesting bacteria.

The Patient

Clinical Symptoms

Symptoms include pain, redness, eyelid swelling, foreign body sensation, photophobia, tearing, blepharospasm, and blurred vision if the corneal lesion involves the visual axis. The pain is often severe and out of proportion to the keratitis and the extent of inflammation present. The accentuated pain may be a result of corneal nerve inflammation; however, the same inflammation may reduce the corneal sensation in some patients.

Clinical Signs

The keratitis may begin as an epithelial haze accompanied by persistent epithelial erosions, punctate staining, pseudodendrites, and elevated epithelial lines. The early presentation may be confined to the epithelium. Later in the infection, a central stromal infiltrate, ring infiltrate, or satellite infiltrates may develop. In addition, scleritis, optic neuritis, uveitis, hypopyon, cataract, increased IOP, preauricular lymphadenopathy, and conjunctival follicles may be present. There is typically an absence of neovascularization. The presence of conjunctival follicles, PA nodes, and corneal hypothesia often lead to a misdiagnosis of herpes simplex keratitis.

Demographics

- Acanthamoeba accounts for <1% of all cases of infectious keratitis.
- While *Acanthamoeba* keratitis can occur in any age group, it is most often found in young adults (median age 29) who are immunocompetent.
- Most cases occur in warmer climates during the summer months.

Significant History

A history of trauma or contact lens wear is important. *Acanthamoeba* has been found in contaminated contact lens solutions, hot tubs, lakes, and swimming pools. Inappropriate use of contact lens solutions, including homemade saline or rinsing of lenses in tap water or bottled water, puts a patient at significant risk.

Ancillary Tests

Confocal microscopy of the infected cornea is possibly the best and most accurate method for identifying *Acanthamoeba*. Unfortunately, the instrument may not be readily available in all areas.

Acanthamoeba can be grown on non-nutrient agar with an overlay of *E. coli*, a known food source for the organism.

The organism can be stained with Gram, Giemsa, or Wright stain; however, these stains may not differentiate *Acanthamoeba* from background cells and tissues. Consequently, the fluorescein conjugated lectins that will visualize both the trophozoites and cysts may become a first line stain.

The chemofluorescent dye, Calcofluor white, is often used to visualize the endocysts; however, the trophozoites, which lack cellulose, will not stain with Calcofluor.

Corneal biopsy is often required to make a definitive diagnosis.

If the patient is a contact lens wearer, the lenses and solutions should be cultured.

The Treatment

Treatment of *Acanthamoeba* keratitis is difficult, often with disappointing results. Success depends on rapid detection and early implementation of a combination of anti-amebic agents. Therapy should be continued for 6 to 8 weeks after resolution, which could extend over 18 months in severe cases.

Acanthamoeba should be suspected in any patient with negative corneal cultures for bacteria, fungus, or virus, or in a patient who is not improving despite aggressive medical therapy.

Topical Therapy

Propamidine isethionate (Brolene) 0.1% (not available in the United States, but available OTC in Europe) and Neosporin drops alternated q15 to 60 min for 3 days (around the clock), followed by the same drops alternated q1h during the day and q2h at night for 4 days. Doses are gradually tapered to qid and dibromopropamidine (Brolene) ointment qhs is used during taper of the Brolene drops.

Polyhexamethylene biguanide (PHMB) 0.02% has been used with good results and is considered another first-line agent. The medication is applied topically q1h until an objective and subjective improvement is noted at which time the drug is tapered in a similar fashion to Brolene and Neosporin. PHMB is often used in combination with Brolene and Neosporin.

Topical antifungals such as miconazole 1% or clotrimazole 1% (q1h), combined with oral ketoconazole (200–400 mg/d) or itraconazole (200 mg/d) have been used with some success in combination with the above drugs.

The role of topical steroids in the treatment of *Acanthamoeba* keratitis remains controversial and in general, is not recommended.

Early penetrating keratoplasty has been suggested. However, recurrence in the graft is not uncommon.

Note: Due to the complexity of these patients, referral to a corneal specialist is often necessary.

DEMODICOSIS
Marcus Piccolo
ICD—9: 373.00

THE DISEASE

Pathophysiology

Demodicosis is an infestation and overpopulation of the lash follicles and accompanying sebaceous glands with the mites *Demodex folliculorum* or *Demodex brevis.* Adult mites migrate to gland orifices, where they copulate. The female mite migrates back into the gland where she deposits her egg. Immature mites eventually migrate to the gland orifice. Infestation results in abnormal function of the glands, including blockage of the orifice, and accumulation of keratin. In addition, the mites may consume the glandular epithelium.

Etiology

Overpopulation of the *Demodex* organisms.

The Patient

Clinical Symptoms

While many patients remain asymptomatic, some will report burning and itching of the eyelid margins. These symptoms are typically worse in warmer weather.

Clinical Signs

Clear keratin sleeves are found around the base of the lashes, which is suggestive of *Demodex* in the follicle. Keratin blockage of the meibomian glands may occur. The organism may act as a vector for bacteria, resulting in a concurrent bacterial blepharitis.

Demographics

Demodicosis increases with age. While this condition is rarely seen in children, 90 to 95% of adults over the age of 45 years have some *Demodex* infestation. The human is a natural host for the organism. Involvement in other areas such as the nose, cheeks, external auditory meatus, and forehead may be present.

Significant History

No particular history exists for demodicosis, although, some infestations have been related to poor hygiene, perioral dermatitis, and rosacea. In fact, there appears to be a clinically significant increase of *Demodex* in patients with rosacea, suggesting that this ectoparasite many be involved in the pathogenesis of rosacea.

Ancillary Tests

The mite is an eight legged, spindle-shaped organism, approximately 0.3 to 0.4 mm long, which can only be viewed with microscopic magnification. Epilation of several lashes, which are then floated on a viscous fluid, can be observed with a light microscope. One to two mites found on 16 epilated lashes (4 lashes from each eyelid) is considered normal. Overpopulation is considered when 6 to 8 mites or more are found on 16 epilated lashes.

The Treatment

Treatment is often problematic, but is aimed at reducing the number of mites in the glands. Some topical agents may be irritable to the eye and may not affect organisms deep within the glands. Application of ether to the lid margins with a cotton-tipped applicator will cause organisms within the glands to migrate to the surface. Repeated scrubs 5 minutes later will kill emerging organisms.

The use of bland ophthalmic ointments or ophthalmic antibiotic ointments may prevent the adult mites from copulating during the night, thereby reducing the population.

PHTHIRIASIS PALPEBRARUM

Nicky R. Holdeman

ICD—9: 132.9

THE DISEASE

Pathophysiology

Phthiriasis palpebrarum is a rare cause of blepharoconjunctivitis produced via an infestation of the eyelids by the crab louse, *Phthirus pubis*. Lice feed solely on human blood by piercing the skin, injecting saliva, and then sucking blood. The fecal material and saliva excreted by the parasite results in an inflammatory response.

Etiology

The crab louse is a six-legged ectoparasite that typically prefers the anogenital area, but may also infest facial hair (i.e., beard, mustache, eyebrows, or eyelashes). Transference to the eye may occur by hand contact from the inguinal area, by contaminated clothing, combs, bedding, or towels, or by sexual activities. Children and infants may acquire the disease by close contact with the chest or axillary hair of an infested parent or caretaker.

The Patient

Clinical Symptoms
- Itching
- Burning
- Conjunctival irritation and injection

Clinical Signs
Gross observation usually reveals a brownish discoloration of the eyelid margins. In severe cases, a mixture of blood from the host and feces from the parasite may appear on the lashes, forming a crust. Cilia may be missing or broken.

Salivary secretion from the lice may produce maculae caeruleae (sky-blue spots), which serve as objective evidence of louse bites. The nits (eggs) are usually visible by gross inspection; however, the adult lice are translucent and may be difficult to see without a biomicroscope (adult lice vary in size from 1.0 to 2.0 mm). Infrequently, marked conjunctival injection, follicular conjunctivitis, preauricular lymphadenopathy, and secondary infection of the lice bites may occur. Rare cases of marginal keratitis have been reported. No association has been made between *P. pubis* and louse-borne systemic disease.

Demographics

In general, pediculosis is uncommon among individuals with good hygiene, although all socioeconomic backgrounds are vulnerable. Most cases of pediculosis pubis are seen at venereal disease clinics, as this disease frequently coexists (~30%) with other STDs. Phthiriasis palpebrarum appears somewhat more common in children, especially those living in unhygienic or crowded conditions.

Significant History

- Any known contact with an infested individual or with infested personal articles (e.g., towels, combs, hats, or clothing)?
- Any known exposure or treatment for other STDs?

Ancillary Tests

Phthiriasis palpebrarum is usually a clinical diagnosis best made by slit-lamp examination. However, if needed, the condition can often be confirmed by plucking a lash and examining it with a light microscope.

On Wood's lamp exam, live nits fluoresce white, empty nits fluoresce gray.

The Treatment

The treatment of phthiriasis palpebrarum is often ineffective and prolonged and the ideal regimen has yet to be established. Recommended treatment modalities include:

1. Mechanical removal of the lice and nits with fine forceps may be attempted, if there is a mild infestation and the patient is cooperative.
2. Careful debridement of the lid margins with an alcohol saturated cotton tip applicator.
3. Application of a bland ointment, (e.g., petroleum jelly, yellow mercuric oxide 1%, Lacrilube), to the eyelids tid for 7 to 14 days to smother the lice and nits.
4. Physostigmine 0.25% (e.g., Eserine) ointment bid for 10 to 14 days. Cholinesterase inhibitors act as a respiratory poison to the lice. Contact with the conjunctiva should be avoided as the anticholinesterase agents can have numerous systemic and ocular side effects.
5. Sodium fluorescein, 20% solution, one or two drops on the lid margins, followed by lice and nit removal with a wet cotton swab. Retreatment in 10 to 14 days if needed.
6. Cryotherapy and argon laser phototherapy may be effective but is not widely used.
7. Rarely, trimming heavily infested lashes may be required.

Note: Pediculicides should never be used to treat eyelash infections.

Recurrences will be high until the primary infestation is resolved. All clothes, sheets, linens, and so on need to be thoroughly washed and dried at high temperatures. The patient, family members, sexual contacts, and close companions should be referred for careful examination and treatment for other sites of infestation.

Contaminated cosmetics should be discarded.

Chapter 10

Immune Disease

ANTERIOR UVEITIS

Richard F. Multack, Milan R. Genge, and Leonid Skorin Jr.

ICD—9: 364.0

THE DISEASE

Pathophysiology

Uveitis refers to inflammation of the uveal tract. Anterior uveitis can be divided into iritis, cyclitis (ciliary body inflammation), and iridocyclitis. Anterior uveitis does not include involvement of the pars plana or the posterior segment. Adjacent, nonvascular structures such as the cornea (keratouveitis) and sclera (sclerouveitis) are often affected secondarily in the inflammatory process.

Anterior uveitis can also be divided by its chronicity. Acute uveitis refers to inflammation that lasts for weeks or a few months and resolves once the attack is over. Chronic uveitis may last for many months or years without clearing completely between exacerbations.

Acute and chronic uveitis can be further subdivided into granulomatous and nongranulomatous that is determined by clinical findings. Granulomatous uveitis presents with large, greasy, "mutton-fat" precipitates on the corneal endothelium with large clumps of inflammatory cells present in the anterior chamber because of exuberant macrophage activity. Nongranulomatous uveitis presents with fine cornea endothelial precipitates and anterior chamber activity.

Etiology

The causes of anterior uveitis are multiple and varied. Recent investigations suggest that uveitis is probably not caused by circulating immune complexes, as it was once believed. Most types of anterior uveitis are sterile inflammatory reactions. Underlying associations include ankylosing spondylitis, Reiter's syndrome, Behçet's disease, trauma, psoriatic arthritis, juvenile rheumatoid arthritis, postoperative iritis, glaucomatocyclitic crisis, intraocular lens-induced UGH syndrome (uveitis-glaucoma-hyphema), Fuchs' heterochromic iridocyclitis, sarcoidosis, and idiopathic causes. Infectious causes of anterior uveitis may include Lyme disease, various viral etiologies, syphilis, and tuberculosis.

The Patient

The signs and symptoms depend on the chronicity of the anterior uveitis and whether it is granulomatous or nongranulomatous.

Clinical Symptoms

The patient with an acute anterior uveitis will complain of ocular pain, red eye, photophobia, epiphora, and blurred vision. Pain from anterior uveitis will often be referred to the eyebrow area. These symptoms may be very mild or absent in chronic anterior uveitis.

Clinical Signs

- Cells and flare in the anterior chamber
- Circumcorneal ciliary flush
- Nongranulomatous: fine keratic precipitates on corneal endothelium and anterior chamber
- Granulomatous: greasy, "mutton-fat" precipitates on corneal endothelium and anterior chamber, with iris nodules (Koeppe-clusters of cells on the pupillary border and Busacca-cells on the anterior iris surface)

Subtle Signs

- Miotic pupil
- Hypopyon
- Hyperemia
- Plastic iridocyclitis: fibrin with sluggish or no movement of cells in the anterior chamber
- Spillover: cells in the anterior vitreous
- Low intraocular pressure secondary to cyclitis
- Elevated intraocular pressure secondary to obstruction of the trabecular meshwork
- Cystoid macular edema
- Posterior synechiae
- Endothelial dysfunction with associated corneal edema
- Fibrin pupillary membrane

Demographics

The incidence of anterior uveitis is 12 per 100,000 people. Most patients affected are from 20 to 50 years of age. The inflammatory period will usually last several days to weeks. It is typically unilateral with a history of previous episodes in either eye. Recurrences are common. Some forms of anterior uveitis, such as acute nongranulomatous uveitis secondary to ankylosing spondylitis and Reiter's syndrome, are more often found in men. Chronic anterior uveitis is more common in women. Immunologic and hormonal differences are thought to underlie some specific types of uveitis.

Seronegative spondyloarthropathies (rheumatoid factor negative) that are associated with acute anterior uveitis are often HLA-B27 positive (located on the short arm of chromosome 6). HLA-B27 is positive in 1.4 to 8% of the general population. In patients who present with acute iritis, up to 60% prove to be HLA-B27 positive. Ankylosing spondylitis, Reiter's syndrome, inflammatory bowel disease, psoriatic arthritis, and postinfectious (reactive) arthritis are all included in this group of diseases.

Behçet's disease is associated with HLA-B51. It is a perivascular inflammation of unknown cause that results in a generalized occlusive vasculitis. The Behçet triad includes a hypopyon with iritis, aphthous stomatitis, and genital ulceration. It is less common in the United States and is more common in Japan and Eastern Europe. Eye findings include retinal vasculitis, retinal hemorrhage, macular edema, retinal necrosis, ischemic optic neuropathy, and vitritis. Systemic signs may include erythema nodosum, nondestructive arthritis, inflammatory bowel disease, ulcerative lesions, and central nervous system strokes.

Glaucomacyclitic crisis (Posner-Schlossman syndrome) is a mild uveitis associated with elevated intraocular pressure, corneal edema, fine keratic precipitates, and a slightly dilated pupil. An association with HLA-B54 has been made with this entity.

Lens-associated uveitis or phacoantigenic endophthalmitis is a presumed immune response to lens protein after violation of the lens capsule.

Pseudophakic uveitis may be seen with closed loop anterior chamber intraocular lenses.

Masquerade syndromes, such as syphilis, may present with an anterior uveitis. Syphilis accounts for 1 to 3% of all uveitis cases. Patients will develop anterior uveitis in 5 to 10% of secondary syphilis cases.

Significant History

- History of ocular trauma or surgery
- Recent viral or bacterial disease
- History of underlying immunologic disease

Ancillary Tests

Ocular assessment includes visual acuity, pupil testing, intraocular pressure, slit-lamp examination, and dilated fundus evaluation.

Laboratory studies: CBC with differential, erythrocyte sedimentation rate, chest x-ray, Lyme titer, antinuclear-antibody, RPR, FTA, PPD, human leukocyte antigen (HLA) typing, angiotension converting enzyme, and serum lysozyme.

The Treatment

As the etiology of anterior uveitis is often unknown, treatment is directed to control the inflammation and prevent damage to uveal vasculature that can result in chronic recalcitrant uveitis or secondary side effects, such as posterior synechiae, cataracts, and glaucoma.

Cycloplegic agents are used to relieve pain, decrease synechiae formation, and reduce the permeability of the iris vasculature. Cyclopentolate or homatropine can be used for mild to moderate inflammation, whereas scopolamine or atropine may be used for more severe inflammation.

Corticosteroids can be applied topically, by periocular injection, or systemically. The steroid therapy should never be stopped abruptly because this may lead to severe rebound in inflammation.

Immunosuppressive agents, such as methotrexate or cyclosporine, may be used in resistant cases.

ANKYLOSING SPONDYLITIS

Tammy P. Than

ICD—9: 720.0M

THE DISEASE

Pathophysiology

Ankylosing spondylitis belongs to a group of seronegative spondyloarthropathies in which the rheumatoid factor is absent. Ankylosing spondylitis is an aggressive inflammatory arthropathy with a predilection for the central skeleton affecting the sacroiliac joint most severely. The joints between the spine and pelvis, and joints between the vertebrae of the spine, eventually may fuse.

Etiology

The etiology is unknown but is thought to be multifactorial. HLA-B27 has been found in 93% of patients with ankylosing spondylitis while present in only 6% of controls. In the absence of HLA-B27, genes for other inflammatory conditions may be important in predisposing individuals. Evidence for this is the greater association with other inflammatory conditions such as Crohn's disease or psoriasis. Alternatively, bacterial and viral infections may trigger ankylosing spondylitis. In particular, *Klebsiella pneumoniae*, commonly found in the gastrointestinal tract, is more common in patients with the disease compared to controls. There appears to be a familial pattern as there is a higher incidence of ankylosing spondylitis if there is a positive history in a first-degree relative.

The Patient

Clinical Symptoms

Symptoms usually begin in the early 20s with an onset rarely after the age of 40. Systemic symptoms begin with intermittent hip and/or lower back pain that are worse at night or after inactivity. Bent posture eases the pain, which improves later in the day and with exercise. There may be pain or tenderness in the ribs, shoulder blades, hips, thighs, shins, and heels. The patient may also complain of fatigue, loss of appetite, and general discomfort. Ocular symptoms include pain, redness, and photophobia if uveitis is present.

The disease in women tends to be less severe than in men and may present with neck pain and breast pain in the absence of lower back pain.

Clinical Signs

Uveitis occurs in about 25% of patients with ankylosing spondylitis presenting as an acute, unilateral, nongranulomatous episode. The ocular manifestations may occur prior to joint and skeletal signs, and ankylosing spondylitis accounts for 10 to 33% of all cases of anterior uveitis.

Early on, limited flexibility of the lower spine is noted. Enthesopathy, new bone formation at the attachment of tendons and ligaments, may be noted. Over time, ankylosing spondylitis progresses to involve the entire spine—lordosis (forward curvature) of the lumbar spine, kyphosis (excessive curvature with convexity backward) of the thoracic spine, and hyperextension of the cervical spine. Other joints are involved in about 33% of cases, most frequently presenting with inflammation of the hips, knees, ankles, and shoulders. Tendons and ligaments can also become inflamed. Cardiac complications include valvular disease (e.g., aortic valve stenosis) and aortitis. Ankylosing spondylitis can affect the bones of the rib cage, reducing lung capacity. Patients may have signs of psoriasis or inflammatory bowel disease.

Demographics

The incidence of ankylosing spondylitis is 0.21% of Americans over the age of 15. The incidence is greatest among Native American Indians and Eskimos, and it is rare in African Americans. The peak age of onset is in the mid-20s, although a juvenile form develops around age 8 to 10 years. The male to female ratio is often overestimated because women are frequently underdiagnosed because the disease manifests less severely in the female gender. The ratio is thought to be 2–3:1 (male:female).

Significant History
- Lower back pain in the morning and after inactivity
- Stooped posture
- Sleeping in a fetal position to minimize pain
- Recurrent unilateral uveitis

Ancillary Tests
- CBC—may reveal mild anemia
- HLA-B27—positive
- Erythrocyte sedimentation rate (ESR)—may be elevated during active stage
- C-reactive protein (CRP)—may be elevated during active stage
- Rheumatoid factor—negative
- Antinuclear Antibodies—negative
- Spine and/or pelvis x-ray—look for Romanus lesion—early radiographic sign indicative of disc margin erosion
- Technetium bone scan—more sensitive than plain film x-rays
- Spine mobility measurements
- Electrocardiogram (EKG)

The Treatment

Exercises to strengthen the back muscles to maintain erect posture; to maintain chest expansion; and to maintain or improve spinal mobility should be part of the patient's daily routine. Heat applied to the joints helps reduce joint pain unless active inflammation is present in which case cold packs are preferred. The patient should be encouraged to sleep on a firm mattress with good neck support. A smoking cessation program, if pertinent, should be a priority. Oral nonsteroidal anti-inflammatory agents are the first line of therapeutic intervention. More aggressive management includes sulfasalazine and other disease modifying antirheumatic drugs such as gold salts, methotrexate, azathioprine, and hydroxychloroquine. Intra-articular corticosteroid injections may be beneficial. Topical corticosteroids and cycloplegics are used to manage the anterior uveitis. Approximately 90% of patients remain fully independent with little or no disability.

BEHÇET'S DISEASE
Tammy P. Ihan
ICD—9: 136.1

THE DISEASE
Pathophysiology

Behçet's disease is a rare, nongranulomatous, obliterative vasculitis that is thought to be immune mediated. Antiendothelial cell antibodies are detected in an increased prevalence; T cells, B cells, and neutrophils are infiltrated perivascularly; and the level of endothelin (ET)-1,2 is increased. It affects arteries and veins, resulting in thrombosis. The disease is chronic and multisystemic, characterized by oral and genital mucocutaneous ulcerations, skin rashes, arthritis, thrombophlebitis, uveitis, colitis, and neurologic symptoms.

Etiology

The exact etiology is unknown; however, immune regulation, immunogenetics, vascular abnormalities, or bacterial or viral infection may play a role in the development of Behçet's disease. An infectious cause may be associated with herpes simplex virus I or *Streptococcus sanguis* in which there is autoimmunity or cross-reactivity between the microbe and the oral mucosal antigens. In countries with a high prevalence of Behçet's disease, HLA-B51 has been found in 72% of patients and appears to predispose patients (especially males) to a more severe disease. The association with HLA-B51 has not been demonstrated in the United States. Other trigger factors may include environmental toxins such as heavy metals or pesticides, English walnuts, Gingko nuts, chocolate, and tomatoes.

The Patient

Clinical Symptoms

Prior to the onset of Behçet's disease, the patient may experience a prodrome and report malaise, weight loss, anorexia, general weakness, and headache. During the disease process, the patient will complain of a painful mouth and genital sores, photophobia with a red and painful eye, and joint pain.

Clinical Signs

Behçet's disease waxes and wanes with periods of exacerbation and remission. As time passes, the recurrence frequency decreases and the severity diminishes.

Ocular signs are present in 75% of patients. Uveitis, which may include a small hypopyon, usually follows the onset of oral ulcers by 3 to 4 years, but ocular disease is the initial presentation in 20% of patients. Late-stage ocular complications include neovascularization, glaucoma, cataracts, retinal detachment, vascular occlusive disease, and optic atrophy. Other potential ocular manifestations are sixth-nerve palsy, hemiparesis, visual field loss, idiopathic intracranial hypertension, internuclear ophthalmoplegia, and complications from intracranial artery aneurysms.

There are two common criteria for the diagnosis of Behçet's disease. The International Study Group (ISG; 1990) criteria require the presence of oral ulceration, which may be a limitation. Therefore, some recommend applying the 1987 criteria from the Japanese group in conjunction with the ISG guidelines (Table 10.1).

Demographics

Behçet's disease has a worldwide distribution and is most prevalent (and more virulent) in the Mediterranean, Middle East, and Far East with an estimated incidence of 14–380/100,000. The prevalence in the United States is 0.33/100,000. The predominant age at diagnosis is in the third to fourth decades, with men affected more often and with a more severe course in some regions. Prognosis is poorer with neurological involvement, where there is a 20% mortality rate after 7 years. Chronic morbidity is usual, with ophthalmic involvement as the leading cause. The effects of the disease appear to be cumulative.

Significant History

- Recurrent oral ulcerations
- Genital sores
- Recurrent uveitis
- Hypopyon

Ancillary Tests

Ocular evaluation includes assessment of the anterior chamber and intraocular pressure. A dilated fundus examination should be performed to rule out occlusive disease, vasculitis, retinal detachment, and optic nerve disease.

▶ TABLE 10.1 Two Criteria for the Diagnosis of Behçet's Disease*

	International Study Group (ISG) Criteria for Diagnosis of Behçet's Disease	Behçet's Disease Research Committee of Japan Criteria	
Major Features	Recurrent oral ulceration (three occurrences within a 12-month period)	Recurrent oral ulcers	
		Skin lesions	Erythema nodosum Subcutaneous thrombophlebitis Folliculitis Acneform lesions Cutaneous hypersensitivity
		Ocular Signs	Uveitis Chorioretinitis
		Genital Ulcers	
Minor Features	Recurrent genital ulceration Ocular involvement (uveitis or vasculitis) Skin lesions Positive pathergy test (see Ancillary Tests under Behçet's Disease)	Arthritis without deformity Gastrointestinal lesions Epididymitis Vascular lesions CNS symptoms	
Diagnosis	1 major + 2 minor	Complete	4 major
		Incomplete	3 major 2 major + 2 minor Typical ocular symptom + 1 major or 2 minor
		Suspected	2 major OR 1 major + 2 minor

Data from Behçet's Disease Research Committee of Japan. Behçet's disease: Guide to diagnosis of Behçet's disease. Jpn J Ophthalmol 1974:18:291–4; and International Study Group for Behçet's Disease. Criteria for diagnosis of Behçet's disease. Lancet 1990;335:1078–80.

There is no diagnostic laboratory test specific for Behçet's disease, but the following may be helpful:

- CBC with differential—anemia observed in some patients with chronic disease
- Erythrocyte sedimentation rate (ESR)—may be elevated during active stage
- C-reactive protein (CRP)—may be elevated during active stage
- Cerebral spinal fluid analysis—protein level elevated
- Rheumatoid factor—negative
- Antinuclear antibodies—negative
- IgA—elevated
- Complement 3 and 4 levels—elevated
- Lipid levels—may be elevated, predisposing the patient to thromboses
- Pathergy test ("skin prick")—outstanding feature of Behçet's disease but infrequently performed; following a needle prick, the puncture site becomes inflamed and

pustular within 24 to 48 hours; test is positive in 24 to 79% of patients with Behçet's disease

The Treatment

There is no established standard therapeutic regimen for Behçet's disease.

Uveitis is managed with topical corticosteroids and cycloplegia. Laser photocoagulation may be used to manage retinal neovascularization. Ocular management may also include cataract surgery and vitrectomy. Skin manifestations are treated with topical corticosteroids or antibiotic solutions. The systemic disease is successfully managed with immunosuppressants such as levamisole, colchicine, dapsone, tacrolimus, azathioprine, chlorambucil, cyclosporine A, and cyclophosphamide. Interferon α 2A and B are useful and are thought to have antiviral, immunomodulatory, and antiproliferative properties. Acyclovir may be effective if the etiology is herpes simplex. Exercise, such as swimming or walking, is beneficial to keep joints strong and flexible.

ATOPIC EYE DISEASE
Christopher Quinn and Leonid Skorin Jr.

SEASONAL ALLERGY
ICD—9: 477.9

THE DISEASE

The conjunctiva is a thin mucous membrane that lines the posterior surface of the eyelids and extends over the globe to the corneal limbus. It has a rich vascular supply and is an important, immunologically active barrier to pathogens. Seasonal allergic conjunctivitis is a mild to moderate manifestation of the immune response of the conjunctiva to a wide variety of antigens. Patients can experience symptoms on a seasonal basis when exposed to antigens or can have symptoms year round (perennial).

Pathophysiology

Once primary exposure and sensitization to antigens occurs, repeat exposure to the antigen initiates the inflammatory cascade. Degranulation of mast cells releases histamine and related chemical mediators. Mast cells migrate into the conjunctival epithelium and are the primary cell type involved in the inflammatory response. These inflammatory mediators induce vasodilation, tissue edema, and nerve stimulation.

Etiology

The clinical manifestations of allergic conjunctivitis are the direct result of the immune response to seasonal exposure to ragweed, pollens, dander, dust, or mold spores.

The Patient

Clinical Symptoms

Patients with seasonal allergic conjunctivitis (SAC) complain of conjunctival hyperemia, tearing, and itching. Symptoms are transient, recurrent, and often follow seasonal patterns.

Clinical Signs

Patients develop variable degrees of conjunctival hyperemia. Conjunctival chemosis can also occur. A papillary conjunctival response can be seen.

Demographics

SAC is a common condition affecting all types of patients.

Significant History

- History of atopy
- Exposure to allergens

Ancillary Tests

Diagnosis is clinical and ancillary testing is not required.

The Treatment

Conservative treatment includes cold compresses, topical lubrication, and vasoconstrictors. Avoidance of antigens known to incite the symptoms is also appropriate. Pharmacologic treatment is the mainstay of therapy in symptomatic patients. Topical vasoconstrictor/antihistamine combinations cause vascular constriction, decrease vascular permeability, and reduce ocular itching by blocking H1 histamine receptors but have a short duration of action. Topical antihistamines competitively bind with histamine receptor sites and reduce itching and vasodilation. Levocabastine hydrochloride 0.05% and azelastine hydrochloride 0.05% are topical-selective H1 histamine receptor antagonists that have shown to be effective in relieving the signs and symptoms of allergic conjunctivitis. Emedastine difumarate 0.05%, a selective H1 antagonist, may be more efficacious than levocabastine in reducing chemosis, eyelid swelling, and other signs and symptoms associated with SAC in both adult and pediatric patients. Olopatidine is a selective H1 histamine antagonist that also has mast cell–stabilizing properties. Olopatadine is effective in reducing the signs and symptoms of allergic conjunctivitis. Olopatadine may more effectively target the subtype of mast cell found in the conjunctiva than other mast cell–stabilizing agents. Ketotifen is also a mast-cell stabilizer that acts as a histamine antagonist. Olopatidine is more effective in relieving itching and redness associated with acute allergic conjunctivitis compared to ketorolac or ketotifen.

Topical mast-cell stabilizers inhibit the degranulation of mast cells that limits the release of inflammatory mediators. Nedocromil 2% has been shown to be an effective treatment for SAC. Pemirolast 0.1% is approved to relieve the itching associated with allergic conjunctivitis and, when used twice a day, is as effective as and more comfortable than nedocromil 2%.

Topical nonsteroidal anti-inflammatory drugs (NSAIDs) offer an alternative treatment option. Ketorolac tromethamine 0.5% and diclofenac sodium 0.1% have been shown to be effective in reducing the signs and symptoms associated with allergic conjunctivitis, although only ketorolac is FDA approved to treat allergic conjunctivitis.

Topical steroids inhibit the inflammatory process (e.g., edema, capillary dilation, and fibroblast proliferation). Steroids are widely employed in the treatment of acute ocular allergic disease. While effective in relieving the acute symptoms of allergy, their use should be limited to the acute suppression of symptoms because of the potential for adverse side effects with protracted use. Chronic unsupervised use of topical corticosteroids can result in the well-documented complications of posterior subcapsular cataract formation and elevated intraocular pressure (IOP). Newly developed "site-specific" steroids have been designed to reduce the complications generally associated with topical steroid use. Loteprednol, available as 0.2% and 0.5% concentrations, has been shown to be an effective treatment as prophylaxis for SAC. Both concentrations of loteprednol have a very low propensity to result in elevated IOP.

Systemic antihistamines may be useful in certain cases of allergic response with associated lid edema, dermatitis, rhinitis, or sinusitis. Care should be exercised in their use because of the sedating and anticholinergic effects of some first-generation antihistamine drugs. Patients should be warned of these potential side effects. Newer, nonsedating antihistamines are less likely to cause sedation but may result in increased ocular surface dryness.

ATOPIC DERMATITIS
ICD—9: 691.8

THE DISEASE

Pathophysiology

Approximately 80% of patients with atopic dermatitis have elevated levels of serum IgE. The level of IgE is most elevated when other intercurrent atopic disorders are present. In addition, defective cell-mediated immunity as manifested by increased susceptibility to viral and fungal infections is also present in atopy.

Decreased numbers and diminished function of T lymphocytes usually correlate with disease activity. Defective chemotactic activity of neutrophils and monocytes is also found.

Also identified in atopic dermatitis is the blockage of β-adrenergic receptors with secondary decrease of intracellular cyclic adenosine monophosphate (leukocyte cyclic AMP).

Etiology

Atopy is a form of hypersensitivity whose immunologic factors relate to potential genetically mediated defects in metabolism or biochemical response to exogenous substances.

The Patient

Symptoms and signs of atopy include dermatitis and keratoconjunctivitis.

Clinical Symptoms

The patient with atopy will complain of intense pruritus (itching) of skin and eyes with partial relief from rubbing.

Clinical Signs

1. **Prominent Signs**
   - Infantile phase (birth to 2 years): facial erythema and crusting; extensor extremity lichenification (leathery induration and thickening); exudative papules on forehead
   - Childhood phase (ages 2 to 12 years): xerosis (dryness) of skin; flexural extremity lichenification
   - Adolescent or adult phase (after 12 years): chronic relapsing dermatitis; immediate skin test reactivity; dermographism
2. **Ocular Signs**
   - Eyelid lichenification
   - Weeping eczematous lesions
   - Eversion or stenosis of lacrimal puncta
   - Dennie-Morgan fold—double lower lid fold
   - Bilateral keratoconjunctivitis
   - Papillary conjunctival hypertrophy
   - Superior corneal shield ulcer
   - Corneal neovascularization
   - Symblepharon
   - Entropion
   - Trichiasis
   - Keratoconus
   - Anterior and posterior subcapsular cataracts in up to 25% of patients

Demographics

The prevalence of atopic dermatitis is from 2 to 5% in the general population. It typically develops before age 5 years (90% of cases) and most often by 1 year of age (60%). There is a family history of atopic dermatitis, asthma, or hay fever in 70% of patients. There is a spontaneous remission rate of 40% by age 5 years.

Significant History
- Chronic, pruritic, erythematous inflammation of the skin
- Asthma
- Allergic rhinitis (hay fever)

Ancillary Tests
- Ocular and skin assessment includes visual acuity, slit-lamp exam, eversion of upper eyelids, and keratometry or corneal topography to identify keratoconus
- Evaluation of hands, extensor, and flexor surfaces for dermatitis and lichenification
- Laboratory studies: Serum IgE level, evaluation of skin test reactivity
- Histopathology of skin samples will show hyperkeratosis, parakeratosis, acanthosis, and intercellular accumulations of fluid. The epidermis and dermis are infiltrated by lymphocytes, monocytes, and macrophages

The Treatment

Skin therapy includes avoiding inciting agents and using moisturizing agents and topical fluorinated corticosteroids, such as triamcinolone or betamethasone and topical antibiotics. In more severe cases, oral corticosteroids, such as high-dose prednisone, may initially be necessary. In chronic cases, low-dose therapy of 5 to 10 mg per day may be sufficient. Oral antihistamines may be of help in cases of severe pruritus.

Ocular therapy may include combination antihistamine/mast-cell stabilizers such as olopatadine 0.1%, two times a day, or mast-cell stabilizers such as lodoxamide 0.1%, four times a day. Topical decongestants may also be of help.

In more severe cases, topical steroids such as loteprednol etabonate 0.2%, four to six times a day, and antibiotic ointment such as erythromycin ointment, three times a day in conjunction with a cycloplegic agent and cool compresses, may relieve many of the ocular symptoms.

ATOPIC KERATOCONJUNCTIVITIS (AKC)
ICD—9: 372.05

THE DISEASE

The conjunctiva is the mucous membrane for the eye and can exhibit a variety of manifestations of immunologic dysregulation and subsequent inflammatory reactions. Atopic keratoconjunctivitis is a rare but potentially sight-threatening condition caused by a complex immunologic response and is nearly always accompanied by corneal involvement.

Pathophysiology

AKC is a complex yet to be fully understood condition that most likely represents the result of both immediate (type I) and delayed (type IV) hypersensitivity reactions. Chronic infiltration of the conjunctiva with T-cells and eosinophils, and the release of their associated inflammatory mediators (cytokines, chemokines), result in the clinical characteristics observed. Neutrophils may also play a role in the inflammatory response. Pathologic changes in the conjunctiva ensue. Toxic eosinophil granule proteins such as major basic protein (MBP) and eosinophil cationic protein (ECP) may accumulate under the epithelial basement membrane and result in the sight-threatening complications of persistent corneal erosions and ulcerations.

Etiology

The etiology of AKC remains unknown.

The Patient

Clinical Symptoms

Patients experience bilateral symmetric itching and tearing. Some patients develop a stringy mucous discharge. In cases of corneal ulceration or erosion, pain and photophobia as well as vision loss may occur. Some patients experience seasonal exacerbations while other patients may be able to identify allergens associated with an increase in symptoms. Late symptoms may include reduced vision from corneal scarring.

Clinical Signs

The conjunctiva develops hyperemia and can become noticeably thickened. A papillary conjunctival reaction is common on the tarsal conjunctiva. The lower eyelids are typically more involved than the upper eyelids. Horner-Trantu's dots may appear as multiple small discreet white spots that form under the epithelial surface at the limbus. These represent accumulations of eosinophils. Chronic tissue changes associated with AKC include conjunctival scarring, fornix foreshortening, and symblepharon formation. Up to 75% of patients develop corneal complications associated with AKC, and these are commonly associated with loss of vision. Corneal findings include persistent keratopathy, corneal neovascularization, corneal scarring, and the development of keratoconus. AKC has also been associated with a higher incidence of cortical cataract formation (10% of cases). Patients with atopic keratoconjunctivitis have depressed T-cell function and may develop staphylococcal blepharitis, meiboimitis, and herpetic keratitis as secondary complications.

Rhegmatogenous retinal detachment (equivalent to traumatic detachment) has been linked to AKC because of vitreal degeneration resulting from excessive eye rubbing because of itching.

Demographics

The age of peak incidence is between 30 and 50 years. Males appear to be more commonly affected then females. It is reported in 25 to 40% of patients with atopic dermatitis.

Significant History

- Previous history of atopy
- History of multiple allergies including those to food, eczema, allergic rhinitis, and asthma
- History of atopic dermatitis

Ancillary Tests

Ocular assessment includes visual acuity, pupil testing, slit-lamp evaluation, tonometry, and dilated fundus examination. Ancillary testing is generally not useful in diagnosing AKC. Conjunctival biopsy can help differentiate AKC from cicatricial pemphigoid. Conjunctival biopsy specimens reveal excessive eosinophils, mast cells, and goblet cells. Conjunctival biopsy specimens can also help to histologically differentiate AKC from cicatricial pemphigoid by the presence of basement membrane antibodies or complement components in cicatricial pemphigoid.

The Treatment

Patient should avoid exposure to any allergen they have identified as suspected to cause exacerbations. Lubrication with nonpreserved artificial tears can help dilute allergens and protect the ocular surface. Cold compresses and topical antihistamines may help control itching. Oral antihistamines may cause additional drying of the ocular surface but may be needed to control intense itching. For acute episodes or during periods of exacerbation, topical and or oral steroids may be required to relieve symptoms. Use of a topical steroid (loteprednol) that is less likely to cause elevated intraocular pressure may be preferred because some patients require prolonged treatment. Topical mast-cell stabilizers and/or combination antihistamine/mast-cell stabilizers should be used as long-term maintenance therapy. Topical cyclosporine has demonstrated effectiveness in reducing the signs and symptoms of AKC in cases that are recalcitrant to traditional treatments. In addition, treatment with topical nonfluorinated steroid cream applied to the skin of the eyelids may be needed to control eczema reactions. Plasmapheresis may be an alternative for patients with severe disease unresponsive to other treatment.

Patients who develop keratoconus may require penetrating keratoplasty for visual rehabilitation. If cataracts develop, cataract extraction may be needed to improve visual acuity.

VERNAL KERATOCONJUNCTIVITIS (VKC)

ICD—9: 372.13 - Vernal conjunctivitis
ICD—9: 370.32 - Limbal and corneal involvement in vernal conjunctivitis

THE DISEASE

The conjunctiva is a thin mucous membrane that lines the posterior surface of the eyelids and extends over the globe to the corneal limbus. It has a rich vascular supply and is an important and immunologically active barrier to pathogens. Immune dysregulation causes a spectrum of conjunctival conditions including vernal keratoconjunctivitis. VKC is a severe conjunctival inflammation that can be associated with sight-threatening corneal complications.

Pathophysiology

VKC is an immunologic disorder that likely involves both type I (immediate) and type IV (delayed-type hypersensitivity) responses. VKC is primarily a Th2 lymphocyte-mediated disease. Mast cells, eosinophils, and their mediators play major roles in producing the clinical manifestation of VKC. In addition to typical Th2-derived cytokines, chemokines, growth factors, and enzymes are overexpressed in the conjunctiva of VKC patients. Furthermore, structural cells such as epithelial cells and fibroblasts are involved both in the inflammatory process and in the tissue remodeling phase, ultimately resulting in the formation of giant papillae (diameter >1 mm). Corneal changes likely result from the effect of inflammatory cells and the release of mediators that are found in high concentrations in the conjunctival epithelium and substania propria.

Etiology

The etiology of VKC is unknown.

The Patient

Clinical Symptoms

Patients with VKC complain of intense bilateral itching. In addition, a stringy, mucus discharge is often present. Visual acuity can be affected, especially if patients experience corneal complications or if mucus strands transiently cross the visual axis. Patients can also report foreign body sensation from large papillae or mucus in the tear film. Symptoms typically wax and wane with periods of exacerbation occurring during warmer spring and summer months and decreased symptoms during fall and winter months.

Clinical Signs

Two forms of VKC are generally recognized, palpebral and limbal. In the palpebral form, large papillae develop on the superior tarsal conjunctiva. The papillae are diffuse and can have flattened tops. In the limbal form, gelatinous nodules form in a thickened limbal conjunctiva. These nodules can have small white dots (Horner-Trantas' dots), which are accumulations of eosinophils. Many patients have both limbal and palpebral VKC. Prominent mucus discharge is often present and can adhere to the giant papillae. In some cases, the discharge can precede the development of giant papillae. The most common corneal finding is punctate keratitis, which can lead to further epithelial breakdown and the development of frank corneal ulceration (shield ulcer). Shield ulcers are typically located in the superior one-third of the cornea and tend to have a horizontally oval shape with sharp borders. Shield ulcers are rarely painful. These ulcers are likely the result of epithelial breakdown from exposure to inflammatory mediators or from direct trauma from the giant papillae. Corneal lesions are found in only 3% of severe forms and up to 50% of palpebral forms of VKC. About 30% of patients who develop corneal involvement will have decreased visual acuity. Patients with VKC also have an increased incidence of keratoconus, pellucid marginal degeneration, and cataracts.

Demographics

VKC is a condition that affects younger patients with peak incidence occurring between ages 8 and 12. Younger patients tend to be predominately male; however, this sex predilection may be reduced with increasing age of onset. The majority of affected patients are under the age of 20 years. The average duration of vernal conjunctivitis is 4 years, and most patients tend to "outgrow" the condition by age 30. The disease is more common in dry, warm climates or in areas with polluted air. In more temperate climates, vernal conjunctivitis tends to be seasonal with symptoms increasing in the spring and decreasing in the fall.

Significant History

- Personal or family history of allergy

Ancillary Tests

Ocular assessment includes visual acuity, pupil testing, slit-lamp evaluation, tonometry, and dilated fundus examination. VKC is a clinical diagnosis.

The Treatment

Treatment of VKC is designed to reduce the potential for sight-threatening complications, minimize the pathologic changes in the conjunctiva, and relieve the patient's symptoms. Cold compresses and lubrication with nonpreserved artificial tears can help protect the ocular surface and offer symptomatic relief in patients with mild disease. Removal of mucus from the conjunctival surface can also provide relief of foreign body sensation.

There are a variety of pharmacologic agents that can be used to modulate the dysfunctional immune response seen in VKC. Topical mast-cell stabilizers produce significant symptomatic relief and, because of their lack of significant adverse effects, are the mainstay of chronic therapy. Lodoxamide and nedocromil have both been shown to be more effective than cromolyn sodium.

In severe cases or during periods of exacerbation, topical steroids should be used as adjunctive therapy. Caution should be exercised with the use of topical steroids because chronic unsupervised use can lead to glaucoma and cataracts. Some patients become "steroid dependent" and may require chronic therapy. In addition, the use of topical steroids in patients with a compromised ocular surface can increase the risk of secondary bacterial or fungal infection. Extreme caution is warranted when using steroids in patients with shield ulcers. Use of a topical steroid that has less of a propensity to cause elevated intraocular pressure may be of value. Topically applied nonsteroidal anti-inflammatory drugs (NSAIDs) are also effective in relieving symptoms in patients with VKC. In patients who have severe disease, topical cyclosporine has demonstrated effectiveness in relieving signs and symptoms of VKC. In patients who are refractory to conventional treatment, a short course of low-dose topical mitomycin-C can improve the signs and symptoms of VKC.

GIANT PAPILLARY CONJUNCTIVITIS (GPC)
ICD—9: 372.30

THE DISEASE

The conjunctiva is a thin mucous membrane that lines the posterior surface of the eyelids and extends over the globe to the corneal limbus. It has a rich vascular supply and is an important, immunologically active barrier to pathogens. Giant papillary conjunctivitis is a severe conjunctival inflammation that occurs most commonly in patients who wear contact lenses.

Pathophysiology

Patients with GPC have an increase in inflammatory cells (lymphocytes, mast cells, eosinophils, plasma cells, basophils) in the epithelium and substania propria of the conjunctiva. GPC represents a delayed type IV hypersensitivity reaction. These cells release a variety of chemical inflammatory mediators that act locally, causing vasodilation, edema, and increased mucus production. Structural cells such as epithelial cells and fibroblasts are involved both in the inflammatory process and in tissue remodeling, ultimately resulting in the formation of giant papillae. Patients who develop GPC have high tear film levels of IgE.

Etiology

The etiology of GPC remains unclear. Evidence exists to suggest an immune response is responsible for the tissue changes seen in patients with GPC. Controversy exists over the cause of the inflammatory response. Evidence exists to suggest the inflammatory response is elicited by an immune reaction to proteins from the lacrimal fluid that are presumably denatured by lens-hygiene solutions and attach to the contact lens when placed in the eye. Deposited on the surface of the lens, these proteins act as antigens, to which antibodies then bind. Mechanical trauma to the upper tarsal conjunctiva is also likely to play a role in the development of GPC.

The Patient

Clinical Symptoms
Patients who develop GPC exhibit a predictable set of symptoms. The patient wears his or her contact lenses without complications for weeks or months and then, suddenly, a problem develops. Most cases are bilateral although unilateral and asymmetric GPC can occur. Patients typically complain of itching, burning, chafing, increased mucus discharge, increased contact lens movement with blinking, decreased contact lens wearing time and blurring of vision when wearing their contact lenses. In severe cases, patients

will complain of eyelid swelling and eyelid drooping. Symptoms are generally absent when contact lens wear is withdrawn.

Clinical Signs
GPC is divided clinically into four stages:

- Stage I. There are no visible changes of the papillae. There may be some minimal mucus and mild itching after the contact lens is removed. The lens comfort is good and vision remains good also.
- Stage II. The papillae are starting to form and enlarge up to a 0.5 mm diameter. There is a moderate amount of mucus and redness of the palpebral conjunctiva. The contact lens will be mildly coated, and wearing comfort is slightly decreased. Visual acuity through the lens remains good.
- Stage III. Papillae have increased to 0.7 mm in diameter. Mucus strands or globs are present, and the contact lens is moderately to heavily coated with a corresponding markedly decreased lens wearing comfort. Vision is variable.
- Stage IV. The papillae have a diameter greater than 0.7 mm, and there is copious mucus discharge with the eyelids stuck together. There is pain on contact lens insertion with excessive movement and often off-center positioning of the lens (high-riding with the lids). Lenses are unwearable, and vision is markedly diminished.

Prominent Signs
- Conjunctival hyperemia
- Mucus discharge causes the eyelids to stick together and limits the mobility of the contact lens during blinking and eye movements
- Giant papillae (cobblestones) of the upper tarsal conjunctiva
- Secondary eyelid edema and ptosis
- Scarring of conjunctiva in advanced cases
- Contact lens coated with a grayish-white film that makes it look dry and dull

Demographics

Most patients are soft contact lens wearers (47.5%) with rigid contact lens wearers being less affected (21.6%). GPC has been reported in patient's ocular prosthesis, exposed sutures from corneal surgery, exposed buckling material from retinal detachment surgery, eyes with corneal deposits of keratin and calcium, band keratopathy, or filtering bleb.

Tear film break-up time, the type of ametropia, and keratometry are not risk factors.

Significant History
- Contact lens wearer
- Improper or poor contact lens hygiene
- History of seasonal allergies
- Younger age

Ancillary Tests

Ocular assessment includes visual acuity, pupil testing, slit-lamp evaluation, tonometry, and dilated fundus examination. Diagnosis of GPC is primarily clinical.

The Treatment

Primary treatment of GPC is to discontinue contact lens wear or eliminate exposure to any offending foreign material. Pharmacologic treatment with topical mast-cell stabilizers can help speed resolution of conjunctival papillae and hasten a return to successful contact lens wear. These agents inhibit the degranulation of mast cells, which limits the release of inflammatory mediators, including histamine, neutrophil and eosinophil chemotactic factors, and platelet-activating factor. In patients who are symptomatic without wearing contact lenses, a short course of topical steroid may be useful in reducing symptoms. Chronic or unsupervised steroid use should be avoided because of the potential for the serious adverse effects such as cataract formation and increased IOP. Loteprednol has been demonstrated to be an effective treatment for GPC and has less of a propensity to cause elevated IOP.

Improved contact lens hygiene, decreased wearing times, and frequent lubrication may also allow limited contact lens wear. When GPC has resolved, using contact lens materials with different wetting properties, edge thickness, and lens design are all strategies for preventing it from recurring. Frequent replacement of contact lenses can also reduce the risk of recurrent GPC.

JUVENILE RHEUMATOID ARTHRITIS (JRA)
Richard F. Multack, Milan R. Genge, and Leonid Skorin Jr.

ICD—9: 714.30

THE DISEASE
Pathophysiology

Juvenile rheumatoid arthritis is an autoimmune disease that results in inflammation of the synovia, an oily fluid that lubricates the joints. It is the most common systemic disease associated with iridocyclitis in the pediatric age group. Risk factors for developing uveitis include a positive antinuclear antibody (ANA), being female, and pauciarticular onset. Uveitis will generally develop within 5 years of the onset of the joint disease. The eye may be white with or without pain. The uveitis is often bilateral. Analysis will often reveal a positive ANA, negative rheumatoid factor (RF), and an elevated erythrocyte sedimentation rate (ESR). Based on the mode of onset of the disease and the extent of joint involvement during the first 6 weeks, the following three subgroups of JRA are recognized:

1. The monoarticular or pauciarticular subgroup involves four or fewer joints and constitutes 68.3% of cases. Type 1 is seen in girls less than 5 years of age who have up to a 25% chance of developing chronic iridocyclitis. Type 2 is seen in older boys and has a

high association with HLA-B27. These patients are likely to develop acute recurrent iridocyclitis. This subgroup has a relatively high risk of developing uveitis.
2. The polyarticular subgroup affects five or more joints at onset and constitutes 21.9% of cases. This subgroup has a moderate risk of developing uveitis.
3. The systemic onset subgroup results in high remittent fever and at least one of the following features: generalized lymphadenopathy, fever of unknown origin, hepatomegaly, splenomegaly, pericarditis, and a transient maculopapular rash, which is most prominent on the trunk and limbs. This subgroup constitutes 6.6% of cases. The risk of developing uveitis in this subgroup is low.

Etiology

The exact etiology of JRA is not known, although various genetic markers have been identified. These include HLA-DR5 and HLA-DPw2.

The Patient

Symptoms and signs, including that of anterior uveitis, depend on which particular subgroup of JRA the patient has. Still's triad of low-grade uveitis, band keratopathy, and cataracts are found more often in pauciarticular JRA, but can be found in any variety. As mentioned earlier, the eye is often white and not inflamed. There may or may not be associated pain, blurring, or photophobia.

Clinical Symptoms
Most children with JRA present with increased irritability, fatigue, exhaustion, and the reluctance to move a swollen and tender extremity or to walk. The child may also complain of blurred vision or may have a white pupil as seen by the parent or teacher. The anterior uveitis associated with JRA may not cause the patient to seek medical attention. The patient may be asymptomatic, and the eye may not show conjunctival inflammation, but the anterior chamber may be greatly inflamed. Unchecked inflammation can lead to choroidal vascular damage, secondary glaucoma because of the formation of peripheral anterior synechiae and/or posterior synechiae, and accelerated cataract formation. A delay in the diagnosis can lead to a poorer prognosis if silent ocular damage is allowed to continue untreated. The long-term outcome will correlate with the severity of the damage present at the time of the initial diagnosis.

Clinical Signs
1. Nonocular Signs
   - Low-grade fever
   - Swollen and tender joint or joints
2. Ocular Signs
   - Clinically silent in up to 50% of cases
   - Nongranulomatous iridocyclitis
   - Dyscoria from posterior synechia
   - Band keratopathy
   - Cataracts—up to 50% of cases

- Secondary glaucoma
- Macular edema and macular folds

Demographics

The peak incidence of JRA is between 1 and 4 years of age, but it can appear throughout childhood. The incidence is approximately 11 cases per 100,000 individuals. The ratio of affected females to males is 2:1. The incidence of bilateral ocular involvement varies between 67 and 89%.

Significant History

- Swollen and tender joints
- White pupil

Ancillary Tests

Ocular assessment includes visual acuity, pupil testing, slit-lamp evaluation, tonometry, and dilated fundus examination.

A screening slit-lamp examination should be performed every 3 months in ANA-positive pauciarticular and polyarticular JRA children whose age of onset was under 7 years. Screenings should be performed every 6 months in pauciarticular or polyarticular JRA children who are ANA negative or whose age of onset was over 7 years of age. Children who develop systemic onset JRA should be examined every 12 months. If no uveitis is discovered after 4 years, the ANA-positive children whose onset was less than 7 years of age can be seen every 6 months, and all patients whose onset was after 7 years of age can be seen annually. After 7 years from the time of onset, all patients are considered to be at low risk for developing uveitis and can be seen yearly from that point onward.

Laboratory studies: The incidence of a positive ANA ranges from 71 to 93% in JRA patients with uveitis, compared with 30% in those without uveitis.

The RF is usually negative. The ESR, C-reactive protein, and immune complexes are useful as nonspecific indicators of disease activity.

The knee is the joint most commonly affected, and a routine knee examination and x-ray can be done in cases where JRA is suspected.

The Treatment

The current trend is to treat even minimal levels of ocular inflammation. It is believed that a chronic, low-grade inflammation can inflict significant damage to the uveal vasculature. More severe and recurrent uveitis requires topical corticosteroids, cycloplegics, periocular injections of depot-steroids, oral nonsteroidal anti-inflammatory agents, oral corticosteroids, or immunosuppressive drugs such as low-dose methotrexate.

Band keratopathy can be removed by scraping or with chelating agents such as disodium EDTA.

Glaucoma is managed as any secondary form of glaucoma. Standard glaucoma surgeries are often unsuccessful. Anti-fibrotics (5-fluorouracil, mitomycin-C) and aqueous drainage devices are usually required.

In those patients who develop cataracts, lensectomy with vitrectomy and no intraocular lens placement may be indicated. Prior to cataract extraction, the eye should be quiet for 3 months, the anterior chamber angle should be evaluated for synechiae, and adequate anti-inflammation and immunosuppressive therapy should be used perioperatively.

PARS PLANITIS
Tammy P. Than

ICD—9: 363.21

THE DISEASE
Pathophysiology

Pars planitis is a chronic inflammation characterized by cells and debris in the vitreous with exudates overlying the peripheral retina, ora serrata, or pars plana ciliaris. Pars planitis is a more specific clinical entity than intermediate uveitis, which is a broad term referring to inflammation of the anterior vitreous with or without the presence of pars plana exudation. Histocompatibility gene typing reveals that HLA-DR15 (suballele of HLA-DR2) is present in 50 to 64% of patients with pars planitis. Increased frequencies of several other human leukocyte antigens have been noted, including HLA-B8, HLA-B51, HLA-DR17, and HLA-DR2, which suggests an immunogenetic predisposition to pars planitis.

Etiology

The etiology and pathogenesis of pars planitis remain unknown. It may be an autoimmune reaction against the vitreous, peripheral retina, and ciliary body. Approximately 55% of cases are idiopathic while 45% of cases are associated with systemic disease. The two most common associations are multiple sclerosis and sarcoidosis. Pars planitis has also been reported in patients with retinitis pigmentosa, cat scratch disease, Epstein-Barr virus, tuberculosis, Lyme disease, ocular lymphoma, and syphilis. The younger age group (5 to 15 years) has been found to have an increased incidence of asthma and atopy. The course and outcome of pars planitis appear to be the same with or without an associated underlying systemic disease. Between 80 and 90% of patients maintain a visual acuity of 20/40 or better in the less involved eye over time.

The Patient

Clinical Symptoms

The symptoms may be so mild that pars planitis may go undetected for several years until young adulthood. The patient may complain of floaters and blurred vision. Pain, photophobia, and ocular redness are usually absent or minimal.

Clinical Signs

The clinical signs, which are bilateral in up to 80% of cases and may wax and wane for 15 to 30 years, include:

- Anterior vitreous cells
- Peripheral retinal snowballs (free-floating yellow-white exudates)
- Snowbanks (layered vitreous exudates over the inferior pars plana and ora serrata)
- Variable degree of peripheral retinal periphlebitis
- Absent or mild anterior chamber reaction

Numerous complications result secondary to pars planitis. The three most common are cystoid macular edema, which is usually the cause of decreased vision; cataracts, either secondary to inflammation or corticosteroid usage; and epiretinal membrane formation. Snowbanks are frequently vascularized, which increases the risk of vitreous hemorrhage and may also cause retinal traction leading to a retinal tear and rhegmatogenous retinal detachment. Other possible findings include retinal or choroidal neovascularization, posterior vitreous detachment, optic nerve edema, open angle glaucoma, and neovascular glaucoma. Anterior segment findings include band keratopathy and infrequent posterior synechiae.

Demographics

Pars planitis is a disease of children and young adults that has a bimodal age distribution with peaks at 5 to 15 years and also at 20 to 40 years. There appears to be a slight predilection for males in the younger group and slightly more females in the older group. The average age of diagnosis is 26 years. Pars planitis accounts for up to 15% of uveitis cases in adults. Prevalence in children is higher, accounting for up to 27% of cases with uveitis.

Significant History

- Insidious onset and may be asymptomatic for several years during childhood
- Increased floaters in younger patient
- Blurred vision in younger patient

Ancillary Tests

Ocular examination requires careful evaluation of the anterior chamber. A significant anterior chamber reaction may be indicative of a diffuse uveitis. A dilated fundus evaluation utilizing binocular indirect ophthalmoscopy with scleral indentation is necessary to visualize snowballs and snowbanks. Fluorescein angiography is useful in detecting subtle macular edema and aids in the diagnosis of neovascularization. Because of the association of pars planitis with other diseases, laboratory testing may include:

- CBC with differential
- Syphilis serology (FTA-ABS and RPR)
- Purified protein derivative (of tuberculin)
- Chest radiograph to rule out sarcoidosis and tuberculosis

- Angiotensin converting enzyme
- Lyme titers
- MRI in patients older than 25 (if other findings and history are suggestive of multiple sclerosis)

The Treatment

Usually no treatment is administered if acuity is good (20/40 or better). However, because of numerous complications, early aggressive treatment is advocated by some if any amount of macular edema is present.

Oral prednisone, dosed 1 mg/kg of body weight, may be prescribed for 2 to 6 weeks followed by a slow taper. Alternatively, periocular corticosteroid injections of methylprednisolone acetate 40 mg or triamcinolone acetonide 40 mg may be administered every 2 to 6 weeks until the resolution of macular edema. Systemic steroids alone manage the inflammation in up to 80% of the cases. Peripheral cryotherapy and peripheral scatter photocoagulation are used to treat neovascularization of the vitreous base. Cryotherapy is not without side effects and has been associated with the development of rhegmatogenous retinal detachments. Pars plana vitrectomy (possibly removing vitreous antigens, inflammatory cells, and inflammatory mediators) may be indicated to remove vitreous opacities or hemorrhages and to reduce or eliminate vitreous traction. If all other treatments prove ineffective, immunosuppressive agents such as methotrexate, azathioprine, chlorambucil, cyclophosphamide, and cyclosporine A may be utilized. Newer therapies such as tacrolimus, etanercept, infliximab, and mycophenolate mofetil have also proven useful. Combined corticosteroids with immunosuppressant therapy may be warranted in severe cases. Cataract surgery, required in up to 20% of cases, is usually recommended once the eye is inflammation free for 3 months prior to surgery. Topical corticosteroids and cycloplegia are used to manage any secondary anterior chamber reaction. Follow-up is every 1 to 4 weeks during acute phase and every 3 to 6 months during chronic phase. Improvement is slow.

REITER'S SYNDROME
Tammy P. Than

ICD—9: 099.3 - Reiter's disease (syndrome)
ICD—9: 372.33 - Conjunctivitis in mucocutaneous disease

THE DISEASE

Pathophysiology

The pathophysiology is uncertain but is thought to be an interaction between bacterial antigens, inflammatory components, and the immune system, combined with a genetic predisposition (HLA-B27). Reiter's syndrome is a seronegative spondyloarthropathy. This syndrome traditionally refers to the triad of arthritis, conjunctivitis, and urethritis; although, a fourth manifestation, mucocutaneous lesions, occurs at high frequency.

Etiology

Reiter's syndrome usually begins after an infection of the genitourinary or gastrointestinal tract. The major enteric bacteria are *Shigella, Salmonella, Campylobacter,* and *Yersinia* while the most common venereal infection is *Chlamydia trachomatis*. The predisposing antigen, HLA-B27, is present in 75 to 90% of cases.

The Patient

Clinical Symptoms

The patient will complain of joint stiffness, heel pain, genitourinary discharge, and skin lesions. Ocular complaints will include mucopurulent discharge, discomfort, red eye, and possibly photophobia.

Clinical Signs

Ocular signs occur in 50% of postvenereal cases and 75% following an enteric infection. Bilateral conjunctivitis is most common and may be observed before or at the onset of arthritis. The second most common ocular finding is acute, nongranulomatous, unilateral anterior uveitis. Ocular complications include cystoid macular edema, epiretinal membrane, optic nerve edema, glaucoma, and cataracts.

Systemic signs include asymmetric arthralgia of the knee, ankle, and toes; sacroiliitis; enthesitis (painful inflammation of tendon or ligament attachment to bone); and talagia (heel pain). The peripheral arthritis is usually acute and migratory. Mucocutaneous lesions are present in 80% of cases and include keratoderma blennorrhagicum (scaling lesions of palms and soles), circinate balanitis (genital ulcers), and painless oral ulcers. Reiter's syndrome may also be associated with nail abnormalities (onycholysis, subungual hyperkeratosis), amyloidosis, aortitis, pulmonary fibrosis, prostatitis, and pulmonary fibrosis.

Complete Reiter's syndrome, present in fewer than 50% of patients, requires manifestation of the triad (arthritis, urethritis, and conjunctivitis). In the absence of the triad, if arthritis is present and at least one other extra-articular feature is present, it is considered incomplete Reiter's syndrome.

Demographics

The exact incidence is unknown but it is thought to be the most common cause of arthralgia in the 20 to 35 age group. The incidence of Reiter's syndrome postvenereal disease is more common in men than women (9:1) with no gender predilection following an enteric infection. This syndrome is more common in Caucasians than African Americans.

Significant History

- History of gastrointestinal disease
- History of genitourinary infection

Ancillary Tests

Ocular evaluation includes a thorough slit-lamp examination of the conjunctiva, cornea, and anterior chamber. A dilated fundus examination is needed to rule out posterior segment complications.

There is no diagnostic test for Reiter's syndrome but the following laboratory tests are useful:

- CBC with differential (leukocytosis is common; mild anemia may be present)
- Erythrocyte sedimentation rate (ESR)—may be elevated during active stage
- C-reactive protein (CRP)—may be elevated during active stage
- HLA-B27
- Rheumatoid factor—negative
- Antinuclear antibodies—negative
- Microimmunofluoresence for *Chlamydia trachomatis*
- Creatinine—elevated
- Radiologic studies corresponding to patients arthralgias

The Treatment

Reiter's syndrome is often not self-limiting and is recurrent and chronic. Antibiotic treatment has not proven effective in shortening the ocular manifestations. The anterior uveitis should be treated with topical corticosteroids and cycloplegics. If Reiter's syndrome is secondary to *Chlamydial* infection, oral azithromycin 1000 mg for one day should be prescribed. The patient's sexual partners should also be treated. The arthralgia is managed with oral nonsteroidal anti-inflammatories, corticosteroids, or immunosuppressive agents. The mucocutaneous lesions respond to corticosteroids, phototherapy, and methotrexate. Physical therapy is also useful.

GRANULOMATOUS UVEITIS
Richard F. Multack, Milan R. Genge, and Leonid Skorin Jr.

ICD—9: 364.3

THE DISEASE

Pathophysiology

A granulomatous uveal inflammation may present acutely or more likely is chronic and insidious in onset. Classification of granulomatous versus nongranulomatous is limited because different doses of the same antigen may produce either appearance. Granulomatous inflammatory cells consist of coalesced macrophages that form large aggregates of cells (up to 1 mm in diameter). These large greasy keratic precipitates are known as "mutton-fat" deposits and are found on the posterior surface of the cornea.

The accumulation of inflammatory cells on the surface of the iris or within its parenchyma also signals granulomatous inflammation. Neutrophils and lymphocytes usually can be found on the iris surface in a random pattern. If they form 1- to 3-mm nodules on the anterior iris, they are known as Busacca's nodules. If they appear near the pupillary border, they are known as Koeppe's nodules. Koeppe's nodules are round or oval, clear cellular aggregates that are actually within the iris itself. Koeppe's nodules are somewhat smaller in size than Busacca's nodules. Iris involvement may also lead to the formation of anterior and posterior synechiae.

Etiology

Granulomatous uveitis can occur in several disease states. These include toxoplasmosis, tuberculosis, sarcoidosis, syphilis, and Vogt-Koyanagi-Harada syndrome (V-K-H syndrome).

- Toxoplasmosis. The organism causing the disease is *toxoplasma gondii*, an intracellular protozoan parasite. It is neurotrophic and attacks the retina as well as other central nervous system tissues. The natural host is the cat.

  Humans are infected by ingestion of contaminated uncooked meat or other foods. Most cases of ocular toxoplasmosis are recurrences of congenitally acquired toxoplasmosis. Women who acquire toxoplasmosis during pregnancy may transmit the trachyzoites to the fetus. This has the potential for severe ocular, central nervous system, and systemic complications.
- Tuberculosis. The organism causing the disease is the acid-fast bacterium *Mycobacterium tuberculosis*, which most commonly involves the lungs but may affect virtually any organ or tissue in the body.
- Sarcoidosis. Antigen-stimulated activated T-helper cells mediate the granulomatous disease of sarcoidosis. The disease reflects an immune response to a still unidentified antigen.
- Syphilis. The organism causing the disease is *Treponema pallidum*, a very fastidious but highly infectious spirochete.
- V-K-H Syndrome. This autoimmune disease results from cellular immunity against melanocytes resulting in inflammation with loss of melanocytes in the uveal tract and skin. The exact triggering agent is not known, although a virus is suspected.

The Patient

Symptoms and signs depend on the underlying cause of the granulomatous uveitis.

Clinical Symptoms

1. Toxoplasmosis
   - Floaters and blurred vision as a result of cells exuding from an active focus of retinitis. Generally at onset, the anterior segment is not inflamed. Granulomatous inflammation with increased intraocular pressure occurs, especially in recurrent disease.
2. Tuberculosis
   - Weight loss, recurrent fevers, cough, night sweats, and blurred vision.

3. Sarcoidosis
   - Dry eye, floaters, photophobia, blurred vision, cough, dyspnea, hemoptysis, wheezing, and joint pain. The eye may be red and painful.
4. Syphilis
   - Painless chancre in primary disease, flu, photophobia, blurred vision in secondary disease, cardiac and neurological changes in tertiary disease.
5. V-K-H syndrome
   - Bilateral decreased vision, pain, photophobia with headache, stiff neck, nausea, vomiting, seizures, paralysis, fever, loss of consciousness, hair loss, hearing loss, and tinnitus.

Clinical Signs

1. Toxoplasmosis
   - Unilateral white-yellow retinal lesion in the posterior pole with overlying vitreal haze. Often an old chorioretinal scar may also be seen adjacent to a new yellow-white lesion. The anterior layers of the retina are more frequently involved; however, deeper layers of the retina can be involved that may take longer for a vitritis to develop. Another presentation of toxoplasma retinitis can be seen as small, punctate peripheral retinal lesions known as punctate outer retinal toxoplasmosis (PORT). Toxoplasmosis infection may also cause disc edema, vitreous precipitate, granulomatous iritis, localized vasculitis, retinal artery or vein occlusion, localized lymphadenopathy, polymyositis, encephalitis, pneumonitis, exanthemas, or psychiatric disturbances. The triad of retinochoroiditis, hydrocephalus, and calcifications in the brain are pathognomonic for congenital systemic toxoplasmosis.
2. Tuberculosis
   - Chronic iridocyclitis, vitreous opacities, yellow-white choroidal lesions, vitritis, papillitis, tubercle formation of the lids, conjunctiva, cornea, sclera and uveal tract, uveal granulomas, choroiditis, granulomatous iritis, lymphadenitis, and pulmonary granulomas.
3. Sarcoidosis
   - Granulomatous iritis with mutton-fat keratic precipitates, vitritis with "snowball" white cells in the anterior/inferior vitreous, "candle wax drippings" or exudates along the retinal vessels, cystoid macular edema, retinal vein sheathing, band keratopathy, nummular corneal infiltrate, corneal endothelial opacification, posterior synechiae, lacrimal gland enlargement, conjunctival nodules, optic disc edema, optic neuritis, facial-nerve palsy, erythema nodosum, arthritis, lymphadenopathy, bilateral hilar adenopathy on chest x-ray, and salivary gland enlargement.
4. Syphilis
   - Congenital syphilis can cause salt and pepper fundus retinal pigment epithelium inflammation, keratouveitis from acute interstitial keratitis, which develops between 5 and 25 years of age, Argyll-Robertson pupil, optic atrophy, failure to thrive, anemia, hepatosplenomegaly, papillomacular rash, and Hutchinson's teeth.
   - Acquired syphilis can cause chancre of conjunctiva and other mucous membranes, nodular or posterior scleritis, perivasculitis and vascular occlusion of retinal arteries and veins, retinitis, cystoid macular edema, granulomatous iritis, neuro-ophthalmic complications, gummas, aortitis, and tabes dorsalis.

5. V-K-H syndrome
- Bilateral mild to severe inflammation, synechiae, hypotony, keratic precipitates, serous retinal detachments, Dalen-Fuchs nodules, granulomatous iritis, vitritis, optic disc edema, alopecia, vitiligo, and poliosis. Choroidal depigmentation creates a characteristic fundus appearance labeled as the "sunset glow" fundus. Areas of focal atrophy and hyperpigmentation can be seen in the healing stages.

Demographics

- Toxoplasmosis. Congenital toxoplasmosis develops after transplacental transmission of the parasite from a recently infected pregnant mother to her fetus. Toxoplasmosis acquired during pregnancy results in half of the infants being born healthy; however, 14% of fetuses develop severe congenital toxoplasmosis if the mother is infected in the first trimester of pregnancy. Of the 3 million babies born annually in the United States, 3,000 have congenital toxoplasmosis. Only about 1% of all cases of toxoplasma retinitis are acquired. Toxoplasmosis accounts for 30 to 50% of all posterior uveitis and 7 to 15% of all uveitis.
- Tuberculosis. In recent years in the United States approximately 25,000 to 30,000 new cases of tuberculosis have been reported annually. The incidence of ophthalmic manifestations is found in approximately 1 to 2% of these new cases. Tuberculosis affects both males and females equally and is seen most often in the 35 to 44 age group.
- Sarcoidosis. Sarcoidosis predominantly affects young adults in the 20- to 40-age range, with Blacks affected 10 times more often than Whites and females more often than males. Up to 3% of all uveitis patients have sarcoid and up to 50% of patients with systemic sarcoid have ocular complications.
- Syphilis. Syphilis occurs equally in both males and females at any age and is responsible for 1 to 3% of all uveitis. Patients who develop secondary syphilis have up to a 10% chance of developing uveitis. There has been a steady rise in overall incidence.
- V-K-H Syndrome. There is a predilection to developing this syndrome in people who are more darkly pigmented and is uncommon in Whites. People of Asian and American Indian ancestry have been shown to be susceptible. It is more common in Japan, where it accounts for 9.2% of uveitis cases. Women are affected more often than men, and most patients are in their second to fifth decade of life at the onset of the disease.

Significant History

Depends on underlying disease process.

Ancillary Tests

- Toxoplasmosis. Complete ocular examination with dilated fundus evaluation, serum antitoxoplasma antibody titer, which should be done in a 1:1 dilution, RPR, PPD (purified protein derivative) with anergy panel, chest x-ray, and HIV testing in high-risk patients.

- Tuberculosis. Complete ocular examination with dilated fundus evaluation, RPR, PPD with anergy panel, chest x-ray. Bronchial washings, gastric washings, sputum cultures, and urine cultures may also be indicated.
- Sarcoidosis. Abnormalities in chest x-rays are found in up to 80% of patients. Serum lysozyme, angiotensin-converting enzyme, serum electrophoresis, and serum calcium help the diagnosis. A gallium scan of the head, neck, and mediastinum may be helpful, but the results are unreliable if the patient is taking any amount of steroid. Biopsy of any conjunctival granuloma or the palpebral lobe of the lacrimal gland when it is enlarged may obviate the need for a transbronchial biopsy.
- Syphilis. RPR or VDRL, microhemagglutination assay-T Pallidum (MHA-TP) and fluorescent treponemal antibody absorption (FTA-ABS). The RPR and VDRL are the nontreponemal tests that indicate active disease or exposure to the bacteria but are insufficient to diagnose syphilis. The FTA-ABS or MHA-TP can confirm the diagnosis. In patients with uveitis and positive serology, asymptomatic neurosyphilis must be ruled out via lumbar puncture. It is important to note that in latent syphilis, the FTA-ABS and VDRL will be positive, but the cerebrospinal fluid (CSF) may be negative, whereas in neurosyphilis the FTA-ABS and CSF will be positive, but the VDRL may be low or negative.
- V-K-H Syndrome. Complete ocular examination with dilated fundus evaluation. There is a strong association between HLA-DR4 and V-K-H syndrome. A CBC with differential, RPR, angiotensin-converting enzyme, and PPD can all be done as a differential. Other testing includes fluorescein angiography, showing multiple focal areas of subretinal leakage in the early phases, and ultrasonography to demonstrate choroidal thickening. Lumbar puncture may identify transient cerebrospinal fluid pleocytosis. Electroencephalography is abnormal in 66% of cases. Magnetic resonance imaging can help differentiate choroiditis from scleritis, and electro-oculograms and electroretinograms can be used to follow the progression of the disease.

The Treatment

- Toxoplasmosis. Treatment depends on the location and severity of the active retinitis. Any retinitis near the macula or optic nerve that threatens central vision and any large exudative lesion should be treated. The anterior uveitis should be treated with topical corticosteroids and cycloplegics.

    Systemic therapy includes sulfadiazine 2 to 4 gm, oral load, then 1 gm orally four times a day for 3 to 6 weeks with clindamycin 150 to 300 mg orally, four times a day, and prednisone 40 to 80 mg orally, daily, begun after the second or third day of antitoxoplasmic therapy until day 10, and then tapered gradually over a period of 4 to 5 weeks. Stop steroids before antitoxoplasma medications. Corticosteroids must be used cautiously or may cause immunosuppression and subsequent microbial proliferation. Pyrimethamine (Daraprim) is also prescribed in an initial loading dose of 75 to 150 mg orally, followed by 25 mg orally bid for 3 to 6 weeks. Pyrimethamine is a folate antagonist that can cause white blood cell and platelet depression as well as megaloblastic anemia. Therefore, 10 mg of folinic acid (leucovorin) can be administered IM or orally to reverse any platelet count below 100,000 mm^3 or folinic acid can be given 3 to 5 mg orally, 2 to 4 times weekly, as a preventive measure.

Trimethoprim-sulfamethoxazole (Septra DS) may be an effective substitute for sulfadiazine, pyrimethamine, and folinic acid. Long-term treatment (up to 20 months) with Septra DS significantly reduces the rate of recurrence of retinochoroiditis in patients with a history of multiple previous recurrences.

- Tuberculosis. Consultation with a pulmonologist is recommended. Treatment includes multiple drug therapy utilizing the following drugs: isoniazid, pyrazinamide, streptomycin, ethambutol, or rifampin. Pyridoxine supplement (vitamin B6) is often given with long-term therapy to prevent deficiencies created by the therapy itself. Corticosteroids may be necessary in conjunction with antimicrobial therapy.

- Sarcoidosis. Consultation with an internist is recommended. Treatment for ocular inflammation includes topical cycloplegics as well as topical, sub-Tenon's injection, and systemic corticosteroids. Retinal neovascularization may require panretinal photocoagulation.

- Syphilis. Penicillin (Penicillin G, 2 to 5 million units, intravenous, every 4 hours for 10 to 14 days). If the patient is allergic to penicillin, doxycycline 200 milligrams orally twice a day or erythromycin 500 mg orally four times a day for 15 days may be used. Topical cycloplegics and corticosteroids are used to treat the anterior uveitis.

- V-K-H Syndrome. The anterior uveitis should be treated with topical cycloplegics and corticosteroids in addition to systemic corticosteroids followed by a slow tapering over 3 to 6 months. Cytotoxic agents, such as cyclophosphamide, chlorambucil, azathioprine, and the cytostatic agent cyclosporine, have all been used successfully to treat V-K-H syndrome.

OCULAR ROSACEA

Christopher Quinn and Leonid Skorin Jr.

ICD—9: 695.3—Rosacea dermatitis
ICD—9: 372.31—Rosacea conjunctivitis

THE DISEASE

Rosacea is a dermatologic condition of unknown etiology. It most likely represents the manifestations of an inflammatory process for which a variety of trigger mechanisms have been identified. Aside from the dermatologic manifestations, a high percentage of patients with rosacea suffer from ocular sequelae. These conditions, when associated with rosacea, are known as ocular rosacea. Rosacea is classified into four subtypes by the National Rosacea Society: erythematotelangiectatic, papulopustular, phymatous, or ocular. Patients may progress from one type or have multiple types simultaneously.

Pathophysiology

Vascular dysregulation with release of inflammatory mediators has been suggested as the underlying pathophysiology.

Tear film disturbances are responsible for the vast majority of subjective complaints and objective findings in ocular rosacea. There is a reduced amount and altered character of the meibomian gland secretions. Also, more than one-third of patients with rosacea have impaired aqueous tear secretion.

Etiology

The etiology of ocular rosacea is unclear and likely to be multifactorial. A variety of "trigger factors" have been identified that exacerbate the signs and symptoms of rosacea. These factors include alcohol consumption, spicy foods, cold weather, hot beverages, sun exposure and other environmental factors, and emotional stress. Some persons may have gastric coinfection with *Helicobacter pylori*, but causation has not been proved. An association with *Demodex folliculorum*, a hair follicle mite that is a permanent ectoparasite in humans, has also been suggested.

The Patient

A classification system of four subtypes was developed by the National Rosacea Society in 2002.

- Subtype 1, erythematotelangiectactic rosacea. Characterized by persistent flushing and redness of the central face. Though common in this subtype, telangiectasia is not essential for its diagnosis. Edema of the central face, burning, scaling, and roughness may also be present.
- Subtype 2, papulopustular rosacea. Characterized by persistent redness, usually of the central face but possible of the perioral, perinasal, and periocular areas, with papules and pustules. Comedones are not present. It may be seen in combination with subtype 1.
- Subtype 3, phymatous rosacea. Characterized by thickness of the skin, enlargement of facial features, and irregular surface nodularities. Rhinophyma may occur.
- Subtype 4, ocular rosacea. Indicates a vascular stage of the disorder. The eyes are watery and bloodshot. Telangiectasia of the conjunctiva and lid margin may be present.

Clinical Symptoms

Rosacea patients complain of episodic central facial flushing (transient erythema) and persistent facial erythema. Some patients report intense stinging associated with the facial flushing. Patients with ocular rosacea exhibit a variety of symptoms most commonly related to blepharitis. Bilateral ocular itching, conjunctival hyperemia, dryness, burning, and foreign body sensation are commonly reported. Ocular irritation is usually worse upon awakening and when performing prolonged visual tasks such as reading, driving, or using the computer. This can cause variable vision with transient improvement after blinking. Ocular symptoms may not be related to the extent of the dermatologic signs.

Clinical Signs

Central facial erythema (redness) and vascular telangiectasia of the face are the primary clinical signs of rosacea. Patients with rosacea may also develop sterile inflammatory papules and pustules on the skin of the face. Patients may also develop rhinophyma, a hypertrophy of the sebaceous glands of the nose. Ocular rosacea is most commonly characterized by the development of chronic posterior blepharitis. The lid margins become thickened, with telangiectatic vessels. Meibomian gland orifices are often inspissated, and tear break-up times are reduced. Patients with rosacea are prone to the development of recurrent chalazia or hordeolum. Low-grade chronic conjunctivitis may occur with or without the presence of blepharitis. Some patients may develop migratory phlyctenular conjunctivitis. Aqueous deficient dry eye can develop as well as episcleritis and iritis. Corneal findings in rosacea are less common but are potentially devastating. Diffuse punctate epithelial erosions can occur as well as inferior infiltrative marginal keratitis. Areas of infiltrate may become vascularized, resulting in corneal scar formation. Repeated episodes of corneal infiltration can result in corneal thinning and perforation.

Demographics

Rosacea affects more than 14 million people in the United States. Rosacea most commonly occurs in patients between the 30 and 50 years of age, and is two to three times more common in females than males. Its incidence peaks between the fourth and seventh decades. It is more likely to occur in fair-skinned individuals of Celtic or northern European ancestry. In rare cases, it affects African Americans. Many persons with rosacea have a history of adolescent acne.

Significant History

- Facial flushing
- Redness of cheeks or nose
- Papules and pustules on cheeks, forehead, and nose

Ancillary Tests

Ocular assessment includes visual acuity, pupil testing, slit-lamp evaluation, Schirmer basal secretion testing, tonometry, and a dilated fundus examination. Rosacea and ocular rosacea are clinical diagnoses. Based on the criteria set by the National Rosacea Society, the diagnosis requires one or more primary features in the central distribution on the face. The primary features are:

- Flushing (transient erythema)
- Nontransient erythema (persistent flushing)
- Papules and pustules, usually in crops, which may be nodular but not comedonal
- Telangiectasia

The Treatment

Patients need to identify and then avoid any potential triggers. Ongoing sun protection is important.

Treatment of rosacea and its ocular manifestations are mostly symptomatic. In patients with significant posterior blepharitis, lid hygiene, which includes warm soaks, gentle massage, and mechanical scrubbing of the lid margin, will often provide relief from itching and burning. Artificial tear supplements can also improve patient comfort.

Nonirritating topical medication known as metronidazole can be used to treat the skin. It is available as a 0.75% formulation used twice daily (cream, gel, lotion) or a 1% formulation used once a day (cream). The key is to use the topical treatment in conjunction with an oral agent to induce remission, then to wean the patient from the oral agent and continue the topical therapy.

Oral antibiotics should be considered for rosacea flares. For patients whose rosacea is in the vascular or more severe stage, antibiotics are the first choice for inducing a remission. These agents work either through antimicrobial means or by changing the chemical composition of meibomian gland secretions. Tetracycline derivatives are the mainstay of therapy. These include: tetracycline 500 mg orally bid, doxycycline 100 mg orally bid, and minocycline 100 mg orally bid.

Pulsed dye lasers and fluorescent pulsed light can be used to manage rosacea-associated skin redness. Telangiectasias are treated with fine-point electrodessication or photocoagulation with pulsed laser. Rhinophyma can be treated with dermabrasion or surgery.

SCLERITIS
Christopher Quinn

ICD—9: 379.00

THE DISEASE

The sclera is the firm, avascular protective outer coat of the eye. The episclera overlies the sclera and provides nutrition and potential inflammatory components to the sclera. Inflammation of the sclera from a variety of reasons is collectively known as scleritis.

Pathophysiology

The pathology of scleritis is dependent on the underlying cause, although all cases of scleritis involve a significant inflammatory response. Intense inflammatory reactions can cause destruction of the collagen of the sclera and destroy its structural integrity. Because scleritis is a potentially destructive condition, it carries a significant risk of blindness. Scleritis is commonly associated with systemic disease and requires systemic treatment. Scleritis can be classified as anterior diffuse, nodular, necrotizing, or scleromalacia perforans. In addition, posterior scleritis can develop. Ocular complications occur in only 13.5% of patients with episcleritis but in 58.8% of patients with scleritis.

Etiology

Scleritis is the clinical manifestation of an intense inflammatory response often associated with systemic inflammatory conditions, especially autoimmune disorders. Rheumatoid arthritis, Wegener's granulomatosis, polyarteritis nodosa, gout, relapsing polychondritis, systemic lupus erythematosus, Reiter's syndrome, Behçet's disease, or Cogan syndrome have all been associated with the development of scleritis. Scleritis less commonly occurs as the result of infection from bacteria, fungi, and viruses. It may also occur following trauma or intraocular surgery such as cataract extraction, pterygium removal, scleral buckling, or strabismus surgery.

The Patient

Clinical Symptoms
Patients with scleritis often report moderate to severe deep boring pain of the affected eye and orbit. The globe can be tender to the touch, and pain can awaken patients during sleep. The pain is only partly relieved with analgesics. The pain is often out of proportion to the other clinical signs. Patients can also develop photophobia and tearing.

Clinical Signs
Patients with scleritis develop significant scleral edema, overlying episcleral congestion and conjunctival hyperemia. Scleral edema results in increased hydration of the sclera, which causes increased scleral transparency. As a result, patients with scleritis can develop a localized area with a blue or violatious hue. These changes are best appreciated during an external scleral examination done in daylight and are an important feature of scleritis. Necrotizing scleritis results in loss of scleral tissue and visible uveal tissue. Patients with posterior scleritis can present with no anterior segment signs, and patients with anterior scleritis can also have posterior scleritis. Posterior scleritis signs can include exudative retinal detachments, uveitis, choroidal folds, hyperopic shift, disc edema, proptosis, extraocular motility disturbances, and lower eyelid retraction with attempted elevation of the eye.

Demographics

Scleritis is most common between the ages of 40 to 60 and occurs more frequently in women than in men.
Scleritis is bilateral, though not necessarily simultaneously, in 40 to 80% of cases with a recurrence rate of up to 70%.

Significant History

A history of eye pain or redness may indicate previous episodes of scleritis. A careful review of systems should be performed because of the high association of scleritis with systemic disease. The most common association is with autoimmune disorders.

Ancillary Tests

Ocular assessment includes visual acuity, pupil testing, slit-lamp evaluation, tonometry, and dilated fundus examination. In addition, B-scan ultrasonography for posterior scleritis and fluorescein angiography (anterior segment for scleritis and fundus for posterior scleritis) may be of benefit.

Because scleritis is often associated with systemic disease, a comprehensive medical evaluation based on the review of systems should be obtained. Additional testing may include, but is not limited to, complete blood count, chest x-ray, rheumatoid factor, antinuclear antibodies, antineutrophil cytoplasmic antibodies (C-ANCA, P-ANCA), HLA typing, uric acid, erythrocyte sedimentation rate, hepatitis B surface antigen, and serology for syphilis (FTA-ABS, MHA-TP).

The Treatment

Treatment of scleritis depends on the severity of the disease and the degree of scleral destruction. Aggressive treatment is required to stop scleral destruction. Topical steroids may help provide some symptomatic relief but are not adequate alone to treat scleritis. Mild cases of scleritis respond well to systemic nonsteroidal anti-inflammatory drugs (NSAIDs). Conventional management held that periocular steroids are contraindicated in the treatment of scleritis, but some patients with non-necrotizing scleritis may benefit from subconjunctival steroid injections. In patients with necrotizing scleritis, oral steroids may be needed to control the inflammation. A high dose of intravenous methylprednisolone may be needed in patients who have necrotizing scleritis, especially if vision is threatened. Oral immunosuppressive agents alone or in combination with steroids may be required to control severe disease. Oral immunosuppressive agents include cyclophosphamide, methotrexate, and azathioprine.

EPISCLERITIS
Christopher Quinn and Leonid Skorin Jr.
ICD—9: 379.00

THE DISEASE

The episclera is a fibroelastic tissue that forms Tenon's capsule and acts as a synovial membrane for smooth movement of the eye. It overlies the sclera. The deep episcleral layer is in close proximity to the sclera and has its own vascular plexus from the anterior ciliary arteries. The superficial episcleral layer with its separate vascular plexus becomes contiguous with the conjunctiva at the corneal limbus.

Episcleritis is a descriptive diagnosis used in patients who have either localized or diffuse episcleral inflammation. Unlike scleritis, episcleritis tends to be a more common, mild, self-limiting, and often recurrent disorder. It typically affects young adults.

Pathophysiology

Inflammation of the superficial episcleral tissue with vascular dilation and perivascular infiltration is seen in patients with episcleritis. There are two clinical types of episcleritis: simple and nodular.

Etiology

The etiology of episcleritis is unclear. Up to one-third of patients with episcleritis can have an associated underlying systemic condition. Conditions associated with episcleritis include atopy, rheumatoid arthritis, systemic lupus erythematosus, polyarteritis nodosa, seronegative spondyloarthropathies, gout, or infections with bacteria, viruses, or fungi.

The Patient

Episcleritis is divided into two clinical types:

- Simple episcleritis: Characterized by sectoral, or rarely, diffuse redness. It resolves spontaneously in 1 to 2 weeks.
- Nodular episcleritis: Characterized by a localized nodule with surrounding injection. It may take longer to resolve than simple episcleritis. Recurrence can cause the underlying sclera to become translucent.

Clinical Symptoms

Patients with episcleritis develop localized or diffuse episcleral hyperemia. The inflammation may be localized sectorally and may overlie the insertion of the medial or lateral rectus muscles. Often the overlying conjunctiva is inflamed as well. Patients can report mild discomfort or pain. If present, pain is described as a mild, usually warm, prickly sensation or a dull ache. This discomfort is usually localized to the eye.

Clinical Signs

Localized or diffuse episcleral edema and vasodilation is observed with slit-lamp examination. The underlying sclera is not edematous. The episcleral blood vessels retain their normal pattern and vasoconstrict with topical phenylephrine. A localized mobile nodule develops in patients with nodular episcleritis. Occasionally patients may develop an associated anterior uveitis. Keratitis can occur in up to 15% of patients.

Demographics

Episcleritis occurs most commonly in the fourth or fifth decade. Women are affected in approximately two-thirds of cases.

Significant History

A previous history of red eye or pain may be an indication of prior episodes of episcleritis. A careful review of systems should be performed because of the occasional association of episcleritis with systemic disease.

Ancillary Tests

Ocular assessment includes visual acuity, pupil testing, slit-lamp evaluation, tonometry, and dilated fundus examination. Additional testing may include but is not limited to chest x-ray, rheumatoid factor, antinuclear antibodies, serum uric acid, erythrocyte sedimentation rate, and syphilis serology (FTA-ABS, MHA-TP).

Topical phenylephrine vasoconstricts superficial episcleral vessels only and can help to differentiate episcleritis from scleritis.

The Treatment

Treatment of episcleritis is generally supportive. Lubrication and cold compresses can provide symptomatic relief. Symptoms and signs generally resolve spontaneously in 7 to 10 days but may last longer, especially in nodular episcleritis. In patients who are significantly symptomatic, treatment with topical steroids may be of benefit. Steroids give temporary relief but may prolong the disease and increase the incidence of recurrence. Frequent intensive topical steroid administration on a short pulsed basis is optimal. In patients in whom symptoms and signs persist, treatment with oral NSAIDS will often offer relief. Oral NSAIDS are preferred to topical steroid administration.

SJÖGREN'S SYNDROME
Alan G. Kabat

ICD—9: 710.2

THE DISEASE
Pathophysiology

Sjögren's syndrome is a multisystem autoimmune disorder with a recognized genetic predisposition that varies among ethnic groups. The disease affects exocrine glands and their associated organ systems, typically involving the eye, mouth and throat, skin, lungs, and genitourinary tract.

Two forms of the condition are recognized. Primary Sjögren's syndrome is generally absent of other autoimmune conditions, while secondary Sjögren's is associated with preexisting systemic inflammatory disorders, such as rheumatoid arthritis, systemic lupus erythematosus, scleroderma, polymyositis, or thyroiditis.

Etiology

In Sjögren's syndrome, exocrine gland epithelial cells display high levels of major histocompatibility complex molecules, triggered perhaps by viral infection or circulating cytokines. These molecules constitute autoantigens; they attract lymphocytes (particularly CD4+ T cells), which infiltrate the glands and subsequently interfere with normal exocrine function.

Research has identified inflammatory cell markers in Sjögren's, although the nature varies depending on the patient. Those of European descent show a link to HLA-B8,

HLA-Dw3, and HLA-DR3; Japanese patients demonstrate HLA-DRw53, while those of Mediterranean descent manifest HLA-DR5 involvement.

The Patient

Patients with Sjögren's syndrome are predominantly adult women. Older patients tend to be more symptomatic. The majority of patients manifest additional systemic auto-immune/inflammatory disorders.

Clinical Symptoms

The most common symptoms involve dry eye and dry mouth. Often the first clinical manifestation of Sjögren's syndrome is keratoconjunctivitis sicca, replete with ocular burning, grittiness, foreign body sensation, and blurred vision. Dry mouth or xerostomia results in complaints of dysphagia, loss of taste, and painful lesions of the lips and tongue. Hoarseness and a dry cough indicate dryness extending to the oropharynx. Other notable symptoms include dry skin or skin rashes, pain or weakness in joints or muscles, numbness or tingling in the extremities, labored breathing, vaginal dryness, difficulty with memory, and general fatigue.

Clinical Signs

1. Nonocular Signs
   - Erythema, cracking and bleeding of lips, gums, and/or tongue
   - Increased incidence of dental caries and periodontal disease, potentially with tooth loss
   - Acquired "smoothness" of the tongue, with loss of normal papillae
   - Bilateral parotid gland and/or submandibular gland enlargement
   - Vasculitic purpura on the lower extremities or erythema multiformlike "target" lesions
2. Ocular Signs
   - Diminished tear meniscus and tear volume (Schirmer or phenol red thread test)
   - Punctate epithelial keratopathy and reduced fluorescein tear break-up time
   - Rose bengal and/or lissamine green staining in the interpalpebral region of the conjunctiva
   - Mucous strands or filaments in the tear film
   - Staphylococcal blepharitis and/or meibomian gland dysfunction

Demographics

Sjögren's syndrome is the second most common autoimmune rheumatic disease in the United States, after rheumatoid arthritis. Prevalence is estimated at between 500,000 and 2 million, the wide range reflecting a lack of uniform diagnostic criteria. More than 90% of patients are female; however, no specific racial predilections have been noted. Sjögren's may be encountered at any age, but onset typically occurs in the fourth to fifth decade. A fair number of patients manifest the disorder in their mid- to late 20s, and pregnancy may actually be a contributory factor.

Significant History

- Keratoconjunctivitis sicca
- Xerostomia
- Rheumatoid arthritis is present in 25 to 50%
- 5 to 8% of patients develop malignant lymphoma as a late complication

Ancillary Tests

Basic ocular assessment includes visual acuity and ocular surface slit-lamp evaluation, including vital dye staining with fluorescein and rose bengal and/or lissamine green. Tear volume assessment may also be helpful in diagnosing keratoconjunctivitis sicca. Cursory examination of the lips, teeth, gums, and tongue may reveal effects of xerostomia. Inspection of the hands may show enlarged metacarpal and phalangeal joints in those with rheumatoid arthritis.

Patients with a diagnosis or significant suspicion of Sjögren's syndrome should be referred for a rheumatologic consultation as well as a comprehensive dental examination.

Laboratory Studies

Minimum serologic testing includes rheumatoid factor, antinuclear antibody (ANA), and antibodies to Sjögren's antigen A (SS-A or Ro) and antigen B (SS-B or La). Of the two, anti-Ro antibodies are more common, found in approximately 75% of patients with primary Sjögren's syndrome and 15% of those with secondary Sjögren's. Anti-La antibodies are present in 40 to 50% of patients with primary Sjögren's, but are rarely seen in the absence of anti-Ro antibodies.

Salivary sialography and scintigraphy, which evaluate salivary gland uptake and outflow rates of various diagnostic agents, may help in revealing xerostomia. However, it should be noted that positive test results are not conclusive for Sjögren's syndrome.

Currently, the single best test to diagnose Sjögren's syndrome is minor salivary gland biopsy, performed on the mucosal surface of the inner lip. Histologic findings include increased focal aggregation of lymphocytes and, to a lesser extent, plasma cells and macrophages.

The Treatment

There is no cure for Sjögren's syndrome, but appropriate therapy may significantly reduce symptoms. Dry eye is best managed with nonpreserved artificial tear preparations, used at least 4 to 6 times daily. Topical cyclosporine A (Restasis™) may offer additional relief for patients with more significant keratoconjunctivitis sicca.

Palliative therapy for xerostomia includes frequent sipping of fluids (preferably water) and use of lozenges throughout the day. Patients should avoid sugary beverages and candies because these may promote tooth decay. Similar to artificial tears, artificial saliva preparations are available for alleviating oral discomfort.

Oral pilocarpine (Salagen™) and cevimeline (Evoxac™) stimulate exocrine glands via parasympathomimetic activity and may offer relief for both dry mouth and dry eye.

Hydroxychloroquine (Plaquenil™) may delay the progression of Sjögren's and reduce the severity of associated symptoms.

OCULAR CICATRICIAL PEMPHIGOID (OCP)
Michael J. Trad

ICD—9: 694.61 - Ocular pemphigus
ICD—9: 372.63 - Symblepharon

THE DISEASE
Pathophysiology

Ocular cicatricial pemphigoid is an insidious disease characterized initially by remissions and exacerbations of a chronic, nonspecific keratoconjunctivitis. It is typically bilateral in its early presentation but, if unilateral, usually progresses to bilateral involvement within 1 to 2 years. OCP may progress through various stages secondary to conjunctival goblet cell destruction, obstruction of lacrimal and accessory lacrimal gland ductules, and mechanical wetting disruption related to inflammatory lid deformities. Ultimately ocular surface keratinization occurs secondary to severe dry eye syndrome.

OCP may present concurrent with, prior to, or in isolation (pure OCP or POCP) from cicatricial pemphigoid (CP), a rare systemic disease. CP, also known as benign mucous membrane pemphigoid, may cause extraocular membrane manifestations such as bullae and subsequent scar formation of the skin, oral cavity, nose, pharynx, larynx, vagina, urethra, and anus.

Etiology

Although not completely understood, OCP is thought to have a multigene predisposition (associated with HLA-DQw7, HLA-B12, and HLA-B27); represent a type II (cytotoxic) ocular hypersensitivity reaction; and possibly involve an environmental stimulus.

The Patient

Clinical Symptoms
Symptoms may include reduced vision, foreign body sensation, photophobia, tearing, ocular redness, lid swelling, and ocular pain.

Clinical Signs
Stages of OCP (may progress over 1 to 3 decades):

- Stage 1—Fibrosis of palpebral conjunctiva, conjunctivitis, keratitis
- Stage 2—Conjunctival shrinkage with fornix foreshortening
- Stage 3—Symblepharon, lagophthalmos, entropion, trichiasis, keratopathy

- Stage 4—Ankyloblepharon and severe dry eye syndrome (other signs may include stenosis, distichiasis, blepharitis, keratitis, corneal perforation, and endophthalmitis)

Demographics

- Occurs at an incidence of one in 12,000 to 60,000 individuals.
- Occurs twice as frequently in women.
- Usually occurs in patients older than 55 years of age (however, do not dismiss the possibility of occurrence in younger individuals).
- 25 to 30% of affected individuals ultimately become blind.

Significant History

Rule out causes of cicatricial conjunctivitis in the differential diagnosis including acne rosacea, acquired epidermal bullosa, adenovirus types 8 and 19, atopic keratoconjunctivitis, β-hemolytic streptococcus, conjunctival lichen planus, diphtheria, herpes simplex keratoconjunctivitis, linear IgA disease, Lyell's syndrome, paraneoplastic pemphigus, Stevens-Johnson syndrome, sarcoidosis, Sjögren's syndrome, squamous cell carcinoma, trachoma, trauma (including chemical burns), and pseudopemphigoid/drug-induced secondary to extended use of topical (timolol, pilocarpine) and systemic (D-penicillamine, practolol) medications.

Ancillary Tests

OCP is usually diagnosed clinically after bilateral conjunctival scarring has occurred and often only in its later stages. Therefore it is critical to have a high degree of suspicion for the disease and recognize one of its earliest clinical signs, subepithelial palpebral fibrosis, to lessen ocular morbidity. Definitive diagnosis involves bulbar conjunctival biopsy (20% of cases may be biopsy negative). Biopsy of palpebral conjunctival tissue is not advocated, however, because of its potential to exacerbate OCP.

Immunopathologic microscopic techniques such as direct immunofluorescence (DIF) and direct immunoelectron microscopy (DIE) aid in identifying linear immune deposits (immunoglobulins and complement) at the level of the epithelial basement membrane.

DIE is the most sophisticated technique and is able to precisely localize the specific basement membrane level involved. Moreover, DIE is able to differentiate OCP (immunodeposition in the lamina densa and lower part of the lamina lucida) from POCP (involvement strictly in the upper lamina lucida region).

The Treatment

Local therapy for associated dry eye syndrome, keratitis, meibomianitis, blepharitis, trichiasis, and distichiasis may be employed. Ocular lubricants, punctal occlusion, warm compresses, lid hygiene, systemic and/or ophthalmic antibiotics, and trichiasis/distichiasis epilation may be beneficial.

Subconjunctival mitomycin-C and steroid injections have also been used to prevent subconjunctival fibrosis progression. Protopic (tacrolimus) ointment, a macrolide immunomodulator drug used in dermatology to treat atopic dermatitis, has also been described in the literature as a potential treatment for OCP (a topical ophthalmic version may be available in the future).

Definitive treatment may necessitate cryotherapy, electrolysis, argon laser photoablation, or surgery. Conjunctival grafts, entropion repair, tarsorrhaphy, and keratoprosthesis have met with limited success, however, even when performed with concomitant systemic immunosuppression.

Systemic immunosuppressive agents represent the best treatment for OCP and are frequently prescribed for a period of at least 1 year. These drugs should be prescribed and monitored by physicians sufficiently knowledgeable of their side effects and potential complications.

For a mild-to-moderate and slowly progressive disease:

- Dapsone 25 mg per day is utilized for 3 days. The dosage is then increased 25 mg/day every 4 to 5 days until the desired result is achieved (typically 400 to 600 mg/day). Some patients, however, may be successfully treated with doses as low as 25 mg every other day.
- A history of allergy to sulfa or glucose-6-phosphate dehydrogenase (G-6-PD) contraindicates dapsone usage.
- A G-6-PD blood test, CBC, and reticulocyte count should be obtained prior to proposed dapsone therapy. CBCs are then repeated weekly when dosages are increased, every 3 to 4 weeks until the CBC is stable, and then every 2 to 3 months thereafter.
- Sulphapyridine may be utilized as a first-line alternative to dapsone.

For a moderate-to-severe and rapidly progressive disease:

- Cyclophosphamide 1 to 2 mg/kg/day may be added to dapsone if necessary. Side effects such as significant myelosuppression, infection, and hemorrhagic cystitis may occur with cyclophosphamide.
- If dapsone is discontinued prior to beginning cyclophosphamide, azathioprine 2 mg/kg/day or methotrexate 7.5 mg once per week may be added as second-line agents.
- Short-term adjunctive therapy with prednisone 1 mg/kg/day may be beneficial in individuals with disease exacerbation.

CORNEAL GRAFT REJECTION

Richard F. Multack and Barry J. Kaufman

ICD—9: 996.51

THE DISEASE

Corneal transplants are done for a variety of clinical pathological reasons. The cornea is considered a "privileged" tissue because it has no blood vessels. The lack of blood vessels protects it to a certain extent from the white blood cells and chemotaxic factors necessary for inflammation leading to rejection. As a result, over 90% of corneal grafts are successful, and some studies report success rates of 97 to 99% over 5 to 10 years.

Pathophysiology

Corneal graft rejection refers to the recognition of donor corneal tissue as antigen by the recipient patient. It can be divided into epithelial, stromal, and endothelial rejection. The vast majority of corneal graft rejections leading to graft failure are endothelial in nature. Cellular immune mechanisms are integral to corneal graft rejection, requiring the sensitization of lymphocytes and monocytes to the graft tissue.

Etiology

While graft rejection is the most common cause of failure of technically successful corneal transplants, certain factors increase the probability that a patient will experience clinical evidence of graft rejection. Patients without any predisposing factors have a 20% chance of experiencing a graft rejection. Up to 65% of patients with corneal vascularization can experience an adverse graft reaction, with 15% losing their grafts to rejection. Pre-existing inflammatory conditions such as herpetic keratouveitis can incite graft rejection. Patients undergoing regrafts have a 30% incidence of graft rejection and shorter intervals between rejection episodes. It is important to recognize that while 90% of graft rejections occur between 1 month and 1 year following surgery, corneal graft rejection is possible through the entire life of the patient. The graft rejection rate is higher for patients with bilateral grafts. It is advisable to wait 1 year if possible between eyes.

The Patient

Clinical Symptoms
- Epithelial rejection can cause foreign body sensation but is usually relatively asymptomatic.
- Endothelial rejection presents with decreased vision, redness, and foreign body sensation.
- Occasionally, if the rejection is more advanced, there can be pain from microcystic epithelial edema.

Clinical Signs
1. Epithelial Rejection
   - An epithelial rejection line occurs, typically across the graft-recipient interface: This jagged line stains with rose bengal; dilated limbal vessels are seen adjacent to the epithelial line; recipient epithelial cells fill in (heaping) behind the epithelial line.
   - An alternate form of rejection manifests by subepithelial infiltrates.
   - Both forms of rejection usually occur within 1 year after surgery.
2. Stromal Rejection
   - This is the least common form of corneal graft rejection.

- A "front" of vessels, infiltrate, and haziness progresses across the stroma.
- The corneal appearance is similar to interstitial keratitis.
3. Endothelial Rejection
   - This is the most common form of graft failure.
   - An endothelial line or "front" of keratitic precipitates form, which is known as Khodadoust line.
   - Stromal edema occurs between the line and the graft-recipient junction.
   - Ciliary flush is most prominent at the origin of rejection.
   - Low-grade anterior chamber reaction is possible.
   - Occasionally, no rejection line or keratitic precipitates are seen.

Significant History

- With no predisposing factors evident, the patient is usually 1-month postcorneal transplant.
- History of recent exposed suture or suture abscess.
- Antecedent inflammatory disease such as bacterial or herpetic keratitis.
- Regraft patient.
- Younger patient (up to third decade).

The Treatment

Corticosteroids are the mainstay of corneal graft rejection treatment. The route of administration depends on the severity of the rejection.

In mild to moderate rejection episodes involving less than one-half of the graft and without predisposing risk factors, hourly instillation of prednisolone acetate 1% drops topically initially is the preferred treatment.

For more severe reactions or in higher risk grafts, initial dosing with 125 to 250 mg of IV methylprednisolone, followed by prednisolone acetate 1% drops topically every half-hour to 1 hour is recommended. Cyclosporine has been used systemically for a variety of ophthalmic conditions including graft rejection. The systemic route of administration results in a great deal of drug-induced systemic side effects. Topical cyclosporine A (Restasis®) has been shown to have a beneficial effect without systemic side effects, particularly when intensive topical corticosteroid therapy might be contraindicated.

SYMPATHETIC OPHTHALMIA (SO)
Nicky R. Holdeman

ICD—9: 360.11

THE DISEASE

Pathophysiology

Sympathetic ophthalmia is a subacute or chronic, bilateral, granulomatous panuveitis that may develop weeks to months after either a penetrating injury ($\approx$0.2%) or intraocular surgery (<0.01%). The condition occurs after trauma to one eye (the exciting eye) that is followed by a latent period of at least 5 to 14 days, with a persistent inflammatory reaction in the non traumatized eye (the sympathizing eye).

SO is a rare disease that has become even more uncommon because of improved surgical repairs of penetrating injuries and early enucleation of injured eyes with no chance of useful vision.

Etiology

The exact etiology of SO is unknown, but it is considered to be a T-cell–mediated autoimmune process. Penetrating ocular injuries are thought to expose "protected" intraocular antigens to the systemic lymphatic system. This antigenic exposure may then incite an autoimmune inflammatory reaction in both the injured and sympathizing eye.

The tissue antigen HLA-A11 is associated with SO.

The Patient

Clinical Symptoms
The earliest symptoms usually consist of photophobia and decreased accommodation because of inflammation of the ciliary body. Other symptoms may include bilateral eye pain, decreased vision, and hyperemia.

Clinical Signs (severity can vary widely)
- Bilateral, granulomatous, anterior uveitis with mutton-fat keratic precipitates
- Edematous iris with possible neovascularization
- Peripheral anterior synechiae
- Glaucoma
- Cataracts
- Small depigmented nodules at the level of the RPE (Dalen–Fuchs nodules)
- Thickening of the uveal tracts (panuveitis)
- Vitritis
- Papillitis, retinal edema, and exudative retinal detachments may occur
- Meningeal inflammation
- Optic atrophy

There may also be signs of vitiligo, dysacusis (pain in the ear from exposure to sound and impairment of hearing), poliosis, and alopecia, but these findings are less common than in V-K-H syndrome.

Demographics

There does not appear to be a true predilection for gender, age, or race. There is a slightly higher incidence of SO in the early decades of life when traumatic injuries are more common and in the elderly when intraocular surgical procedures are more frequent.

There is also a slightly higher incidence in males, probably because men sustain more ocular injuries; however, the risk of SO is <1% for an eye with penetrating trauma.

Significant History

The patient with SO will have a history of a perforating corneal ulcer, ocular injury, or ocular surgery usually associated with uveal prolapse. The inflammation typically develops 4 to 8 weeks after the inciting event (range 5 days to 50 years) with 70% of cases occurring within the first 3 months and 90% of cases occurring within the first year.

Because sarcoid, tuberculosis, and syphilis can cause a granulomatous panuveitis, the patient should be questioned regarding pulmonary problems and sexually transmitted diseases.

There have been rare cases of SO associated with cyclocryotherapy, ocular radiation procedures, cataract surgery, and vitrectomy.

Ancillary Tests

The diagnosis of SO is primarily based on the history of ocular injury or ocular surgery and the appropriate clinical findings.

Fluorescein angiography and/or B-scan ultrasonography may help to confirm the diagnosis. ERG and EOG may assist in establishing the severity of disease and help to monitor the response to therapy, but are rarely indicated.

If the diagnosis of SO is not readily apparent, one should consider a chest x-ray, RPR, FTA-ABS, and ACE level to exclude other uveitic syndromes.

The Treatment

Prompt and aggressive use of cycloplegics and anti-inflammatory therapy can improve the visual outcome. The concentration and dosage of steroids will depend on the severity of the condition and should be slowly tapered as the condition improves. Intraocular pressures must be closely monitored.

For moderate-to-severe cases, one should consider:

- Cycloplegic agents (scopolamine 0.25% tid).
- Prednisolone acetate 1% q1 to 2 hours.
- Subconjunctival or sub-Tenon's injections of soluble steroids, such as 4 mg of dexamethasone 2 to 3 times per week, may be given in the initial phase of therapy.
- Systemic steroids are recommended on a daily basis, beginning with a high dose of oral prednisone (1 to 2 mg/kg/day) for 1 to 2 weeks. Steroids should then be gradually tapered to a maintenance dose of 15 to 20 mg per day, and in the absence of systemic complications, treatment should be maintained several months after the inflammation has cleared.

If the patient fails to respond to corticosteroid therapy or if steroid therapy is contraindicated, then other immunosuppressive drugs such as methotrexate, cyclosporine, chlorambucil, cyclophosphamide, azathioprine, and the like have benefited some patients.

Exacerbations of SO are unpredictable, and lifetime observation of the patient is necessary.

Enucleation of the impaired eye should prevent SO if performed within 9 days of the inciting injury or surgery. The importance of enucleating the exciting eye after the onset of symptoms in the sympathizing eye remains controversial, but should be performed if the eye has no potential for recovery, is cosmetically unacceptable, or is painful. Evisceration causes a greater risk of SO than enucleation.

FUCHS' HETEROCHROMIC IRIDOCYCLITIS (FHI)
Nicky R. Holdeman

ICD—9: 364.21

THE DISEASE
Pathophysiology

Fuchs' heterochromic iridocyclitis is a nongranulomatous, chronic, low-grade iridocyclitis associated with iris stromal atrophy, heterochromia, posterior subcapsular cataract formation, and open angle glaucoma. While evidence suggests that an immune mechanism may underlie the pathogenesis of FHI, the stimulus for this immune response is still unknown.

Etiology

The etiology of FHI has not been fully established. An association with congenital ocular toxoplasmosis is suspected; however, there are conflicting opinions. Herpes simplex virus (HSV) DNA has been isolated from the aqueous humor of an eye with FHI, suggesting that HSV may play a role in the pathogenesis of this disorder.

Currently, the etiology of the syndrome is still under investigation.

The Patient
Clinical Symptoms
Because of the insidious nature of this disease, the patient may either be asymptomatic or may present with complaints of decreased vision or glare secondary to cataract formation. Patients usually have minimal inflammatory symptoms but on occasion may report mild ocular discomfort or ciliary spasm type pain.

Clinical Signs
The classic triad of signs in FHI are iris heterochromia, cataracts, and keratic precipitates (KP). However, iris heterochromia is seen in only 40 to 90% of patients and is no longer considered an essential feature in the diagnosis.

The KP on the corneal endothelium in FHI are diffuse and have a stellate shape with interspersed wispy filaments. KP are seen in 83 to 96% of patients. Other findings may include:

- Vitreous opacities ($\approx$66% of patients)
- Fine vessels on the iris surface and anterior chamber angle ($\approx$20 to 30% of patients); neovascular glaucoma rarely if ever occurs

- POAG ($\approx$25 to 60% of patients)
- Mild to no anterior chamber reaction
- Hyphema
- Macular edema

FHI is mainly unilateral with 10 to 15% of patients demonstrating bilateral disease.

Note: Unilateral, transparent, multiple iris nodules without synechia may be observed and could be especially helpful in the diagnosis of FHI in African Americans when heterochromia may not be obvious.

Demographics

There is no evidence of hereditary, sexual, or racial predisposition. The age at diagnosis is usually between 20 to 60 years with a mean of about 40 years. Because FHI is often asymptomatic, the diagnosis is frequently delayed until visual symptoms develop.

Significant History

Has the patient noted a change in iris color? (Typically about 50% of patients with iris heterochromia are aware of a difference in color between the eyes. Ten to 15% may report a congenital heterochromia.)

The affected eye is usually lighter in color; however, patients with dark irides may have the darker eye involved as the iris pigment epithelium is visible through an atrophic iris stroma.

There should be no history of acute inflammatory symptoms or of ocular trauma.

No systemic features have been observed.

Ancillary Tests

The diagnosis of this disease is based mainly on history and clinical appearance. Atypical presentations may justify excluding inflammatory conditions such as syphilis, TB, and so on, as well as other entities that present with heterochromia (i.e., iridocorneal endothelial [ICE] syndrome, glaucomatocyclitic crisis, congenital Horner's syndrome, herpetic infection, iris melanoma, intraocular foreign body, and ocular medications). Most of these conditions are easily excluded.

The Treatment

Because most patients with FHI rarely complain of symptoms secondary to ocular inflammation, no treatment is often required. Cycloplegia is usually not needed because synechiae formation is rare. Topical corticosteroids are occasionally useful but should be reserved for patients in whom keratitic precipitates obstruct the visual axis. Patients with FHI frequently become refractory to topical steroids, and steroids can exacerbate cataract formation and glaucoma, the two most common complications that result in a reduction of vision.

Cataracts develop in most, if not all, patients with FHI. The opacity is posterior subcapsular and can quickly advance, even in relatively young patients. Most patients undergoing cataract extraction do well, but complications are typically greater when compared to the general population.

Glaucoma occurs in up to 60% of patients with FHI and may be a result of trabeculitis, rubeosis, hyphema, lens-induced angle closure, and/or as a response to steroids. The development of glaucoma is an ominous complication, as intraocular pressures frequently become unmanageable with medical therapy and surgery often has only moderate success.

ORBITAL INFLAMMATORY PSEUDOTUMOR
Joseph W. Sowka

ICD—9: 376.11

THE DISEASE

Pathophysiology

Orbital inflammatory pseudotumor is a nonspecific inflammatory process of unknown etiology. The term is used to describe any idiopathic inflammatory lesion that simulates a neoplasm within the orbit. It presents as a unilateral orbital mass lesion with compressive effects to orbital structures with evidence of inflammation and infiltration. It is believed to be a self-limiting disease and, while benign in nature, can cause serious ocular damage and possibly vision loss from optic nerve compression.

Depending upon the histological characteristics, orbital inflammatory pseudotumor can be subdivided into different types: granulomatous, lymphoid, sclerosing, vasculitic, and eosinophilic.

Etiology

Mechanisms ranging from autoimmunity to infectious to poor wound healing have all been proposed to account for the development of orbital inflammatory pseudotumor. The inflammatory infiltrate is composed of polymorphic leukocytes, lymphocytes, plasma cells, and fibrovascular tissue. Granulomatous orbital pseudotumor is characterized by histiocytes and multinucleate giant cells. Well-formed noncaseating granulomas may be present. Granulomatous inflammatory orbital pseudotumor has been linked with Tolosa Hunt syndrome and may well be the same disease, though Tolosa Hunt syndrome typically occupies the cavernous sinus while orbital pseudotumor occupies the orbit. Sclerosing orbital pseudotumor has proportionately greater interstitial connective tissue than inflammatory cells.

Inflammatory orbital pseudotumor gives the clinical impression of a benign or malignant lesion; however, only inflammatory tissue is present. Macroscopically, orbital inflammatory pseudotumor appears as a pink, firm, rubbery lesion. Pseudotumors can affect any structure within the orbit and may be confined to only one structure (e.g., lacrimal gland).

The Patient

Inflammatory orbital pseudotumor may occur in any age group without racial or gender predilection. The presentation is usually acute, though chronic forms do exist. Typically, the patient complains of an acute unilateral onset of pain, swelling, and proptosis. Vision may be reduced.

Clinical Symptoms
- Orbital pain
- Vision loss
- Swelling
- Diplopia
- Unilateral
- Recurrent

Clinical Signs
- Proptosis
- Swollen eyelid
- Increased orbital pressure
- Palpable orbital mass
- Motility restriction
- Perineuritis
- Disc edema or atrophy

Demographics

Studies have shown inflammatory orbital pseudotumor to occur in ages from 4 to 80. There is no racial or gender predilection.

Significant History

The patient will manifest acute onset of orbital and retro-orbital pain. The patient may feel a fullness or pressure on the globe. There are no specific precipitating conditions, but the patient may have a history of systemic autoimmune disease such as systemic lupus erythematosus, rheumatoid arthritis, and diabetes.

Ancillary Tests

Orbital inflammatory pseudotumor is a diagnosis of exclusion. Neoplastic disease must be ruled out. The differential diagnosis includes orbital cellulitis, thyroid ophthalmopathy, sarcoidosis, lymphoid tumor, lymphangioma, and metastatic carcinoma.

The diagnosis of inflammatory orbital pseudotumor is largely a clinical one. High resolution CT scanning will demonstrate soft tissue swelling. Contrast enhanced MRI is clinically superior to CT scanning and remains the test of choice. Because of potential damage to orbital structures, biopsy is not typically done.

In that this is a diagnosis of exclusion, the following tests should be run:

- Complete blood count
- Erythrocyte sedimentation rate
- Antinuclear antibodies
- Anti-dsDNA
- Antineutrophil cytoplasmic antibodies (C-ANA, P-ANCA)
- Rapid plasma reagin
- Serum protein electrophoresis

The Treatment

Inflammatory orbital pseudotumor is very steroid responsive with remission of signs and symptoms within days. In fact, steroid responsiveness is considered a diagnostic feature of this disease. However, in that malignancies are also steroid responsive to some degree, this should not be taken as an absolute diagnostic test. Oral prednisone 60 to 80 mg daily with slow taper is advocated. Radiation therapy may work in those who are not steroid responsive or can be used adjunctively. Other immunosuppressant agents have achieved some anecdotal success.

Chapter 11

Lacrimal Disorders

DACRYOADENITIS
Andrew Mick

ICD—9: 375.00

THE DISEASE
Pathophysiology

Dacryoadenitis is a disease characterized by inflammation and enlargement of the lacrimal gland. Depending on the clinical characteristics and etiology, it is classified as acute, chronic, or granulomatous.

Etiology

Underlying causes of dacryoadenitis include infectious diseases, inflammatory disorders, malignancies, and benign enlargements.

ACUTE DACRYOADENITIS
Andrew Mick

ICD—9: 375.01

THE DISEASE
The Patient

Clinical Symptoms
- Sudden onset of pain in the superior temporal orbit
- Upper eyelid is swollen, red, and tender to the touch
- Secondary red, irritated eye with occasional tearing and itching
- If severely inflamed, double vision in attempted superior gaze

Clinical Signs
- Usually unilateral, but can be bilateral
- Eversion of the upper eyelid reveals an enlarged, inflamed lacrimal gland
- Palpebral, orbital, or both lobes of the lacrimal gland may be involved

- Chemosis of surrounding conjunctiva with an occasional follicular response
- Erythema/edema of upper temporal eyelid: "S-shaped" ptosis
- Mucopurulent discharge may be present, especially if bacterial
- Tender palpable ipsilateral preauricular nodes
- Occasional proptosis with mild extraocular muscle (EOM) disruption

Demographics

Acute dacryoadenitis is a rare disorder usually of infectious etiology. It is most common in children and young adults, but all ages can be affected. Route of infection can be blood borne, transconjunctival, transneuronal, or through direct inoculation from trauma. The most common causative agents are viruses including mumps, Epstein-Barr (mononucleosis), herpes simplex, and rarely HIV. Bacterial dacryoadenitis is less common and often accompanies traumatic inoculation. Frequently recovered organisms include *Straphylococcus sp.*, *Streptococcus sp.*, and *Neisseria* gonorrhoeae. Inflammatory disorders such as sarcoidosis, Wegener granulomatosis, and Crohn's disease usually manifest as chronic or bilateral dacryoadentis, but must be ruled out. Rarely neoplastic etiologies including leukemia and lymphoma present as acute dacryoadenitis.

Significant History
- Recent and rapid onset of symptoms
- Occasional fever

Laboratory Tests
- CBC with differential (leukemia, lymphoma).
- Culture any discharge on blood agar (most bacteria) and chocolate agar (*Haemophilus sp.*, *Neisseria* gonnorrhoeae).
- Computed tomography (CT), magnetic resonance imaging (MRI), or orbital ultrasound to delineate extent of tissue involvement. Scanning especially indicated if there is presence of proptosis, limited EOM motility, or decreased vision.
- Appropriate blood titers for suspected viral etiologies (mumps, Epstein-Barr, HIV).

The Treatment

Bacterial: Broad-spectrum antibiotics should be initiated until cultures can better direct therapy. Appropriate choices would include:

- Amoxicillin/clavulanate 500/125 mg bid
- Cephalexin 250 to 500 mg qid
- If penicillin/cephalosporin sensitive, Azithromycin: 500 mg daily × 3 days (Tri-Pak) or 250 mg bid × 1 day, then daily × 4 days (Z-Pak)
- Severe presentations or pediatric cases should be referred for possible hospitalization with IV drug therapy

Viral:

- Cool compresses
- Topical lubricants
- Appropriate analgesic as needed
- Herpetic: Acyclovir 400 mg 5×/day (simplex) or 800 mg 5×/day (zoster), Valacyclovir 1000 mg tid, Famciclovir 500 mg tid

CHRONIC/GRANULOMATOUS DACRYOADENITIS
Andrew Mick

ICD—9: 375.02

THE DISEASE

The Patient

Clinical Symptoms
- Chronic or recurrent swelling and redness of the upper lid
- Occasional pain and double vision

Clinical Signs
- Localized mass in the lateral upper eyelid area
- Occasional proptosis with downward displacement of the globe
- EOM restrictions

Etiology

Chronic/granulomatous dacryoadenitits has a variety of etiologies. Causes include inflammatory disorders (sarcoidosis, Wegener granulomatosis, Crohn's disease), infectious (tuberculosis, mumps, HIV, syphilis), and neoplastic (leukemia, lymphoma).

Significant History
- Symptoms/signs of systemic infectious, inflammatory, or neoplastic disease

Laboratory Tests
- CBC with differential (leukemia, lymphoma).
- Suspected sarcoidosis: Chest x-ray, serum angiotensin converting enzyme (ACE).
- Suspected Wegener granulomatosis: Sinus/chest x-ray, antineutrophil cytoplasmic antibody (ANCA) test, erythrocyte sedimentation rate (ESR), C-reactive protein (CRP).
- Suspected Crohn's disease: History of characteristic symptoms (weight loss, chronic diarrhea, abdominal pain), hematocrit/hemoglobin (GI bleeding), ESR, x-ray with barium, abdominal CT.

- Presumed tuberculosis: PPD with anergy panel.
- Presumed syphilis: RPR or VDRL and FTA-ABS.
- HIV serology.
- Orbital CT, MRI, or ultrasound to delineate extent of tissue involvement. Scanning especially indicated if there is presence of proptosis, limited motility, or decreased vision.
- Lacrimal gland biopsy.

The Treatment
- Treatment will depend on underlying cause of the chronic dacryoadenitis and will involve referral to appropriate subspecialist for evaluation.

DACRYOCYSTITIS
Andrew Mick

ICD—9: 375.30

THE DISEASE
Pathophysiology

The disorder is characterized by acute or chronic infection or inflammation of the lacrimal sac. Complete or partial obstruction of the nasolacrimal duct is often the precipitating event, prior to infection. Obstruction can result from developmental anomalies, nasal/sinus disease, trauma, neoplasm, dacryolith formation, or systemic inflammatory disease.

Etiology

Acute (ICD—9: 375.32)

- Lacrimal stenosis that results in secondary acute and severe infection
- Most commonly cultured bacteria are gram-positive cocci: *Staphylococcus aureus*, *Staphylococcus epidermidis*, *Streptococcus* pneumoniae
- Less common gram-negative bacteria: *Pseudomonas aeruginosa*, *Escherichia coli*
- Rarely anaerobic bacteria are cultured: *Actinomyces israelii*, *Propionibacterium acnes*
- Rarely fungi are cultured: *Aspergillus sp., Candida sp*

Chronic (ICD—9: 375.42)

- Partial or complete blockage of the nasolacrimal that results in secondary chronic infection
- Similar flora to acute dacrocystitis are often cultured including gram positive (*Staphylococcus a., Staphylococcus e., Streptococcus p.*), gram negative (*Pseudomonas a., E. coli*), or fungal (*Aspergillus sp., Candida sp.*)

The Patient

Clinical Symptoms
Acute

- Significant pain, redness, and swelling over the lacrimal sac
- Tearing and discharge
- Occasional fever

Chronic

- Tearing may be the only symptom in many cases
- Occasional swelling
- Discomfort with local digital pressure

Clinical Signs
Acute

- Edema and hyperemia overlying the lacrimal sac. Swelling concentrated under the medial canthal ligament
- Mucopurulent discharge may be expressed from the punctum
- A localized abscess may be present with breakthrough to the surface
- Occasional preauricular and submandibular swollen lymph nodes

Chronic

- Epiphora
- Local swelling over lacrimal sac
- Regurgitation of mucopurulent material with digital pressure

Demographics

Acute

- Diagnosis can be made in all age groups. The highest incidence is in middle-aged adults, with women and Caucasians more commonly afflicted.

Chronic

- Associated with congenital nasolacrimal obstruction in infancy
- In the elderly, dacryocystitis often occurs secondary to involutional stenosis or scarring of the nasolacrimal drainage system

Significant History
- Tearing
- Discharge
- Chronic conjunctivitis
- Chronic sinusitis or current upper respiratory tract infection

Laboratory Tests
- Culture-expressed discharge on blood (all bacteria), chocolate (children: *Haemophilus sp.*), Thioglycolate (aerobic and anaerobic), Sabouraud's (fungal), and Lowenstein-Jensen (*Mycobacterium sp.*)

- CT scan of orbit and sinuses if there is no immediate improvement with therapy to rule out widespread pathology or neoplasm

The Treatment

Broad-spectrum antibiotics that have coverage for the common bacterial causative agents should be initiated until cultures can better direct therapy. Appropriate choices would include:

- Amoxicillin/clavulanate 500/125 mg bid
- Cephalexin 250 to 500 mg qid
- If penicillin/cephalosporin sensitive: Azithromycin 500 mg daily × 3 days (Tri-Pak) or 250 mg bid × 1 day, then daily × 4 days (Z-Pak)
- Severe presentations or pediatric cases should be referred for possible hospitalization with IV drug therapy
- Warm compresses
- Analgesic therapy is important because there is often significant pain. Appropriate therapy includes:
  1. For mild pain: Acetaminophen 500 mg q4–6h, Ibuprofen 400–600 mg q4–6 h, Naproxen 250–500 mg bid
  2. For moderate pain: Acetaminophen with codeine (30 mg codeine) 1 to 2 tablets q4–6 h
  3. For severe pain: Acetaminophen (500 mg) with hydrocodone (5 mg) q4–6 h, Ibuprofen (200 mg) with hydrocodone (7.5 mg) q4–6 h, Acetaminophen (325 mg) with oxycodone (10 mg) q4–6 h
- Consider incision with nonresolving dacryocystitis with abscess
- Febrile or pediatric cases with systemic disease should be referred for possible hospitalization with IV drug therapy

CANALICULITIS

Andrew Mick

ICD—9: 375.31 - Acute canaliculitis, lacrimal
ICD—9: 375.41 - Chronic canaliculitis

THE DISEASE

Pathophysiology

The disorder is characterized by infection or inflammation of the canaliculi.

Etiology

Infectious agents include bacteria, fungi, and viruses. Common causative organisms include bacteria (*Actinomyces israelii*, *Propionibacterium propionicum*), fungi (*Candida sp.*, *Aspergillus sp.*), and viruses (*Herpes simplex*). Canaliculitis is rarely associated with punctal plug occlusion.

The Patient

Clinical Symptoms
- Irritation, redness, and swelling over medial portion of eyelids
- Tearing and discharge

Clinical Signs
- Mucopurulent discharge or concretions expressed from punctum
- Conjunctivitis more severe nasally
- Erythematous area around punctal openings
- Periocular skin vesicles (herpes simplex)

Demographics

Canaliculitis can affect all ages but is more common in older adults and elderly populations.

Significant History
- Chronic/recurrent conjunctivitis
- Epiphora
- History of herpetic eye disease

Laboratory Tests
- Culture any discharge from punctum on blood (all bacteria), chocolate (children: *Haemophilus sp.*), Thioglycolate (aerobic and anaerobic bacteria), and Sabouraud's (fungi)

The Treatment
- Cultures positive for bacteria: Polymyxin B/Trimethoprim oph. sol. qid
- Cultures positive for fungus: Natamycin 5% oph. susp. qid
- Suspected herpetic infection: Trifluridine 1% oph. sol. qid
- Removal of debris in canaliculus with irrigation
- Permanent scarring/stenosis may require surgical intervention

EPIPHORA

Andrew Mick

ICD—9: 375.20

THE DISEASE

Pathophysiology

The presentation of excessive tearing can be because of lacrimal hypersecretion or failure of the lacrimal system to adequately drain the tears. The four primary mechanisms are:

- Dry eye or other secondary causes of reflex hypersecretion of tears

- Blockage within the lacrimal drainage apparatus or punctal malposition
- Secondary hypersecretion of the lacrimal gland due to mechanical effects
- Primary hypersecretion of the lacrimal gland

Etiology
- Dry eye: Dryness produces ocular irritation that results in subsequent hypersecretion of tears
- Secondary hypersecretion from environmental irritants (smog, dust, or pollen) or mechanical irritants (trichiasis, entropion, or ectropion) can also produce irritation and induce hypersecretion
- Primary hypersecretion: There are many etiologies that can produce direct stimulation of the lacrimal gland. These include:
  1. Dacryoadenitis
  2. Viral infections: mumps, Epstein-Barr, herpes zoster
  3. Bacterial infections: *Straphylococcus sp.*, *Streptococcus sp.*, *Neisseria* gonorrhoeae, *Mycobacterium tuberculosis*
  4. Inflammatory conditions: sarcoidosis, thyroid ophthalmopathy, Wegener granulomatosis, Sjögren's syndrome
- Use of topical or systemic parasympathomimetic agents
- Tumors of the lacrimal gland

Blockage of the Lacrimal Drainage System
Blockage of lacrimal drainage can be congenital or acquired and occur proximally or distally within the system (see Figure 11.1).

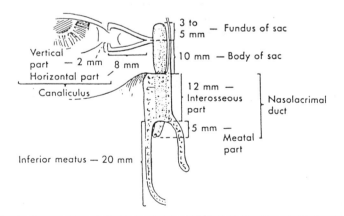

FIGURE 11.1. Lacrimal excretory system. (From Jones LT. The Cure of Epiphora Due to Canalicular Disorders, Trauma and Surgical Failures on the Lacrimal Passage. *Trans Am Acad Ophthalmol Otolaryngol* 1962;66:506.) (Previously used in *Ocular Therapeutics Handbook: A Clinical Manual.* 1st ed. Onofrey, Skorin, Holdeman, p. 274.)

Congenital Structural Blockage
ICD—9: 375.55 or 743.65

The most common congenital causes of nasolacrimal obstruction include:

- Failure of the distal end of the duct to completely canalize during development
- Lack/malformation/membranes of one or more puncta
- Lack/malformation/membranes of the canaliculi
- Congenital tumors of the lacrimal sac:
  1. Mucocele
  2. Hemangioma
  3. Dermoid
- Membrane/cyst in the nasolacrimal duct

Acquired Structural Blockage
ICD—9: 375.56

Acquired nasolacrimal duct obstruction in adults is most often caused by age-related anatomical changes or low-grade infection or inflammation of the lacrimal drainage system.

Proximal end blockage can be caused by a variety of disorders:

- Lid ectropion results in eversion of the punctum away from the tear lake. Ectropion can be caused by any chronic inflammation/infection (blepharitis, allergic conjunctivitis), scarring (chemical burns, skin disease), facial nerve palsy, age-related changes to the lid anatomy, or history of blepharoplasty.
- Megalocaruncles: Enlarged caruncle that extends to the level of the lower punctum. Presence of excess tissue results in pushing of the punctum away from its appositional location with the tear lake.
- Punctal stenosis (scarring/narrowing/occlusion).
- Canalicular stenosis (scarring/narrowing/occlusion). Chronic infection/inflammation in addition to some topical and systemic medications have been associated with canalicular scarring (i.e., topical timolol, systemic docetaxel, systemic 5-fluorouracil).

Distal end blockage also has numerous etiologies:

- Etiologies of lacrimal sac and nasolacrimal duct obstructions: dacryocystitis, dacryolith formation, cysts, mucocele, neoplasms

The Patient

Clinical Symptoms
- Watering of one or both eyes, with or without periocular pain
- Pain, redness, and swelling around lacrimal sac or upper lid
- Foreign body sensation

Clinical Signs
- Negative Jones I or II tests
- Asymmetric dye disappearance test
- Increased lacrimal tear lake

- Lid, punctum, caruncle abnormalities
- Tender swollen lacrimal gland or sac area
- Expression of purulent material from the punctum

Demographics

Epiphora can present in all age groups.

Significant History

- Persistent tearing
- Recurrent sinusitis or dacryocystitis
- Swelling or pain over lacrimal sac
- History of facial trauma or lid surgery

Laboratory Tests

- Culture any discharge if infectious etiology is suspected on blood (all bacteria), chocolate (children: *Haemophilus sp.*), Thioglycolate (aerobic and anaerobic bacteria), and Sabouraud's (fungi)
- Suspected thyroid disease: Serology for T_3, T_4, TSH
- Suspected sarcoidosis: Chest x-ray, serum angiotensin converting enzyme (ACE)
- Suspected Wegener granulomatosis: Sinus and chest x-ray, antineutrophil cytoplasmic antibody (ANCA) test, erythrocyte sedimentation rate (ESR), C-reactive protein (CRP)
- Suspected Sjögren's syndrome: Consistent history (dry mucus membranes, enlarged salivary or parotid glands), ESR, complete blood count (CBC), rheumatoid factor (RF), antinuclear antibodies (ANA)
- Dacryocystography (DCG)
  1. Conventional DCG: Contrast medium is passed through canaliculus and nasolacrimal system and imaged with computed tomography (CT), sequential radiographic images, or fluoroscopy
  2. Magnetic Resonance DCG: A more dilute contrast medium is used and ionizing radiation is avoided in the imaging of the nasolacrimal system
- CT: Axial and coronal views allow visualization of bony lacrimal canal, nasal cavity, and sinuses. CT is indicated if there is a history of trauma and sinus surgery or if there is concern about the presence of a tumor in the area.

Other Diagnostic Tests

- If infectious, inflammatory, or neoplastic lacrimal duct obstruction is not suspected, the following sequence of testing is indicated. (See Lacrimal Tests and Procedures for more detail.)
  1. Dye disappearance test confirms asymmetric production/or drainage of tears.
  2. Tear break-up time (TBUT), Schirmer testing, phenol red thread testing, rose bengal dye staining, or lissamine green dye staining are performed to rule out dry eye or other irritations as a causative factor.

3. Careful questioning of the patient regarding environmental irritants and examination of the lids, lashes, and adnexa for signs of secondary causes of hypersecretion (blepharitis, trichiasis). Examination and palpation in the area of the lacrimal sac looking for signs of infection, inflammation, or neoplasm.
4. Careful examination of the lid and punctum position in relationship to the globe and tear lake. If no observable cause of hypersecretion is found and the puncta are in apposition to the globe, a diagnosis of lacrimal system blockage is made.
5. Jones I Test performed. A negative test confirms, but does not localize the blockage.
6. Jones II Test performed. If test is positive and dye is retrieved from nasal cavity, the blockage is distal in the lacrimal system. If the test is positive and clear fluid is retrieved from the nasal cavity, the blockage is at the puncta or canaliculi. Failure to retrieve clear fluid or dye signifies complete blockage.

The Treatment

Punctal Malposition
ICD—9: 375.51

- Presence of ectropion or entropion that leads to malposition of the punctum and subsequent epiphora should be referred to an oculoplastic surgeon. Numerous blepharoplasty techniques have been developed with a high rate of success in repositioning the punctum within the lacrimal lake. Carunclectomy can be performed if underlying cause of punctal malposition is megalocaruncle.

Congenital Obstruction
ICD—9: 375.55 or 743.65

- Treat any suspected infection of the nasolacrimal system.
- Massage lacrimal sac from the common canalicular junction down to the ampulla. Ten strokes four times a day are recommended. This technique is best accomplished while feeding the infant. The vast majority of obstructions spontaneously resolve within the first year.
- Lacrimal probing from 6 to 12 months is extremely successful. The longer probing is delayed, especially beyond 12 months, the lower the success rate. Probing before 6 months carries inherent risks of anesthesia to the neonate.
- Children who do not respond to lacrimal probing are candidates for balloon dacryocystoplasty, silicone tube intubation, or dacryocystorhinostomy.

Acquired Obstruction
ICD—9: 375.56

- Treat any active infection with topical or systemic antibiotics (see Dacryocystitis/Canaliculitis).
- If negative Jones I Test, attempt to irrigate lacrimal drainage system. To rule out punctal/canalicular stenosis, dilate structures prior to irrigation.
- If irrigation of the nasolacrimal system fails, initiate further workup or refer patient to oculoplastic surgeon for evaluation.

▶ **TABLE 11.1** Commercially Available Non-dissolving Punctal Plugs. Numerous Companies Have Dissolving Punctal Plugs

Company	Product Name	Material	Sizes (mm)
Alcon (Ft. Worth, TX)	Tears Naturale	Silicone	.4, .5, .6, .7, .8
Ciba Vision (Duluth, GA)	Tear Saver	Silicone	.4, .5, .6, .7, .8,
	Tear Saver Low Flow	Silicone	.5, .6, .7, .8
Eagle Vision (Memphis, TN)	Eagle Flex Plug	Silicone	.4, .5, .6, .7, .8, .9, 1.0, 1.1
	Eagle Plug	Silicone	.4, .5, .6, .7, .8
	Eagle Low Controller	Silicone	.5, .6, .7, .8
FCI (Marshfield Hills, MA)	Ready-Set Plugs	Silicone	.4, .5, .6, .7, .8, .9,1.0
	PVP Perforated	Silicone	.7, .9
Lacrimedics (Eastwood, WA)	Herrick (Intracanalicular)	Silicone	.3, .5, .7
Medennium (Irvine, CA)	Smart Plug (Intracanalicular)	Acrylic	One Size
Oasis (Glendora, CA)	Soft Plug	Silicone	.4, .5, .6, .7, .8
Surgical Specialists (Reading, CA)	Ultra Plug	Silicone	.4, .5, .6, .7, .8
Odyssey (Memphis, TN)	Parasol	Silicone	Small ($\sim$.3–.5) Med. ($\sim$.6–.8)
	Plus	Silicone	Small ($\sim$.4–.5) Med ($\sim$.6–.7) Large ($\sim$.7–.8) XL ($\sim$.8+)

Hypersecretion
ICD—9: 375.21

- Manage dacryoadenitis if present (see Dacryoadenitis)
- Get rheumatology consult if sarcoidosis, Wegener granulomatosis, or Sjögren's disease is suspected
- Correct any trichiasis
- Manage ocular surface disease (OSD): Dry eye (artificial tears, punctal occlusion Table 11.1), allergic conjunctivitis (see Atopic Eye Disease), blepharitis (see Blepharitis)

OCULAR SURFACE DISEASE
Andrew Mick

ICD—9: 375.15

THE DISEASE

Pathophysiology

The physiology of the ocular surface is dependent upon a variety of cells whose purpose is to maintain the tear film. The tear film itself has numerous functions including creating a smooth refracting surface, transporting nutrients to the avascular cornea, and protecting the tissues from infection. Stability of the tear film is primarily under neural control and is influenced by hormones, systemic medications, emotions, dietary intake (specifically vitamin A), and a variety of environmental factors. The tear film was originally believed to be composed of three layers, but now is generally considered to contain only two. The most superficial is the thin lipid layer, which is secreted by the meibomian glands that are located within the upper and lower lids. The lipid layer serves to decrease the rate of evaporation of the tear film. Under the lipid layer is the thick aqueous-mucin gel layer. The aqueous component of this layer is produced by the main and accessory lacrimal glands. The mucin component of the layer, which is believed to be most concentrated closest to the surface epithelium, is primarily secreted by the conjunctival goblet cells. The aqueous-mucin layer allows for even wetting of the ocular surface in addition to being a barrier to foreign materials. It also contains antimicrobial proteins, nutrients, and growth factors, which further aid the superficial epithelium. The tear film is smoothed and refreshed by the blink of the lids.

While commonly referred to as simply dry eye, any abnormality to the composition or quantity of tears, disruption of the normal eyelid anatomy, or dysfunction of the blink mechanism can result in tissue damage and inflammation. Regardless of initiating events, the surface epithelium and tear film of all patients with ocular surface disease show uniform characteristics. There is an increase of the tear osmolarity as the deficiency of the aqueous component concentrates the tear film. The increased osmolarity and overall dryness results in damage to the cornea and conjunctiva and elicits an inflammatory response. The role of inflammation is evidenced by an increased number of lymphocytes and inflammatory cytokines in the tears of patients with ocular surface disease and is the basis behind the usage of topical steroidal and immunosuppressive therapies in dry eye patients.

Etiology

Ocular surface disease (or dry eye) can be classified into two main groups that have different etiologies but often have overlap in the final injury and inflammation pathways. These two categories are evaporative tear loss and aqueous deficiency.

Evaporative Tear Loss

The main cause of evaporative tear loss is blockage or a deficiency in the production of the normal lipid layer by the meibomian glands. With the loss of the stabilizing lipid layer, the aqueous component of the tear film is lost at a higher rate. Meibomian gland dysfunction can occur in isolation, but often accompanies dermatologic disorders such as acne rosacea (see Ocular Rosacea) and seborrheic dermatitis. Staphylococcal and seborrheic blepharitis (see Bacterial Blepharitis/Meibomianitis) also can influence the stability of the tear film by producing toxins and lipases that irritate the corneal epithelium and induce an inflammatory response. The lipid layer can also be influenced by the placement of a contact lens into the tear film, abnormalities in the blink mechanism, or prolonged exposure secondary to disrupted lid anatomy.

Aqueous Deficiency

This form of ocular surface disease is primarily caused by a decrease in the secretion from the primary and accessory lacrimal glands and subsequent deficiency in the aqueous component of the tear film. Classically this condition is caused by Sjögren's syndrome, but other etiologies exist.

Sjögren's Syndrome

Sjögren's syndrome is a generalized systemic autoimmune disease characterized by lymphocytic infiltration of the exocrine glands. In primary form, the glands throughout the body are affected, resulting in keratoconjunctivitis sicca, xerostomia (dry mouth), and dryness to other mucus membranes including the nose and vagina. Secondary Sjögren's syndrome has the same signs in addition to a systemic autoimmune disorder (see Sjögren's syndrome).

Non-Sjögren's Syndrome

Other less common causes of decreased aqueous layer production by the lacrimal glands exist. Disruption of the neuronal secretion control can occur after surgical procedures such as LASIK. Damage of the accessory conjunctival glands and ducts of the primary gland can result from scarring processes in disorders such as trachoma, ocular cicatricial pemphigoid, Stevens-Johnson syndrome, and chemical burns. Infiltrative diseases, such as sarcoidosis and lymphoma, can result in destruction of the glands. Systemic medications such as oral contraceptives, β-blockers, antihistamines, tricyclic antidepressants, and benzodiazepines can depress aqueous tear production as well.

The Patient

Clinical Symptoms
- Foreign body sensation
- Gritty, burning, or soreness of the eyes
- Red eyes
- Photophobia
- Discharge on the lashes
- Worsening of symptoms in windy areas, arid environments, or air conditioning

Clinical Signs
- Conjunctival injection
- Punctate epithelial defects (concentrated inferiorly and in the interpalpebral zone)
- Decreased height of inferior tear meniscus
- Mucus debris in the tear film
- Increased blink rate
- Decreased TBUT
- Fluorescein and vital dye staining
- Positive Schirmer test

Demographics

The incidence of dry eye increases with age and is extremely common in the elderly. The condition is more prevalent in woman, especially in the postmenopausal period.

Dry eye is a common sequelae of a variety of autoimmune diseases. Those people who live in dry environments or whose work requires prolonged near or computer tasks are often afflicted. Contact lens wearers also have a higher rate of dry eye symptoms.

Significant History
- Bilateral (may be asymmetrical)
- Long-standing
- Symptoms often worse in the morning
- Symptoms exacerbated by smoke, wind, heat, low humidity, prolonged near or computer work
- Taking systemic β-blockers, antihistamines, tricyclic antidepressants, benzodiazepines, or oral contraceptives
- Additional systemic symptoms that might signal the presence of Sjögren's syndrome or other autoimmune disease

Ancillary Tests (see Lacrimal Tests and Procedures)
- TBUT
- Fluorescein stain
- Vital dye stain (Rose Bengal, Lissamine Green)
- Schirmer test
- Phenol red thread test

The Treatment

After careful examination of the eye and eyelids is undertaken and appropriate additional tests have been performed, treatment should be initiated to address the underlying cause of the ocular surface disease. Any lid anatomical variant or dysfunction in the blink mechanism should be referred to an oculoplastics specialist. Contact lens wearers should consider changing lens materials, decreasing wear time, or discontinuing wear. Avoidance of contributing environmental factors such as wind, smoke, fumes, and air conditioning should be discussed. If suspected underlying autoimmune disease is present, a rheumatology consult is indicated.

Evaporative Tear Loss
The usual cause of evaporative tear loss is a disorder of the lipid layer and subsequent decrease in the aqueous component of the tear film. The main cause of lipid layer dysfunction is meibomian gland disease and blepharitis. These disorders often respond well to simple lid hygiene and warm compresses, but topically applied antibiotic ointment or oral doxycycline may be required. It has been proposed that oral supplements containing omega-3 fatty acids (Flaxseed oil, fish oil) may enhance the quality of the lipid layer, but true efficacy and safety have not been extensively studied.

- Warm compresses and lid hygiene done twice daily
- Artificial tears four times a day. (Nonpreserved formulations are always preferred and should be used if more than four times a day dosing is required to relieve symptoms.) (See Ophthalmic lubricants.)

- Lubricating ophthalmic ointment at bedtime
- Consider erythromycin, bacitracin, or polymyxin B/trimethoprim ophthalmic ointment at bedtime
- Consider doxycycline 100 mg orally, two times a day for 4 weeks, then taper

Aqueous Deficiency

In this disorder, the main problem is a deficiency in the aqueous component of the tear film. Consequently, the treatment focuses on replacing lost tears, conserving present tears, and controlling the secondary inflammation.

Mild

- Artificial tears four times a day. (Nonpreserved formulations are always preferred and should be used if more than four times a day dosing is required to relieve symptoms.)
- Lubricating ophthalmic ointment at bedtime

Moderate

- Lubricating ophthalmic gels four times a day
- Nonpreserved artificial tears four times a day to every 30 minutes
- Nonpreserved ophthalmic ointment at bedtime
- Consider punctal occlusion (see Table 11.1)

Severe Ocular Surface Disease

- Nonpreserved artificial tears every 2 hours to every 30 minutes
- Nonpreserved ophthalmic ointment at bedtime
- Punctal occlusion or cauterization
- Consider mild topical steroid: Fluoromethalone alcohol 0.1% suspension: four times a day; Loteprednol etabonate 0.2% suspension: four times a day
- Consider immunosuppressant: Cyclosporine ophthalmic emulsion 0.05%: two times a day
- Heavy mucus strands, consider mucolytic agent: Acetylcysteine 10%: four times a day
- The use of a room humidifier
- Tight-fitting goggles
- Consider tarsorrhaphy

LACRIMAL TESTS AND PROCEDURES

JONES TEST I AND II
Andrew Mick

Purpose

To determine the patency of the nasolacrimal drainage system.

Procedure

1. Jones I

- Instill copious fluorescein dye into the conjunctival sac.
- Instruct the patient to wait 5 minutes and to blink normally.
- After 5 minutes, have the patient occlude the contralateral nostril and blow the ipsilateral nostril into a white facial tissue. Examine the facial tissue for the presence of fluorescein dye. The use of the slit lamp with a cobalt blue filter or a Burton lamp may aid in detection of the dye.
- Check for fluorescein again a few minutes later.
- If no dye is visible on the facial tissue after several attempts, place a cotton-tipped applicator in the nostril at the inferior turbinate and examine for dye.

Interpretation

- Positive Jones I Test: Dye is recovered and there is no blockage.
- Negative Jones I Test: Dye is not recovered and blockage is present. No additional information regarding the location of blockage is gained.

2. Jones II

- If Jones I Test is negative, then Jones II Test is done immediately after to localize the blockage.
- Rinse excess fluorescein from conjunctival sac.
- Irrigate the lacrimal system through the inferior punctum using a lacrimal cannula.
- Have the patient occlude the contralateral nostril and blow the ipsilateral nostril into a white facial tissue. If no dye or fluid is seen on the tissue with the slit lamp or Burton lamp, place a cotton-tipped applicator in the nostril at the level of the inferior turbinate. Examine the applicator for dye.

Interpretation

- Negative Jones II Test: No dye or fluid is retrieved. Total blockage
- Positive Jones II Test: Dye is retrieved. Blockage is at distal end of lacrimal system
- Positive Jones II Test: Clear fluid is retrieved. Blockage is at the punctum or upper canaliculus

DYE DISAPPEARANCE TEST
Andrew Mick

Purpose

To determine the patency of the nasolacrimal system

Procedure

- Instill equal amounts of fluorescein dye into the conjunctival sacs of both eyes
- After 5 minutes, evaluate the loss of dye from each eye

Interpretation

- Most valuable in cases of unilateral epiphora. Asymmetric loss of dye points to a nasolacrimal obstruction on the side of the eye with the most retained fluorescein
- This test is a nonlocalizing test of nasolacrimal system blockade

TEAR BREAK-UP TIME (TBUT)
Andrew Mick

Purpose

To evaluate the quality of the tear film.

Procedure

- Instill a small amount of fluorescein into the conjunctival sac
- Position the patient into the slit lamp and instruct him or her to give a full blink and then to refrain from blinking
- Measure time to the development of dark spots in the precorneal tear film

Interpretation

- A TBUT of less than 10 seconds is considered abnormal and a sign of poor tear film quality

SCHIRMER TEST I AND II/BASIC SECRETION TEST
Andrew Mick

Purpose

- Schirmer Test I: A measurement of total tear production that includes both reflex and basal components
- Schirmer Test II: A measurement of the reflex component of total tear production
- Basic secretion test: A measurement of the basal component of total tear production

Procedure

1. Schirmer I
   - Fold commercially available Schirmer test strip approximately 3 to 5 mm from the tip. Place strip over the lower lateral lid margin of an unanesthetized eye. Care should be taken to minimize irritation to the eye when positioning the strip. The patient can be instructed to look up to minimize irritation and to blink as needed.
   - After 5 minutes, measure the amount of strip wetting.
2. Schirmer II
   - Place strips as directed for Schirmer I.
   - Stimulate nasal mucosa with cotton-tipped applicator for 10 to 15 seconds.
   - After 2 minutes, measure the amount of strip wetting.

3. Basic Secretion Test
   - Instill topical anesthetic into both eyes. Blot excess anesthetic and wait until anesthetic irritation subsides.
   - Place strips as directed for Schirmer I.
   - After 5 minutes, measure the amount of strip wetting.

Interpretation
1. Schirmer I
   - Normal wetting is 10 to 30 mm in 5 minutes
   - <10 mm of wetting is abnormal
2. Schirmer II
   - <15 mm wetting in 2 minutes indicates failure of reflex secretion
3. Basic Secretion Test
   - <10 mm wetting in 5 minutes is abnormal

PHENOL RED THREAD TEST
Andrew Mick

Purpose

To measure total tear production including basal and reflex tearing. It is a direct measurement of tear quantity. The phenol red thread test is beneficial because of its short testing time and increased patient comfort.

Procedure
- Place the cotton thread coated with phenol red over lateral half of inferior lid. The threads have a 3 mm folded end to aid in positioning
- The thread is kept in place for 15 seconds with the patient blinking normally
- As the tears are drawn down the thread, the phenol red turns from yellow to red allowing for easy visualization
- The entire length of the red portion is measured including the 3 mm intrapalpebral portion

Interpretation
- A measurement of <10 mm wetting is considered abnormal

ROSE BENGAL DYE TEST
Andrew Mick

Purpose

To measure damage to the ocular surface secondary to dry eye or other causes.

Procedure
- Instill rose bengal dye into the lower conjunctival sac
- Examine ocular surface with white light from the biomicroscope

Interpretation
Mucus and devitalized epithelial cells stain with rose bengal stain. The pattern and extent of staining reveal the amount of surface damage. Rose bengal also lightly stains healthy cells and is mildly toxic to the epithelium. The dye has been shown to be weakly virucidal. Application of rose bengal dye is often accompanied with a complaint of stinging and irritation.

LISSAMINE GREEN DYE TEST
Andrew Mick

Purpose

To measure damage to the ocular surface secondary to dry eye or other causes.

Procedure
- Instill lissamine green dye into lower conjunctival sac
- Examine ocular surface with white light from the biomicroscope

Interpretation
Mucus and devitalized epithelial cells are stained by lissamine green dye. The pattern and extent of staining reveal the amount of surface damage. Lissamine green may be less irritating to the eye than rose bengal stain.

PUNCTAL DILATION
Andrew Mick

CPT: 68801

Purpose

To provide a punctal opening adequate for tear drainage or to facilitate insertion of a lacrimal cannula or punctal plugs.

Procedure
- Place a drop of anesthetic into the eye (proparacaine 0.5% or lidocaine 4%). An anesthetic-soaked cotton-tipped applicator may also be placed over the punctum for 15 seconds.
- The patient should be supine with head firmly against the headrest.

- Insert thin end of lacrimal dilator vertically approximately 2 mm into punctal opening, and rotate the instrument between the thumb and forefinger.
- Insert the larger end of the dilator, and rotate in a similar manner.
- Bring the dilator into a horizontal position, passing it into the canaliculus while applying lateral traction to the lower lid. Continue to rotate the instrument for about 10 to 15 seconds.
- When completed, remove the dilator in a reverse fashion, following the anatomy.

Other Punctal Procedures

When repeated dilation fails to alleviate punctal stenosis, more permanent options should be considered.

- Perforated punctal plugs: Plugs that hold punctum open and allow tear flow through central channel. Often fail because of residue buildup in the central orifice.
- Snip punctoplasty (one, two, and three-snip): Scissors are used to widen punctal orifice opening communication into the punctum and upper canaliculus.
- Punch punctoplasty: Specially designed punches are used to open communication into the punctum and upper canaliculus.
- Retropunctal cautery: Cautery to bulbar conjunctival mucosa at base of punctum/canaliculus results in traction on the wall of the punctum and subsequent reestablishment of patency.

LACRIMAL IRRIGATION
Andrew Mick

CPT: 68801

Purpose

To test the patency of the nasolacrimal drainage system and possibly clear minor obstructions. Lacrimal irrigation should not be performed during active dacryocystitis.

Procedure
- Dilate the punctum (see earlier: Punctal Dilation).
- Insert the cannula (usually-23 gauge blunted needle with syringe) 2 mm vertically into the lower punctum. Then bring the cannula horizontal, inserting it up to 8 mm horizontally to the common canaliculus.
- Depress the plunger, and attempt to pass the saline or balanced salt solution through the lacrimal system.

Interpretation
- If the patient tastes/feels solution in back of the mouth or throat, the system is patent or a minor obstruction was cleared.

- If solution exits the superior punctum, a blockage likely exists in the area of the common canaliculus or lacrimal sac.
- If solution exits the inferior punctum where the cannula is inserted, a blockage likely exists in the inferior canaliculus.
- Presence of blood may indicate the presence of a tumor.
- Failure to irrigate may indicate need for surgical consultation for obstruction removal.

LACRIMAL PROBING
Andrew Mick

CPT: 68810

Purpose

The therapeutic removal of any blockage within the canaliculus, lacrimal sac, or nasolacrimal duct.

Procedure
- Place a drop of anesthetic into the eye (proparacaine 0.5% or lidocaine 4%). An anesthetic-soaked cotton-tipped applicator may also be placed over the punctum for 15 seconds.
- Patient should be supine with head firmly against the headrest.
- Insert lacrimal probe 2 mm. vertically into the punctum.
- While rotating gently, position the probe horizontally and pass it nasally until a hard stop is reached.
- Raise probe vertically to reach the lacrimal sac and gently pass it down.
- Do not force the probe against a hard stop.

DACRYOCYSTOGRAPHY (DCG)
Ryan M. Hogan

CPT: 68850

Purpose

The purpose of this test is to identify the location of a nasolacrimal obstruction as well as provide information as to the possible cause of the obstruction.

Procedure
- Patient is put in the supine position and trial radiographic films are taken to verify proper technique and view any bony abnormalities that may be present

- Several drops of topical anesthetic are applied to the cul de sac and the lower punctum is dilated
- A small catheter or cannula is carefully inserted approximately 5 to 7 mm into the lower canalicular system, following the natural anatomy
- The catheter is taped into place and radiographic contrast material is slowly and steadily injected into the lacrimal system
- As the media is being injected, sequential radiographic images are taken to assess lacrimal drainage flow and timing of flow

Interpretation

The images provided allow you to locate the obstruction (high, mid, or low level), as well as provide exquisite detail of the nasolacrimal system morphology. Dacryocystography is especially useful in helping to visualize diverticula, fistulas, polyps, foreign bodies, masses, and stones (dacryolithiasis). It will often pinpoint the specific problem, making it easier to determine a proper corrective course of action. Because of this, it is especially useful in surgical planning.

DACRYOCYSTORHINOSTOMY
Andrew Mick
CPT: 68720

Purpose

To relieve nasolacrimal obstruction that fails to clear with probing or irrigation by creating a communication between the lacrimal sac and the nasal cavity.

Procedure

1. External Dacryocystorhinostomy (DCR)
   - The external approach is the most commonly used and often requires general anesthesia.
   - External DCR has a success rate of over 90% and is the procedure of choice for the treatment of acquired nasolacrimal duct obstruction.
   - An incision is made in the area between the medial canthus and the bridge of the nose.
   - The lacrimal sac is located and an incision is made in its medial wall.
   - A new communication directly between the medial lacrimal sac and the lateral nasal cavity is created through the lacrimal bone.
   - Mucosal flaps are sometimes created from the lacrimal and nasal systems to create an epithelium-lined fistula.
   - Removable silicone tubing is placed in the new communication to inhibit closure from scarring. The use of antimetabolites (mitomycin-C) has also been advocated to control scarring at the surgical site.
2. Endoscopic Dacryocystorhinostomy (DCR)
   - Endoscopic Nasal DCR

- An endoscopic guided transnasal approach is used to create the ostium from the nasal cavity to the lacrimal sac therefore eliminating the cutaneous scar and allowing for excellent visualization of intranasal pathology. The ostium can be made with laser energy or standard incision.
- Once the ostium is formed, antimetabolites and stents may be utilized to prevent closure of the ostium.
- Even with stent placement success rates are slightly less than external DCR.
- Complications include bleeding from the middle turbinate and stent displacement.
- Endoscopic Transcanalicular DCR
  - An endoscopic guided laser passes through the canaliculus to reach the ostium site.
  - Advantages include laser energy being directed away from the globe, short duration of treatment, decreased recovery time, reduced bleeding, and the need for only local anesthetic.
  - Initial studies have shown a lower success rate than external and endoscopic nasal DCR.
- Lacrimal Sump Syndrome
  - Rare complication of DCR in which the surgical ostium is placed too high.
  - Results in the formation of a blind pouch, which collects stagnant tears and can produce recurrent dacryocystitis and epiphora.

CONJUNCTIVODACRYOCYSTORHINOSTOMY (CDCR, JONES TUBE PROCEDURE)
Andrew Mick

CPT: 68750

Purpose

This procedure bypasses the proximal lacrimal drainage system by creating a direct communication between the caruncle and the nasal cavity. CDCR is the standard treatment for canalicular obstruction and is the primary procedure after failure of conventional dacryocystorhinostomy. It is ideal for traumatic and herpetic obstruction.

Procedure

- An incision is created in the caruncle that passes directly into the nasal cavity. Visualization of the anatomy can be done directly through the surgical site or assisted with nasal endoscopy.
- Tubing is placed at the caruncle passing into the nasal cavity.
- The use of antimetabolites may be used to limit scarring.
- Complications are common and include tube extrusion, tube obstruction, patient discomfort, and infection.

BALLOON DACRYOCYSTOPLASTY (DCP)
Ryan Hogan
CPT: 68815

Purpose

Treatment to relieve incomplete nasolacrimal duct obstruction. Often performed in patients over 12 months of age that failed to clear with conservative treatment and initial probing and irrigation.

Procedure
- General anesthesia is indicated for children, but the procedure can be performed on adults with local anesthesia.
- Punctal dilation and Bowman probing are performed.
- Bowman probe is withdrawn and the balloon catheter is inserted through the upper punctum until it reaches a hard stop on the floor of the nose.
- The balloon is positioned halfway between the terminal end of the lacrimal duct and the nasal cavity and then inflated to 8 atmospheres with saline for 90 seconds. It is then deflated and inflation is repeated for 60 seconds.
- After deflating the second time the catheter is then moved to the proximal lacrimal duct, as indicated by the markings on the probe. The inflation-deflation process is repeated as discussed earlier.
- After the final complete deflation, the balloon catheter is removed with a rotating movement and patency is confirmed with irrigation of fluorescein stained saline.
- Silicone tubes may then be inserted.
- After the surgery the patient is put on a combination of steroids and antibiotics both topically and systemically, as well as a nasal decongestant spray. These drugs are very important to ensure proper healing and prevent scarring.

SILICONE TUBE INTUBATION
Ryan M. Hogan
CPT: 68815

Purpose

Silicone tube intubation is used to maintain the integrity and patency of the nasolacrimal system. The tissue heals around the silicone tubing, leaving an adequate passageway for lacrimal drainage (once the tubes are removed). It is often performed after a failed probing, postcanalicular and/or punctal trauma, or after lacrimal surgery (most commonly DCR).

Procedure

- General anesthesia is usually used for all patients.
- Punctal dilation and lacrimal probing are performed.
- Intubation apparatus consists of two stainless steel intubation probes with 1-foot of 0.025-inch silicone tubing connecting the two probes.
- The intubation probe is inserted into the superior punctum and is advanced through the nasolacrimal system into the nasal cavity.
- Once the probe is in the nasal cavity, a metal groove director is inserted beneath the inferior meatus. The groove director helps to confirm proper placement and is used to grasp the small bulbed end of the intubation probe.
- The groove director is then carefully withdrawn from the nose, pulling the probe with it.
- The procedure is repeated through the lower punctum leaving a small loop between the two puncta.
- The intubation probes are then cut from the silicone tubing and the loose ends are kept in place by tying them together with multiple square knots.
- An optional suture can then be used to secure the knot to the lateral wall of the nasal vestibule.
- Following intubation, the patient is started on a steroid-antibiotic solution qid for 1 to 2 weeks until the first follow-up visit.
- The tubes are usually removed around 6 months.
- The silicone tubes serve no drainage purpose. They are used to maintain the integrity of the passageway until the body has healed and is able to remain patent on its own.

Chapter 12

Ocular Trauma

BLUNT TRAUMA
Andrew Mick

THE DISEASE
Pathophysiology

Trauma to the eye from a blunt object results in a concussive shock wave throughout the orbit and globe. The mechanical forces exerted on the globe have the potential to produce damage in all orbital structures.

Common causes include fistfights, airbags, golf balls, baseballs, and bungee chords. Rocks and snowballs are common causes of blunt trauma in children. Greater damage often occurs with smaller objects because the force is more concentrated into the orbital structures. Smaller objects are also able to fit within the protective orbital rim. Larger objects dissipate a large amount of their force into the bones of the face and orbital rim.

The Patient
Significant History
- Recent eye trauma

Clinical Symptoms
1. Pain
   - Sharp and sectoral: Corneal abrasion, laceration of conjunctiva or lid
   - Dull aching: Orbital blowout, retrobulbar hemorrhage
   - Photophobia: Traumatic iritis
2. Watery discharge
3. Double vision
   - Entrapment of extraocular muscles
   - Damage to controlling cranial nerve
   - Retrobulbar hemorrhage
4. Decreased vision
   - Damage to cornea, iris, lens, retina, or optic nerve
   - Intraocular bleeding: Hyphema or vitreous hemorrhage

Clinical Signs

1. Acuity
   - Visual acuity should always be checked prior to performing your examination or other clinical testing.
2. Extraocular muscles (EOMs)
   - Check for restriction of EOMs. Restriction may indicate muscle entrapment secondary to an orbital fracture or damage to controlling muscle. Retrobulbar hemorrhage can also produce restriction of movement of the globe.
3. Lids
   - Ecchymosis and swelling. Make sure to check for lid lacerations and rule out injury from a sharp or penetrating object. Crepitus or subcutaneous emphysema, the introduction of air into periocular tissues, suggests orbital blowout fracture.
4. Globe
   - Examine globe for rupture: Rupture can occur with blunt trauma, but is more commonly associated with smaller, sharp objects. Rupture can take place within the cornea, the corneal-limbal junction, or the sclera. Ruptures within the cornea may be associated with a more favorable outcome because of absence of retinal involvement.
   - Conjunctival laceration.
   - Subconjunctival hemorrhage.
5. IOP
   - Low IOP may indicate a rupture of the globe, retinal detachment, or iridocyclitis.
   - High IOP may result from intraocular hemorrhage, inflammation, or lens subluxation into the anterior chamber.
6. Cornea
   - Abrasion: Only superficial epithelial layer involved.
   - Laceration: Deeper structures involved without full thickness wound.
   - Perforation: Full thickness wound.
7. Anterior chamber
   - Check for signs of intraocular inflammation, bleeding, or change in normal anatomical position of tissues.
8. Grading anterior uveitis
   - Subclinical: No cells or flare
   - Trace: Any cells or barely noticeable flare
   - Grade 1: 5 to 10 cells
   - Grade 2: 11 to 20 cells
   - Grade 3: 21 to 50 cells
   - Grade 4: Cells too numerous to count, fibrinous/plasmoid aqueous
9. Hyphema: Bleeding within the anterior chamber
   - Microhyphema
     - No layering of red blood cells in the inferior angle
     - Visible red blood cells suspended throughout the anterior chamber
   - General Hyphema
     - Grade I: <1/3 of the anterior chamber
     - Grade II: 1/3 to 1/2 of the anterior chamber

- Grade III: >1/2, but <Total
- Grade IV: Total (100%) hyphema (a.k.a. 8-ball hyphema)

10. Iris
   - Iridodialysis: Iris disinsertion at scleral spur
   - Sphincter or dilator muscle tears
   - Transillumination defects: Possible site of intraorbital foreign body entrance

11. Lens
   - Subluxation
   - Anterior segment displacement
   - Opacification: Secondary to trauma or penetrating foreign body

12. Vitreous
   - Posterior vitreous detachment
   - Vitreous hemorrhage: Greatly increases the chance of retinal detachment or tear

13. Retina
   - Retinal detachment
       - One of the most serious complications of blunt trauma to the eye is a retinal tear or detachment. Pre-existing retinal holes or breaks predispose the injured patient to greater risk of detachment. Retinal dialysis is a severe form of detachment in which there is a disinsertion of the sensory retina at the ora serrata. Late-phase detachments can occur as a result of vitreal syneresis. Patients exhibiting vitreal hemorrhage following blunt trauma have a greater risk of having a concurrent retinal tear or detachment.
   - Traumatic macular hole
       - The exact pathogenesis of traumatic macular holes is not completely elucidated. Blunt trauma to the globe produces stress especially on areas of strong vitreal retinal adhesion including the fovea. The initial equatorial expansion of the globe when the trauma occurs causes a forward and flattening of the posterior pole. Immediately after, the posterior pole rebounds to its normal anatomical position, resulting in a tangential traction at the fovea.
   - Commotio retinae
       - The shock wave produced by blunt trauma can result in a clinical picture similar to that seen in retinal edema. The retinal whitening actually represents fragmentation of the photoreceptor outer segments. The course is variable as the cells regenerate, but complete resolution can occur.

14. Choroid
   - Choroidal rupture
       - The mechanical forces exerted upon the globe during an episode of blunt trauma have the ability to deform the globe. Tissues that are less dense or less elastic have a greater propensity to rupture. The choroid commonly ruptures because it is less dense than the sclera and less elastic than the retina. Direct ruptures of the choroid occur at the point of impact, whereas indirect ruptures occur opposite the point of impact. Choroidal rupture can also occur secondary to shock waves from a high velocity, grazing object passing adjacent to the globe (chorioretinitis sclopetaria).
       - Regardless of etiology, these lesions represent ruptures of the inner choroid and overlying RPE, and are usually curvilinear and concentric to the optic

nerve. Acutely, they may be associated with subretinal hemorrhage or serous detachment of the retina. Upon resolution of the subretinal fluid, the rupture takes on the characteristic yellowish appearance with associated RPE hyperplasia.

■ If the rupture is not located centrally, vision often returns to normal. Patients with choroidal rupture should be monitored for choroidal neovascularization (CNVM) that can occur at the site of the rupture well after the acute trauma.

15. Optic nerve
   ■ Traumatic optic neuropathy
      ■ Indirect damage to the optic nerve secondary to blunt trauma is fortunately relatively rare. It is caused by the translation of force through the orbital bones or the displacement of the globe into the optic nerve. Acutely the optic nerve can appear normal, but there usually is a functional deficit. Progressive atrophy can develop over several weeks. The following clinical signs can help to make the diagnosis: decreased visual acuity, sluggish or absent pupillary responses, afferent pupillary defect, color vision deficits, visual field defects.
      ■ The most common site of injury to the nerve is in the intracanalicular portion, which is fixed to the rigid canal at the orbital apex. Another cause of damage may be the compression of the nerve or its blood supply secondary to post-traumatic inflammation.
   ■ Avulsion
      ■ It is possible for the optic nerve to be avulsed from the globe following severe frontal trauma. During certain forms of trauma, the globe may rotate or be pulled forward. These extreme forces result in tearing of the lamina cribrosa and nerve fibers at the disc margin. Over time, fibrous proliferation fills in the area surrounding the avulsion site.

Demographics

Blunt trauma is more common in males than females and has a higher prevalence in the younger age groups. Work environments and recreational activities that put eyes at risk of trauma also increase the prevalence of injuries.

Ancillary Tests

■ Binocular indirect ophthalmoscopy should be performed to evaluate the vitreous, retina, choroid, and optic nerve. Scleral indentation should be avoided in the presence of hyphema.

■ Tonometry should be done to rule out elevated IOP secondary to inflammation, hyphema, or synechiae formation. Low IOP should raise suspicion of globe rupture or retinal detachment.

■ Gonioscopy should be performed within the first month post-trauma to rule out angle recession or anterior synechiae formation. Gonioscopy should be avoided with hyphema to prevent rebleeding.

■ Screen Black patients for sickle cell disease if hyphema is present.

- Seidel Testing allows for visualization of fluid leakage from suspected penetrating injury to the globe.
- Forced duction tests should be performed if EOM restrictions persist to differentiate between mechanical resistance and paresis.
- Infraorbital nerve testing can signal presence of orbital fracture.
- Computed tomography (CT) scanning is the standard of care and is capable of detecting subtle orbital fractures or ruptures of the globe. CT can also identify metallic foreign bodies, but does not image stone, glass, or wood well.
- Magnetic resonance imaging (MRI) offers more detail of soft-tissue damage resulting from trauma. The presence of metallic foreign bodies must be ruled out prior to MRI scanning.
- Orbital ultrasonography (B-scan) is inexpensive, quick, and quite useful in detecting a ruptured globe or retinal detachment through hazy media or cataract.
- Fluorescein angiography may be ordered to rule out choroidal rupture.

The Treatment

1. Corneal abrasion
   - Antibiotic coverage
     - Noncontact lens wearer: Polymyxin B/trimethoprim oph sol qid
     - Contact lens wearer needs anti-Pseudomonal coverage: moxifloxacin, gatifloxacin, ofloxacin, ciprofloxacin, tobramycin qid
   - Cycloplegia
     - Cyclopentolate 1% tid
     - Scopolamine 0.25% bid
   - Bandage contact lens
   - Debridement of loose epithelium
2. Orbital fracture
   - Broad-spectrum antibiotic therapy
     - Amoxicillin/clavulanate 500/125 mg bid
     - Cephalexin 250 to 500 mg qid
     - Azithromycin 250 mg bid × 1 day, then qd × 4 days
   - Cool compresses/ice packs
   - Appropriate analgesics
     - Mild pain: acetaminophen 500 mg q4–6 h, ibuprofen 400 to 600 mg q4–6 h, naproxen 250 to 500 mg bid
     - Moderate pain: acetaminophen with codeine (30 mg codeine) q6 h
     - Severe pain: acetaminophen (500 mg) with hydrocodone (5 mg) q4–6 h, ibuprofen (200 mg) with hydrocodone (7.5 mg) q4–6 h, acetaminophen (325 mg) with oxycodone (10 mg) q4–6 h
   - Refer for surgical evaluation immediately
     - Oculocardiac reflex present: Bradycardia, heart block, nausea, vomiting
     - Orbital floor fracture with muscle/soft tissue entrapment: High risk of secondary ischemia, especially in children
     - Early/severe enophthalmos present or severe facial asymmetry
     - Cerebral spinal fluid rhinorrhea
     - Large fractures (>1/2 floor) or any involving the roof or orbital apex

- Refer for surgical evaluation within 1 month
  - Forced duction testing is positive or the patient experiences persistent diplopia
  - There is at least 3 mm of persistent enophthalmos present
- Observe
  - Diplopia only in extreme gazes
  - Minimal cosmetic change

3. Hyphema
   - General and microhyphema management guidelines
     - Bedrest with only bathroom privileges
     - Elevate head to at least 30° at all times, asleep and awake
     - No NSAIDs or any aspirin-containing medications
     - Protective eye shield with holes to allow for detection of decreased acuity
     - Topical steroids: Prednisolone acetate 1% qid
     - Cycloplegia: Scopolamine 0.25% bid, atropine 1% qd
     - Order lab tests for sickle cell disease/trait in African American patients
     - Monitor and treat elevated IOP over 24 mm Hg. IOP may be elevated in hyphema patients secondary to trabecular meshwork obstruction by red blood cells, inflammatory debris, or peripheral synechiae. A large, central clot can also induce secondary pupillary block. Elevated IOP can result in damage to the optic nerve and blood staining of the cornea. β-blockers should be the first line of therapy in the absence of contraindications. Prostaglandin analogs should not be used to avoid adding to the inflammatory response. Miotics increase vascular permeability and increase the risk of posterior synechiae. Carbonic anhydrase inhibitors are contraindicated in sickle cell disease due to acidification of anterior chamber.
     - Daily ocular evaluation, including visual acuity, tonometry, and slit-lamp evaluation. Patient should return immediately if there is a decrease in vision or change in symptoms.
   - A more severe hyphema or a noncompliant patient may require hospitalization. While hospitalized, activity can be more closely monitored, and antifibrinolytic agents (aminocaproic acid 50 mg/kg q4 h) may be administered. Patients in which hospitalization should be considered:
     - Large hyphema: Greater than 1/3 anterior chamber
     - Uncooperative patients
     - Children: Amblyopia risk with persistent hyphema
     - Presence of rebleeding
     - Patient utilizing anticoagulant therapy
     - Sickle cell disease/trait patients
     - Medically uncontrolled IOP
   - Reasons to refer hyphema patient for consideration of surgical removal of blood
     - IOP extremely elevated and not responsive to topical therapy
     - Grade III or IV hyphema lasting 6 days: Risk of corneal blood staining
     - Children with persistent hyphema: Amblyopia risk

4. Traumatic uveitis
   - Treatment guidelines:
     - Subclinical: Cyclopentolate 1% qid

- Grade 1: Homatropine 5% tid, prednisolone acetate 1% tid
- Grade 2: Homatropine 5% qid, scopolamine 0.25% bid, prednisolone acetate 1% qid
- Grades 3 and 4: Atropine 1% bid–qd, scopolamine 0.25% tid.–bid; prednisolone acetate 1% q5 min–q2 h; consider steroid ointment qhs: Vasociden or cetapred (sulfacetamide/prednisolone); Pred-G (gentamicin/prednisolone); tobradex (tobramycin/dexamethasone)
- Presence of elevated IOP associated with iritis: β-blockers are first line of therapy; selective α_2–agonists; topical carbonic anhydrase inhibitors; no prostaglandin analogs: May promote inflammation; no miotics: increased vascular permeability and posterior synechiae formation

5. Lens subluxation
    - If there is subluxation of the lens into the anterior chamber, there may be a marked increase in IOP secondary to pupil block. Prior to referral for repositioning or removal of the lens, the following should be done to decrease IOP:
        - Cycloplegia with appropriate agent
        - Treat IOP with β-blocker, α-agonist, topical or oral carbonic anhydrase inhibitor (acetazolamide 250 qid, 500 mg sequel bid, methazolamide 25 mg bid), or oral hyperosmotic agent (isosorbide 1 to 3 gm/kg, not metabolized to glucose)
6. Ruptured globe
    - Advise patient to not touch, rub, or squeeze eyes. Position eye shield, and advise the patient to not consume any food or water. Immediately transport patient to ophthalmic surgeon for surgical repair.
7. Commotio retinae
    - This condition is a common sequelae of blunt trauma and represents local damage and disruption to the photoreceptor outer segments. The prognosis with uncomplicated commotio retinae is excellent, and vision often returns to normal. More extensive damage to the photoreceptors manifests in RPE mottling and atrophy that may result in functional deficits. There is no specific treatment for this condition.
8. Retinal tears and detachments
    - A primary reason for conducting a thorough evaluation of the eye is to detect retinal tears and detachments. If the posterior pole cannot be visualized because of media opacity, then a B-scan ultrasonography should be performed to evaluate for retinal detachments. An afferent pupil defect may be an early indicator of possible detachment. Patient should be referred for retinopexy or vitreal-retinal surgery as the extent of damage warrants.
9. Choroidal rupture
    - There is no specific treatment for choroidal rupture. Those involving the center of the macula have a very poor prognosis for return of normal vision. The clinician must be alert for the development of a choroidal neovascular membrane (CNVM) at the site of RPE disruption. A CNVM can occur within 6 months of the injury or years later. If a patient with a history of choroidal rupture develops new symptoms of decreased acuity or metamorphopsia, a fluorescein angiogram should be

performed. A CNVM in choroidal rupture patients should be comanaged with a retinal specialist.

10. Optic nerve trauma
   - The most commonly accepted treatment of optic nerve trauma is the administration of IV steroids, usually methylprednisolone. The optimal dose and duration of treatment is not completely elucidated and will vary with extent of damage and treating physician.
   - Surgical decompression of a damaged optic nerve canal may be undertaken if necessary.
   - There is no treatment for avulsion of the optic nerve.

CORNEAL ABRASION
Andrew Mick

THE DISEASE
Pathophysiology

The cornea is composed of five distinct layers, including the epithelium, Bowman's membrane, stroma, Descemet's membrane, and the endothelium. A defect in the most superficial layer, the epithelium, is classified as a corneal abrasion.

Any object that strikes the cornea can produce a superficial abrasion. Common causes are fingernails, tree branches, mascara brushes, and paper cuts.

The Patient
Significant History
- Trauma from vegetative matter: Increased risk of fungal infection
- Contact lens wear: Increased risk of bacterial infection, especially *Pseudomonas*
- Paper cuts or fingernail injuries: Increased risk of recurrent erosion after resolution
- High-speed foreign body or associated blunt trauma: Increased risk of penetrating injury

Clinical Symptoms
- Pain/foreign body sensation
- Lacrimation
- Light sensitivity

Clinical Signs
- Positive fluorescein staining of defect
- Negative Seidel Test
- Mild anterior chamber reaction
- Swollen eyelid

The Treatment

- Cycloplegia: Cyclopentolate 1% qid–bid, homatopine 5%, tid–bid, scopolamine 0.25% bid
- Noncontact lens wearers:
  - Polymyxin B/trimethoprim oph sol qid
  - Polymyxin B/bacitracin oph ung qhs
- Contact lens wearers: *Pseudomonas* coverage
  - Moxifloxacin, gatifloxacin, ofloxacin, ciprofloxacin, levofloxacin, tobramycin oph sol qid
  - Ciprofloxacin, tobramycin, polymyxin B/bacitracin ung qhs
- Consider a tight-fitting low-powered soft contact lens applied overnight to decrease lid-cornea interaction and facilitate epithelial healing of large or extremely painful abrasions.
- Consider topical NSAID to decrease pain: Ketorolac or diclofenac oph sol.
- Appropriate analgesics for pain:
  - Mild pain: Acetaminophen 500 mg q4–6 h, ibuprofen 400 to 600 mg q4–6 h, naproxen 250 to 500 mg bid
  - Moderate pain: Acetaminophen with codeine (30 mg codeine) q6 h
  - Severe pain. Acetaminophen (500 mg) with hydrocodone (5 mg) q4–6 h, ibuprofen (200 mg) with hydrocodone (7.5 mg) q4–6 h, acetaminophen (325 mg) with oxycodone (10 mg) q4–6 h.
- Reevaluate until reepithelialized; monitor for infection or recurrent erosion

RECURRENT CORNEAL EROSION

Andrew Mick

THE DISEASE

Pathophysiology

Damage to Bowman's membrane, the basement membrane of the epithelium, prevents normal adherence of the epithelium. This results in a weakened area of epithelium that regularly sloughs off. Bilateral anterior corneal dystrophies (Epithelial Basement Membrane Dystrophy, Meesmann's Dystrophy, Reis-Bucklers' Dystrophy) can result in a similar clinical presentation.

Etiology

Recurrent epithelial defects secondary to poor adherence to the basement membrane. Commonly caused by prior injury to the cornea.

The Patient

Significant History
- History of corneal trauma
- Previous episodes of similar symptoms

Clinical Symptoms
- Recurrent pain and foreign body sensation, most prominent upon awakening
- Lacrimation
- Light sensitivity
- Decreased vision

Clinical Signs
- Negative and/or positive corneal staining with fluorescein dye
- Injection of conjunctiva
- Mild anterior chamber reaction
- Presence of anterior corneal dystrophy

Demographics

Anterior Corneal Dystrophies
1. Epithelial Basement Dystrophy (Map Dot Dystrophy)
   - Most cases not inherited, may show autosomal dominant pattern
   - Intricate pattern of dots and lines throughout the epithelium
   - Most commonly seen in adults between 40 and 70 years
2. Meesmann's Dystrophy
   - Autosomal dominant inheritance
   - Intraepithelial cysts especially concentrated in the interpalpebral space
   - Most commonly presents in first to second decade
3. Reis-Bucklers' Dystrophy
   - Autosomal dominant inheritance
   - Honeycomb appearance of central epithelium
   - Usually presents in first to second decade with painful erosions

Ancillary Tests

None.

The Treatment

Initial Therapy
- Cycloplegia: Cyclopentolate 1% tid, homatropine 5% bid
- Polymyxin B/trimethoprim oph sol qid, polymyxin B/bacitracin oph ung qhs
- Copious artificial tears and ophthalmic lubricants

- Consider tight-fitting bandage contact lens if erosion is large or patient is extremely symptomatic
- Follow closely until reepithelialized

After Reepithelialization
- Nonpreserved artificial tears during the day, lubricating ung qhs
- Consider 5% NaCl ung qhs × 4 to 6 weeks, then as needed

Failure to Reepithelialize
- Anesthetize eye with proparacaine 0.5%.
- Remove abnormal/loose epithelium with sterile forceps.
- Apply bandage contact lens and treat as directed in the "After Reepitheliaztion."

Continued Recurrence
- If a large area of the cornea is involved, preferably not in optic axis, remove abnormal epithelium with forceps. Apply micropuncture therapy (multiple punctures through Bowman's membrane) with 23-gauge needle. Apply bandage lens and treat as directed earlier.

Other Treatment Options
- If treatment zone is large or if affected area is in the optic axis, the patient should be referred for superficial keratectomy or phototherapeutic keratectomy (PTK).

SUPERFICIAL OCULAR FOREIGN BODY
Andrew Mick

THE DISEASE
Pathophysiology

A variety of materials in the environment can easily embed themselves into the cornea or conjunctiva. Evaluation of the type of material and its precise location in the eye is necessary to determine appropriate management.

Etiology

Drilling, chopping, and sanding can produce particles that can become entrapped in superficial layers of the eye. Wind-borne particles are another source of this injury.

The Patient
Significant History
- Report of getting something in the eye or employment/environment that entails exposure to debris.
- Report of high-speed foreign body increases risk of penetrating injury.

Clinical Symptoms
- Foreign body sensation
- Lacrimation
- Photophobia

Clinical Signs
- Corneal FB tracks
- FB embedded in the cornea/conjunctiva
- Accumulation of mucous around FB
- Metallic corneal/conjunctival rust ring if material is oxidized
- Secondary iritis

Demographics

Most cases of superficial foreign bodies occur in association with occupations that involve exposure to projectiles including carpentry, metal working, and mechanics. Recreational activities and outside environments may also predispose patients to this type of injury.

Ancillary Tests
- If the foreign body was high speed in origin, there is increased suspicion of intraocular penetrance
  - Careful examination of the fundus with ophthalmoscopy and anterior chamber with gonioscopy
  - CT/MRI/Ultrasound scanning

The Treatment
- Careful history to find type of material and speed introduced
- Careful slit-lamp evaluation with single, and if necessary, double-lid eversion
- Conjunctival FB
  - Remove FB with cotton-tipped applicator moistened with sterile saline. If embedded, use proparacaine 0.5% or lidocaine 4% prior to removal to anesthetize the eye. Remove FB with a spud or jewelers forceps.
- Nonmetallic corneal FB
  - Anesthetize with one drop of proparacaine 0.5%.
  - Remove with spud tool, taking care to minimize damage to the epithelium.
  - Polymyxin B/trimethoprim oph sol qid.
  - Cycloplegia: Cyclopentolate 1%, homatropine 5% can be instilled if there is a secondary uveitis.
- Metallic corneal FB
  - Anesthetize with one drop of proparacaine 0.5%.
  - Remove as much material as possible with spud tool.
  - Remove rust ring with Alger brush.

- Cycloplegia: Cyclopentolate 1%, homatropine 5% or scopolamine 0.25% if marked inflammation.
- Follow closely until reepithelialized.

INTRAOCULAR/INTRAORBITAL FOREIGN BODY
Andrew Mick

THE DISEASE
Pathophysiology

Small high-speed foreign bodies have the force to penetrate the ocular tissues and lodge themselves anywhere within the orbit or globe. The majority of these foreign bodies are metallic and inorganic (bullets, pellets, shrapnel), but the organic materials (wood) are more likely to cause severe infection and inflammation.

Etiology

A history of hammering metal on metal, grinding metallic objects, or being in the vicinity where such work is being performed increases the possibility of an intraocular foreign object. A child falling on an object is also a common cause.

The Patient

Significant History
- Struck in eye with high-speed projectile
- Delayed onset of ocular or orbital inflammation and a history of periocular trauma

Clinical Symptoms
Patient may be asymptomatic or present with:

- Aching pain
- Light sensitivity
- Decreased vision
- Double vision
- Increased tearing

Clinical Signs
1. Intraocular foreign body
   - Chemosis
   - Corneal laceration
   - Anterior or posterior segment cell and flare
   - High or low IOP

- Hyphema
- Cataract
- Irregular pupil
- Iris tears
- Subconjunctival hemorrhage
- Vitreous hemorrhage
- Retinal detachment
2. Intraorbital foreign body
   - EOM limitation or pain on eye movement
   - Ecchymosis/laceration of eyelid
   - Orbital cellulitis
   - Ptosis
   - Palpable mass

Ancillary Tests

- CT scan.
- B-scan ultrasonography if full fundus examination is not possible with ophthalmoscopy or if initial CT scan is normal with a high suspicion of orbital foreign body. Nonmetallic, inorganic (glass, plastic), and organic (wood) materials are not imaged well with CT.
- MRI only if metallic object can be completely ruled out.

The Treatment

1. Intraocular foreign body
   - If an intraocular foreign body is discovered, the patient should be advised to not consume any food or water and should be immediately transported to an ophthalmic surgeon for removal of the foreign object.
2. Intraorbital foreign body
   - Broad spectrum antibiotics
     - Amoxicillin/clavulanate 500/125 mg bid
     - Cephalexin 250 to 500 mg qid
     - Azithromycin 250 mg bid × 1 day, then 250 mg qd × 4 days
   - Consider tetanus prophylaxis
   - Appropriate analgesics:
     - Mild pain: Acetaminophen 500 mg q4–6 h, ibuprofen 400 to 600 mg q4–6 h, naproxen 250 to 500 mg bid
     - Moderate pain: Acetaminophen with codeine (30 mg codeine) q6 h
     - Severe pain: Acetaminophen (500 mg) with hydrocodone (5 mg) q4–6 h, ibuprofen (200 mg) with hydrocodone (7.5 mg) q4–6 h, acetaminophen (325 mg) with oxycodone (10 mg) q4–6 h
   - Surgical removal of foreign body will depend on location and extent of secondary complications. Inflammation, infection, cosmetic disturbance, or functional deficit necessitates removal. Nonreactive foreign bodies that result in no complications or those where surgical intervention would cause risk of morbidity may be observed.

CONJUNCTIVAL/CORNEAL LACERATIONS
Andrew Mick

THE DISEASE
Pathophysiology

Trauma to the globe from a sharp object or grazing forces from blunt objects can result in lacerations of the conjunctiva or cornea. By definition, the globe is not penetrated.

Etiology

Lacerations can be produced by a variety of objects (fingernails, broken glass, forks, knives, sharp tools, fish hooks).

The Patient
Significant History
- Trauma involving sharp object or being "poked in eye" with any object

Clinical Symptoms
- Eye pain
- Reduced vision
- Light sensitivity
- Increased tearing

Clinical Signs
1. Conjunctival laceration
   - Break within conjunctival tissue: Seen with direct light or with fluorescein staining
   - Conjunctival hemorrhage
   - Direct observation of sclera
2. Corneal laceration
   - Variable thickness corneal defect: Seen with direct light or fluorescein staining
   - Larger lacerations may have varying amounts of wound gape

Demographics

Most cases of conjunctival or corneal lacerations occur in association with occupations that involve exposure to trauma (carpentry, metal working, and mechanics). Recreational activities and inadvertent poking of the eye by children are also common causes.

Ancillary Tests
- Seidel Testing to rule out full-thickness perforation
- Gentle tonometry away from laceration site if possible: Low IOP signals possible globe penetration

- Thorough examination by slit lamp to rule out flat anterior chamber: Signals possible full-thickness penetration
- Full retinal examination with ophthalmoscopy to rule out intraorbital foreign body, globe rupture, or retinal damage.
- B-scan ultrasonography if full extent of the retina is not visible because of media opacity or if intraorbital foreign body is suspected.
- CT scan of globe and orbit to allow for better differentiation of damage or localization of suspected foreign body.

The Treatment

Conjunctival Laceration
- Broad-spectrum antibiotic ointment (tobramycin, polymyxin B/trimethoprim, ciprofloxacin)
- Cycloplegia: Cyclopentolate 1% or homatropine 5%
- Pressure patch for 24 hours
- Monitor closely for infection

Corneal Laceration-Partial Thickness without Wound Gape
Option #1
- Broad-spectrum antibiotic ointment (tobramycin, polymyxin B/trimethoprim, ciprofloxacin)
- Cycloplegia: Cyclopentolate 1% or homatropine 5%
- Pressure patch for 24 hours
- Monitor closely for infection

Option #2
- Tight-fitting bandage contact lens
- Fluoroquinolone antibiotic qid (moxifloxacin, gatifloxacin, levofloxacin, ofloxacin, ciprofloxacin)
- Cycloplegia: Cyclopentolate 1% or homatropine 5%
- Recheck daily

Appropriate Analgesics
- Mild pain: Acetaminophen 500 mg q4–6 h, ibuprofen 400 to 600 mg q4–6 h, naproxen 250 to 500 mg bid
- Moderate pain: Acetaminophen with codeine (30 mg codeine) q4–6 h
- Severe pain: Acetaminophen (500 mg) with hydrocodone (5 mg) q4–6 h, ibuprofen (200 mg) with hydrocodone (7.5 mg) q4–6 h, acetaminophen (325 mg) with oxycodone (10 mg) q4–6 h

Corneal Laceration with Wound Gape or Suspicion of Globe Penetration
- Large lacerations with wound gape often require suturing. A plastic or metal shield should be applied and patient transported to an ophthalmic surgeon.

- Conjunctival or corneal lacerations that are associated with a shallow anterior chamber, positive Seidel Test, or any other sign of possible globe penetration should also have shield applied and patient immediately sent to an ophthalmic surgeon.

PERIORBITAL ANIMAL BITES
Andrew Mick

THE DISEASE
Pathophysiology

Tissue damage occurs from the initial bite or infection/inflammation, resulting from oral pathogens of the attacking animal.

Etiology

Periorbital bites can occur from a wide variety of animals. The most common animals involved are household pets, especially dogs and cats.

The Patient
Significant History
- Recent attack from animal and subsequent damage to periocular tissues

Clinical Symptoms
- Pain
- Bleeding
- Reduced acuity
- Double vision

Clinical Signs
- Globe rupture
- Corneal/conjunctival/lid laceration
- Ecchymosis of adnexal tissues
- Enophthalmos
- Traumatic uveitis
- Hyphema
- Iris sphincter/dilator tears
- Traumatic cataract
- Retinal detachment/choroidal rupture

Demographics

The majority of periocular animal bites occur in young children, but any age group can be affected.

Ancillary Tests
- Seidel Test to rule out globe rupture
- Careful slit-lamp and ophthalmoscopy examination to rule out intraorbital damage
- Computed tomography (CT) scanning to rule out facial/orbital bone fracture
- Magnetic resonance imaging to elucidate extent of soft tissue damage

The Treatment
- Immediate copious irrigation for the wound
- Initiate broad-spectrum systemic antibiotics directed at the multiple common oral flora of attacking animal. Recommended antibiotics include amoxicillin/clavulanate 500/125 mg bid, cephalexin 250 to 500 mg bid, clindamycin 150 to 450 mg qid, ciprofloxacin 500 mg bid
- Initiate postexposure prophylaxis for rabies
- Check tetanus immunization status
- Appropriate analgesia:
  - Mild pain: Acetaminophen 500 mg q4–6 h, ibuprofen 400 to 600 mg q4–6 h, naproxen 250 to 500 mg bid
  - Moderate pain: Acetaminophen with codeine (30 mg codeine) q4–6 h
  - Severe pain: Acetaminophen (500 mg) with hydrocodone (5 mg) q4–6 h, ibuprofen (200 mg) with hydrocodone (7.5 mg) q4–6 h, acetaminophen (325 mg) with oxycodone (10 mg) q4–6 h
- Minor conjunctival/corneal lacerations (see Conjunctival/Corneal Lacerations)
- Traumatic iritis (see Blunt Trauma)
- Hyphema (see Blunt Trauma)
- Eyelid lacerations, periocular skin lacerations, and corneal lacerations with wound gape require suturing for closure. Patient should be transported to ophthalmic surgeon.
- Orbital/facial bone fractures may require surgical intervention. Patient should be referred for evaluation if fractures detected with imaging studies (see Blunt Trauma).
- Globe rupture is an extreme emergency. Advise patient to not touch, rub, or squeeze eyes. Position eye shield, and advise patient not to consume any food or water. Immediately transport patient to ophthalmic surgeon.

ULTRAVIOLET INDUCED INJURY
Andrew Mick

THE DISEASE

Pathophysiology

Ultraviolet (UV) radiation produces local cell death, resulting in inflammation and sloughing of the affected tissue.

Etiology

Exposure to natural or artificial UV radiation source.

The Patient

Significant History

- Recent exposure to artificial or natural source of UV radiation. Activities that have a high amount of direct and reflected UV exposure include sunbathing (natural or tanning salon), snow or water skiing, and fishing.

Clinical Symptoms

- Burning/aching pain
- Headache
- Reduced acuity
- Light sensitivity
- Increased tearing
- Foreign body sensation

Clinical Signs

- Loss or disruption of corneal and conjunctival epithelium
- Epithelial/stromal edema
- Hyperemia/chemosis
- Anterior uveitis
- First- or second-degree burns of the lids and surrounding skin of the face

Ancillary Tests

None necessary.

The Treatment

- Cool compresses: Do not apply ice directly to the eye. Put ice into pan of water and soak washcloth in cooled solution. Apply cooled cloth to the affected area.
- Cycloplegia: Cyclopentolate 1% qid–bid or homatropine 5% tid–bid.
- Antibiotic: Polymyxin B/trimethoprim oph sol qid.
- If extremely symptomatic or presence of more severe anterior chamber reaction, consider antibiotic/steroid suspension qid vasociden or cetapred (sulfacetamide/prednisolone), Pred-G (gentamicin/prednisolone), tobradex (tobramycin/dexamethasone).
- Appropriate analgesia:
  - Mild pain: Acetaminophen 500 mg q4–6 h, ibuprofen 400 to 600 mg q4–6 h, naproxen 250 to 500 mg bid
  - Moderate pain: Acetaminophen with codeine (30 mg codeine) q6 h

- Severe pain: Acetaminophen (500 mg) with hydrocodone (5 mg) q4–6 h, ibuprofen (200 mg) with hydrocodone (7.5 mg) q4–6 h, acetaminophen (325 mg) with oxycodone (10 mg) q4–6 h
- Keep burned skin clean and dry.
- Comanage with patient's physician as needed.
- Do *not* patch eye with burned lids.

THERMAL BURNS
Andrew Mick

THE DISEASE
Pathophysiology

Infrared-or thermal energy–induced damage to tissues.

Etiology

Cigarettes, hot metal or oil, and curling irons are common causes of this type of injury.

The Patient
Significant History
- Recent exposure to fire, heated metal, or electrical discharge

Clinical Symptoms
- Burning/aching pain
- Headache
- Reduced acuity
- Light sensitivity
- Increased tearing
- Foreign body sensation

Clinical Signs
- Loss or disruption of corneal epithelium
- Epithelial/stromal edema
- Hyperemia/chemosis
- Anterior uveitis
- First- or second-degree burns of the lids and surrounding skin of the face

Burn Classification
- First degree: Reddened swollen skin
- Second degree: Skin blisters
- Third degree: Charring of deeper layers occurs

The Treatment

- Remove any foreign material (ash or cinder).
- Carefully debride necrotic epithelium.
- Cycloplegia: Cyclopentolate 1% qid–bid or homatropine 5% tid–bid.
- Antibiotic solution: Polymyxin B/trimethoprim oph sol qid.
- If extremely symptomatic or presence of more severe anterior chamber reaction, consider antibiotic/steroid suspension qid Vasociden or cetapred (sulfacetamide/prednisolone), Pred-G (gentamicin/prednisolone), tobradex (tobramycin/dexamethasone).
- Appropriate analgesia:
  - Mild pain: Acetaminophen 500 mg q4–6 h, ibuprofen 400 to 600 mg q4–6 h, naproxen 250 to 500 mg bid
  - Moderate pain: Acetaminophen with codeine (30 mg codeine) q6 h
  - Severe pain: Acetaminophen (500 mg) with hydrocodone (5 mg) q4–6 h, ibuprofen (200 mg) with hydrocodone (7.5 mg) q4–6 h, acetaminophen (325 mg) with oxycodone (10 mg) q4–6 h
- Keep burned skin clean and dry.
- Comanage with patient's physician as needed.
- Do *not* patch eye with burned lids.

TRAUMATIC HYPHEMA

Anastas F. Pass

ICD—9: 364.41

THE DISEASE

Pathophysiology

A traumatic hyphema results from the direct action of blunt trauma to the globe or the shock waves created by the sudden compression and decompression of the cornea. A traumatic hyphema is often associated with a post-traumatic iridocyclitis and a relatively nonreactive pupil because of iris inflammation. A hyphema typically occurs from a rupture of the iris or ciliary body vessels. In a mild presentation, red blood cells can be observed in the anterior chamber without layering. In a severe case, the anterior chamber may fill with blood. The former presentation is termed a *microhyphema* and the latter an *"eightball"* or *total hyphema*. When hyphema is categorized into the four main groups (Grades I–IV), approximately 60% of the hyphemas are Grade I, and less than 10% form total "eight-ball" hyphemas.

Etiology

The most common cause of traumatic hyphema is blunt injury to the eye by bungee cord straps, air guns, sports injuries, motor vehicle accidents, and falls. Microhyphemas and low-grade hyphemas may be self-limiting; however, because of the potential of poor visual outcomes, all hyphemas should be examined and monitored closely. The presentation of a hyphema may be presumed to be from trauma, but a careful history is still crucial to help differentiate a "spontaneous" hyphema as may occur in neovascularization of the iris (rubeosis) secondary to diabetes or in neoplastic presentations. In a pediatric patient, juvenile xanthogranuloma (JXG) is an uncommon but important cause of spontaneous hyphema.

The Patient

Clinical Symptoms
- Pain-orbital and/or periorbital
- Blurred or reduced vision

Clinical Signs
- Blood in the anterior chamber by gross inspection or by biomicroscopic assessment
- Hyphema—if blood has layered or is in the process of layering in the anterior chamber
- Microhyphema—if only free-floating red blood cells are seen by biomicroscopy
- The face and ocular adnexa may show observable signs of injury
- The patient may be lethargic or somnolent (somnolence may also be indicative of neurological complications in patients sustaining closed head trauma)

Note: Blunt trauma may result in damage to multiple areas of the eye and head. The extent of injury will depend on the type and magnitude of force encountered during the injury. A comprehensive exam is required in all cases.

Significant History
- The patient will typically report a history of trauma to the eye. It is critical that the specific etiology be identified in order to assess the ocular complications associated with a particular injury. It is also critical to consider the possibility of globe rupture in every case.
- Notation of the patient's drug allergies and medications (especially anticoagulants and antiplatelets) is necessary.
- Blood dyscrasias should be noted.
- Pre-existing ocular and systemic disorders should be noted. Certain ocular conditions (such as prior cataract extraction with IOL, PKP, keratoconus, RK, etc.) may predispose the patient to more severe damage. Concurrent medical disorders (such as asthma, CHF, sickle cell disease, nephrolithiasis, etc.) could influence medical mangement of the hyphema.

Demographics
- Male:Female 3:1.
- 70 to 75% of those that present with traumatic hyphema are under the age of 20 years.
- Increased incidence of falls occurs more in the elderly population.

Ancillary Tests

Assessment of a traumatic hyphema includes a gross inspection to rule out facial fractures, neurologic damage, and/or an occult rupture of the globe. Best visual acuity (pinhole or refraction if acuity is reduced), confrontation fields, pupil assessment, measurement of the layered blood with the head in an upright position, anterior segment and lens assessment, IOP measurement, and a dilated fundus evaluation should all be performed. Direct pressure should not be applied to the globe (e.g., palpation, gonioscopy, scleral indentation, etc., are usually deferred for 3 to 4 weeks).

Note: A "reverse pupil" testing technique may be required because of trauma and inflammation of the iris or if the pupil in the eye with a hyphema is not visible. Though a true APD (implicating an optic neuropathy) is rarely caused solely by a hyphema, a false APD may be noted in cases of sluggish iris activity or where the hyphema covers the pupil; the hyphema acts as an extremely dense neutral density filter.

Laboratory Studies
- Lab testing depends on the individual patient: Tests may include a CBC with differential, PT, PTT, bleeding time, platelet count, creatinine, liver function tests, and/or an electrolyte panel.
- If the patient is African American, a sickle cell prep and hemoglobin electrophoresis should be performed to identify those with the sickle cell trait or disease.
- If a dilated fundus view is not possible, a B-scan ultrasound may be performed to detect subluxed lenses, vitreous hemorrhages, and/or retinal detachments. Ultrasonography should not be performed unless globe perforation has been excluded.
- A CT scan is indicated in cases of significant facial trauma and to rule out orbital fractures, optic nerve injury, and intracranial bleeds. Many cases of blunt injury are also associated with penetrating trauma; a CT scan may be necessary to exclude an intraocular or intraorbital foreign body.

The Treatment

Treatment of a traumatic hyphema may vary, depending on the presentation (Table 12.1) and the subjective determination of patient compliance. here is controversy regarding treatment paradigms, primarily including the use of aminocaproic acid and corticosteroids. A multicentered clinical trial attempted to assess the clinical viability of aminocaproic acid. The study, however, had to be discontinued because of lack of an appropriate number of study subjects. Though the study was terminated, trends seemed to demonstrate that topical aminocaproic acid (administered q6 h × 5 days) was safe in the appropriate population and that the incidence of rebleeding was reduced. Aminocaproic acid is an antifibrinolytic agent that reduces the chance of a rebleed by slowing the lysis of the clot from the initial bleed. The use of aminocaproic acid is contraindicated in patients with sickle cell hemoglobinopathies, intravascular clotting disorders, pregnancy, heart disease, liver disease, and kidney disease.

▶ **TABLE 12.1 Hyphema: Grading and Clinical Presentation**

Hyphema Grade	Amount of Blood in the Anterior Chamber	Treatment
Microhyphema	Only red blood cells visible in the anterior chamber (there is no layering of the blood cells)	Daily observation for ≈1 week, cycloplegia, tempered activity, analgesics (prn), antiemetic (prn), head elevated when resting, consider oral or topical aminocaproic acid.
Grade I	Less than 1/3 of the anterior chamber	Avoid antifibrinolytics (aspirin, naproxen sodium).
Grade II	From 1/3 to 1/2 of the anterior chamber	Hospitalization with the head inclined ≈30° to 40°, cycloplegia, shield the affected eye,
Grade III	From 1/2 to near total filling the anterior chamber	topical steroid can be used to reduce inflammation.
Grade IV	Total anterior chamber filled with blood ("eight-ball" hyphema)	For elevated IOP, the use of brimonidine, prostaglandins, and topical CAI's can be very effective along with topical β-blockers, apraclonidine, and oral CAI's. Consider the use of aminocaproic acid (if not contraindicated in the patient), antiemetic (prn), surgical intervention (prn).

Hospitalization may be indicated for children, for more severe cases, or when it is felt that the patient may be noncompliant with instructions for care. Outpatient care can be administered in an otherwise healthy, compliant individual without complicating injury and presenting with a low-grade hyphema.

Microhyphema or Low-Grade Hyphema (I)
- The patient should be observed daily for at least 1 week to verify that a microhyphema is not layering or that a low-grade hyphema is resolving. IOPs and visual acuity should be recorded each day. Rebleeding may occur, which is most common from the second to the fifth day post-trauma, and often represents a poorer visual prognosis. Predictive factors for a rebleed include:
  - Initial VA <20/200
  - Care initiated >24 hours after the injury
  - Elevated IOP on presentation
  - >1/3 of the AC filled with blood on the initial visit
- The patient should be cyclopleged with 0.25% scopolamine or 1% atropine two to three times a day for 5 days. A dilated fundus assessment should be attempted at the initial visit; however, the dilation may be minimal and the view less than ideal. Subsequent internal exams may be more productive.
- Topical steroids will reduce post-traumatic inflammation, decrease congestion of the iris vessels, and reduce the chance of rebleeding.
- The patient should be instructed to limit activity for at least 5 days. Infrequently, sedation may be required.

- The patient should avoid salicylates (aspirin) and other NSAIDs with antiplatelet activity such as naproxen sodium; the antiplatelet effect of these products tends to increase the incidence of rebleeding.
- If the patient has significant pain, analgesics may be considered (e.g., acetaminophen with or without narcotics).
- If the patient presents with nausea, oral or rectal antiemetics (e.g., trimethobenzamide) may be prescribed. Nausea may cause emesis, which could exacerbate the hyphema by transitory increased vascular pressure with vomiting.
- When the patient is at rest or in the supine position, the head should be elevated approximately 30° to 40° to facilitate layering of the hyphema and to lower the venous pressure in the eye. During sleep, the head should be elevated and supported in a manner to restrict movement.
- The involved eye should be protected with an eye shield, but not pressure patched.
- The use of oral aminocaproic acid (Amicar) or topical aminocaproic acid (Carpogel) may be considered if not contraindicated for the patient's use. The dosage suggested orally is 50 mg/kg q4 (not to exceed 30 g per day) × 5 days. For topical aminocaproic acid, the dosage suggested is q6 h × 5 days.

Hyphema (Grades II to IV)
- All of the aforementioned procedures should be initiated.
- The patient with a severe hyphema should be considered for hospitalization and limited to bed rest with the head inclined by 30° to 40°.
- The eye should be shielded for protection.
- The use of topical steroids may be employed to minimize intraocular inflammation (e.g., 1% prednisolone acetate every 2 to 4 hours).
- For elevated IOP, the use of α-agonists (brimonidine), prostaglandins, and/or topical carbonic anhydrase inhibitors can be very effective. As always, the use of topical β-blockers (qD), apraclonidine 0.5% bid, or oral carbonic anhydrase inhibitors (e.g., acetazolamide 500 mg orally every 12 hours) can also be administered as needed to control IOP.

Note: Acetazolamide should not be administered to patients with sickle cell trait or disease as it may promote sickling of the RBCs in the anterior chamber.

- Analgesics, sedatives, and antiemetics considered as noted previously.
- In a severe presentation, surgery may be required to minimize the damage from the hyphema (i.e., corneal blood staining, prolonged and/or severe elevated IOP). Considerations for surgical evacuation of blood in the anterior chamber include:
  - An IOP >50 mm Hg for 4 days or 35 mm Hg for >7 days, despite medical management.
  - In sickle cell patients, even a mild IOP elevation (25 mm Hg) may produce significant consequences for a poor visual prognosis. An IOP >25 mm Hg for 1 day should be considered for surgery.
  - Complete hyphema ("eight-ball" hyphema) lasting 5 days.
  - Prolonged clot duration (50% hyphema for >1 week), which places the patient at risk for developing peripheral anterior synechia.
  - Blood staining of the cornea.

Long-Term Care

- Restraint from excessive physical activity for approximately 3 weeks. Patients should not stoop, lift heavy objects, or bend below the waist.
- IOP measurements should be conducted at periodic intervals (monthly for the first 6 months, followed by quarterly visits for the remainder of the year) and an elevated IOP appropriately treated.
- Gonioscopy should be performed after approximately 3 to 4 weeks to assess the integrity of the iridocorneal angle.
- Dilated fundus examination with scleral indentation should also be conducted after approximately 3 weeks to rule out any peripheral retinal tears.
- Protective eye wear (polycarbonate lenses) should be dispensed.
- Follow-up care if complications arise (e.g., traumatic cataract).
- Yearly evaluation to exclude angle recession glaucoma.

Chapter 13

Ocular Emergencies and Urgencies

SUDDEN VISION LOSS

Anastas F. Pass

ICD—9: 362.34—Amaurosis fugax
ICD—9: 368.10—Transient visual obscuration
ICD—9: 368.11—Sudden visual loss
ICD—9: 368.12—Transient visual loss

THE DISEASE

Pathophysiology

Sudden vision loss may indicate a serious vascular disorder, and as such should be recognized as an ocular emergency. Long-standing vision loss may not be recoverable and may be a precursor to cerebrovascular accidents. The spectrum of sudden vision loss includes local and benign causes (e.g., retinal migraine or acephalgic migraine) (Table 13.1); however, these are to be considered diagnoses of exclusion. Vascular anomalies that give rise to vision loss are not only sight threatening, but may be life threatening as well. When discussing vision loss, transient or otherwise, it should be remembered that there are various categories of vision loss with specific diagnostic coding.

- Transient Visual Obscuration (TVO)—Not a complete loss of vision but a "white-out" or "grey-out" of vision that can present unilaterally or bilaterally. It is most commonly associated with papilledema related to increased intracranial hypertension and lasts seconds to minutes. The TVO may be precipitated by Valsalva maneuver or simply by standing up.
- Amaurosis Fugax—A very brief loss of vision (typically unilateral) of seconds to minutes.
- Transient Vision Loss (TVL)—A rapid loss of vision (unilateral or bilateral) of minutes to longer. Commonly, TVL lasts 2 to 15 minutes, but by convention, less than 24 hours in duration.

Etiology

Vision loss, when it is acute and transient (amaurosis fugax or transient vision loss), should be considered secondary to a vascular disorder until proven otherwise.

▶ TABLE 13.1 Clinical Differentiation of Common Etiologies Involving Transient Vision Loss

Etiology	Clinical Symptoms	Clinical Signs	Significant History	Diagnostic Procedures
Embolus	TVL from seconds to permanent (CRAO) Typically lasting 30 sec (amaurosis fugax)	Usually none Emboli may be visible (either cholesterol, fibrin-platelet, or calcific)	Previous episodes of TVL History of cardiac or carotid disease Neurologic/sensorium	NaFl angiography (retinal) Carotid duplex Echocardiogram
Hyperviscosity syndromes	Blurred vision TVLs of varying times Visual field scotomas Visual hallucinations Headache	Darkening and tortuosity of the retinal vessels "Box carring" of the blood column Disc edema	Reported inherited or acquired hemoglobin abnormalities Pulmonary disease Cong. heart disease Cystic kidney disease	CBC with differential Platelet count Lipid profile Echocardiogram Kidney function
Inflammatory (neuritis)	Decreased vision TVLs of varying times Flashing lights Orbital or periorbital pain Pain on eye movement	Fundus may appear normal (RON) Blurred disc margins Elevated ONH Central scotoma on field testing	Previous episodes Tick bite (Lyme disease) History of MS (self or familial) Ataxia or paresthesia Uhtoff's phenomenon	Monitor V/As, pupils, and visual fields CBC, SED rate, FTA-Abs, RPR, ANA, PPD, chest film, Lyme titer Immunoassay of CSF
Headache	Headache Scintillating vision, TVL Peripheral or central visual field loss Photophobia Nausea	Typically no apparent ocular abnormality May manifest dilated pupil during episode May manifest (+) APD during episode	History of migraines Aura occurs after headache (R/O AVM)	Thorough history Neurologic exam MRI or MRA Lumbar puncture; initial pressure and CSF assessment
Disc edema	Blurred vision TVLs of varying times Headache Diplopia	Blurred disc margins Elevated ONH Drusen of the ONH Enlarged blind spot Tortuosity of the retinal vessels	Pain at base of neck, unrelenting or wakens from sleep (R/O mass) History of headaches Female, obese, 15–35 yrs of age Hypertensive Tetracyclines, steroids, or vitamin A	Vision field testing Ultrasound (B-scan) Blood profile, blood pressure MRI or MRA Lumbar puncture

TVL, transient vision loss; AVM, arteriovenous malformations; ONH, optic nerve head; RON, retrobulbar optic neuritis; APD, afferent pupillary defect; CBC, complete blood count; ANA, antinuclear antibodies; PPD, purified protein derivative MRI, magnetic resonance imaging; MRA, magnetic resonance angiography; CSF, cerebrospinal fluid.

Retinovascular and/or cerebrovascular accidents may be caused by emboli that can occlude the retinal arterial supply (twig, branch, or central) or the cerebrovascular circulation (carotid or vertebral-basilar). These occlusions may be temporary or fleeting, causing little or no retinal damage or may result in long-standing retinal nonperfusion and permanent sight loss.

Blood dyscrasias, dyslipidemia, hyperviscosity syndromes, sickle cell disease, syphilis, systemic hypertension, idiopathic intracranial hypertension, diabetes mellitus, as well as inflammatory conditions (e.g., giant cell arteritis [arteritic ischemic optic neuropathy]) can also lead to occlusion of the arterial system. The same diseases may also produce optic nerve head edema, resulting in vision loss. Connective tissue diseases and the vasculitidies (giant cell arteritis, polyarteritis nodosa, Takayasu's arteritis) have also been implicated in vision loss. Arteritic ischemic optic neuropathy typically presents as a painful vision loss and should also be considered a medical emergency.

Other etiological considerations include Uhtoff's phenomenon (associated with MS or Leber's optic neuropathy), antiphospholipid antibody syndrome, BRVO/CRVO, venous stasis retinopathy, papillophlebitis, vasospastic amaurosis fugax, recurrent hyphema, orbital tumors, and ocular ischemic syndrome.

Local causes, such as disc drusen, retinal detachment, and/or maculopathies, may result in sudden vision loss (or vision obscurations). Other considerations, as diagnoses of exclusion, include migrainous (scintillating) vision loss, acute angle closure glaucoma, or compressive lesions of the visual pathway.

The Patient

Symptoms and signs will vary depending on the circulatory system involved. Following is a list of classic findings involving the retinal (R), carotid (C), and vertebral-basilar (VB) arteries as well as inflammatory (I) causes.

Causes—Clinical Symptoms
- R/C/VB—Decreased vision, visual field defects or vision loss (complete or incomplete); typically unilateral. If bilateral, consider VB disorders.
- R—Flashing lights
- C—Hemisensory loss
- C/VB—Diplopia
- C/VB—Dysphasia
- VB—Loss of equilibrium (ataxia)
- VB—Weakness of the extremities (hemiplegia)
- I—Pain (head, scalp tenderness, neck, periorbital)
- VB—Most likely bilateral involvement (visual, motor, cerebellar)

Clinical Signs
Prominent signs include:

- Decreased acuity; typically unilateral (bilateral vision loss is an uncommon occurrence). With presentation of bilateral vision loss, one should assume a vertebral-basilar vascular anomaly (compression, embolus, occlusion), space occupying lesions, or a migrainous event; the latter on an exclusionary basis.

- Retinal emboli may be visible and can be divided into three main categories:
  1. Fibrin-platelet—which originate in the heart or large vessels or from a thrombus. This form of embolus rarely results in retinal infarction.
  2. Cholesterol "Hollenhorst" plaque—which typically originate from a plaque forming at the carotid bifurcation
  3. Calcific—which originate from cardiac valves and associated with rheumatic heart disease. This form of embolus will result in occlusion with infarction of the retina.
- "Boxcarring" of blood flow (hyperviscosity syndromes)
- Retinal nonperfusion and edema (as in artery occlusion)
- Vein occlusion
- Tortuous vasculature
- Retinal arteriolar narrowing, focal constrictions, venous nicking

Subtle signs include:

- Subtle relative afferent pupillary defect
- Disc elevation/edema
- Nerve fiber layer infarct(s)
- Sensorium changes
- Horner's pupil (possible in long standing atherosclerosis and carotid dissection)

Demographics

By radiographic studies, 56 to 100% of patients with CRAO demonstrate carotid occlusive disease. Individuals ≥40 years old demonstrate the highest incidence of CRAO. The mean presentation is in the sixth decade of life.

Men have a higher incidence of CRAO, retinal occlusive disease, and transient vision loss (associated with atherosclerotic plaques) than do women; however, the incidence in postmenopausal women is equal to that of men. Life expectancy of patients with CRAO is 5.5 years, compared to 15.4 years for an age-matched population without CRAO.

Individuals with retinal infarcts and emboli have a risk of stroke of 3% per year. Patients with transient vision loss have a risk of stroke of 2% per year. (By comparison, patients *without* carotid artery disease [atherosclerosis] have a risk rate of 0.1% per year.)

Patients who report episodes of transient vision loss have a high incidence of dyslipidemia (60%) as well as ischemic heart disease (25%). The National Institute of Neurological Disorders and Stroke reports that approximately one-third of individuals who experience a transient vision loss will experience an acute stroke in the "near" future. However, the most common cause of death in patients with TVL/AF is cardiac disease and not stroke.

Incidence of retinal vascular occlusion is rare in children and young adults; however, the presence of transient vision loss and/or retinal occlusive disease in this group should be suspect for mitral valve prolapse, rheumatic heart disease, systemic lupus erythematosus, migrainous events, and recurrent hyphema. In patients younger than 40 years, an embolus from the heart is the most common cause of (central) retinal arterial occlusion. There is also suspicion that the use of oral contraceptives may cause transient vision losses in susceptible patients. Other entities in young patients include mitochondrial myopathy-encephalopathy-lactacidosis-stroke (MELAS), moyamoya disease, and in migrainous cerebral autosomal dominant arteriopathy with subcortical infarcts and leukoencephalopathy (CADASIL).

Significant History
- Previous report of a transient ischemic attack or stroke
- Long-standing atherosclerosis
- Cardiovascular anomalies (mitral valve prolapse, prosthetic valves, vasculitis, patent foramen ovale [PFO], polycythemia, thrombocytosis)
- Arterial hypertension
- Diabetes mellitus
- Dyslipidemia
- Family history of transient ischemic attacks, vascular occlusive disease, or migraines
- Oral contraceptives
- Smoker

Ancillary Tests
- Ocular assessment for transient vision loss would include best visual acuity, pupil assessment, dilated fundus examination, and visual field assessment.
- Laboratory studies: erythrocyte sedimentation rate, C-reactive protein level, CBC with differential, platelet count, lipid profile, ANA, anticardiolipin, antiphospholipid antibody, and lupus anticoagulant.
- Noninvasive testing: blood pressure, carotid auscultation, cardiac evaluation (electrocardiogram, Holter monitor, echocardiogram), carotid duplex ultrasound, brain CT/MRI (consider magnetic resonance angiography [MRA] as a noninvasive carotid arterial evaluation), ophthalmodynamometry, or oculoplethysmography (for ocular perfusion pressures).
- Invasive testing: IV retinal fluorescein angiography may show the presence of embolic particles in areas of vessel leakage. Carotid angiography should be limited to those patients who will undergo carotid surgery (with >90% stenosis).

The Treatment

Transient Vision Loss
- No immediate treatment is typically warranted; however, identifying the underlying etiology will determine the appropriate mode of therapy. A Westergren sedimentation rate (ESR) and C-reactive protein (CRP) should be ordered immediately in every elderly patient to exclude a diagnosis of giant cell arteritis (GCA) even if pain is not elicited. A combination of ESR and CRP gives the best specificity (98%) in detection of giant cell arteritis. If GCA is suspected, high-dose steroids (i.e., prednisone 80 to 100 mg orally every day) should be initiated and a temporal artery biopsy should be performed within 1 week. IV methylprednisolone therapy is also used to treat GCA.

If GCA is confirmed, the patient will be on a maintenance dose of prednisone (5 to 7 mg orally every day).

- Treatment is often limited to prevention; as with cardiac or carotid disease. Prophylactic initiation of an antifibrinolytic agent (e.g., aspirin 80 mg orally every day), other NSAIDs with antiplatelet activity such as naproxen sodium, calcium channel blockers, or ticlopidine have been suggested.
- In profound carotid occlusive disease, surgical intervention may be warranted.
- If the patient is a cigarette smoker, cessation is essential.

ACUTE ANGLE CLOSURE GLAUCOMA
G. Richard Bennett and Michael B. Caplan

ICD—9: 365.22

THE DISEASE
Pathophysiology

Acute angle closure glaucoma is characterized by a rapid and large increase in the intraocular pressure, resulting from a sudden blockage of the anterior chamber angle.

Etiology

Angle closure can be precipitated by several different mechanisms. The most common cause is pupillary block. A resistance to flow of aqueous humour develops between the iris and lens that causes pressure to increase in the posterior chamber. This causes the peripheral iris to bow forward, which obstructs the anterior chamber angle and causes the intraocular pressure to rise rapidly. Conditions that place the pupil in a mid-dilated position (i.e., eyedrops to dilate the pupil, dim illumination, and/or anticholinergics such as antihistamines or antipsychotics) maximize lens/iris touch and can precipitate pupillary block in patients with a narrow anterior chamber angle.

Acute angle closure can also occur because of plateau iris syndrome in which the peripheral iris obstructs outflow without pre-existing pupillary block (see section on plateau iris).

Secondary causes of acute angle closure include posterior synechiae formation (chronic inflammation or neovascular membranes) or anterior displacement of the lens-iris diaphragm (central retinal vein occlusions, scleral buckles, panretinal photocoagulation, posterior segment tumors, choroidal detachments, or posterior misdirection syndrome).

The Patient

Clinical Symptoms
Symptoms on presentation include ocular pain, lacrimation, frontal headache, nausea, vomiting, photophobia, seeing colored halos around lights, and decreased vision.

Patients can have a history of similar symptoms, suggesting prior episodes of intermittent angle closure.

Clinical Signs
- Decreased vision
- Conjunctival injection
- Corneal microcystic edema
- Shallow anterior chamber (deeper centrally than peripherally)
- Mid-dilated pupil (pupil may be miotic if acute angle closure is secondary to posterior synechiae formation) and significantly elevated intraocular pressure

Other signs that may be present include:

- Glaukomflecken (anterior subcapsular lens opacities)
- Iris atrophy (generalized or sectorial)
- Mild cells and flare in the anterior chamber
- Optic disc edema

Gonioscopy will demonstrate closure of the anterior chamber angle and usually a narrow angle in the contralateral eye.

Demographics

Groups at higher risk to develop acute angle closure glaucoma include: hyperopes, Whites greater than Blacks, women greater than men, people of Pacific Rim ancestry, Eskimos (from Canada, Greenland, and Alaska), and those who have had acute angle closure in the other eye. The most frequent age range is 55 to 65 years old. Acute angle closure glaucoma is estimated to occur in 0.1% of Whites.

Significant History

Acute angle closure in the other eye, hyperopia, recent dilation or use of antihistamines or antipsychotic medication, Eskimo or Asian ancestry, previous episodes of blurred vision, and colored halos around lights.

Ancillary Tests
- Gonioscopy
- A-Scan ultrasonography (anterior chamber angle depth)
- Stereo disc photography (once it is safe to dilate)
- Baseline visual fields

The Treatment

The initial management is aimed at lowering the intraocular pressure and breaking the pupillary block. The patient's health status, habitual medications, and medical conditions should be considered prior to administering any topical or oral medications.

Initial Medical Therapy

- Place the patient in a supine position to allow the lens to locate posteriorly
- Topical β-blocker (one drop timolol 0.5%, levobunolol 0.25% to 0.5%, or carteolol 1.0%)
- Topical steroid (1% prednisolone acetate one drop q15 min $\times$ 4)
- Topical apraclonidine, one drop 0.5% to 1.0% or brimonidine 0.15% to 0.2%
- Oral or intravenous acetazolamide (250 to 500 mg orally or IV—not oral sequels)
- Oral or intravenous osmotic agent: One of the following may be indicated (may not be tolerated if the patient is experiencing nausea or vomiting):
  1. Oral isosorbide 45% 1.0–1.5 g/kg (preferred in diabetics)
  2. Oral glycerol 50% 1.0–1.5 g/kg
  3. IV mannitol 20% 1–2 g/kg over 45 minutes
- Pilocarpine 1 to 2%, one to two drops after IOPs are lower than 40 mmHg in cases of phakic pupillary block.

Note: Pilocarpine should be used with caution because it may increase the pupillary block by causing forward displacement of the lens/iris diaphragm and is ineffective at elevated IOPs. Analgesics and antiemetics may also be required to control pain and vomiting. Gonioscopy should be repeated once the IOP is reduced to ensure that the angle is open.

Subsequent Management

- Angle-closure glaucoma is a surgical disease and appropriate surgical care is indicated. Cases of pupillary block require a peripheral iridotomy or iridectomy. If the intraocular pressure is successfully reduced with medical therapy, then postpone the iridectomy for a few days and continue the appropriate medications (topical β-blocker twice a day, pilocarpine 1 to 2% four times a day, apraclonidine 0.5 to 1.0% two to three times a day, or brimonidine 0.15 to 0.20% twice a day, prednisolone acetate 1% as indicated, and acetazolamide 250 mg orally four times a day or 500 mg sequels orally twice a day).
- Use pilocarpine 0.5 to 1.0% four times a day in the contralateral eye, if the angle is narrow, until a peripheral iridectomy is performed.
- If the intraocular pressure cannot be controlled in cases of pupillary block with medical therapy, then attempt laser peripheral iridotomy (or surgical iridectomy) as soon as possible. In cases of angle closure secondary to anterior displacement of the lens/iris diaphragm, consider argon laser gonioplasty to help lower the intraocular pressure.
- If acute angle closure glaucoma persists despite a patent peripheral iridectomy, plateau iris syndrome may be present (see section on plateau iris).
- Iridoplasty and immediate paracentesis may be appropriate in some cases.
- If the intraocular pressure remains elevated after a peripheral iridectomy is performed, medical treatment or filtration surgery may be necessary. Goniosynechialysis may also be helpful if chronic angle closure develops.
- Cataracts frequently develop after acute angle closure glaucoma and may need extraction.

CHEMICAL INJURIES

Anastas F. Pass

ICD—9: 940.2—Alkali burn of the cornea and conjunctival sac
ICD—9: 940.3—Acid burn of the cornea and conjunctival sac

THE DISEASE

Pathophysiology

Alkaline

The effect of lipophilic alkaline material (pH >10) on the cornea may be extremely invasive. As cellular destruction begins in the presence of high pH substances, secondary sequelae may occur that prolongs the alkaline injury. These sequelae often make the treatment more difficult and may result in sight-threatening complications.

Destruction to the cornea and contiguous tissues is dependent on the alkaline material involved. The ultimate effect of alkaline compounds is related to the number of hydroxyl (OH) groups. Additional OH ions increase the pH and the destructive capabilities of the compound. The alkaline substance reacts with the fatty acids of the cornea and converts these units to soaps (soponification) as well as denaturing the collagen. This reaction results in cellular destruction and perpetuates corneal penetration.

Injuries to the adnexal, corneal, conjunctival, and intraocular tissues can create multiple problems in the management of an alkaline burn. Some alkaline material can penetrate into the anterior chamber within 15 minutes, involving the iris, lens, and other intraocular structures, perpetuating further damage. The clinician must be aware of intraocular conditions (secondary glaucoma, cataracts, uveitis), as well as periocular damages (lid destruction and/or appositional anomalies, symblepharon and/or ankyloblepharon).

Acid

An acidic injury (pII <4) may present in similar fashion as an alkaline burn. With sufficient quantity and concentration, an acid burn can be as severe as an alkaline injury; however, an acid burn is *usually* limited to the superficial layers of the cornea. An exception to this rule would be hydrofluronic acid (HF), which can cause liquifaction necrosis in a similar mechanism as an alkaline material.

As the proteins within the epithelial and superficial stromal layers coagulate in the presence of acidic compounds, a barrier is established, minimizing or halting destruction to the inner layers. Though superficial corneal opacification and tissue damage can be extensive, the resolution from an acid burn can be equally dramatic.

Injuries to the adnexal, corneal, conjunctival, and intraocular tissues must again be addressed. The clinician should monitor for intraocular damages as well as periocular trauma (see earlier).

Etiology

Alkaline

Alkaline chemicals are found in the home as well as the work site. Ammonia (a cleaning agent), ammonium hydroxide (a fertilizer), sodium hydroxide (lye), and calcium hydroxide (lime) are common causes of ocular alkaline injuries. Ammonia penetrates quickly and deeply as can ammonium hydroxide, the latter being considered one of the most severe alkaline injuries. Lye (which is found in cleaning agents and drain cleaners) and lime (used in construction and building materials) are less severe, but may still cause considerable damage to the cornea. Lime-containing material, though it does not penetrate the corneal stroma well, can persist in the conjunctival fornices prolonging contact to the eye.

Acid

Acid injuries occur less frequently than alkaline burns, as stronger acids are not as common in households and are more limited to the work site. An exception would be automobile-battery accidents involving sulfuric acid. The most common acids include sulfuric acid, hydrochloric acid, nitrous acid, and acetic acid. Many of these acids are used in dilute solutions; however, given an adequate concentration or volume, severe ocular destruction can occur. With blast injuries, such as a car battery explosion, it is essential to exclude extraocular and intraocular foreign bodies in addition to managing the burn.

The Patient

Clinical Symptoms

A cursory history and inspection will obviate the reason for the patient's presentation. Treatment precludes an extensive history or detailed assessment because of the nature of this emergent condition. The patient will often report:

- Severe pain
- Halos around lights
- Reduced vision
- Photophobia

Clinical Signs

Significant signs include:

- Corneal opacification (the greater the degree of opacification, the more severe the burn)
- Limbal ischemia (the greater the degree of limbal ischemia, the more severe the burn)

  Associated signs include:

- Conjunctival edema, injection, hemorrhage
- Anterior chamber reaction
- IOP elevation
- Lid margin involvement/palpebral involvement

- Periocular skin and oral mucosal burns
- Breathing or swallowing difficulties (aspiration or ingestion of the chemical)

Demographics

- Incidence/Prevalence in the United States: Estimated 300/100,000/year.
- Predominant Age: Between age 18 and 65. One study indicated that the average age of patients with ocular burns is 36 years.
- Predominant Gender: Male > Female.

Significant History

- The patient will report a foreign substance being introduced to the eye.
- *After* copious lavage has been initiated, the patient may be questioned as to the etiology of the compound, time of the injury, and previous treatment.
- A family member or coworker may also be questioned regarding the source of the chemical and other details of the accident.

Ancillary Tests

There are no laboratory studies that are necessary in the immediate management of the chemical burn; however, in-office pH measurement of the tears in the conjunctival fornices is useful in determining neutralization of the chemical compound. Additional tests and procedures can be obtained at a later time to assess collateral damage caused by the chemical injury.

- After several minutes of lavage with sterile isotonic saline solution, the pH of the tears should be tested with litmus paper. If a neutral reading is not obtained, lavage should continue. If neutral, the pH should be retested in 30 minutes, as there may be a gradual change in pH that would necessitate supplemental irrigation.
- Additional information should be obtained, including vital signs, visual acuity, and intraocular pressure (IOP may be more accurately obtained and without causing additional damage to the cornea by pneumotonometry or TonoPen).
- Document corneal clarity and limbal ischemia. Limbal ischemia is a negative prognostic indicator.
- Examine the skin, lid margins, conjunctiva, anterior chamber, and lens.
- Verify that particulate matter is not present in the conjunctiva or periocular skin. Residual material should be removed using a moistened cotton-tipped applicator, fine-tipped forceps, or Kimura spatula. Double eversion of the superior lid may be required to fully assess the fornix for damage and/or residual material. Maintaining a sample may be helpful in identifying the material via laboratory analysis if the patient does not know the substance causing the injury.
- Superficial damage to the corneal epithelium can be quite extensive; partial debridement may be necessary to assess the extent of corneal involvement and to remove necrotic tissue. This material may be cultured if there is concern of a secondary bacterial infection.

▶ **TABLE 13.2** Classification and Prognosis for Chemical Burn Damage of the Cornea

Grade (Thoft's Classification)	Prognosis
I. Corneal epithelial damage No limbal ischemia	Good
II. Corneal haze Limbal ischemia <1/3 of limbus	Good

III. Total loss of corneal epithelium
     Stromal haze obscuring iris details
     Ischemia 1/3 to 1/2 of limbus
	Guarded

IV. Corneal opacity
     View of iris or pupil obscured
     Limbal ischemia >1/2 of limbus
	Poor*

*At risk for perforation or phthisis.

The Treatment (Tables 13.2, 13.3, and 13.4)

Immediate Treatment

- In cases involving chemical injuries, the most important initial care that can be provided is immediate irrigation with any available appropriate source (tap water, shower, water fountain, artificial tears) by the patient or by a coworker or family member that may be with the patient). If you or your office is contacted, instructions of immediate and copious irrigation should be given, including irrigation of the eye in transit to the health-care facility.
- When the patient presents to the health-care facility, continue or initiate irrigation immediately even prior to determining visual acuity. Irrigation should continue with sterile isotonic saline solution or lactated Ringers solution until litmus paper becomes neutral with the tears (checked approximately every 5 to 10 minutes).
- Instill a topical anesthetic to facilitate irrigation and to relieve pain. Instillation should be repeated as needed (every 15 to 20 minutes) during lavage.
- Neutralizing lid function, by inserting a lid speculum, may be necessary.

▶ **TABLE 13.3** Hughes' Classification of Chemical Injury

Mild	Erosion of corneal epithelium Faint haziness of cornea No ischemic necrosis of conjunctiva or sclera	Prognosis good
Moderately severe	Corneal opacity blurs iris detail Minimal ischemic necrosis of conjunctiva or sclera	Prognosis good to guarded
Very severe	Blurring of pupillary outline Significant ischemic necrosis of conjunctiva or sclera	Prognosis guarded to poor*

*At risk for perforation or phthisis.

Subsequent Treatment: Alkaline

- Examine the conjunctival tissues and fornices for particulate matter. Any remaining material must be removed.
- Cycloplegia, 5.0% homatropine (three to four times per day), or 0.25% scopolamine (two to three times per day) are recommended.
- *Do not* instill phenylephrine-containing solutions. The vasoconstrictive action may exacerbate limbal ischemia.
- Administer a broad-spectrum antibiotic ointment (i.e., erythromycin, polymyxin B/bacitracin) two to four times a day. It may also be advisable to instill a flouroquinolone such as moxifloxacin hydrochloride 0.5% or gatifloxacin 0.3%.
- If an IOP rise is noted, administer topical β-blockers (timolol 0.5% twice a day, levobunolol 0.5% twice a day), topical carbonic anhydrase inhibitors (dorzolamide 2% three times a day), or oral carbonic anhydrase inhibitors (acetazolamide 250 mg orally four times a day or methazolamide 25 to 50 mg orally two to three times a day) as needed.
- Though topical corticosteroids may increase the risk of microbial involvement and effect stromal wound healing, they may be considered to decrease the inflammatory response. Use of corticosteroids (prednisolone acetate 1% every 2 to 4 hours) should be guarded and the patient monitored closely for adverse effects. The use of corticosteroids should generally be limited to the first 10 –to 14 days. Beyond this time, the risk of corneal ulceration increases as a result of the rise in collagenase production. After the first 2 weeks, it may be advisable to substitute progestational steroids (medroxyprogesterone 1%), NSAIDs, or both, if anti-inflammatory agents are still required.
- Collagenase inhibitors (i.e., topical acetylcysteine 10 to 20% every 4 hours or oral tetracycline 250 mg orally four times a day) may be considered. The use of collagenase inhibitors should be started 7 to 10 days after the initial injury. They should not be used in severe burns or in association with topical ascorbate.
- 10% sodium citrate solutions and 10% ascorbate solutions may also be employed. The use of these solutions should be limited to late aspects of the treatment regime (21 days postinjury). Ten percent ascorbic acid has been suggested to help in increasing the production of collagen. It has also been suggested that ascorbic acid reduces the incidence of corneal perforation postinjury.
- Pressure patch the patient, and follow up no later than 24 hours. It may be advisable to reassess the patient later in the evening if the injury occurred in the morning.
- Oral analgesics may be prescribed as needed (acetaminophen 650 mg orally three to four times a day; ketoprofen 25 to 50 mg orally every 6 to 8 hours). Narcotic analgesics may be indicated in severe cases.
- Topical analgesics, such as diclofenac (four times per day), may be considered as an adjunct to treatment. It should be noted that idiopathic corneal melting has been reported with generic diclofenac and should therefore be avoided.

Subsequent Treatment: Acid

- Debridement of devitalized corneal epithelium improves observation of the cornea and facilitates healing of the epithelium.
- Cycloplegia, 0.25% scopolamine three to four times a day is recommended.

▶ TABLE 13.4 Therapeutic Timeline for Chemical Burns

Emergent Care	Intermediate Care	0–7 Days	7–21 Days	First Year	Long-Term Care
Lavage, copious and continuous	Sweep of fornices to remove any particulate matter	Sweep fornices daily to remove any particulate matter and to break any adhesion formation	Cease (taper) the use of topical steroids at this point to minimize the risk of ulceration due to increased collagenase production	Periodic sweeps of fornices to break any adhesion formation	Consultation for keratoplasty
Instillation of anesthetic	Debride superficial devitalized tissue	Continuation of the intermediate care regimen	If re-epithelialization does not occur, consider systemic steroids (prednisone 20–40 mg/d or medoxyprogesterone 1% q1–2 h)	Continue the use of tear substitutes	
Use of lid speculum	Corticosteroid therapy to be initiated. Use of 1% prenisolone or 0.1% dexamethasone q1–4 h	Consider the use of fibronectin or epidermal growth factor	Consider cyanoacrylates for small persistent defects; keratoplasty for large persistent defects	Consideration of limbal stem cell transplantation	
Sweep of fornices to remove any particulate matter	Control elevated IOP with appropriate ocular hypotensives	Consider the use of ascorbate and/or citrate	Continue the use of fibronectin or epidermal growth factor to d 21	Conjunctival flap to maintain the eye	
Continuation of lavage until pH has neutralized	Administer cycloplegic agents. DO NOT use any phenylephrine-containing solutions. Use of 0.25% scopolamine or 1% atropine bid–tid	Monitor closely and conservatively	Continue the use of ascorbate and/or citrate to d 21	Management of trichiasis	

Verification of pH neutrality. Reinstitute lavage if pH creeps back into alkaline or acidic range.	Instillation of antibiotics therapy (use of broad spectrum solutions and ointments)	Use of a bandage contact lens (disposable) to protect ocular surface from lid action	Monitor closely and conservatively	Reconstruction of any lid abnormalities	Restoration of vision
Paracentesis and aqueous exchange if necessary	Pressure patch and follow-up within 24 h (or sooner)	Use of tear substitutes to maintain surface hydration	Continue the use of bandage contact lens and tear substitutes	Consider retinoic acid to promote goblet cell function	
Initiate immediate care	Control external ocular inflammation	Prevention of adhesion or symblepharon formation	Prevention of adhesion or symblepharon formation	Prevention of adhesion or symblepharon formation	
Reducing the degree of damage from exposure	Control IOP	Prevention of ulceration	Prevention of ulceration	Prevention of ulceration	
Stabilize pH	Control internal ocular inflammation	Promotion of re-epithelialization	Promotion of re-epithelialization	Promotion of re-epithelialization	
	Control for bacterial or fungal involvement	Maintain lubrication of the eye	Promote the stromal integrity	Promote the stromal integrity	
	Control for corneal melt or ulceration		Maintain lubrication of the eye	Maintain lubrication of the eye	

- *Do not* instill phenylephrine-containing solutions. The vasoconstrictive action may exacerbate limbal ischemia.
- Administer a broad-spectrum antibiotic ointment (i.e., erythromycin, polymyxin B/bacitracin) or a broad-spectrum antibiotic solution (levofloxacin 0.5%, or gatifloxacin 0.3%) four times a day.
- Sterile, nonpreserved tear substitutes should be used liberally if the patient is not pressure patched.
- Pressure patch the patient, and follow up no later than 24 hours. It may be advisable to reassess the patient later in the evening if the injury occurred in the morning. A collagen shield or therapeutic soft contact lens may be considered.
- Though topical corticosteroids may increase the risk of microbial involvement and effect stromal wound healing, they may be considered to decrease the inflammatory response. Use of corticosteroids (prednisolone acetate 1% every 2 to 4 hours) should be guarded and the patient monitored closely.
- If an IOP rise is noted, administration of topical β-blockers, topical carbonic anhydrase inhibitors, or oral carbonic anhydrase inhibitors should be employed as described earlier.
- Oral analgesics may be prescribed as needed.

Moderate to Severe Presentation
- After initiation of treatment (described earlier), admission to a hospital may be in the patient's best interest to more carefully monitor IOP and healing anomalies.

Long-Term Care
- Long-term management should attempt to minimize symblepharon formation and to promote re-epithelialization of the cornea. This care includes artificial tears, bandage contact lens, tarsoraphy, and/or conjunctival stem cell grafting. Sterile, topical autologous serum may help promote healing of corneal epithelial defects, especially if the patient develops a neurotrophic keratopathy.
- Surgical intervention may be needed to address oculoplastic concerns, an opacified cornea, or secondary glaucoma. Lamellar keratoplasty or penetrating keratoplasty may be considered within a year after corneal vascularization has stabilized.

Note: Whenever possible, try to identify the type of chemical or chemicals that have caused the injury to the patient and the manner in which the chemical was introduced to the eye. It is not uncommon that a coworker, friend, or relative that accompanies the patient may be a more reliable historian given the traumatic event.

When classifying the extent of the chemical injury, Tables 13.2 (Thoft's Classification) and 13.3 (Hughes' Classification) offer a guide for documentation. Though Thoft's criteria may allow for better differentiation of the extent of damage (and ultimate prognosis), many worker's compensation providers rely on the Hughes' Classification. Both classification systems are provided for the reader's benefit.

When the offending chemical is identified, it is suggested that the practitioner access information about this chemical from an Internet site that provides MSDS (Material Safety and Data Sheets) information and place a copy of the appropriate MSDS in the patient's record. Examples of web sites with this information are:

- http://msds.ehs.cornell.edu/msdssrch.asp
- http://www.msds.com/SearchPage.asp
- http://www.msdsonline.com/
- http://www.msds.com/

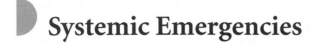

Chapter 14

Systemic Emergencies

SYSTEMIC EMERGENCIES IN AN OFFICE-BASED PRACTICE

Nicky R. Holdeman

Most of the problems encountered by an eyecare provider are not life threatening, but many conditions can become serious if not identified early and managed appropriately. Therefore, every health-care practitioner should be prepared to properly oversee various office emergencies until professional help arrives (i.e., manage iatrogenic complications, initiate resuscitative efforts, stabilize the patient, and make prompt referrals). In addition, one should be able to assess, in most cases, whether a person is experiencing a true emergency, thus summoning Emergency Medical Services (EMS) appropriately.

Emergency preparedness will vary depending on the type of practice, the transport time to an emergency facility, the types of medications used, and the types of procedures performed. However, there are basic steps each office should take to prepare for emergencies. These steps include:

1. Posting current emergency numbers in various locations throughout the office
2. Keeping a first aid kit and other medical supplies readily available
3. Learning and practicing first aid and CPR—basic life support with defibrillator (AED) training or advanced cardiac life support
4. Preparing and rehearsing emergency procedures with your office staff
5. Ensuring that your office address numbers are posted and easy to read for emergency personnel

Note: The best tool to reduce the risk of an emergency in a private office is knowing the patient's medical history. The doctor should establish a complete baseline history on all new patients and update the record on all return patients. A comprehensive history should incorporate the patient's current medications (including nonprescription drugs, vitamins, dietary supplements, home remedies, and medications not prescribed to the patient); allergies (medications and/or environmental agents); past and current medical conditions; previous surgeries/hospitalizations; and family history. The patients most likely to have complications are the elderly, those with advanced comorbid conditions, those taking multiple medications, and those with a history of previous complications. Recognizing and recording any predisposing history may help to avoid problems, or help to recognize them early should problems occur.

EQUIPMENT

A standard first aid kit will typically contain an antiseptic ointment, small bandages, scissors, tweezers, Band-Aids, gauze pads, and adhesive tape. In addition, one may consider equipping the office with:

- O_2 (E-size portable cylinder) with a low flow regulator
- Pocket face mask with one-way valve
- Nasal cannula
- Ambu bag
- Examination gloves
- Stainless steel basins
- Stethoscope
- Sphygmomanometer with several size cuffs
- Cold/hot packs
- Thermometer
- Glucometer
- 4 × 4 pads
- Skin cleanser (Hibiclens, Betadine)
- Syringes (IM 3cc disposable; SC tuberculin)
- Tourniquets
- Automated external defibrillator (AED)

OFFICE EMERGENCY DRUGS

Protocols should be established for common office emergencies, especially those resulting from iatrogenic complications of medications and procedures. Recognition and prompt action lead to appropriate management. Several in-office drugs should be readily available, assuming the proper level of training. These medications include:

- Ammonia capsules
- Glucose tablets/paste
- Bulk saline
- Epinephrine preloaded syringe (AnaKit/EpiPen)
- Albuterol
- Dexamethasone, hydrocortisone, or methylprednisolone
- Diazepam
- Diphenhydramine
- Glucagon
- Nitroglycerin

In general, emergencies should be referred immediately by the best means possible to a qualified acute care facility. Occasionally, it is unclear whether a patient requires an EMS unit or whether they can be referred to a physician's office for further management. Some *general guidelines* to consider would be calling for an ambulance if the victim:

- Is unconscious, confused, or seems to be losing consciousness
- Has trouble breathing or is breathing in a strange way

- Has persistent chest pain or pressure
- Has pressure or pain in the abdomen that does not go away
- Has seizures, a severe headache, or slurred speech
- Appears to have been poisoned
- Has injuries to the head, neck, or spine
- Has severe bleeding
- Has the possibility of broken bones
- Has paralysis or inability to move

When summoning EMS, it is important to follow several basic rules. Each caller should:

- Identify himself or herself
- Supply necessary information to the dispatcher, such as:
  1. The exact address where the victim is located
  2. The telephone number at the scene of the incident
  3. What happened to the victim
  4. The person(s) involved
  5. The condition of the victim
  6. The care being given
  7. Any special instructions for the drivers
- Hang up last, allowing the dispatcher to hang up first
- Return to offer further assistance

Last, it is usually helpful (and courteous) to the EMS and the receiving facility to have a copy of any relevant medical information from the referring practitioner. However, copying records should never delay prompt transport of an emergent patient.

HYPOGLYCEMIA
Nicky R. Holdeman
ICD—9: 251.2

THE DISEASE
Pathophysiology

Hypoglycemia is a condition in which glucose is moving out of the bloodstream and into cells more rapidly than it is being produced. Because glucose normally furnishes 98 to 100% of the brain's energy needs, hypoglycemia may result in permanent brain damage or death if emergency care is not provided immediately.

"Clinical hypoglycemia" is described as a low blood glucose along with the symptoms and signs consistent with hypoglycemia. While the classic definition of hypoglycemia is a plasma glucose less than 60 mg/dL after an overnight fast or less than 50 mg/dL after a meal, the actual modicum of glucose needed to maintain the brain cells is poorly defined and will vary among different individuals.

▶ **TABLE 14.1** Causes of Hypoglycemia

Reactive (Postprandial) Hypoglycemia
  Alimentary
      postgastrectomy
      functional (increased vagal tone)
  Occult adult onset diabetes mellitus
      delayed insulin release because of B-cell dysfunction
  Hereditary fructose intolerance
  Idiopathic
Fasting Hypoglycemia
  Hyperinsulinism
      pancreatic B-cell tumor
      surreptitious insulin injection or sulfonylureas
  Extrapancreatic neoplasms
  Islet cell hyperplasia
  Adrenocortical insufficiency
  Growth hormone deficiency
  Glucagon deficiency
  Hepatic failure
  Renal failure
  Autoimmune
      anti-insulin antibodies (release-bound insulin)
      antireceptor antibodies (act as agonists)
  Ethanol
  Other medications
      β-blockers, pentamidine, disopyramide, and so on

Etiology

Hypoglycemia may occur for many reasons (see Table 14.1). Most commonly, hypo-glycemia results from oral hypoglycemic agents, or a relative excess of exogenous in-sulin in insulin-treated diabetic patients. As intensive (or tight control) therapy increases in order to reduce the well-known complications of diabetes mellitus, the incidence of both mild and severe hypoglycemia (i.e., blood glucose <30–35 mg/dL) will also increase.

The Patient

Clinical Symptoms
■ Headache
■ Hunger
■ Shakiness
■ Visual disturbances (blurred vision, diplopia)
■ Tingling and numbness in the extremities
■ Dizziness

- Profuse sweating
- Speech difficulties
- Difficulty concentrating, confusion
- Pounding heart (palpitations)

Clinical Signs
- Hypotension
- Tachycardia
- Full and bounding pulse
- Diaphoresis
- Pale skin coloration
- Tremors
- Incoordination
- Muscle weakness or paralysis
- Dilated pupils
- Anxiety, nervousness, combativeness, or irritability
- Disorientation or changes in personality
- Convulsions, syncope, and/or coma in late stages

Note: In insulin-treated diabetics, it may be difficult to distinguish patients in ketotic hyperglycemia from those with severe hypoglycemia. In contradistinction to severe hyperglycemia, patients with severe hypoglycemia will have no unusual odor on the breath, will manifest normal or depressed respirations, and will appear adequately hydrated. However, if in doubt, administer glucose to the patient in these situations.

Significant History

Because the majority of cases of hypoglycemia result from the effects of exogenous insulin or oral hypoglycemic agents, diabetics should be carefully questioned. The clinician should ask the following:

- Have you eaten today? If so, did you eat less than your doctor recommended?
- Have you taken your insulin today?
- Have you taken your insulin and skipped a meal?
- Have you vomited a meal after taking your insulin?
- Has your diabetes medication(s) or your insulin dosage recently been increased?
- Have you recently worked or exercised strenuously?
- Do you vary the sites of insulin injection?

Because drugs other than insulin and conditions besides diabetes may also cause or contribute to clinical hypoglycemia, patients should be questioned regarding:

- Renal failure
- Hepatic disease
- Pancreatic tumors (B-cell tumors)
- Excessive ethanol intake
- Aspirin overdose
- Use of β-blockers, pentamidine, or disopyramide

Demographics

The signs and symptoms of hypoglycemia manifest at varying levels among different individuals. Hypoglycemia is much less common among insulin-treated type 2 diabetic patients than among type 1 patients. Insulin shock may occur more often in children because of their broadly varied activity and diet.

Ancillary Tests

Determine the patient's blood glucose by in-office glucometer.

The patient should be referred to his or her primary physician for further evaluation. The physician will differentiate whether the patient has reactive hypoglycemia (e.g., early DM, idiopathic, etc.) or fasting hypoglycemia (e.g., insulinoma, extrapancreatic neoplasms, hepatic or renal failure, insulin reactions, adverse side effects of various medications, ethanol abuse, etc.). Testing to detect or exclude these conditions will be performed as deemed appropriate.

The Treatment

The definitive treatment of hypoglycemia will be determined by identifying the specific underlying disease. However, emergency in-office care may include the following procedures.

If the patient is conscious, give a commercially prepared glucose paste or tablet. Orange juice with two teaspoons of sugar, sugar-containing soft drinks, corn syrup, honey, jelly, sugar cubes, or hard candy will help to increase the carbohydrate level.

The goal is to raise the patient's blood glucose to a minimum level of 70 to 80 mg/dL. It takes about 15 minutes for the carbohydrates to be digested and to enter the blood stream as glucose.

Gels or liquids should never be forced into the mouths of unarousable patients because of the risk of aspiration.

If the patient is unconscious, make sure there is an adequate airway and administer oxygen if available. If properly trained, the patient should have an indwelling catheter placed in a large vein (e.g., brachial vein) and given 50% dextrose in water, 50 mL at 10 mL/min. Most patients regain consciousness within 5 to 10 minutes.

If an IV cannot be established, the patient should be given 0.5 to 1.0 mg of glucagon injected IM or SC in the deltoid or anterior thigh.

Oral gel glucose (Glutose 15) may be applied for oral mucosal absorption as long as it does not obstruct the airway.

Transport immediately to the hospital, even if the patient seems to be completely recovered. Patients with hypoglycemia secondary to oral hypoglycemic agents should be monitored for 24 to 48 hours because hypoglycemia may recur.

Note: A diabetic patient who has a sudden change in mental function or level of consciousness is more likely to be hypoglycemic than hyperglycemic. Consequently, if the patient is a known or suspected diabetic, and insulin shock cannot be excluded, when in doubt, give glucose!

CHOKING/AIRWAY OBSTRUCTION
Nicky R. Holdeman

ICD—9: 934.9

THE DISEASE
Pathophysiology

The organs of the body require a continuous supply of oxygen in order to survive. Thus, an acute obstruction of the airway by foreign material poses a potential life-threatening emergency. Without a patent airway and adequate gas exchange, other resuscitative measures will usually not be successful. Respiration may be interrupted by either obstruction or compression.

Etiology

Choking is a common breathing emergency. Aspiration of any foreign material may cause asphyxia if the substance aspirated is large or the cough reflex is impaired. However, one of the most common obstructions of the upper airway is by food. This condition, often referred to as a "cafe coronary," could easily occur in an office setting.

The Patient

The clinical presentation of a choking individual will depend on whether the airway is partially or completely blocked and on the site of obstruction. In general, one should look for the following symptoms or signs.

Clinical Symptoms
- Clutching the throat with one or both hands (the universal distress signal for choking)
- Coughing/gagging
- Wheezing
- Difficulty talking

Note: A partially blocked airway can become completely obstructed. A person whose airway is totally blocked can't speak, cough forcefully, or breathe.

Clinical Signs
- Tachypnea
- Labored breathing with inadequate movement of air
- Stridor
- Substernal notch retraction
- Agitation or lethargy
- Cyanosis

- Rapid pulse initially, then decreased pulse
- Cardiac arrest

Significant History

History of an aspiration event may be absent in 30 to 50% of patients. Lack of a positive history often delays diagnosis, so foreign bodies should be suspected, especially in children as the airway is smaller. Aspiration of food is more likely to occur in the following patients.

- Intoxicated individuals
- Those with swallowing difficulties
- Older individuals (75 or over)
- Patients with poor dentition
- Denture wearers (difficulty to sense whether food has been fully chewed)
- Those who eat while excited or laughing
- Those who play or run with food in the mouth
- Those who use sedative drugs

Demographics

More than 3,000 deaths annually are because of choking.

While most airway obstruction because of foreign bodies occurs between the ages of 1 and 5 years, more adults than children die each year as a result of choking.

Ancillary Tests

Lab testing per se is not indicated. Ultimately, the patient may have plain radiographic films, fluoroscopy, or endoscopy to assist in the diagnosis of airway obstruction.

If a foreign body is not recovered, the patient should undergo radiological imaging for localization.

The Treatment

Management of foreign bodies in the airway is dictated by the location of the object and the age and condition of the patient.

If the choking person is coughing, do not interfere; the normal reflexes will often clear the airway. Allow the patient to assume a position that is comfortable and that facilitates respiration.

O_2, if available, should be administered to all patients with foreign body aspiration.

If there is total obstruction, the Heimlich maneuver should be attempted in patients 1 year or older. In younger children, back blows and chest thrusts are recommended. Continue maneuvers until the airway has cleared or the patient loses consciousness.

If the foreign body is visible, the airway may be cleared with a manual sweep. Blind sweeps are not recommended, especially in infants and young children.

If there is no success at clearing the airway and if the patient loses consciousness, EMS should be activated for assistance. In the meantime, place the patient in a supine position; tilt the head backward and continue to attempt to open the airway; check for respiratory sounds and ventilate if possible; perform abdominal thrusts.

If these methods are unsuccessful, a surgical airway (access to the airway by tracheotomy) may be necessary.

Ultimately, the patient may require removal of the foreign body under general anesthesia with a laryngoscope or bronchoscope.

SYNCOPE
Nicky R. Holdeman
ICD—9: 780.2

THE DISEASE
Pathophysiology

Syncope, or fainting, is a sudden and transient loss of consciousness because of inadequate cerebral blood flow and oxygenation. It must be distinguished from epileptic seizures, transient ischemic attacks, vertigo, hysteria, and hypoglycemia.

Etiology

An attempt to establish the etiology of syncope is important because the symptom is common and potentially fatal. While the list of possible causes is long and diverse, the major categories include:

- Vasovagal (vasomotor) syncope—because of excessive vagal tone resulting in a decrease in both arterial pressure and heart rate. Accounts for 21% of syncopal episodes.
- Orthostatic (postural) hypotension—another type of vasomotor syncope. May result from multiple factors such as certain drugs (e.g., antihypertensives), neuropathies (e.g., diabetes mellitus), hypovolemia, or spinal cord injuries. Orthostasis is estimated to cause 9% of syncopal events.
- Cardiogenic syncope—involves a wide range of conditions and diseases including dysrythmias, cardiomyopathies, conduction disorders, aortic stenosis, acute myocardial infections (AMI), or cardiac tamponade. Cardiac conditions account for 10% of syncopal events and has a 2–3 fold increase in all cause mortality.

The Patient

In general, syncope will be characterized by a loss of consciousness, unresponsiveness, loss of postural tone, and spontaneous recovery. However, certain symptoms and signs will often manifest depending on the underlying cause. Because vasovagal episodes are the most common entity seen in outpatient facilities, the following descriptors pertain to this particular type of syncope.

Clinical Symptoms

Brief prodrome of nausea, dizziness, light-headedness, weakness, sweating, salivation, and blurred vision. The prodrome usually lasts from 10 seconds to a few minutes.

Clinical Signs

Initially, tachycardia, hypotension, and pallor are seen. These signs are soon followed by bradycardia, pupillary dilation, weak pulse, diaphoresis, and transient loss of consciousness. Abnormal movements that may mimic a seizure are often noted, but urinary incontinence and tongue biting is rare.

Demographics

Vasovagal disorders are very common and occur in all age groups, affecting men and women equally. Syncope, from all causes, accounts for about 1 to 6% of hospital admissions and about 3% of emergency room visits. Five to 20% of adults will have one or more episodes of syncope by age 75.

Significant History

The evaluation for syncope depends heavily on a careful history if the underlying cause is to be discovered. Witnesses to the event may provide additional insight. The clinician should obtain the following information:

- The events leading up to the syncopal episode (e.g., coughing, urinating, defecating) Syncope with exertion suggests a cardiac cause
- The patient's posture before syncope (e.g., vasovagal syncope does not occur when the patient is horizontal but cardiac syncope can occur in any position)
- Prodromal manifestations (e.g., syncope with marked sweating and tachycardia is likely the result of hypoglycemia, whereas syncope with mild sweating, nausea, and bradycardia is more often a result of a vasovagal episode, especially in circumstances provoking strong emotion. Syncope of sudden onset with brief or no premonitory symptoms suggest a cardiac cause.)
- Were there focal neurologic signs (e.g., neurologic abnormalities such as a motor or sensory loss may suggest transient cerebral ischemia (TIA) and prompts a search for emboli or thrombosis)?
- Is there a family history of syncope (e.g., a family history of syncope suggests migrane, epilepsy, or vasovagal attacks)?
- Does the patient have any underlying diseases?
- Is he or she taking any medications (e.g., several classes of drugs have a predisposition to syncope)?
- Has he or she recently ingested drugs or alcohol?

Ancillary Tests

In addition to a careful history, a thorough physical examination and ECG are important procedures in determining a diagnosis. Depending on the outcome of these standard procedures, a given patient may also require hematology testing and blood chemistries (e.g., CBC, electrolytes, glucose, toxicology), cardiac studies (e.g., transtelephonic ECG, echocardiogram, stress testing, electrophysiologic studies [EPS]), neurologic investigations (e.g., EEG, CT, or MRI of the head), and/or psychiatric evaluation (e.g., exclude anxiety, depression, alcohol and drug abuse).

Unfortunately, even after careful evaluation and testing, the cause of syncope will be determined in only 63% of patients.

The Treatment

Because syncopy itself is not a disease but can indicate a wide range of conditions and disorders, the ultimate treatment will be directed toward the underlying etiology. In-office care for syncope should include the following:

- If the person has not yet fainted but becomes pale, begins to perspire, and feels faint, have the patient sit and lower his or her head to a level between the knees or carefully help place him or her in a recumbent position.
- If the patient has already fainted, lower the victim to the ground, position him or her on his or her back, and elevate the legs 8 to 12 inches. (Get the patient's toes above their nose.)
- Loosen any tight clothing, such as a tie or collar, that may restrict free breathing or impinge on the carotid sinus.
- Check to make sure the patient is breathing. Establish an airway and administer O_2, 2 to 3L/min, by nasal canula if the patient is conscious.
- Place crushed ammonia capsule under the nose.
- Monitor for vomiting and possible aspiration. If the patient vomits, place the victim on his or her side.
- Check vital signs; initiate appropriate emergency care.
- Apply cold compresses to forehead or back of neck.
- Do not give the victim anything to eat or drink unless hypoglycemia is suspected and the victim is fully conscious.
- Check for any injuries that may have been sustained during a fall and treat them appropriately.
- Keep the victim from getting chilled or overheated.
- If the patient manifests abnormal movements or has a seizure, do not hold or restrain the person or place anything between the teeth. Cushion the victim's head and prevent bodily injury by removing nearby objects. Seizure-like movements are not uncommonly seen in syncopal patients.
- Do not allow a person who has fainted to get up after regaining consciousness. Syncope may recur, especially if the patient stands within 30 minutes after the attack.
- Transport the patient to the emergency room for further management and observation.

Note: Vasovagal syncope has an excellent prognosis, and the risk of death is not increased by these events.

ANAPHYLAXIS (ANAPHYLACTIC SHOCK)
Nicky R. Holdeman

ICD—9: 995.0

THE DISEASE

Pathophysiology

Shock is a clinical syndrome defined by an inadequate blood flow and transport of oxygen to organs and tissues. When the body's organs do not receive blood, they fail to function properly, and the potential for irreversible tissue damage occurs. Anaphylaxis, a form of shock, is a serious and potentially catastrophic IgE-mediated, Type 1 allergic reaction to a foreign antigen. Initial exposure to an antigen may result in specific IgE antibodies to that antigen. On re-exposure, the antigen can bind the IgE antibodies on the surface of mast cells and basophils. This cross-linking can result in degranulation and release of vasoactive substances and chemotactic factors such as histamine, tryptase, and other mediators of inflammation into the systemic circulation. These mediators result in vasodilatation, increased vascular permeability, and smooth muscle contraction, producing the clinical symptoms of anaphylaxis.

Anaphylactoid reactions are clinically similar to anaphylaxis, but may occur after the first exposure of certain drugs or contrast agents. These reactions are not IgE mediated but are rather because of direct activation of mast cells and basophils by certain substances.

Etiology

A growing number of agents can cause anaphylaxis, including proteins (e.g., antiserum, insulin, ACTH), enzymes (e.g., insect venoms), pollen (e.g., grass, ragweed), food (e.g., eggwhite, rice, raw milk, nuts, seafood, chocolate), diagnostic agents (e.g., NaFl), antibiotics (e.g., penicillin, tetracyclines), latex products, and/or exercise. In rare cases of anaphylaxis, an etiologic "trigger" agent is never identified.

The Patient

After exposure to the offending agent, the clinical features of anaphylaxis can begin within seconds or take as long as an hour to develop. However, the spectrum of symptoms may range from mild to fatal within minutes. The most commonly affected organ systems are the skin, GI tract, respiratory tract, and cardiovascular system. Isolated urticaria and angioedema are more common forms of anaphylaxis with a better prognosis. Ominous signs and symptoms are those of progressive respiratory and circulatory failure.

Clinical Symptoms
Symptoms vary, and rarely does one patient develop all the symptoms.

- Itching (particularly of the nose and hands)
- Sneezing/coughing

- Watery eyes and nose
- Skin rash
- Sense of throat closing, hoarseness (laryngeal edema)
- Feeling of warmth (flushed skin)
- Throbbing in the ears
- Nausea/vomiting
- Crampy abdominal pain
- Light-headedness
- Shortness of breath or labored breathing (bronchospasm)
- Feeling of substernal pressure
- Sense of agitation or of impending doom

Clinical Signs

- Erythema and angioedema of the skin (painless, deeper, subcutaneous swelling, often involving the periorbital, circumoral, and facial regions. Represents vasodilation and escape of plasma into tissues and results in a decrease of effective plasma volume, which is a major cause of shock).
- Pruritis
- Urticaria (large, irregularly shaped pruritic, erythematous wheals)
- Conjunctival injection, lacrimation
- Rhinorrhea
- Coughing, hoarseness, stridor
- Dyspnea, tachypnea, wheezing
- Cyanosis
- Tachycardia, hypotension, arrhythmias
- Vomiting, diarrhea
- Incontinence
- Dizziness, weakness, syncope, seizures

Note: Primary cardiovascular collapse can occur without respiratory symptoms.

Demographics

Anaphylaxis may occur in any patient regardless of race, sex, or age. The severity of an individual's response is dependent on the rate, amount, and site of mediator release, as well as preexisting medical conditions (e.g., asthma, cardiovascular disease). Generally, the shorter the time before symptoms appear after exposure, the greater the risk of a fatal reaction. Patients with immediate allergic reactions are at risk for shock and respiratory arrest.

Significant History

The signs and symptoms of anaphylactic shock are acute, generalized, and often extreme. In cases precipitated by an obvious cause, there is seldom any question as to the diagnosis. The history is most useful in the area of prevention.

Clinicians should inquire carefully about any history of drug allergies before giving any medications.

Anaphylaxis in a patient being treated with topical or oral β-blockers, may be refractory to epinephrine and selective β-agonists.

Patients with significant atopy (allergic skin rashes, hay fever, asthma) are at greater risk for anaphylactoid reactions.

Patients with a history of anaphylactic reactions to insect venom, or other environmental agents, should be identified.

Patients with a history of anaphylaxis should wear a medical alert bracelet.

Ancillary Tests

Ancillary testing would be most useful in helping to distinguish other medical emergencies that may clinically mimic anaphylaxis, such as a primary cardiac event. On the other hand, physical assessment is very important, and it is incumbent on the provider to document and verify hemodynamic and respiratory stability before, during, and after procedures.

The clinician should continually check:

- Airway viability (respirations should be full and 12 to 20/min)
- Pulse rate (pulse should be strong and between 60 to 100/min)
- Capillary refill (skin color should return in 2 seconds after compression)
- Adequate perfusion (normal level of consciousness)
- Skin color (cyanosis indicates a lack of adequate O_2)
- Skin temperature (skin should feel normal in temperature)
- Blood pressure (hypotension is often a late sign of shock)

The Treatment

Anaphylaxis is a medical emergency that demands immediate recognition and treatment to prevent morbidity or death from respiratory failure, circulatory collapse, or both. EMS should be activated immediately and treatment should begin as soon as anaphylaxis is suspected; do not wait until it is fully developed.

1. Secure an open airway.
2. Place the patient in a recumbent position with the feet elevated about 8 to 12 inches. (Trendelenburg position.)
3. Administer 100% oxygen at 4 to 8 L/min and ventilate manually if indicated.
4. Epinephrine 1:1000 solution in an adult dose of 0.3 to 0.5 mL (0.3 to 0.5 mg) injected SC or IM in the anterolateral thigh. IM administration is faster and less variable in effect than SC injection. Repeated injections can be given every 15 to 20 minutes when necessary. Epinephrine is an antagonist to the effects of the chemical mediators on smooth muscle, blood vessels, and other tissues.
5. IV infusion of large volumes of fluid (saline or lactated Ringer's) is essential in hypotension, to replace the loss of intravascular plasma into tissues.
6. Inhalation of β_2-agonists, such as albuterol, are effective for bronchospasm (wheezing and dyspnea).
7. Glucagon, 0.03 to 0.05 mg/kg IV bolus over 1 minute, may be beneficial for resistant hypotension caused by concurrent beta-blockade therapy.
8. Diphenhydramine 50 mg IM or IV.

9. Hydrocortisone 100 to 250 mg IV push (up to 5 to 10 mg/Kg), methylprednisolone 60 mg IV push, or dexamethasone 4 mg IV push to prevent late phase recurrence of symptoms.
10. Monitor vital signs (blood pressure, heart rate, respirations).
11. Maintain the patient's normal body temperature.
12. Keep the patient quiet and still.
13. Give the patient nothing by mouth.
14. Transport the patient rapidly to the nearest emergency department. Even if the patient is improving, he or she is at risk for a late phase reaction 2 to 12 hours later, that can be more severe than the initial reaction. All patients with anaphylaxis should be monitored for at least 6 hours after apparent recovery and sometimes up to 24 hours.

After appropriate treatment, prevention is of the utmost importance. Detection and avoidance of the offending (triggering) agent will reduce the chances of future life-threatening episodes. Any person with anaphylaxis should be instructed in the use of emergency epinephrine and have an autoinjector epinephrine kit (*EpiPen*) readily available at all times.

ASTHMATIC ATTACK/BRONCHOSPASM
Nicky R. Holdeman

ICD—9: 493.9

THE DISEASE
Pathophysiology

Asthma is a disorder of the tracheobroncheal tree characterized by periodic bronchospasm and hypersecretion of mucus, with intervals of relative good health. Numerous inflammatory mediators, such as histamine, bradykinin, chemotactic factors, prostaglandins, and leukotrienes appear to play a pivotal role. The release of these products results in airway edema and narrowing, hyperemia, and increased secretion of mucus. Ultimately, the reactions result in expiratory airway obstruction and air trapping.

Etiology

Most asthmatic patients can be placed into one of two clinical categories.

Extrinsic asthma, or "allergic" asthma occurs in patients who are predisposed to respond to certain antigens by producing IgE antibodies. Reactions are often triggered by environmental irritants (e.g., dust, pollen, molds, animal dander, etc.), are typically seasonal, and occur most often in children.

Intrinsic asthma or "nonallergic" asthma is characterized by the absence of external triggers of bronchospasm, although exacerbations often accompany respiratory infections. Intrinsic asthma is most common in adults, is not seasonal, but is often chronic. These patients have normal serum levels of IgE; however, they may demonstrate bronchial hyperactivity to inhaled fumes, cigarette smoke, emotional stress, exercise, or cold air.

The Patient

Clinical Symptoms

- Cough
- Dyspnea/labored breathing
- Wheezing
- Chest tightness
- Sputum production
- Nocturnal attacks

Patients with extrinsic asthma may also complain of rhinitis, sneezing, nasal obstruction, conjunctivitis, or other allergic symptoms. Symptoms are usually progressive and occur over a period of hours or days.

Clinical Signs

- Wheezing and respiratory distress
- Prolonged expiration
- Hyperresonance
- Decreased breath sounds
- Tachycardia
- Use of accessory respiratory muscles
- Anxiety
- Flaring of the nares
- Barrel chest (hyperinflation)
- Cyanosis

Note: Wheezing is a whistling sound made by air partially blocked by narrowed airways. If the asthma attack is severe, air cannot flow and the wheezing may stop. This scenario is a life-threatening emergency requiring immediate treatment.

Demographics

- Asthma has an estimated prevalence of 4 to 8% of the population; there are 10 million new cases each year.
- Asthma may manifest at any age, but 50% of cases are children under 10.
- The onset of extrinsic asthma is usually before 30.
- There may be a slight female predominance in adults, whereas there is a male predominance in children under 10.

Significant History

The history may be crucial for determining the patient's prognosis and proper management. The clinician should obtain the following information:

- Are the patient's symptoms worse in the early mornings (i.e., nocturnal exacerbations)?
- Are the symptoms episodic or chronic?
- Are there other coexisting allergic disorders?
- Is the patient on medications for asthma? If so, is he or she compliant?
- Are there known precipitating factors?

Ancillary Tests

While in-office testing is generally not applicable, these patients frequently undergo tests and procedures that are useful in the management of asthma. This workup may involve:

- Spirometry—used to judge the severity of an attack and monitor the response to therapy. Peak flow testing can help track the progress of a patient's asthma treatment.
- Chest x-ray—usually is normal or may show mild hyperinflation, flattened diaphragms, or atelectasis. Used also to exclude foreign body aspiration, pneumothorax heart failure, and so on.
- CBC—note active infection and eosinophilia.
- Allergy testing.
- Exercise tolerance testing.

In more severe cases, arterial blood gasses, pulse oximetry, ECG, and sputum analysis may be indicated.

The Treatment

Because the onset of symptoms is seldom abrupt, most asthmatic events seen in an office setting would be considered mild attacks. The goals of therapy would be to improve oxygenation, relieve bronchospasm, and increase ventilation. One should perform the following steps:

- Position the patient upright or as is comfortable for the patient.
- Maintain an airway; breathe for the patient if necessary.
- Administer humidified O_2, 2 to 3 L/min, via nasal canula.
- Monitor vital signs; proceed with CPR, if necessary.
- Keep the patient calm, as stress may worsen the attack.
- Often the patients will have a bronchodilator (e.g., β_2-agonist) in the form of a metered-dose inhaler (MDI). Assist them in properly inhaling these drugs. May repeat after 10 to 20 minutes if needed.
- Transport to the nearest appropriate facility if the patient's condition deteriorates.

Once in the Emergency Department, asthmatic patients will often undergo pulmonary function tests to assess airflow before and after therapy. Pharmacologic management frequently involves:

- β_2-agonists (e.g., albuterol, terbutaline)

- Anticholinergic agents (e.g., ipratropium, atropine)
- Corticosteroids (e.g., beclomethasone, prednisone)
- Methylxanthines (e.g., theophylline)
- Cromolyn sodium
- Magnesium sulfate

CHEST PAIN (ANGINA PECTORIS AND ACUTE MYOCARDIAL INFARCTION)
Nicky R. Holdeman

ICD—9: 413—Angina pectoris
ICD—9: 410.9—Myocardial infarction

THE DISEASE
Pathophysiology

Chest pain is one of the most common symptoms for which a patient seeks medical attention. The list of potential causes is both long and diverse. It is often difficult to establish, particularly in an office setting, the exact etiology of the pain. Therefore, it is usually wise to regard every adult with chest pain as a potential heart attack victim.

Two types of coronary artery disease, arteriosclerosis and atherosclerosis, are responsible for 97% of all acute myocardial infarctions (AMI), the remainder being because of coronary vasospasms and other rare etiologies. Atherosclerotic plaques develop when fatty substances and other debris are deposited on the intimal lining of the arterial wall. An AMI may then result from decreased blood flow, stasis, hemorrhage, or thrombus formation secondary to coronary occlusion.

Angina pectoris is a symptom and usually occurs in patients with coronary artery disease (CAD). Angina is typically precipitated by physical exertion or emotional stress but can manifest if the coronary arteries have abnormal spasms (Prinzmetal's angina). Angina may be exacerbated by anemia, hypoxemia, systemic hypertension, hyperthyroidism, and tachyarrhythmia. In essence, angina occurs when the heart's demand for oxygen exceeds the oxygen available.

Etiology

Chest pain may result from many causes, some of which are relatively benign, others may be life threatening. Chest pain can occur secondary to pulmonary problems, (e.g., pleurisy, pneumothorax, embolism, pneumonia), gastrointestinal disorders (e.g., esophagitis, duodenal ulcer, pancreatitis, cholecystitis), or musculoskeletal abnormalities (e.g., costochondritis, rib fractures).

Cardiovascular diseases, however, account for the majority of serious pains originating from the chest. While conditions such as pericarditis, aortic dissection, and valvular disease may produce thoracic pain, angina and AMI are the most common causes of cardiovascular symptoms.

The Patient

Clinical Symptoms

It is generally impossible, in an outpatient facility, to differentiate the pain of angina pectoris and the pain of an AMI. In fact, patients may not describe a pain but rather a sensation of tightness, squeezing, burning, indigestion, or ill-defined discomfort. Typically, the most common symptoms of heart disease include:

- Dyspnea
- Cough
- Chest pain (precordial pressure or heaviness)
- Palpitations
- Light-headedness
- Nausea
- Fatigue

Most patients (80 to 90%) with an AMI have chest discomfort that is substernal and may radiate to the neck, left shoulder, and left upper arm. Occasionally, pain may occur in atypical areas such as the right arm, right shoulder, wrist, back, or epigastrium. Some patients report pain only in the jaw or in the teeth.

It should also be noted that up to 25% of myocardial infarction patients have no chest pain at all, especially the elderly or diabetic individuals. These patients are at increased risk for delays in seeking medical attention, less-aggressive treatments, and mortality.

For many patients, sudden collapse is the first symptom of a cardiac event.

Clinical Signs

The signs of myocardial infarction vary depending on the extent of cardiac damage and how the autonomic nervous system responds to the damage. Physical findings will therefore vary and none are specific or diagnostic of an AMI. Interpretation depends on the entire clinical picture and, in many cases, diagnostic testing. Common signs of an AMI may include:

- Diaphoresis
- Cool and pale skin
- Possible cyanosis
- Weakness
- Anxiety
- Gallop rhythm
- Variable blood pressure and pulse (pulse may be thready)
- Syncope
- Dysrhythmias

In patients with an uncomplicated MI, there may be no abnormal findings on physical examination, or the heart rate and blood pressure may be elevated. In some patients, an increase in vagal tone may result in bradycardia or hypotension. Heart failure is usually accompanied by hypotension and tachycardia.

Note: Most cases of sudden cardiac death (SCD) result from dysrhythmias. Tachyarrhythmia and ventricular fibrillation are the most common disturbances in survivors of SCD.

Significant History

The history may be helpful in revealing symptoms and conditions that increase the likelihood of certain causes of chest discomfort and in identifying known risk factors for coronary artery disease.

In patients suspected of having heart-related pain, one should obtain the following information:

- When the pain started
- What initiated the pain (i.e., exercise, emotional stress, or was the patient at rest)?
- Description of the pain (sharp pain seldom indicates a cardiac etiology)
- Where does it hurt?
- Does the pain radiate? If so, where does it radiate?
- What lessens the pain (i.e., rest, nitrates)?
- Is there a history of heart disease?
- Are there any associated symptoms?

The clinician should also ascertain all known cardiac risk factors that predispose an individual to CAD. The major risk factors include:

- Family history of CAD, especially before the age of 55
- Poorly controlled diabetes mellitus
- Age (>50)
- Sex (males > females)
- High serum cholesterol and triglycerides
- Systemic hypertension
- Smoking
- Sedentary lifestyle
- Obesity

Demographics

It is estimated that over 70,000,000 Americans suffer some form of cardiovascular disease, which is the leading cause of death in North America. The most common problem is CAD leading to angina pectoris and eventually AMI.

Angina is the presenting symptom of CAD in 38% of men and 61% of women. CAD is more predominant in males than females. Almost 500,000 Americans die each year of cardiovascular disease before they reach a hospital.

Ancillary Tests

While in-office testing of patients with chest pain is limited to physical exam findings, these patients often require extensive studies to determine the underlying cause.

The initial evaluation of a patient with chest pain usually includes an ECG and chest radiograph. Other studies will depend on the history and physical examination of a particular patient.

The Treatment

Patients with chest pain (especially those with severe pain, those with pain lasting longer than 10 minutes, and those with pain that persist during rest) require prompt medical care. In-office management should include the following measures:

- Call emergency medical services—dial 911 in most cities.
- Assess for airway, breathing, and circulation; assist as necessary.
- If the patient is not allergic to aspirin, administer 162 mg or 325 mg (chewed and absorbed in mouth) at once regardless of whether thrombolytic therapy is being considered or whether the patient has been taking aspirin.
- Be calm and reassuring to relieve patient anxiety.
- Help the patient to rest comfortably.
- Loosen restrictive clothing.
- Begin O_2, 3 to 6 L/min by nasal prongs or 15 L/min with a face mask.
- Help the patient with his or her medications or administer nitroglycerin, 0.2 to 0.6 mg SL. Repeat in 5 minutes if chest pain is not relieved. (Nitroglycerin is a smooth muscle relaxer and vasodilator. Overall, the drug helps balance myocardial O_2 supply and demand, and pain relief often occurs within 2 to 3 minutes.)
- Monitor vital signs continuously; proceed with CPR if indicated.
- Conserve body heat but do not overheat.
- Transport by EMS immediately to the nearest facility, especially if the pain has not responded to three nitroglycerin tablets or has lasted more than 15 minutes.

Thrombolytic therapy has been shown effective in reducing mortality and myocardial damage when started within 3 to 6 hours after the onset of infarction. Many heart attack victims delay getting care and rationalize that their symptoms are a result of muscle soreness or indigestion. Do not let their denial influence your decision to call for emergency care.

Note: While AEDs are not necessarily considered standard of care for every private office, they do provide an efficient method of delivering defibrillation to persons experiencing out-of-hospital cardiac arrest. It is highly recommended that health-care providers and first responders be trained to operate these life-saving devices, and to have immediate access to an AED in case of a cardiac emergency.

Chemical and Bioterrorism

INTRODUCTION
Andrew R. Buzzelli and Leonid Skorin Jr.

Bioterrorism is the unlawful use, or threatened use, of chemicals, microorganisms, or toxins to produce death or disease in humans, animals, or plants. The act is intended to create fear and/or intimidate governments or societies in the pursuit of political, religious, or ideological goals. Biological warfare has been part of the human arsenal of weapons from almost the start of recorded military history. We can turn back as early as 400 BC to discover arrows dipped into the fluids of decomposing bodies to inflict biologic as well as mechanical destruction on their intended victims. The 14th-century siege of the Crimean city of Kaffa (now in Ukraine) was aided by an epidemic of plague when the attacking Tartar force catapulted cadavers of plague victims into the city. In 1995, the Aum Shinrikyo apocalyptic cult in Japan attempted on several occasions to spread terror by means of sarin gas, botulinum toxin, and anthrax. Biological terrorism is a public health event. Chemical terrorism, which is a Haz-Mat event, usually escalates quickly into a public health event.

Bacteria are unicellular, self-sustaining etiologic elements in a pathologic process causing destruction, tissue invasion, and toxin production. The weaponization of bacteria as well as viruses will depend on availability, ease of production, lethality, stability, and infectivity. The selected agent can be aerosolized in particle size designed to contaminate the respiratory apparatus. Weaponization can also be accomplished by food and water contamination and contact with infected individuals. The method of disease transmission will vary with the selected agent and terrorist access to a specific population. The difficulty in diagnosing and treating the victims owing to the delayed onset of agent infectivity is a perfect platform for the warfare objectives of the terrorist— *death, disease, and fear.*

The health-care provider must be alert for unusually large numbers of ill patients with unusual disease profiles for a given region. In the absence of intelligence reports, the provider must alert local and federal public health agencies to the possible existence of a chemical or biological attack. The incubation period between attack and clinical symptoms is a valuable clue in identifying an agent. Particular agents demonstrate unique incubation times.

Travel, employment, and unusual illnesses among friends, family members, and the community are crucial links in making the diagnosis and instituting treatment. Frequently, pneumonia is associated with an aerosol attack of one of these agents. It is the inhalation forms of these diseases that are life threatening. Providers should be aware when acute respiratory distress manifests in large numbers of a previously healthy population, particularly in urban areas.

The single-celled, self-reproducing natures of bacteria make them prime candidates for waging war by both disease and terror. The bacterial disease agents produce varying disease presentations. Our lack of experience with these infections in our current populations is further complicated by the fact that these bacteria can be developed into different weapons-grade organisms. The identical argument can be advanced for the selection of viral weapons. Ease of transmission, high contagion rates, and treatment unavailability are all attractive elements for the terrorist.

Chemical nerve agents, also known as nerve gas, can be liquid or vapor. They are spread primarily by aerosol devices or explosive charge. The March 1995 attack in the Tokyo subway system used a colorless and odorless gas, an organophosphate known as sarin. That attack killed 11 people and injured more than 5,500 others, hospitalizing 1,200.

The Centers for Disease Control and Prevention (CDC) catalog the critical biologic agents by category, according to their ability to affect and disrupt a population. Category A agents gain their notoriety as weapons of mass destruction because of their established ability to infect the target, affect mass casualties, and escalate public fear to civil disturbance. Specifically, Category A agents are: (a) moderately easily disseminated or transmitted from person to person; (b) result in moderate morbidity with low mortality rates and have the potential for major public health impact; (c) could cause widespread panic and social disruption; and (d) require enhanced disease surveillance and diagnostic capabilities. Anthrax, plague, tularemia, smallpox, botulism, and viral hemorrhagic fevers are among the agents in this category. The World Health Organization (WHO) estimates agents such as *Bacillus anthracis* and *Francisella tularensis* have the potential, under favorable conditions, to kill or disable 125,000 people in a community of 500,000 exposed victims.

Category B agents are not as viable for use in bioterrorism because of their limited ability to spread infection and diminished casualty counts for the enemy. The characteristics of Category B agents are: (a) moderately easily disseminated or transmitted from person to person; (b) result in moderate morbidity with low mortality rates and have the potential for major public health impact; (c) could cause panic and social disruptions; and (d) require specific enhancement of CDC's diagnostic capacity and enhanced disease surveillance. Category B agents include Alpha viruses, ricin, and foodborne and waterborne diseases. Salmonella, a foodborne disease, has already been utilized in a 1984 bioterrorist attack in a small Oregon town called The Dalles. A religious cult known as the Rajneeshees used *Salmonella typhimurium* to poison residents before a crucial election in hopes of taking over the local county government. Category B agents still require disease surveillance and public health response.

Category C agents are perhaps the most ominous of the bioweapons. Category C agents include emerging pathogens that could be engineered for mass dissemination in the future because of: (a) availability; (b) ease of production and dissemination; and (c) potential for high morbidity and mortality rates and major health impact. These include the Nipah and Hanta viruses, the tickborne hemorrhagic fever and encephalitis viruses, yellow fever, and multidrug-resistant tuberculosis. They are the gathering storms on the horizon of micro-organisms, which are as of yet unutilized or undeveloped for the bioterrorist armory. Ominous, not because of their lethality, but because we will be unaccustomed to their characteristics and penetrance as a result of the science of genetic engineering. They may become the greatest challenges yet to the development of our technologies of surveillance and detection and the emergence of our medical treatment protocols.

The ophthalmologist or optometrist may be the first practitioner the patient seeks for care. Single-doctor office sites in rural areas and hospitals in more metropolitan areas may be quickly overcome with casualties and unable to handle the surge. Your treatment resources, both personnel and material, may be quickly exhausted. Your decision may have to be to initiate postexposure treatments for known infected victims and abandon attempts at the more time- and resource-consuming preferred initial treatments. Ensuring that current and future health professionals are well versed in the potential threats of chemical and bioterrorism is a vital step in protecting and serving the public.

BACTERIAL AGENTS
Andrew R. Buzzelli

ANTHRAX (BACILLUS ANTHRACIS)
ICD—9: 022.9

THE DISEASE
Pathophysiology

Anthrax, long considered conquered in Western civilization, has gained a new notoriety by its successful use in attacks against the American public in the new millennium. Inhalation anthrax destroys the tracheobronchial nodes. The circulatory collapse, inherent in cutaneous anthrax caused by these toxins, results in tissue necrosis and sets the stage for death owing to bacteremia. Aerosol delivery is the most likely weaponized form of the agent, but there are many methods of attack, as demonstrated by the U.S. postal attacks of 2001.

Etiology

Bacillus anthracis is an aerobic, nonmotile, gram-positive rod, capable of spore formation. The *anthracis* spore is transported within alveolar macrophages to regional lymph nodes. They vegetate, within the macrophage, producing both lethal and edema toxins. Both toxins also consist of PA (protective antigen) that activates to inhibit an immune response to the bacteria and facilitate their transport across the cell membrane. These trivirulent factors are preliminary to septicemia and toxic shock.

Anthrax disease is transmitted by inoculation (cutaneous anthrax), inhalation (inhalation anthrax), and ingestion (gastrointestinal anthrax). It is normally contracted from anthrax-infected animals or -contaminated food products. *Bacillus anthracis* is a Category A bioterrorism agent.

The Patient

Clinical Symptoms
Cutaneous Anthrax
- The lesions are most common to the eyelids on facial infection. They initiate as 1- to 2-cm red papules and evolve into edematous, necrotic, bullous lesions. The base of the lesion is characterized by the dark black eschar (hence its name from the Greek word *Anthrakis* or *coal*).
- Cicatrization and ectropion
- Exposure keratitis
- No pain, itching, swelling
- Clear fluid discharge
- Red skin, congested conjunctiva
- Preseptal cellulitis
- Epiphora

Inhalation Anthrax
- Chills and sweats
- Fatigue and malaise
- Nonproductive cough
- Nausea
- Dyspnea
- Severe sternal chest pain
- Headache

Clinical Signs
- Incubation period of 7 days (range 2 to 60) for inhalation; 10 days (range 2 to 12) for cutaneous. This incubation period has previously been characterized by an early improvement for 1 or 2 days during the first stage of the disease. Providers should be aware that this did not occur in patients infected with inhalation anthrax during the bioterrorist attacks of 2001.
- Fever
- Tachycardia
- Acute preseptal cellulitis from inoculation
- Enlarged mediastinum on computed tomography (CT)/magnetic resonance imaging (MRI)
- Bilateral pleural effusions on CT
- Epileptic convulsions may occur with disease progression to hemorrhagic meningitis

Demographics

Traditionally, anthrax infection occurs with the handling of animal fluids or hides that are contaminated. Vaccines have led to the eradication of the disease from those with occupational exposure. Inhalation anthrax has a mortality rate of 90%, but untreated inoculation anthrax will produce death from septicemia in 25% of the cases. The high mortality rate may be because of the compilation of the statistical data in the 20th century before the advent of antibiotics. The U.S. Post Office and Sverdlovsk, Russia, infection incidents indicate a lower mortality rate.

Significant History

- International disease surveillance reports
- Occupational exposure to sheep, cattle, horses, or their products
- Rapid onset of febrile illness
- High-profile individuals at high risk for terrorist attack

Ancillary Tests

- Gram stain of the blood and blood cultures
- Chest x-ray
- Gram stain and culture of lesion discharge in cutaneous anthrax (dry swab)
- Punch biopsy of the cutaneous lesion
- ELISA (enzyme-linked immunosorbent assay) for IgG, IgM
- SGOT/SGPT
- PCR (polymerase chain reaction) gene amplification
- Direct IFA (immunofluorescence assay) microscopy
- Throat or nasal swab
- Smear from cerebral spinal fluid (if meningeal signs present), lymph nodes, and spleen
- Lumbar puncture
- Tests should be performed through the end of the disease stage because the agent may be present after the symptoms manifest

The Treatment

Inhalation Anthrax

Either ciprofloxacin 400 mg IV every 8 to 12 hours or doxycycline 200 mg IV loading followed by 100 mg IV every 12 hours. Either of these can be combined with additional IV antimicrobial therapeutic agents (e.g., clindamycin).

This will be followed by oral administration of ciprofloxacin 500 mg p.o. every 12 hours for 60 days or doxycycline 100 mg p.o. every 12 hours for 60 days. The 60-day regimens are the total treatment amount for both oral and IV administration.

The oral drug treatment portion of the regimen for inhalation anthrax will be the schedule for cutaneous anthrax infection, mass-casualty resource exhaustion, prophylactic protection, or confirmed exposure. Recommendations can also be found for extending the treatment to 100 days or adding 3 doses of the anthrax vaccine to the 60-day treatment regimen. Only ciprofloxacin has Food and Drug Administration (FDA) approval for postexposure intervention.

Vaccination should commence with the start of IV drug therapy. Anthrax Vaccine Absorbed is administered in 0.5 mL subcutaneous injections over a period of 0, 2, and 4 weeks and at 6, 12, and 18 months with an annual booster. There is very little flexibility in the administration schedule. Ophthalmic providers should take particular note that headache and blurred vision were the predominant adverse reactions to the vaccine.

Topical lubricants are utilized when periorbital edema is interfering with lid mechanics and threatening an exposure keratitis.

Provider Precautions

When cutaneous anthrax is suspected, barrier isolation precautions are sufficient to protect against transmission of the disease. Contamination by infected patient contact has not been demonstrated in previous attacks. The crucial protective element is the immediate notification of public health authorities, including those local, state, and national, to begin disease monitoring.

PLAGUE (YERSINIA PESTIS)
ICD—9: 020.9

THE DISEASE
Pathophysiology

This pandemic of the Middle Ages traces its roots back to early biblical times. This history of fear accompanying the Black Death plays a prominent role in the terrorist arsenal. The organism causes death through infection in secondary organ systems. The infection may be classified as bubonic (site of the inoculation), pneumonic (lungs), or septicemic (blood). The bubo is the inflamed lymph node, located primarily in the groin area, which is a conglomerate of the infectious organisms and hence its designation as bubonic plague. Pneumonic plague arises directly from blood infection or by inhalation.

Etiology

This bacterium exists as a gram-negative coccobacillus with a characteristic bipolar staining. Plague travels through lymphatic channels to regional lymph nodes. Bacterial multiplication secretes cytotoxins into the local tissue and blood, where the secondary infection engulfs organs, including lungs, liver, and brain.

The normal route of transmission to a human host is through fleas, which transport the disease from rodents. The patient contracting the disease may then develop a secondary pneumonic plague. This individual now becomes a vector for respiratory spread of primary pneumonic plague. The absence of buboes is a distinguishing diagnostic factor of a primary pneumonic plague.

The most common terrorist delivery system would be through direct contact with suicide disease carriers and inhalation. Infection could be expected within 6 days of the attack. There is an aerosol delivery option available, but the disease organism is unstable and subject to rapid decay when exposed to environmental factors such as sunlight. Yersinia pestis is a Category A bioterrorism agent.

The Patient

Clinical Symptoms
- Chills
- Cough
- Headache
- Dyspnea
- Chest pain

- Abdominal pain
- Nausea
- Hemoptysis

Clinical Signs
- 2- to 8-day incubation period (2- to 6-day range for pneumonic plague; 2 to 8 days for bubonic plague)
- Bloody sputum
- Erythema
- Enlarged, painful, infected lymph nodes up to 10 cm in diameter (buboes)
- Fever
- Tachypnea
- Infiltrates visible on chest x-ray
- Cyanosis
- Leukocytosis
- Large display of polymorphonuclear cells

Demographics

Plague is still present, particularly in the western United States, with fleabite being the mode of transmission. A 50-kg attack would produce an infection rate of 150,000 victims, including 36,000 fatalities, in a population of 5 million inhabitants. The mortality rate is 60% for untreated bubonic plague and 100% for untreated pneumonic plague. Early treatment improves the survival rate dramatically. The lack of rapid detection systems for this disease is especially problematic for the provider, who must link sudden increases in patients presenting with severe pneumonia and sepsis in a nonpredictive environment.

Significant History
- Recent exposure to rodents (i.e., rats, squirrels, prairie dogs)
- Living or recently traveling in the southwestern United States

Ancillary Tests
- Giemsa, Wayson, or Wright show bipolar staining of lymph node aspirates
- Culture sputum, blood, buboes, and lymph node aspirates
- Throat and nasal swab
- Chest radiograph demonstrates pulmonary consolidation and infiltrates
- ELISA for IgG, IgM, and polymerase chain reaction
- Indirect fluorescent antibody test
- Always continue retrospective lab analysis into the convalescent stage because the organism and antibodies may be present only after the disease resolves

The Treatment

Streptomycin 1 gram IM bid for 10 days or gentamycin 5 mg/kg IM or IV daily for 10 days or 2 mg/kg loading dose followed by 1.7 mg/kg IM or IV tid. If neither of these treatment protocols is available, then start doxycycline 100 mg IV bid for 10 days or 200 mg IV daily or ciprofloxacin 400 mg IV bid for 10 days.

The discontinuation of vaccine production for plague removes this as one of the treatment options.

Dosage adjustment should be done for children, pregnant women, and immunosuppressed patients. When mass-casualty situations are encountered, oral therapy becomes the only reasonable treatment regimen. This includes either doxycycline 100 mg p.o. bid for 7 days or tetracycline 500 mg p.o. qid for 7 days or ciprofloxacin 500 mg p.o. bid for 7 days.

This is also the supportive oral pharmacology for citizens suspected of being exposed to a bioterrorist attack, but who are currently asymptomatic. They should be closely monitored for any developing fever or cough.

Provider Precautions

The health-care worker is at risk for development of the disease through respiratory fluid. Strict patient respiratory isolation and provider maximal droplet precautions are mandatory. Vaccines are in the early developmental stages and unavailable for prophylaxis.

TULAREMIA (FRANCISELLA TULARENSIS)
ICD—9: 021.9

THE DISEASE
Pathophysiology

Tularemia has many manifestations dependent on the route of infection it takes in the host. It is a highly infective pathogen, devastating the patient with as few as 10 organisms. The bacterium multiplies within macrophages, spreads to regional lymph nodes, and promotes focal tissue necrosis in the lungs and pleura, spleen, liver, and kidneys.

Oculoglandular tularemia is a particular inoculation tularemia. The main ophthalmic consideration is the associated follicular conjunctivitis. The conjunctival lesion is a proliferation of epithelioid cells with an infiltration of mononuclear cells presenting as an infective granuloma. An oculoglandular infection and general disease are followed by sepsis and meningitis.

Pneumonia is commonly manifested in the patient with tularemia (pneumonic tularemia). The type A form of the organism, although not capable of spore formation, is the most common in the United States and will survive in moist soil, hay and straw, and decaying animals.

Etiology

This coccobacillus is an aerobic, nonmotile, gram-negative organism. The infective organism is a colony of small encapsulated bacillus. Tularemia has a route of infection through inoculation and mucosal membrane contamination (ulceroglandular tularemia, glandular tularemia, oculoglandular tularemia, oropharyngeal tularemia) or by inhalation (typhoidal tularemia, pneumonic tularemia).

Human transmission is most frequently from rabbits and squirrels. These and other small mammals are infected via intermediary transmission of deerflies, mosquitoes, and ticks. Humans, in turn, are infected through bites, direct contact of tissue or fluid, or inhalation. The biologic warfare capability of this bacterium is through aerosolization, with febrile illness onset 3 to 5 days postattack. *Francisella tularensis* is a Category A bioterrorism agent.

The Patient

Clinical Symptoms

The provider should match the specific clinical symptoms with the suspected tularemic clinical syndrome.

- Severe headache
- Ocular itching
- Ocular pain
- Pharyngitis
- Fever
- Chills
- Otitis media
- Coryza (acute rhinitis)
- Dry cough

Clinical Signs

- Incubation period of 3 to 5 days (range 1 to 14 days)
- Pleural effusion on chest x-ray
- Bloody sputum
- Hilar lymphadenopathy

Conjunctival Tularenesis

- Necrotic conjunctival ulcers
- Lymphadenopathy
- Lid edema
- Swollen lymph nodes on the affected side including parotid, preauricular, submaxillary, and cervical
- Unilateral, inflamed, chemotic conjunctiva with small yellow granulomas (1 to 5 mm) presenting more on the tarsal than bulbar conjunctiva
- Straw-colored, muco-watery discharge and resultant corneal toxicity

Demographics

The disease is amenable to aerosol weaponization as typhoidal tularemia. A 50-kg attack can be expected to yield a 250,000 infective rate and 19,000 fatality rate in a population of 5 million inhabitants. The untreated fatality rate from such a biological attack will be 5% for ulceroglandular disease and 35% for typhoidal disease.

Significant History

- Hunters in contact with infected squirrels and rabbits that gain the infection through environmental contaminants or insect bites
- Occupational exposure from farming or butchering
- Disease prevalence shows tendencies to southcentral and western United States

Ancillary Tests

- Mediastinal lymphadenopathy on chest x-ray
- Elevated retrospective titers (usually the safest and most accurate diagnostic entity)
- IFA (immunofluorescence assay)
- ELISA
- PCR assay (polymerase chain reaction)
- Throat or nasal swab
- Blood and sputum culture
- Fluorescent antibody tests on lymph node smears

The Treatment

Streptomycin 1 gram q12 h IM for 10 to 14 days or gentamycin 3 to 5 mg/kg/day IM or IV for 10 to 14 days.

The oculoglandular form should also be treated with ciprofloxacin 1 drop every hour for 3 days then qid for 7 days or moxifloxacin 1 drop every hour for 3 days then qid for 7 days.

An experimental vaccine, limited to exposed laboratory personnel, is not currently available to the general public. Prophylaxis can be administered to individuals who are known victims of an attack. The treatment is doxycycline 100 mg p.o. bid for 2 weeks or ciprofloxacin 500 mg p.o. bid for 2 weeks. Dosage adjustment should be observed for pediatric, pregnant, and immunocompromised patients.

Provider Precautions

Universal precautions for health-care workers are adequate protection from contamination. Tularemia does not act as a person-to-person infective agent. Vaccination is unnecessary, unless laboratory personnel routinely handle the agent.

VIRAL AGENTS

Gregory G. Hom

SMALLPOX

ICD—9: 050.0—Variola major
ICD—9: 999.0—Vaccinia (complications of medical care, NEC)
ICD—9: 323.5—Postvaccinial encephalitis

THE DISEASE

Pathophysiology

Smallpox is a DNA virus from the orthopox virus family. The virus is transmitted from person to person via inhalation of respirable particles, direct skin contact, or contact with fomites.

Smallpox was declared globally eradicated in 1980. The CDC has designated smallpox a Category A bioterrorism agent.

There are two distinct strains of variola that lead to different clinical manifestations. Classical smallpox disease is caused by the variola major strain while variola minor causes a milder set of symptoms.

The incubation of smallpox is about 12 days, with a range of 10 to 14 days. During incubation, an intense process of viral replication occurs, with no overt clinical symptoms.

Etiology

There are nine poxviruses that can cause disease in humans. Four of them are known to cause infection of the eye or adnexa, including variola virus (the virus that causes smallpox) and vaccinia virus (the virus used in the smallpox vaccine).

The Patient

The smallpox patient will exhibit symptoms and signs that are different from a patient suffering from complications of the smallpox vaccine.

Diagnosis of complications from smallpox vaccination is supported by a history of recent smallpox vaccination or, in some circumstances, close contact with another individual who recently received the vaccine.

Clinical Symptoms and Signs
Complications of Smallpox

The prodromal phase is characterized by a high fever of sudden onset that lasts several days, accompanied by malaise, prostration, and headache. At this stage, the mucous membranes of the oropharyngeal region become infected with the virus and the patient is at the highest level of infectiousness. The virus creates a rash in the mucosa of the mouth and pharynx (the enanthematous stage), which develops into the exanthematous stage within 2 days. The exanthematous stage is a result of the virus invading the capillary epithelium of the dermal layer in skin, leading to the characteristic skin response. At first, the lesions appear on the face and forearms and eventually appear on the trunk and legs.

The dermal manifestations of smallpox begin as a maculopapular rash, which evolves into a vesicular and gradually pustular response. Pustular lesions are round, firm, and deeply embedded in the skin. The pustules produce scabs that separate from the skin about 10 days later, leaving behind a small pitted scar.

Hemorrhagic smallpox is the most serious form of smallpox. In addition to the characteristic skin lesions, patients with hemorrhagic smallpox will also experience bleeding from body orifices and widespread ecchymosis. Subconjunctival hemorrhages will occur in nearly every case.

In terms of the ocular effects of smallpox, the skin of the eyelids is affected in the same manner as other areas of skin on the face. When lesions have resolved, pitting of the skin, trichiasis, symblepharon formation, or other lid deformities may occur.

Conjunctivitis can occur in smallpox and even precede the prodromal fever stage. Pustules and phlyctenules can also occur on the conjunctiva, and patients may experience pain, lacrimation, and photophobia. Conjunctivitis typically becomes apparent at about the fifth day and resolves when the systemic disease clears.

Corneal involvement is marked by infiltrates that appear before the skin rash. Keratitis, corneal ulceration and perforation, secondary bacterial infection, hypopyon, and panophthalmitis can occur. Scarring of the cornea, including disciform scarring late in the disease, can result in blindness.

Rare ocular complications include chorioretinitis, optic neuritis, dacryocystitis, iridocyclitis, and secondary glaucoma.

Complications of Smallpox Vaccine

A smallpox vaccine is available that contains the vaccinia virus, an orthopox virus. The vaccine is administered in the deltoid area of the arm by multiple punctures of the skin with a bifurcated needle.

The vaccinia virus contained in the smallpox vaccine is an active virus capable of causing infection. Vaccinial infection can occur if other parts of the body are touched subsequent to touching the vaccination site. Infection can also be spread from person to person.

Individuals with predisposing conditions are at increased risk for developing complications from the vaccine. Eczema vaccinatum occurs in one to two cases per 100,000 immunizations and produces fever and generalized vaccinial lesions. Individuals with a history of atopic dermatitis are at increased risk for developing eczema vaccinatum. Progressive vaccinia—a dissemination of ulcerative vaccinial lesions throughout the body—occurs primarily in immunocompromised patients.

Other serious systemic complications of vaccinia include encephalitis (at an approximate rate of 3 cases per million vaccinations) and myocarditis (occurring in approximately 1 in 10,000 vaccinations). Upward of 25% of vaccinees with encephalitis die and 25% have permanent residual central nervous system (CNS) effects. Patients with postvaccinial encephalitis may experience headache and photophobia. Patients who experience postvaccinial cardiac illness report shortness of breath, palpitations, and chest pain.

The ocular complications of vaccinia infection include blepharitis, canaliculitis, conjunctivitis, and keratitis. Blepharitis lesions undergo vesicular and pustular stages and can produce severe swelling and erythema, which can mimic orbital cellulitis. Conjunctivitis can affect both the papillary and bulbar conjunctiva. A thick membrane can cover the lesions and lead to symblepharon formation. Follicles are rarely present in vaccinial conjunctivitis. Obstruction of the lacrimal canaliculus can occur following an active conjunctival vaccinia infection. Keratitis is thought to occur in about one in one million vaccinations and can range from mild punctate keratitis to disciform keratitis and potentially progress to perforation.

Epidemiology

There is a seasonal variation in the frequency of smallpox infection, with the highest incidence occurring in winter and spring.

Fewer than 3% of cases of smallpox progress to hemorrhagic smallpox, but nearly all die within the first 7 days of illness. The incidence of hemorrhagic smallpox is thought to be much higher in pregnant women.

The overall case fatality rate for smallpox is about 30%.

Historically, upward of 9% of smallpox patients will develop an ocular complication. Approximately 1 of every 40,000 vaccinees will experience an ocular complication from vaccinia.

Ancillary Tests

Direct viewing of microscopic signs can aid in diagnosis. Direct scrapings of vaccinia lesions may contain eosinophilic inclusion bodies known as Guarnieri bodies, as well as polymorphonuclear cells.

Electron microscopy will reveal the characteristic brick shape of variola or vaccinia viruses.

The Treatment

Suspected cases of smallpox must be reported immediately to public health authorities.

There is no treatment approved by the FDA for orthopox viruses.

If a person exposed to smallpox receives the smallpox vaccine within 3 days after exposure, a milder form of smallpox will result; in some cases, postexposure vaccination can avert smallpox disease altogether.

For smallpox disease, supportive care, including adequate hydration and nutrition, can aid in survival.

Because of the contagious risk of smallpox, strict respiratory and contact isolation of infected patients is necessary. In addition, all health-care providers caring for smallpox patients need to use airborne and contact precautions.

Adverse effects of the vaccinia vaccine are mainly self-limiting. More severe complications, however, may benefit from intramuscular treatment by vaccinia immune globulin (VIG). VIG is available from the CDC under Investigational New Drug protocols.

Treatment regimens for ocular complications of vaccinia are based on strategies employed in other viral diseases: treating the active viral infection followed by judicious use of topical steroids to minimize inflammatory damage to the cornea.

VIG is not recommended for the treatment of any cases of vaccinia with corneal involvement, as VIG has been shown experimentally to produce persistent corneal clouding. The risk of corneal scarring with VIG must be weighed on a case-by-case basis against the beneficial treatment of underlying and potentially fatal vaccinial complications.

Topical antiviral agents, such as trifluridine 1%, are recommended (as an off-label use) in the treatment of keratitis and/or blepharoconjunctivitis. The recommended dosing is 9 times a day for 2 weeks. Application of topical antibiotic ointment as prophylaxis against secondary bacterial infections is also recommended. Systemic antivirals, such as cidofovir, are being considered as possible treatments for complications of orthopox infections.

VIRAL HEMORRHAGIC FEVER
ICD—9: 065—Arthropod-borne hemorrhagic fever
ICD—9: 060—Yellow fever

THE DISEASE

Pathophysiology

Viral hemorrhagic fever is a syndrome that is caused by a diverse group of RNA viruses belonging to one of four families: Filoviridae (which includes Ebola and Marburg viruses), Arenaviridae (which includes Lassa fever), Bunyviridae (which includes Rift Valley fever), and Flaviviridae (which includes yellow fever). Transmission of hemorrhagic fever viruses usually occurs by contact with animal reservoirs, contaminated animal excreta, or arthropod vectors (mosquitoes and ticks).

As the name implies, viral hemorrhagic fever involves hemorrhaging in addition to a febrile illness. The bleeding is thought to occur as a result of damage to the vascular endothelium.

The CDC has designated hemorrhagic fever viruses as Category A bioterrorism agents.

The Patient

Clinical Symptoms and Signs

The incubation period for viral hemorrhagic fever ranges from 4 to 21 days. Initial signs and symptoms include fever, nausea, vomiting, cough, and headache. A nonpruritic maculopapular skin rash typically appears at day 5. The full-blown hemorrhagic stage is accompanied by jaundice (particularly with yellow fever), renal failure, and cardiovascular dysfunction. Death occurs between days 7 to 16 as a result of hypovolemic shock and multiorgan necrosis.

Initial ocular signs may be limited to conjunctival injection and may progress to subconjunctival hemorrhaging, uveitis, retinal vasculitis, and retinal hemorrhaging. Once the illness has progressed to the hemorrhaging phase, nearly every case will present with subconjunctival hemorrhaging on the papillary and/or bulbar conjunctiva.

Ancillary Tests

Diagnosis of viral hemorrhagic fever is confirmed either by detection of viral antigens in bodily fluids or the presence of antibodies to the virus. Viral isolation and identification is of limited diagnostic value because such procedures can take 10 days or more to perform and because they must take place in a biosafety level 4 laboratory.

Enzyme-linked immunosorbent assays are utilized to detect viral antigen. Polymerase chain reaction is also a common diagnostic test for these agents. IgM and IgG antibodies to the viruses can aid in diagnosis, but are typically not detectable until the patient is already into the recovery phase of the illness.

Epidemiology

Because the viral hemorrhagic fever is represented by a diverse collection of viruses, mortality rate can vary from less than 1% for some viruses to upward of 90% for the Ebola virus.

The Treatment

Treatment is generally supportive care to help maintain fluid and electrolyte balance, and blood pressure and volume. Patients undergoing rehydration therapy often develop pulmonary edema. Other interventions include mechanical ventilation, renal dialysis, and antiseizure therapy on an as-needed basis.

There are no antiviral drugs approved for treatment of hemorrhagic fever viruses. However, ribavirin may exhibit activity against a select few of the hemorrhagic fever viruses (especially in the early stages of Lassa fever) and could be administered under Investigational New Drug protocols. Other antimicrobials can be administered to prevent secondary infection on an as-needed basis. There is no specific treatment for the ocular sequelae.

ENCEPHALITIS
ICD—9: 062—Mosquito-borne viral encephalitis
ICD—9: 323.5—Postvaccinial encephalitis

THE DISEASE
Pathophysiology

Viral encephalitis is a condition that is characterized as inflammation of the brain secondary to a viral infection. The swelling is caused by an influx of inflammatory infiltrates of lymphocytes and neutrophils. Vascular changes, including vascular necrosis, can also occur in some instances. Meningitis can coexist with some cases of encephalitis.

The majority of infections caused by these viruses cause typical viral "flu-like" symptoms: fever, headache, and myalgia. The neurological sequelae vary greatly depending upon the etiologic agent.

Incubation periods for the viral encephalitides can range from as little as 2 days and up to 10 days. Some cases have been documented to occur as soon as 12 hours after known exposure.

The encephalitis viruses identified as potential bioterrorist agents are designated as Category C agents by the Centers for Disease Control and Prevention. Category C is reserved for any "emerging" pathogen for which the bioterrorist potential has not been fully characterized.

Etiology

Viral encephalitis is caused by a number of viruses. These include Alphaviruses (a family of RNA viruses that include eastern, western, and Venezuelan equine encephalitis viruses) and Flaviviridae (a family of RNA viruses, including West Nile virus). These viruses are transmitted by mosquitoes, but some viruses are also considered to be highly infectious by aerosol.

The Patient

Diagnosis of viral encephalitis is supported by a history of recent mosquito bites; however, the potential aerosol release of the viruses as a biological weapon may cause disease in the absence of contact with infected arthropods.

Diagnosis of postvaccinial encephalitis is supported by a history of receiving the smallpox vaccination approximately 7 to 15 days prior to the onset of symptoms.

Clinical Symptoms and Signs

The eastern equine encephalitis initially presents with high fever, headache, myalgia, and photophobia. The symptoms may persist or perhaps even improve somewhat for several days before the symptoms worsen to include dizziness, vomiting, frontal headache, and neck stiffness. Nystagmus, gaze deviation, and sluggish pupil response may occur along with flaccid or spastic paralysis, hemiplegia, or aphasia. Patients can lapse into coma and death can result.

Western equine encephalitis typically begins with headache, fever, dizziness, and myalgia. As the disease worsens, the dizziness worsens as well and is accompanied by vomiting, drowsiness, neck stiffness, cranial nerve palsy, convulsions, and hemiplegia. The disease can progress to coma.

Venezuelan equine encephalitis has a relatively abrupt onset of illness with sudden chills, headache, and fever. The headache tends to be severe and is exacerbated by bright lights or small movements of the eyes or neck. Severe dizziness, nausea, and vomiting frequently occur, as well as conjunctival injection. Cranial-nerve palsy and motor weakness occur occasionally, as well as coma.

West Nile virus infection will produce a fever of abrupt onset, headache, backache, and myalgia. About half of all cases of West Nile virus will have a roseolar or maculopapular skin rash on the face and trunk. Weakness and tremor or seizures will occur in more serious cases. From an ocular standpoint, West Nile virus can cause eye pain, optic neuritis, anterior uveitis, vitritis, and chorioretinitis.

Postvaccinial encephalitis is characterized by headache, fever, drowsiness, and vomiting. Serious cases can manifest themselves with paralysis and incontinence, as well as convulsions and coma. The patient will present with a history of receiving the smallpox vaccination 7 to 15 days prior to the onset of symptoms. Although there is no correlation between the central nervous system and ocular sequelae, the presence of vaccinial blepharoconjunctivitis or keratitis may aid in the diagnosis of postvaccinial encephalitis.

Ancillary Tests

Diagnosis of viral encephalitis is confirmed either by detection of the actual virus or viral antigens in bodily fluids, or the presence of antibodies to the virus. However, some viruses are cleared rapidly by the body, so detection of the virus can be difficult.

IgM specific to the encephalitis virus in question can be helpful in diagnosis. Upward of 90% of patients with encephalitis virus infection will have detectable levels of IgM. The levels of IgM can persist over 6 months, so the presence of IgM is not necessarily suggestive of acute infection unless the presence of encephalitic symptoms supports the suspicion.

Cerebrospinal fluid (CSF) pressure is often increased. Protein level in the CSF is mildly to moderately elevated but glucose levels are normal.

In the encephalitic phase, radiological imaging may reveal brain swelling.

Epidemiology

The Alphaviruses are transmitted across a broad geographic range of the Western Hemisphere. The eastern variety is rarely seen west of Texas, and the western variety is rarely seen east of Illinois. The Venezuelan variety is mainly limited in distribution to Mexico, Central America, and the northern part of South America.

West Nile virus, though native to the Middle East, has been found in nearly every region of the United States.

Generally, children and the elderly appear to be more likely to develop encephalitis after being bitten by an infected mosquito.

Case fatality rates range from 1% for Venezuelan equine encephalitis to about 10% for western equine encephalitis and upward of 30% for eastern equine encephalitis. In the United States, case fatality rates for West Nile virus have remained at about 12%.

The case fatality rate of postvaccinial encephalitis is approximately 25%.

The Treatment

No effective therapeutic agents exist, and treatment is limited to supportive care, including maintenance of airways and proper electrolytes and fluid balance. Patients must be monitored for secondary infections, especially pneumonia.

TOXINS
Thomas J. Kelly, Jr.

BOTULINUM TOXIN
ICD—9: 005.1

THE DISEASE

Pathophysiology

Botulinum toxins are a group of seven related neurotoxins produced by the spore-forming bacillus *Clostridium botulinum* and two other Clostridia species. The clinical syndrome of botulinum intoxication is called botulism.

Autonomic effects of botulism are manifested by typical anticholinergic symptoms and signs: dry mouth, ileus, constipation, and urinary retention. The onset of symptoms is 12 to 36 hours after exposure. There is variable onset depending on route of absorption. Inhalation has longer onset of action whereas ingestion of *botulinum* has a shorter onset. Recovery follows only after the neuron develops a new axon, which can take months. Death frequently results from respiratory failure. Botulinum toxins do not cross the blood brain barrier and therefore do not cause central nervous system disease or symptoms.

Toxicology

Botulinum toxin is the most toxic compound per weight of agent known to man. Up to 50% of animals will perish with only 0.001 micrograms of toxin per kilogram of body weight. Botulinum type A is 15,000 times more toxic by weight than VX gas and 100,000 times more toxic than sarin (see the section on Nerve Agents). These large proteins are easily denatured by environmental conditions such as air, sunlight, heat, and chlorine.

Several countries and terrorist groups have weaponized botulinum. It is feasible to deliver botulinum toxins as an aerosolized biological weapon. A more common method is through contaminated food. Botulinum toxin is a Category A bioterrorism agent.

The Patient

The occurrence of an epidemic of afebrile, alert, well-oriented patients with progressive symmetrical descending flaccid paralysis, dilated, fixed pupils, and diplopia strongly suggests botulinum toxin intoxication.

Clinical Symptoms
- Blurred vision from mydriasis
- Diplopia
- Dry mouth

Clinical Signs
- Dilated and fixed pupils—50%
- Cranial nerve palsies
- Ptosis
- Difficulty speaking and swallowing
- Absent gag reflex
- Variable skeletal muscle weakness
- Cyanosis or narcosis because of CO_2 retention from respiratory failure

The Treatment

Respiratory failure as a result of paralysis of respiratory muscles is the most prominent feature of botulinum intoxication and the usual cause of death. Supportive care of respiratory function and hypotension is life saving. Hydration, nasogastric suction for ileus, bladder catheterization, prevention of infection, and decubitus ulcers are mandatory. Recovery may take 3 to 12 months, during which time patients require ongoing intensive nursing care.

Botulinum antitoxin neutralizes circulating toxins in patients with progressive symptoms. Three different types of antitoxin are available in the United States. Botulinum antitoxin is very effective when given before the onset of symptoms. If the antitoxin is delayed until after the onset of symptoms, it does not protect against respiratory failure. A pentavalent toxoid vaccine is available under Investigational New Drug protocol for pre-exposure prophylaxis.

RICIN
ICD—9: 988.2

THE DISEASE

Pathophysiology

Ricin is a potent protein cytotoxin derived from the beans of the Castor plant (*Ricinus communis*). When ricin is inhaled as a small aerosol particle, the toxin produces pathologic changes within 8 hours. Ricin causes cell death by blocking intracellular protein synthesis. Severe respiratory symptoms are followed by acute hypoxic respiratory failure in 36 to 72 hours. When given intravenously, the toxin may cause disseminated intravascular coagulation, microcirculatory failure, and multiple organ failure.

Toxicology

Ricin is made up of two hemagluttinins and two toxins. The toxins are heterodimers with molecular weights of about 66,000 daltons. Ricin can be prepared in liquid or crystalline form, or it can be lyophilized to make a dry powder. It can be disseminated as an aerosol, injected into a target, or used to contaminate food or water on a small scale.

The entire Castor bean plant is toxic if chewed, although the beans contain the highest concentration of the poison in the plant. The lethal dose of ricin in adults is 1mg/kg. Two to four seeds cause severe illness but are not fatal. Eight seeds provide a fatal dose.

Ricin is less potent than botulinum toxin but is more potent than cobra venom and much more potent than cyanide. Ricin is inactivated by chlorine.

Ricin is a Category B bioterrorism agent because it is generally considered to be less important in terms of risk for a mass bioterror attack than Category A agents such as botulism, anthrax, smallpox, plague, and other highly lethal agents.

The Patient

The clinical picture of ricin intoxication depends on the route of exposure and the dose of ricin inhaled, ingested, or injected.

Clinical Symptoms and Signs
Oral Ingestion
- Dilated pupils
- Nausea and vomiting
- Bloody diarrhea
- Local hemorrhage
- Hypotension
- Circulatory failure, death

Inhalation
- Fever
- Chest tightness
- Cough, dyspnea
- Nausea
- Arthralgias
- Profuse sweating
- Lung inflammation
- Pulmonary edema

Injection
- Local muscle necrosis
- Tachycardia
- Swollen lymph nodes
- Shock
- Anuria
- Abdominal pain, vomiting, diarrhea (sometimes bloody)
- Death

Ancillary Tests

Ricin exposure can be diagnosed with specific enzyme-linked immunosorbent assay testing on nasal smears, serum, and respiratory secretions within 24 hours of exposure. Immunohistochemical stains of tissue may be used where available to confirm the diagnosis. Confirmation of exposure can be obtained with paired acute and convalescent antibody response. Polymerase chain reaction can detect Castor bean DNA in most ricin preparations. A chest x-ray is helpful in determining whether the patient has acute respiratory distress syndrome.

The Treatment

Medical management of ricin poisoning depends on the route of exposure. There is no specific treatment available, so therapy is supportive. With pulmonary exposure, appropriate respiratory support is required. This may include oxygen, intubation, ventilation, positive end-expiratory pressure, hemodynamic monitoring, and anti-inflammatory (corticosteroids) agents. Vigorous treatment of pulmonary edema is indicated.

Gastrointestinal (GI) intoxication is managed by vigorous gastric lavage, use of cathartics, volume replacement of GI fluid losses, and electrolyte replacement.

Protective masks are effective in preventing aerosol exposure. No vaccine is available.

CHEMICAL POISONS
Thomas J. Kelly, Jr.

MUSTARDS
ICD—9: E997.2

THE DISEASE
Pathophysiology

The mustards are a group of chemical warfare agents consisting of sulfur mustards and nitrogen mustard. Only sulfur mustard, in various forms, has been used in chemical warfare. These agents are included in a class of chemical warfare agents referred to as blister agents or vesicant agents. These agents burn and blister skin or other part of the body they contact. The mustards are highly reactive and combine readily with proteins, DNA, or other molecules. They impair the function of the respiratory tract when inhaled and cause nausea, vomiting, and diarrhea when ingested. When absorbed, they damage the hematopoietic system. Delay in decontamination of only a few minutes results in irreversible tissue damage. While the effects of exposure to mustard are incapacitating, the mortality rate is low. During World War I, the death rate was less than 5% of those who received medical treatment. Death usually occurred between the fifth and tenth days and was usually caused be pulmonary failure or infection.

Toxicology

Sulfur mustard is an oily liquid with odor of mustard, onion, or garlic or no odor at all. Mustard is soluble in organic solvents, oils, and fats and easily penetrates skin, mucous membranes, and clothing. Sulfur mustard is a persistent agent at low temperatures and vaporizes at high temperatures. Mustard gas has predominately been employed as a vapor rather than liquid because the vapor is three times more toxic than an equal concentration of cyanide gas.

The LCt50 (the product of concentration times the time in minutes that is lethal to 50% of adults exposed by inhalation) is 1,500 mg-min/mm^3. The LCt for airway injury is 100 to 200 mg-min/m^3. The median incapacitating dose of the vapor is 200 mg-min/m^3. An LCt of 12 to 70 mg-min/m^3 produces ocular damage. The lethal dose is approximately 100mg/kg.

The Patient

The mustards injure skin, eyes, mucous membranes, respiratory system, GI tract, and the hematopoietic system. Exposure of skin to liquid mustard produces burns that may be superficial to full thickness. Contact with the vapor usually causes first- or second-degree burns while contact with the liquid typically causes second- and third-degree burns. There is a latent or sign-free period of several hours that may occur after skin exposure. The burns may appear deceptively mild and superficial initially but may progress over a 24- to 72-hour period to bullae, and partial or full-thickness burns. The latent period may cause rescuers to delay decontamination.

Clinical Symptoms and Signs
Ocular
- Ocular pain
- Miosis
- Chemosis, corneal burns, edema, ulceration
- Blindness

Respiratory Tract
- Copious nasal and upper airway secretions
- Sore throat, cough, hoarseness, shortness of breath, and respiratory distress
- Hemorrhagic inflammation of airways
- Pulmonary edema and respiratory failure if inhaled dose is very high

Gastrointestinal Tract
- Pain
- Nausea, vomiting
- Diarrhea
- Bleeding

Hematopoietic System
- Bone marrow suppression
  - Leucopenia
  - Anemia
  - Thrombocytopenia

The Treatment

Immediate decontamination is the most important intervention. The patients' clothing and jewelry must be removed and the skin immediately washed with alkaline soap and water. A 0.5% solution of hypochlorite is preferred because it inactivates sulfur mustard. Once the mustard has become fixed to the tissues, its effects become irreversible. Immediate copious irrigation of the eyes with saline, or water if saline is not available, is necessary.

There are no specific antidotes available to treat mustard toxicity. Treatment of the specific effects of mustard is necessary. Severe burns require irrigation, debridement, and topical antibiotics. Mustard gas burns are especially painful, and adequate pain relief is required.

Ocular burns require aggressive treatment. Copious irrigation with saline, topical antibiotic eye drops, mydriatics, and topical corticosteroids are indicated to treat severe burns.

Administration of granulocyte colony-stimulating factor or filgrastim (Neupogen) may be necessary for the treatment of neutropenia caused by mustard toxicity of the hematopoietic system.

Chemical burns cause less fluid loss than thermal burns. Fluid and electrolyte loss should be monitored closely and replaced as necessary.

Protection against the effects of mustard requires full protective clothing and respirators. The respirator itself will protect the eyes and airways. Those performing decontamination must take precautions since they are at risk for dermal contact of mustard from those affected.

NERVE AGENTS
ICD—9: E997.2

THE DISEASE

Pathophysiology

The nerve agents are a group of chemical warfare agents that have chemical structures similar to the organophosphate pesticide malathione. They exert their biological effects by inhibiting acetylcholinesterase enzymes. The nerve agents are divided into two classifications based on volatility and persistence: the G-series including tabun (GA), sarin (GB), and soman (GD), and the V-series including VX gas and several other less-known agents. The G agents are volatile at room temperature and are more effective as gases. The V agents are less volatile and tend to remain in a liquid state in the environment.

Nerve agents phosphorylate and inactivate butyrylcholinesterase in the plasma, red blood cell acetylcholinesterase, and the acetylcholinesterase at cholinergic receptors in tissues. Acetylcholine, the neurotransmitter at the receptor site, cannot be hydrolyzed by acetylcholinesterase. Acetylcholine accumulates at the nicotinic (skeletal muscle and ganglia) and muscarinic (smooth muscle and glands) receptors and other receptors in the CNS. Nerve agents initially stimulate the tissue but ultimately paralyze cholinergic neurotransmission. The nerve agents may also antagonize gamma-amino butyric acid (GABA) neurotransmission and stimulate glutamate N-methyl-D-aspartate (NMDA) receptors. These may be involved in nerve agent–induced seizure activity and other CNS symptoms. The nerve agents are the most toxic of the known chemical warfare agents.

Toxicology

The toxicity of the nerve agent is dependent on the route of exposure and the relative volatility of the agent. The toxicity of the nerve agents is measured in two forms, the LCt50 and the LD50. The LCt50 is the inhalation dose that results in death in 50% of the individuals so exposed. The LD50 is the dose absorbed through the skin that results in death in 50% of the victims. The LCt50 (the lethal concentration of vapor in mg-min/m3) of sarin is 100 while the LD50 on skin is 1700 mg. The large difference in the lethal dose of sarin is because of its volatility. The G-series agents tend to evaporate rather than penetrate the skin. Clothing or other occlusives will prevent evaporation and promote absorption through the skin. VX, on the other hand, has the consistency of motor oil and evaporates very poorly. It therefore is much more lethal than the G agents when in contact with the skin. The LCt50 of VX when inhaled is 10 mg-min/m^3, and the LD50 of dermal exposure is 10 mg.

The Patient

The onset of symptoms and the manifestations of these symptoms depend on the route of exposure and the dose.

Vapor Inhalation

The signs and symptoms occur within seconds to minutes. Exposure to a small amount of sarin vapor may cause ocular symptoms such as miosis, blurred vision, eye pain, and conjunctival injection. Exposure to a high concentration of sarin vapor may result in loss of consciousness after only one breath, respiratory arrest, and death.

Liquid Exposure

Liquid agents (VX) easily penetrate skin and clothing. Minimal exposure consisting of a droplet on skin may cause local sweating and muscle fasciculation, followed by nausea, vomiting, diarrhea, and generalized weakness.

Severe liquid exposure may cause symptoms in 1 to 30 minutes. An exposed individual may rapidly lose consciousness; suffer convulsions; and exhibit generalized muscular fasciculation, flaccid paralysis, copious secretions from nose, mouth, and lungs, bronchospasm, apnea, and finally death.

Clinical Symptoms and Signs
Ocular
- Miosis
- Blurred vision, dim vision
- Tearing, redness

Central Nervous System
- Headache
- Irritability
- Nervousness
- Fatigue
- Insomnia
- Memory loss
- Slurred speech
- Vertigo
- Loss of consciousness

- Seizures
- Apnea
- Death

Respiratory Tract
- Rhinorrhea
- Copious bronchial secretions
- Dyspnea
- Bronchoconstriction
- Respiratory failure

Cardiovascular
- Bradycardia
- Heart block
- Ventricular arrhythmias

Gastrointestinal Tract
- Nausea, vomiting
- Abdominal cramping
- Diarrhea
- Fecal incontinence

Skeletal Muscle
- Muscle twitching and fasciculation
- Generalized fasciculation
- Flaccid paralysis

Physical Signs
The physical signs depend on the amount and route of exposure. Small vapor exposure causes miosis, rhinorrhea, and pulmonary signs. Large vapor exposure causes copious secretions, generalized muscular fasciculation, seizures, loss of consciousness, apnea, cyanosis, hypotension, and bradycardia just before death.

Small liquid dermal exposure causes few physical signs. Sweating and blanching of the skin at the site of exposure as well as localized muscular fasciculation may be present soon after exposure. Large liquid dermal exposure causes diaphoresis, nausea, vomiting, diarrhea, generalized weakness, loss of consciousness, seizures, generalized fasciculation, flaccid paralysis, and apnea.

Miosis is a useful sign after exposure to vapor but does not occur after skin exposure with liquid unless the dose is large or the exposure is near or in the eye.

The Treatment

Decontamination
Vapor exposure does not require decontamination. Remove victim from closed, contaminated area and provide fresh air.

Liquid exposure requires immediate decontamination to prevent further absorption of the agent.

- Remove all clothing and jewelry
- Wash body with soap and water
- Wash body with 0.5% hypochlorite solution

Medical Management
- Atropine sulfate 2 mg IV or IM every 2 to 5 minutes up to 20 mg per day
- Pralidoxime chloride (protopam chloride) 600 mg
- Diazapam (valium) 10 mg IM
- Anticholinergic eye drops (tropicamide, homatropine, atropine)

No other known chemical agent produces muscular twitching and fasciculation, rapidly progressing pupil constriction, and characteristic muscarinic, nicotinic, and CNS manifestations as cited earlier. Rapid diagnosis and treatment are critical in the event of accidental release of a military nerve agent or terrorist attack.

Chapter 16

Systemic Disease and the Eye

DIABETES MELLITUS (DM)

Nicky R. Holdeman

ICD—9: 250.00

THE DISEASE

Pathophysiology

Diabetes mellitus involves a complex sequence of events that often evolve over many years. It is characterized by a broad array of abnormalities and frequently results in long-term vascular and neurologic complications. Pathologic changes may lead to systemic hypertension, renal failure, blindness, autonomic and peripheral neuropathy, amputations of the lower extremities, myocardial infarctions, and strokes.

The most notable feature of the disease is a disordered metabolism of glucose leading to an inappropriate hyperglycemia. Elevated blood glucose results from either an absolute deficiency of insulin secretion, a reduction in its effectiveness, or both. Chronic hyperglycemia is presumed to cause tissue damage by glycation of proteins and/or excess production of polyol compounds from the metabolism of glucose.

There are two major types of DM: Type 1 (formerly insulin-dependent diabetes mellitus—IDDM) and type 2 (formerly noninsulin-dependent diabetes mellitus—NIDDM). Other forms of diabetes mellitus exist but are beyond the scope of this section. Each form of DM has a distinct etiology, clinical presentation, and course.

Note: The terms and acronyms IDDM and NIDDM are no longer used since the names are based on pharmacological treatment rather than causative considerations. The new classification system recognizes that DM results from different mechanisms, with the common end point being hyperglycemia.

Etiology

Type 1

Type 1 diabetes mellitus results from the gradual destruction of pancreatic beta cells, associated with lymphocytic infiltration of the pancreas (termed insulitis), and often the production of autoantibodies such as anti-islet cell autoantibodies (ICAs) and autoantibodies to insulin (IAAs). There is evidence that a precipitating event, possibly a toxic insult, viral illness, or diet supplementation with gluten-containing foods before age 3 months, any of which may initially damage the beta cells of the pancreas, followed by autoimmune destruction of the remaining beta cells in genetically predisposed persons. Clinical diabetes occurs when roughly 90% of the beta cells have been destroyed, which can be quite rapid in infants and children and slower in adults. Circulating insulin is virtually absent, thus these patients are dependent on exogenous insulin for survival. Ketosis is common in patients with poor glucose control.

Note: Preliminary studies suggest that treatment with immune system modulating agents and/or specific monoclonal antibodies soon after diagnosis may protect and prolong the period of beta cell function. Further studies will determine whether this type of intervention will yield long-term benefits.

Type 2
The exact etiology of type 2 diabetes mellitus continues to be debated. Some patients with type 2 diabetes show normal insulin levels, and autopsy studies have revealed only a minor reduction in islet cell mass as compared with nondiabetic individuals. Clinically, patients with type 2 diabetes demonstrate an insulin resistance with a defect in compensatory insulin secretion. These patients may exhibit reduced numbers of insulin receptors, increased hepatic glucose production, impaired glycogen synthesis, elevated levels of glucagon, decreased peripheral glucose uptake, abnormal patterns of insulin secretion, or a combination of these conditions. Ultimately, it is the beta cell response to insulin resistance that determines the evolution to type 2 DM. Circulating endogenous insulin is usually sufficient to prevent ketoacidosis but inadequate to prevent hyperglycemia.

Note: Combination therapy using oral antidiabetic agents with different mechanisms of action is becoming the standard of care to meet glycemic treatment goals; however, insulin is sometimes required in the management of type 2 diabetes.

It is now believed that about two million Americans currently diagnosed with type 2 diabetes may actually have latent autoimmune diabetes in adults (LADA), or type 1.5 DM. This condition appears to be a hybrid or "stealth" type of diabetes, which progresses slower in its attack and destruction of insulin-producing beta cells than type 1. Patients with LADA cannot normalize their blood glucose with oral antidiabetic agents, thus require insulin injections.

The Patient

Clinical Symptoms (see Table 16.1)
Some cases of DM (especially type 2) are diagnosed at an asymptomatic stage as a result of a screening program, routine blood tests, or an eye examination. Compared with type 1 patients who commonly present with acute symptoms, individuals with type 2 diabetes are much more likely to have no symptoms or fewer symptoms, as the hyperglycemia develops gradually. Patients may report the classic syndrome of polyuria, polydipsia, polyphagia, unexplained weight loss, weakness, and fatigue; however, these symptoms are typically associated with marked hyperglycemia as seen in type 1 patients.

Clinical Signs (see Table 16.1)
The physical findings will vary depending on the type of DM, the severity of insulin deficiency, and the duration of the disease. Examination may reveal systemic

▶ **TABLE 16.1 Clinical Features of Diabetes Mellitus⁺**

* Polyuria	Upper body fat deposits
* Polydipsia	Cardiovascular complications
* Polyphagia	Large babies (>9 lbs.)
* Weight loss	Pregnancy complications
* Fatigue	Systemic hypertension
* Weakness	Impotence
* Dry mouth	Skin infections
* Postural hypotension	Retinopathy/Blurred vision
Pruritus	Cranial-nerve palsies
Vulvovaginitis	Thrush
Neuropathy	Balanitis
Lipoprotein abnormalities	Periodontal disease

⁺Note: While many of these signs and symptoms may occur in both type 1 and type 2 diabetes, those conditions indicated with an asterisk (*) are most commonly detected in type 1 disease and associated with marked hyperglycemia. Retinopathy may be detected in over 20% of type 2 patients at the time of initial diagnosis and may predate the diagnosis of diabetes by up to 6 years. Early detection, improved delivery of care, and better self-management are key strategies for preventing diabetes-related complications. (For every 1% decrease in the HbA$_{1c}$ there is a 35% reduction in risk of diabetic complications.)

hypertension, neuropathy, periodontal disease, vaginitis, skin abnormalities, arteriopathy, blurred vision, retinopathy, nephropathy, and/or increased susceptibility to infections. Diabetics also have a much higher risk for cardiovascular disease, abnormalities in lipid metabolism (dyslipidemia), and vascular thrombosis.

Ocular manifestations of DM occur frequently and careful examination with appropriate treatment can often reduce the ophthalmic complications (see Table 16.2). Visual impairment resulting from diabetic retinopathy predicts a high mortality rate, particularly from cardiovascular diseases and stroke.

Demographics

The estimated lifetime risk of developing DM for individuals born in 2000 is 32.8% for males and 38.5% for females. DM is the fifth deadliest disease in the United States and is believed to be underreported both as a condition and as a cause of death. It is estimated that 17% of all deaths in the United States are related to diabetes.

The incidence, target population, and genetics differ between type 1 and type 2 (see Table 16.3).

It is estimated that 18 million people in the United States have DM and that the number of patients with diabetes will double every decade.

- Type 1 diabetes affects one in 250 persons in the United States. Approximately 10,000 to 15,000 new cases are reported each year.
- Type 1 diabetes is less common among Black and Asian populations.
- Type 2 diabetes has an overall prevalence of 6.6% in the United States. 800,000 new cases are reported each year; many patients are unaware of their disorder at the time of diagnosis.

▶ TABLE 16.2 Ocular and Periocular Manifestations of Diabetes Mellitus

Glaucoma	Possibly increased incidence of POAG
Pupils	Light-near dissociation
Refraction	Fluctuations in refractive errors
Cornea	Hypesthesia, corneal abrasions, poor epithelial healing
Iris	Neovascularization of the iris (NVI). Obtain retinal consult within 2–4 days. PRP may prevent development of neovascular glaucoma, Ectropian uveae
Lens	Premature cataracts
Ciliary body	Thickening of the basement membrane
	Premature presbyopia
Extraocular muscles	III, IV, VI nerve palsies (mononeuropathy)
Vitreous	Detachment, hemorrhages
	—treat a pre-retinal and/or vitreous hemorrhage as high-risk proliferative diabetic retinopathy. Obtain retinal consult within 24–48 hours.
Optic nerve	Ischemic optic neuropathy
	Neovascularization of the disc (NVD)
Macula	Diabetic maculopathy is the most common cause of visual loss in diabetes and may be exudative, edematous, or ischemic
	Clinically significant macular edema (CSME)
	—thickening of the retina at or within 500 microns from the center of the macula,
	—hard exudates at or within 500 microns from the center of the macula if there is thickening of the adjacent retina,
	—zone or zones of retinal thickening, one disc area or larger, any part of which is within one disc diameter of the center of the macula.
	CSME may be present at any stage of diabetic retinopathy and should be treated with focal or grid photocoagulation. Intravitreal injection of triamcinolone acetonide shows promise for the treatment of diabetic macular edema that is unresponsive to laser photocoagulation. Obtain retinal consult within a 2- to 4-week period.
Retina	Mild to moderate non-proliferative retinopathy; no CSME
	—microaneurysms, intraretinal hemorrhages (dot or splinter shaped), retinal edema, soft exudates,
	—follow every 6–12 months depending on extent of lesions.
	Severe nonproliferative retinopathy (pre-proliferative); no CSME
	—increased intraretinal hemorrhages and exudates, venous beading and loops, intraretinal microvascular abnormalities (IRMA), cotton wool spots, large areas of capillary nonperfusion;
	—eyes with hemorrhages in all four quadrants; or venous beading in two or more quadrants; or IRMA in one or more quadrants are considered to have severe NPDR. Patients with two or more of these characteristics have very severe NPDR;
	—obtain retinal consult within 3–4 weeks and follow every 2–4 months

(continued)

▶ **TABLE 16.2 Ocular and Periocular Manifestations of Diabetes Mellitus (Continued)**

Proliferative retinopathy; no CSME —neovascularization of the disc (NVD), —retinal neovascularization elsewhere (NVE), —preretinal or vitreous hemorrhage, —requires PRP, —obtain retinal consult within 2–4 days if high-risk characteristics are present. Retinal detachments —tractional, —rhegmatogenous, —obtain retinal consult within 3–5 days. Other vision-threatening retinal conditions that are more prevalent in the patient with diabetes include: —branch retinal vein occlusion, —central retinal vein occlusion, —branch retinal artery occlusion, —central retinal artery occlusion, —anterior ischemic optic neuropathy, —diabetic papillopathy.
Patients > 10 years of age with type 1 diabetes should have an initial dilated and comprehensive eye examination within 3 to 5 years after the onset of diabetes and at least every year thereafter. Patients with type 2 diabetes should have an initial dilated and comprehensive eye examination shortly after diagnosis and at least every year thereafter.

- Type 2 diabetes is more common in Native Americans, African Americans, and Hispanic Americans. This same population has a three- to sixfold higher incidence of end-stage renal disease than in Caucasians.
- Type 2 diabetes increases with age, lack of physical activity, and obesity. Individuals who have a body mass index (BMI) >30 are at 10 to 20 times greater risk.
- Type 2 diabetes occurs more frequently in women with prior gestational diabetes mellitus; these women have a 20 to 50% chance of developing diabetes over 5 to 10 years.

Diabetic retinopathy is the leading cause of new cases of blindness in patients 25 to 74 years of age. Each year, 12,000 to 24,000 people lose their sight because of diabetes. African Americans are twice as likely to suffer from diabetes-related blindness.

Significant History

- Age (type 2 DM is more common in people >45 years of age)
- Family history of DM in a first-degree relative; if family history is positive for DM, determine age of onset, whether it was associated with obesity, and form of treatment. Family history is much stronger in type 2 (70 to 80%) versus type 1 (20%)
- Unexplained weight loss (type 1) or visceral obesity (type 2)

▶ **TABLE 16.3** **Comparison of the Essential Features of Type 1 and Type 2 Diabetes Mellitus**

	Type 1	*Type 2*
Other Names (outdated terms)	IDDM, juvenile onset, growth onset, ketosis-prone	NIDDM, adult onset, maturity onset, ketosis-resistant
Age of onset	Usually under 35 but can occur at any age	Usually over 35 but the incidence is rapidly increasing in children
Nutritional status at onset	Usually nonobese	Usually obese
Symptoms	Polyuria, polydipsia, polyphagia	Frequently none
Ketosis	Common, unless diet, insulin, and exercise are coordinated properly	Uncommon except in the presence of infection or stress
Endogenous insulin secretion	Severe deficiency to absent	Moderate deficiency; may be in excess but relatively ineffective because of obesity (i.e., insulin resistance)
Associated lipid abnormalities	Dyslipidemia increases with age	Cholesterol and triglycerides frequently elevated
Insulin requirements	Always necessary	Needed in 20–30% of patients
Insulin resistance	Occasional	Almost always
Oral agents	Sometimes efficacious	Frequently efficacious
Diet	Mandatory along with insulin supplementation	Diet alone frequently adequate to control blood glucose
HLA association	DR3, DR4	None
Family history of DM in a first-degree relative	≈20%	≈70–80%
Identical twins	≈50% concordant	≈100% concordant
Islet cell autoantibodies (ICAs) or insulin autoantibodies (IAAs)	Autoantibodies are detected in 85–90% of patients.	Absent
Association with other autoimmune diseases	Frequent	None

- Physical inactivity
- Polyuria, polydipsia, polyphagia
- Chronic or recurrent infections
- Gestational diabetes or having delivered a baby weighing >9 pounds
- Long or highly irregular menstrual cycles
- Member of a high-risk ethnic population
- Systemic hypertension, smoking, dyslipidemia, use of oral contraceptives, or other factors that increase cardiac risk

Ancillary Tests

A diagnosis of DM in nonpregnant adults is appropriate in one of three circumstances, each of which must be confirmed on a subsequent day:

- Symptoms of diabetes plus casual plasma glucose concentration ≥200 mg/dL (11.1 mmol/1). Casual is defined as any time of day without regard to time since last meal. The classic symptoms of diabetes include polyuria, polydipsia, and unexplained weight loss.
- Fasting plasma glucose (FPG) ≥126 mg/dL (7.0 mmol/l). Fasting is defined as no caloric intake for at least 8 hours. If the FPG level is over 126 mg/dL on more than one occasion, further evaluation of the patient with a glucose challenge is unnecessary.
- 2-h plasma glucose (PG) ≥200 mg/dL during an oral glucose tolerance test (OGTT).

Note: Because of the difficulties in performing and interpreting OGTTs, it is not recommended for routine use and is being replaced by documentation of fasting hyperglycemia.

If a diagnosis of DM is made, other baseline tests should be performed. These tests may reveal coexistent disorders, document pre-existing target organ damage, and help guide future assessments. These tests include:

- Fasting plasma triglycerides
- Total cholesterol, HDL cholesterol, LDL cholesterol
- Electrocardiography (ECG)
- Renal function studies
- Peripheral pulses
- Neurologic, podiatric, and eye examinations

Self-monitoring of blood glucose is a critical component of managing diabetes; however, standard glucometers are invasive, painful, and provide only periodic measurements. An automatic glucose biographer (GlucoWatch) can provide three readings per hour, for up to 12 hours, by using reverse iontophoresis to collect glucose samples through intact skin. The wearer can also set alerts for high and low glucose levels.

Minimed, another continuous glucose monitoring system (CGMS), utilizes a temporary sensor inserted into subcutaneous tissues.

While both of the devices provide additional information on glycemic control, neither is intended to replace traditional fingerstick B.G. measurements, but rather should be used as an adjunct.

Thus, a reliable outpatient blood-testing system should be used, as most studies confirm that conventional home glucose monitoring is associated with better glycemic control, especially in insulin-treated diabetics. Of course, the accuracy of data obtained by any glucose monitoring system requires proper instruction of the patient in sampling and measuring procedures as well as in proper calibration of the instruments.

Glycosylated hemoglobin (HbA$_{1c}$) reflects metabolic control and state of glycemia over the preceding 8 to 12 weeks and is directly proportional to the concentration of free glucose in the blood. This test is not currently recommended for the initial diagnosis of diabetes but does provide a unique method of assessing and monitoring diabetic management. Three to four HbA$_{1c}$ measurements a year are usually sufficient. Ideally, these levels should be maintained in the nondiabetic range (<6.05%); however, levels <7.0% are good.

Urine strips are a precise and convenient method to detect glucosuria (Diastix are sensitive to as little as 0.1% glucose in urine). However, the renal threshold for plasma glucose is approximately 180 mg/dL, thus urine glucose is not the method of choice for monitoring diabetic control.

Urine testing for ketones (Acetest or Ketostix) is important for type 1 diabetics when they are ill, under stress, or when their blood glucose exceeds 240 mg/dL.

The Treatment

The patient should be referred to his or her primary-care physician for systemic management. Currently, the treatment objectives for both type 1 and type 2 are similar and that is to maintain glycemic control as close to normal as possible. Treatment strategies are individualized based on the type of diabetes and the specific requirements of each patient. The treatment of DM involves lifestyle adaptations such as diet, exercise, and self-monitoring of blood glucose. Medications include oral antidiabetic agents (such as the sulfonylureas, biguanides, alpha-glucosidase inhibitors, thiazolidinediones, and the meglitinides) (see Table 16.4) as well as various parenteral insulin preparations (see Table 16.5). It is important to note that many type 2 patients who start on oral agents will eventually require insulin to maintain adequate glycemic control. Insulin therapy may also abate the expense, side effects, and inconvenience of taking multiple oral drugs several times a day.

Note: Incretin hormones are being investigated for their therapeutic potential in the treatment of type 2 DM. Many of these agents target physiologic defects not addressed by current medications and may prove useful in the management of type 2 diabetes.

Coexistent disorders such as obesity, systemic hypertension, and/or dyslipidemia need to be addressed as they may increase the risk and accelerate the progression of diabetic complications (i.e., retinopathy, neuropathy, nephropathy, and peripheral vascular disease). If no contraindications exist, enteric coated aspirin (81 to 325 mg per day) is recommended in diabetic adults with evidence of macrovascular disorders and/or in patients with increased risk factors for cardiovascular disease.

The Diabetes Control and Complications Trial (DCCT) demonstrated that "tight" metabolic control, geared toward maintaining near normal glucose levels, had a definite and beneficial effect on the development and progression of long-term diabetic microvascular complications. In addition, the Epidemiology of Diabetes Interventions and Complications (EDIC) study showed the reduction in the risk of progressive retinopathy and nephropathy resulting from intensive therapy persisted for at least 4 years, despite increasing levels of blood glucose. While patients with type 2 DM were not included in the DCCT or EDIC studies, there was no reason to believe that the effects of at least "moderate" control of blood glucose levels would not also benefit this patient population. As a point in fact, reports from the U.K. Prospective Diabetes Study (UKPDS) showed that intensive therapy in the total group of type 2 diabetics did indeed reduce diabetes related microangiopathic organ damage by 25%. In addition, intensive antihypertensive therapy showed beneficial effects on virtually all diabetes-related complications.

The most serious complication of tight metabolic control of blood glucose is hypoglycemia, which can potentially result in central nervous system (CNS) damage. However, the consistent effects of intensive therapy in reducing long-term diabetic complications seem to outweigh the efforts and costs involved in such treatment and the increased risk of hypoglycemia. On the other hand, the weight gain that can potentially occur with

▶ TABLE 16.4 Oral Antidiabetic Drugs

Drug	Tablet Size	Daily Dose	Duration of Action	Peak Action
Tolbutamide (Orinase)	250 and 500 mg	0.5–3 g in 2 or 3 divided doses	6–12 hours	3–5 hours
Tolazamide (Tolinase) (Tolamide)	100, 250, and 500 mg	0.1–1 g as single dose or in 2 divided doses	12–24 hours	4–8 hours
Acetohexamide (Dymelor)	250 and 500 mg	0.25–1.5 g as single dose or twice daily dosage	12–24 hours	2–4 hours
Chlorpropamide (Diabinese)	100 and 250 mg	0.1–0.5 g as single dose	24–60 hours	3–6 hours
Glyburide (Dia*β*eta, Micronase)	1.25, 2.5, and 5 mg	1.25–20 mg as single dose or in 2 divided doses	16–24 hours	2–6 hours
Glyburide— micronized (Glynase PresTab)	1.5, 3, and 6 mg	1.5–18 mg as single dose or in 2 divided doses	12–24 hours	2–3 hours
Glipizide (Glucotrol)	5 and 10 mg	2.5–40 mg as single dose or in 2 divided doses before meals	10–24 hours	1–3 hours
Glipizide—GITS (Glucotrol XL)	2.5, 5, and 10 mg	Up to 20 mg daily as a single dose	Up to 24 hours	6–12 hours
Glimeperide (Amaryl)	1, 2, and 4 mg	1–8 mg as single dose	Up to 24 hours	2–3 hours
Metformin (Glucophage)	500, 850 and 1,000 mg	1–2.55 g. One tablet with meals 2 or 3 times daily	6–12 hours	2–3 hours
Metformin (Glucophage XR)	500 mg	0.5–2.0 g once per day	Up to 24 hrs	4–8 hrs
Acarbose (Precose)	50 and 100 mg	75–300 mg in 3 divided doses with first bite of food	4–6 hours	1 hour
Miglitol (Glyset)	25, 50, and 100 mg	25–100 mg 3 times per day before meals	4–6 hours	2–3 hours
Repaglinide (Prandin)	0.5, 1, and 2 mg	0.5 to 4 mg taken with meals	2–4 hours	1 hour
Nateglinide (Starlix)	60 and 120 mg	60–120 mg 3 times daily before meals	1–3 hours	1 hour
Rosiglitazone (Avandia)	2, 4, and 8 mg	4–8 mg as a single dose once daily or in divided doses	15–25 hours	1–2 hours
Pioglitazone (Actos)	15, 30, and 45 mg	15–45 mg once daily	Up to 24 hours	2–3 hours
Metformin/Glyburide (Glucovance)	250 mg/1.25 mg 500 mg/2.5 mg 500 mg/5.0 mg	500 mg/5 mg tablets Two tablets twice daily with meals	See individual drugs	See individual drugs
Rosiglitazone/ Metformin (Avandamet)	1 mg/500 mg 2 mg/500 mg 4 mg/500 mg	One tablet bid with meals May dose 8 mg/2000 mg per day	See individual drugs	See individual drugs

▶ **TABLE 16.5** Human Analog Insulin Preparations

Preparation	Onset	Peak	Duration	Concentration
Rapid-acting Insulin				
Insulin lispro (Humalog)	15 min	30–90 min	6–8 h	U100
Insulin aspart (NovoLog)	15 min	1–3 h	3–5 h	U100
Short-acting Insulins				
Regular	30–60 min	2–3 h	8–12 h	U100
Regular (concentrated)	30–60 min	2–3 h	8–12 h	U500
Velosulin (buffered regular)	30–60 min	2–3 h	8–12 h	U100
Semilente	60–90 min	5–10 h	12–16 h	U100
Intermediate-acting Insulins				
Humulin N/Novolin N	2–4 h	4–10 h	10–16 h	U100
Lente	1–2.5 h	7–15 h	24 h	U100
Humulin L/Novolin L	2–4 h	4–12 h	12–18 h	U100
NPH	60–90 min	4–12 h	24 h	U100
Premixed Insulins				
70% NPH/30% regular (Humulin 70/30)	30–60 min	Dual	10–16 h	U100
50% NPH/50% regular (Humulin 50/50)	30–60 min	Dual	10–16 h	U100
75% NPL/25% lispro (Humalog Mix 75/25)	5–15 min	Dual	10–16 h	U100
70% NP/30% aspart (NovoLog Mix)	5–15 min	Dual	10–16 h	U100
Long-acting Insulins				
Ultralente, Humulin U	4–8 h	10–30 h	>36 h	U100
Insulin glargine (Lantus)	1.1 h	No peak	24 h	U100

Note: Continuous infusion of insulin (insulin pump) usually achieves slightly better glycemic control than does an optimized-injection regimen. However, it is not clear whether insulin pumps are cost-effective and they are usually reserved for patients in whom injection regimens do not provide adequate control.

intensive therapy may adversely effect blood pressure and lipid profiles. Unless properly managed, these changes could possibly offset the benefits of better glycemic control in some patients.

Note: Intensive regulation of blood glucose is difficult at best, and glycemic controls should always be realistic. In some patients (e.g., small children, the elderly, those with advanced renal disease), the criteria for optimal control may need to be adjusted upward as the detrimental risks of hypoglycemia may outweigh the benefits of tight glycemic control. However, in general, rigorous management of blood glucose, comorbid conditions, and other risk factors should be considered in all patients regardless of their age.

Ophthalmic management of retinal disease involves the use of focal or grid laser treatment for clinically significant macular edema (see Table 16.2) and pan-retinal photocoagulation for retinopathy of high-risk characteristics. High-risk characteristics include:

- NVD >1/4 the disc area in size, on or within 1 DD of the optic disc
- Any amount of NVD if accompanied by a fresh preretinal or vitreous hemorrhage
- NVE >1/2 the disc area, with a fresh vitreous or preretinal hemorrhage

▶ **TABLE 16.6** International Clinical Diabetic Retinopathy (DR) Disease Severity Scale

Proposed Disease Severity Level	Finding Observable with Dilated Ophthalmoscopy
No apparent DR	No abnormalities
Mild nonproliferative DR	Microaneurysms only
Moderate nonproliferative DR	More than "mild" but less than "severe"
Severe nonproliferative DR	Any of the following:
	Twenty or more intraretinal hemorrhages in four quadrants
	Definite venous beading in two or more quadrants
	Prominent intraretinal microvascular abnormalities (IRMA) in one or more quadrants and no neovascularization
Proliferative DR	One or more of the following:
	Definite neovascularization
	Preretinal or vitreous hemorrhage

One should also keep in mind that diabetic retinopathy may progress more rapidly in some patients and that various risk factors may increase the chances for the development of retinal complications. The risk of retinal complications in diabetics increases with:

- Duration of disease
- Uncontrolled systemic hypertension
- Pregnancy
- Cataract surgery or YAG capsulotomy
- Carotid disease
- Poor glycemic control (9 years exposure to a HbA_{1c} of 8% yields the same risk of retinopathy as 2.5 years exposure to a HbA_{1c} of 11%)
- Proteinuria

▶ **TABLE 16.7** International Clinical Diabetic Macular Edema (ME) Scale

Proposed Classification	Findings Observable on Dilated Ophthalmoscopy*
Diabetic Macular Edema Absent	No retinal thickening or hard exudates in posterior pole
Diabetic Macular Edema Present	Some retinal thickening or hard exudates in posterior pole
If diabetic macular edema is present, it can be categorized as follows:	
Diabetic Macular Edema Present	• Mild Diabetic Macular Edema
	Some retinal thickening or hard exudates in posterior pole, but distant from the macula
	• Moderate Diabetic Macular Edema
	Retinal thickening or hard exudates approaching the center of the macula, but not involving the center
	• Severe Diabetic Macular Edema
	Retinal thickening or hard exudates involving the center of the macula

*Hard exudates are a sign of current or previous macular edema. Diabetic macular edema is defined as retinal thickening, which requires a three-dimensional assessment best performed by a dilated examination using slit-lamp biomicroscopy and/or stereo fundus photography.

- Strenuous exercise (proliferative diabetic retinopathy is a relative contraindication to strenuous exercise, since strenuous exercise could potentially precipitate a vitreous hemorrhage)

Note: The grading scales in Tables 16.6 and 16.7 represent a "proposed" classification system introduced by the Diabetic Retinopathy Task Force. The new *International Clinical Disease Severity Grading Scale for Diabetic Retinopathy and Diabetic Macular Edema* represents a simplified version of the Early Treatment of Diabetic Retinopathy Study (ETDRS) classification.

SYSTEMIC HYPERTENSION
Nicky R. Holdeman

ICD—9: 401.1

THE DISEASE
Pathophysiology

Systemic hypertension is a multifactorial disease produced by an array of pathogenetic mechanisms; it is not a single disease entity. Essential hypertension appears to involve a complex interaction between the central nervous system, the kidneys, and the renin-angiotensin-aldosterone system. Systolic hypertension in the elderly is usually because of age-related reductions in the elasticity and compliance of large- and medium-sized arteries.

Etiology

In 90 to 95% of cases, no cause can be established (primary or essential hypertension). Causes of secondary hypertension (5 to 10% of all cases) include:

- Drug induced or drug related
- Renal parenchymal disease
- Renal artery stenosis
- Primary aldosteronism
- Cushing's syndrome and chronic steroid therapy
- Pheochromocytoma
- Coarctation of the aorta
- Pregnancy (gestational hypertension)
- Hyperparathyroidism
- Hyperthyroidism
- Hypercalcemia
- Acromegaly
- Sleep apnea

Blood pressure rise and hypertension are *not* inevitable consequences of aging; however, isolated systolic hypertension (ISH) frequently occurs in individuals over 50. ISH is defined as a systolic blood pressure (SBP) of 140 mm Hg or more and a diastolic blood pressure (DBP) less than 90 mm Hg. ISH is related to loss of arterial elasticity (or compliance) because of atherosclerosis and is often more recalcitrant to treatment than essential hypertension. ISH is the most frequent form of uncontrolled hypertension in the United States; thus, clinicians should focus equally on the management of systolic and diastolic hypertension.

A pulse pressure (difference between peak SBP and DBP) >60 mm Hg is a significant risk factor for heart failure and may be a slightly stronger determinant of cardiovascular risk than SBP. As the population of the United States ages, elevated SBP and parallel widening of pulse pressure will become more commonplace. Consequently, older patients should be carefully monitored and their blood pressure treated appropriately.

The Patient

Clinical Symptoms

The majority of hypertensive individuals are *asymptomatic* until there is an end-organ deficit. The major target organ damage (TOD) caused by systemic hypertension occurs in the heart, brain, kidneys, peripheral arteries, and the retinas. Elevated blood pressure may produce vague complaints such as suboccipital headaches, palpitations, facial flushing, lightheadedness, or fatigue. Accelerated hypertension may produce visual disturbances.

Clinical Signs

Clinical findings will depend on the etiology of the hypertension, duration, severity, and total effect on target organs. The physical examination should inspect for known causes of high blood pressure, assess the presence and extent of target organ damage and cardiovascular disease, and identify other risk factors or concomitant disorders. One should look for the following signs:

- Elevated blood pressure (see Table 16.8) in accordance with the recommended techniques for in-office blood pressure measurements
- Hypertensive retinopathy (see Table 16.9)
- Left ventricular heave (established disease)
- Abdominal bruits (renovascular disease)
- Delayed or absent femoral artery pulses or leg pressure <20 mm Hg below the forearm pressure (coarctation of aorta)
- Truncal obesity with pigmented striae (Cushing's syndrome)
- Sweating, flushing, tachycardia, orthostasis (pheochromocytoma)
- Diminished or absent peripheral arterial pulsations (peripheral vascular disease)
- Carotid bruits (vascular disease), distended neck veins (right heart failure), or enlarged thyroid (hyperthyroidism)
- Pulmonary rales (left heart failure)
- Neurological deficits

Untreated hypertension can result in heart failure (HF), myocardial infarction (MI), cerebral vascular accidents (CVA), nephrosclerosis, retinopathy, and/or aneurysmal formation. Clinicians should also recognize that a "high normal" blood pressure is more akin to high blood pressure than it is to a normal blood pressure. Patients with this

▶ **TABLE 16.8   JNC 7 Classification of Blood Pressure for Patients Age 18 Years or Older*⁺**

BP Classification	Systolic, mmHg		Diastolic, mmHg
Normal	<120	and	<80
Prehypertension	120–139	or	80–89
Stage 1 hypertension	140–159	or	90–99
Stage 2 hypertension	≥160	or	≥100

*Classification assumes two or more readings on two or more occasions, separated by 2 or more minutes.
*When the systolic and diastolic blood pressures fall into different categories, the higher category should be selected to classify the individuals' blood pressure status.
⁺For patients under the age of 18, the definition of systemic hypertension takes into account age and height by sex. A child whose blood pressure is higher than that of 95% of other children of similar age, weight, and height is "hypertensive." Prehypertension is defined as an average SBP >/ = 90th and <95th percentiles (http://pediatrics.aappublications.org/).

condition should be informed that they may be at increased risk for cardiovascular disease, even at BP levels traditionally not considered to be hypertensive. For example, patients with a systolic BP of 120 to 139 mm Hg or a diastolic of 80 to 89 mm Hg are considered prehypertensive and require lifestyle modifications to prevent CVD. An estimated 45 million Americans fall into this grouping.

Note: Ambulatory blood pressure monitoring (ABPM) is indicated in some patients, especially when "white coat hypertension" is suspected. These ambulatory BP values are often lower than in-office readings and can sometimes be used to alter therapy.

Demographics

Systemic hypertension is the number 1 modifiable risk factor for cardiovascular disease in the world.

In the United States, over 65 million adults have elevated blood pressure; 30% are unaware they have hypertension. Another 45 million American adults are prehypertensive.

▶ **TABLE 16.9   Classification of Hypertensive Retinopathy**

Stage	Ophthalmoscopic Appearance
I	Minimal narrowing or sclerosis of arterioles
II	More definite narrowing of retinal arterioles, focal constrictions, sclerosis, A-V nicking
III	Grade-II findings plus localized arteriolar spasm, hemorrhages, exudates, cotton wool spots, retinal edema
IV	Findings in group III plus optic disc swelling

Note: Occasionally, patients with systemic hypertension will develop a central or branch occlusion of an artery or vein, neovascular complications, focal areas of choriocapillaris nonperfusion (Elshnigs spots), and/or lobular areas of choroidal infarction (Siegrest streaks).
Patients with hypertensive retinal microvascular abnormalities are at increased risk for stroke and coronary heart disease, independent of the presence of other known risk factors.

Onset of essential hypertension is usually between 25 and 55 years of age. Prevalence of hypertension* and cardiovascular disease is greater in (or increases with):

- Age (>55 years for men; >65 years for women)
  Two in three adults older than 65 have hypertension and normotensive adults older than 55 have a 90% lifetime risk of developing elevated BP
- African Americans more than Whites (38% vs. 29%)
- Family history of systemic hypertension or early cardiovascular disease
- Increased Na intake
- Obesity (BMI ≥30)*
- Sedentary lifestyle
- Excessive consumption of alcohol
- Smoking
- Lower socioeconomic class
- Dyslipidemia* (including a low HDL)
- Diabetes mellitus* (or glucose intolerance)
- Men and postmenopausal women
- Sleep disordered breathing (SDB) and sleep apnea

(*Components of the metabolic syndrome. Each component should be appropriately treated.)

Significant History

- Known duration and levels of elevated blood pressure. (The risk of CVD, beginning at 115/75 mmHg, doubles with each increment of 20/10 mm Hg.)
- Patient history of cardiovascular or cerebrovascular disease, renal disease, sexual dysfunction, diabetes mellitus, dyslipidemia, peripheral vascular disease, or gout.
- Personal history of alcohol and tobacco abuse; weight change; exercise activities; salt, fat, and caffeine intake; emotional stress; and environmental factors.
- Family history of systemic hypertension, early cardiovascular disease, stroke, dyslipidemia, diabetes mellitus, or renal disease.
- Medicational history of all drugs used, including illicit drugs and over-the-counter medications, as well as results and side effects of previous antihypertensive treatments.
- Symptoms suggesting secondary hypertension (see earlier).

Ancillary Tests

Most lab tests are normal in uncomplicated essential (primary) hypertension. The following tests are usually performed prior to initiating therapy in order to assess end-organ damage, to screen for secondary causes of systemic hypertension, and to determine the presence of other cardiovascular risk factors.

- CBC (anemia or polycythemia)
- Urinalysis (primary renal disease)
- Serum creatinine (primary renal disease)
- Serum K+ (hyperaldosteronism)

- Fasting plasma glucose (diabetes/pheochromocytoma)
- Plasma lipids (should include total cholesterol, HDL, LDL, and triglycerides)
- Electrocardiography (left ventricular hypertrophy)
- Serum uric acid (gout)
- Chest x-ray (cardiac enlargement)
- Blood calcium (parathyroid disease)

Optional tests include creatinine clearance, 24-hour urinary protein, thyroid function tests, and limited echocardiography. If symptoms, physical examination, or initial lab tests suggest a secondary cause of hypertension, further studies may be indicated.

The Treatment

The patient should be referred in a timely manner (see Table 16.10) to a primary care physician for appropriate and aggressive management of both systolic and diastolic hypertension. The goal of therapy is to reduce the complications of high blood pressure by the least intrusive means possible. Authorities agree that patients with repeatable diastolic blood pressures >90 mm Hg and systolic pressures >140 mm Hg should be treated. However, the risk for cardiovascular disease is determined not only by the level of blood pressure but also by the presence or absence of target organ damage or other risk factors such as diabetes mellitus or dyslipidemia. Consequently, therapy should be initiated based on individual risk stratification. (See Table 16.11.)

Note: It is recommended to measure the BP lying, seated, and standing, with at least 2 to 3 minutes between each position. The standing SBP should be below 140 mm Hg, but not below 120 mm Hg, especially in the elderly patient. These readings ensure that the BP is lowered sufficiently to minimize the risk of heart, brain, and kidney damage, but not so low as to potentially exacerbate perfusion pressure to vital tissues such as the optic nerve.

Nonpharmacologic therapy (or lifestyle modifications) has been shown to be effective in lowering blood pressure at little cost and with minimal risk. Lifestyle modifications not only decrease BP, but they can also enhance antihypertensive drug efficacy and

▶ **TABLE 16.10 Recommendations for Follow-up Based on Initial Set of Blood Pressure Measurements for Adults**

Systolic		Diastolic	Follow-up Recommended*
<120	and	<80	Recheck in 1–2 years
120–139	or	80–89	Recheck in 6–12 months
140–159	or	90–99	Confirm within 1–2 months
160–179	or	100–109	Evaluate or refer to source of care within 2 weeks
≥180	or	≥110	Evaluate or refer to source of care immediately or within 1 week depending on clinical situation

*The follow-up schedule should be modified according to previous blood pressure measurements, other cardiovascular risk factors, or target organ disease.
+Individuals in the 130/80 to 139/89 mm Hg BP range are at twice the risk to develop systemic hypertension as those with lower values. Lifestyle modifications and self-measurement of BP should be encouraged.

▶ **TABLE 16.11 High Blood Pressure Guidelines***

	No Risk Factors	*Minor Risk*	*Major Complications*
Blood pressure stages (readings in millimeters of mercury)	**Risk group A** No risk factors, no target organ damage (TOD) or clinical cardiovascular disease (CCD)	**Risk group B** At least one risk factor, not including diabetes; No TOD/CCD	**Risk group C** TOD/CCD and/or diabetes, with or without other risk factors
Prehypertension (120–139/80–89)	Lifestyle modification	Lifestyle modification	Possible drug therapy for those with heart failure, kidney damage or diabetes+
Stage 1 hypertension (140–159/90–99)	Drug therapy++	Drug therapy	Drug therapy
Stage 2 hypertension (160 or greater/100 or greater)	Drug therapy+++	Drug therapy	Drug therapy

*Guidelines of risk and treatment recommend lifestyle modification for all groups at all stages.
+Patients with chronic kidney disease or diabetes mellitus should have a BP goal of <130/80 mm Hg. Combinations of two or more drugs are usually needed to achieve the target BP.
++May be controlled with one drug; thiazide-type diuretics are indicated for most patients without high-risk conditions or compelling indications for another class of drugs.
+++Most patients require a two-drug combination, one of which should usually be a thiazide-type diuretic. Other antihypertensive agents should be employed to address specific high-risk conditions (i.e., heart failure, post-MI, diabetes, chronic kidney disease, recurrent stroke prevention, and/or high coronary disease risk).

decrease cardiovascular risk. Thus, the guidelines of risk and treatment recommend lifestyle modifications for all groups at all stages. This management often includes:

■ Weight reduction, if overweight (a normal body mass index [BMI], between 18.5 and 24.9)
■ Reduced alcohol and/or tobacco consumption (tobacco avoidance should be promoted)
■ Reduced sodium, saturated, and total fat intake
■ Increased aerobic activity (30 to 45 minutes per day most days of the week)
■ Adequate dietary intake of K^+, Ca^+, and Mg (diet rich in fruits, vegetables, and low-fat dairy products)

If blood pressure cannot be controlled with the previous modalities, drug therapy is required. The major classes of drugs, which are often employed in a "stepped care" approach, include:

■ Diuretics (i.e., HCTZ, furosemide, chlorthalidone, triamterene)
■ β-blockers (i.e., propranolol, nadolol, metoprolol, atenolol)
■ ACE inhibitors (i.e., captopril, lisinopril, enalapril, ramipril)
■ Calcium channel blockers (i.e., verapamil, amlodipine, felodipine, nifedipine)
■ Angiotensin II receptor blockers (i.e., losartan, valsartan, irbesarten, condesartan)

Note: Thiazide-type diuretics are the most effective first-line treatment for preventing the occurrence of cardiovascular disease morbidity and mortality. They should be preferred for first-step antihypertensive therapy for most patients, unless there are compelling indications for a different class of drugs.

Other classes of drugs are available and may be used in certain cases.

- Central α-agonists (i.e., clonidine, reserpine, guanfacine, methyldopa)
- α-blockers (i.e., prazosin, terazosin, doxasozin)
- direct vasodilators (i.e., hydralazine, minoxidil)
- combined α- and β-blockers (i.e., carvedilol, labetalol)

Note: Many patients with systemic hypertension will require two or more antihypertensive agents to effectively control their blood pressure, especially if their untreated BP is more than 20/10 mm Hg above the goal BP. Unfortunately, about one-half of all patients who are prescribed antihypertensive medications discontinue therapy by the end of the first year. It is therefore imperative that all health-care providers measure each patient's BP and reinforce the importance of lifestyle modifications and proper blood pressure control at each visit.

DYSTHYROID DISEASE AND OPHTHALMOPATHY
Nicky R. Holdeman

ICD—9: 376-21

THE DISEASE
Pathophysiology

Dysthyroid ophthalmopathy (and Graves' disease) appears to be an autoimmune disorder with antibodies directed against orbital antigens (and thyroid thyrotropin receptors). The mechanism by which thyroid-stimulating antibodies bind to and activate the thyrotropin receptor is not known. The majority of patients ($\approx$80%) with autoimmune thyroid disease will, however, eventually develop some form of thyroid eye disease (TED), also called thyroid-associated ophthalmopathy (TAO). About 90% of patients with ophthalmopathy have hyperthyroid disease; the remainder have autoimmune hypothyroidism or are euthyroid at presentation.

Etiology

The major abnormality in thyroid ophthalmopathy is inflammation and enlargement of the orbital tissues, particularly the extraocular muscles. Exophthalmos and optic nerve compression are caused by deposition of mucinous edema, proliferation of fibroblasts, and accumulation of lymphocytes within the muscles, resulting in an increase in orbital connective tissue and fat. Orbital venous obstruction and capillary collapse as a result of inflammation and cigarette smoking contribute significantly to the clinical manifestations of TAO by affecting oxygen delivery to the orbit.

The Patient

Clinical Symptoms

The clinical presentation of the thyrotoxic patient and thyroid ophthalmopathy may be extremely variable. The actual features relate to the age of onset, the duration of the condition, and the degree of hormone excess. The general symptoms of thyrotoxicosis (hyperthyroidism) are sweating, increased appetite, weight loss, nervousness, hyperdefication, heat intolerance, restlessness, irritability, insomnia, exertional dyspnea, fatigue, weakness, tremor, palpitations, decreased menstrual flow in women, pruritus, and warm, moist skin. With increasing age, weight loss and anorexia become more common, whereas irritability and heat intolerance are less common.

The onset of ocular manifestations may be acute or quite gradual. The symptoms of thyroid eye disease often include eyelid retraction or stare, ocular irritation, retrobulbar pressure, eyelid swelling, photophobia, diplopia, and/or decreased vision. Fortunately, only a small percentage of patients experience severe consequences such as persistent diplopia or optic neuropathy. It is important to remember, however, that ophthalmic symptoms and signs can occur prior to the systemic manifestations of thyroid disease in about 20% of patients.

Clinical Signs

Signs of thyrotoxicosis may include a diffusely enlarged thyroid (often with overlying bruit), warm skin, thinning and loss of hair, tachycardia or atrial fibrillation, muscle wasting, tremors, hyperreflexia, palmar erythema, onycholysis, and rarely high output heart failure.

The characteristic findings in thyroid eye disease include lid retraction, conjunctival injection and chemosis, superior limbic keratoconjunctivitis, periorbital edema, proptosis (either unilateral or bilateral), restricted eye movements, elevation of intraocular pressure, resistance to retropulsion of the globe, exposure keratopathy, pupillary defects, acquired color vision deficits, and/or visual acuity loss (Table 16.12). Graves' ophthalmopathy usually involves both orbits, although an asymmetry may be present. A small number of patients (5 to 11%) show no progression to bilateral disease and have only unilateral involvement.

Graves' ophthalmopathy typically goes through three phases—progression, stabilization, and perhaps improvement. In fact, spontaneous improvement of mild ophthalmopathy is seen to occur in approximately 60% of patients. However, unpredictable and sudden worsening of ophthalmopathy can occur at any time, independent of antithyroid therapy.

Thyroid patients frequently develop eye findings that mimic dry eye, conjunctivitis, cellulitis, allergic reactions, episcleritis, myositis, EOM nerve paresis, orbital tumors, AV malformations, Parinaud's syndrome, and so on. Clinicians must maintain a high index of suspicion for the varied ophthalmic signs that may indicate thyroid disease.

Demographics

Graves' disease is the most prevalent autoimmune disorder in the United States, affecting 2.2% of the population.

▶ TABLE 16.12 "NO SPECS" Classification of Graves' Orbitopathy

Class	Characteristics
0	**N**o physical signs or symptoms
1	**O**nly signs (i.e., lid retraction, stare)
2	**S**oft tissue signs and symptoms (i.e., conjunctival injection, conjunctival and lid edema, lacrimation)
3	**P**roptosis (upper limits of normal is approximately 22 mm in Caucasians and 24 mm in African Americans there should be no more than a 2-mm difference between the two eyes).
4	**E**xtraocular muscle involvement (i.e., restrictions, adhesions)
5	**C**orneal involvement (i.e., stippling, ulceration, scarring)
6	**S**ight loss (i.e., optic disc changes, field loss, reduced acuity)

Source: Van Dyk JHL: Orbital Graves' disease: A modification of the "NO SPECS" classification. *Ophth* 1981;88:479–483.
Note: While the NOSPEC mnemonic is often helpful in directing the eye examination, it is not useful in predicting the course of disease or in guiding treatment.

Graves' disease may occur in men or women at any age; however, it is much more common in women than men (8:1), in part the result of the modulation of the autoimmune response by estrogen. The onset of disease is usually between the ages of 30 and 60. The clinical course of dysthyroid ophthalmopathy is likely to be more severe in men, older patients, and those with a family history of thyroid disease.

Among patients with hyperthyroidism, 60 to 80% have Graves' disease. There appears to be an increased risk of Graves' disease during pregnancy, but conversely, there is often a spontaneous remission of hyperthyroidism in the last trimester, in which case therapy can be stopped.

Graves' disease may be associated with other diseases that have autoantibody production such as lupus, multiple sclerosis, pernicious anemia, scleroderma, vitiligo, myasthenia gravis, inflammatory bowel disease, type 1 diabetes mellitus, rheumatoid arthritis, and/or alopecia areata.

The severity of eye disease frequently does not correlate with the degree of thyrotoxicosis, although ophthalmopathy tends to be more severe in cigarette smokers and patients in whom hyperthyroidism is poorly controlled.

The prevalence of Graves' disease is similar among Whites and Asians, and it is lower among Blacks.

Significant History

Graves' disease has a familial tendency; however, genes make only a moderate contribution to susceptibility of Graves' disease. Approximately 20% of those affected have a family history of thyroid disease.

Risk factors for ophthalmopathy may include therapeutic irradiation of the neck and/or smoking.

There is a higher incidence ≈90% of ophthalmopathy in patients with hyperthyroidism; however, eye findings may occur in an euthyroid or even hypothyroid patient.

Note: ≈10% of orbitopathy patients remain euthyroid, further complicating confirmation of the clinical diagnosis.

Ancillary Tests (Table 16.13)

Many drugs can affect thyroid function tests. It is imperative to know all the medications the patient is taking to avoid misinterpretation of the test results.

Thyroid function tests (TFTs)—the typical thyroid panel often includes a T_3 resin uptake (T_3RU), total serum thyroxin (T_4), and a free thyroxin index (FT_4I or T_7). Serum-free T_4 and T_3 are available but may be difficult to obtain and expensive to perform. However, 5 to 10% of hyperthyroid patients will only manifest an elevated serum T_3, a condition called "T_3 toxicosis." Serum triiodothyronine (T_3) should be measured if the thyrotropin (TSH) level is low but the thyroxin level is normal (see later).

Sensitive serum thyroid stimulating hormone assays (s-TSH)—particularly useful in the diagnosis of hypothyroidism but is also employed in diagnosing hyperthyroidism. While rare exceptions exist, the presence of a normal serum thyrotropin (TSH) concentration nearly always excludes a diagnosis of hyperthyroidism. The highly sensitive TSH assays are considered by most to be a viable screening test for thyroid disease, but thyroid hormone concentrations and clinical presentation should be used to determine severity of disease. One approach to the laboratory investigation of suspected hyperthyroidism is as follows.

Order a serum thyrotropin (immunometric s-TSH) assay:

- If normal (0.3 mIU/L to 3.0 mIU/L), hyperthyroidism is excluded (except in rare cases of a TSH-producing pituitary tumor or a pituitary resistance to thyroid hormone)
- If low, order a free T_4 (thyroxin) level
- If T_4 is high, hyperthyroidism confirmed
- If T_4 is normal, order a free T_3 (triiodothyronine)
  - If the free T_3 level is high, T_3 toxicosis is confirmed
  - If the free T_3 level is normal, the patient may have subclinical hyperthyroidism, evolving Graves' disease, toxic nodular goiter, and the like. Tests should be repeated in 2 to 3 months.

Thyroid scans (^{123}I)—useful for studying thyroid nodules. Functioning ("hot") nodules are rarely malignant while nonfunctioning ("cold") nodules could indicate malignancy.

Thyroid stimulating immunoglobulins (TSIg)—can be used to distinguish Graves' disease from other forms of hyperthyroidism. TSIgs are typically present in patients with Graves' disease (>80%) but are not usually required for diagnosis, especially when eye disease occurs in patients with known hyperthyroidism. Although TSIgs cause Graves' hyperthyroidism, the serum antibody concentrations are often very low and are even undetectable in a few patients. When the diagnosis is unclear clinically, the presence of a high serum concentration of thyroid peroxidase antibody, present in about 75% of patients with Graves' hyperthyroidism, may provide evidence of Graves' disease.

▌ **TABLE 16.13   Tests Employed in the Evaluation of Patients with Thyroid Abnormalities**

Test	Purpose	Methodology	Comments
Total serum T_4 (Thyroxin)	T_4 level	Enzyme-linked immunosorbant assay (ELISA) Radioimmunoassay (RIA)	Detects >90% of cases of hyperthyroidism Affected by alterations in the thyroxine-binding globulin (TBG) level and can be misleadingly high or low Free T_4 (FT_4) makes up only a fraction of T_4 level (0.04%)
Resin T_3 uptake (RT_3U)	Assessment of free T_4	Binding of labeled T_3 to resin versus patient's serum	Clarifies whether alterations in T_4 are the result of thyroid pathology or alterations in T_4-binding proteins
Free T_4 (free thyroxine)	Assessment unbound T_4	Equilibrium dialysis	Directly measures FT_4 Independent of TBG levels
Serum T_3 (Triiodothyronine)	T_3 level	Radioimmunoassay	Used for detecting hyperthyroidism, especially T_3 toxocosis in which T_3 is elevated but T_4 is within normal limits Not to be confused with RT_3U
Radioactive iodine uptake (RAIU)	Extent of thyroid function	Measurement of percentage uptake of iodine tracer dose after given time	Normal range must be determined for each population district Difficult to distinguish low values from low-normal values when dietary iodine is high Hyperthyroidism does not always cause high iodine uptake
Thyroid-stimulating hormone (TSH) (also called thyrotropin)	Serum TSH level: an index of thyroid status	Immunoradiometric assay (IRMA) Chemiluminescent assay (ICMA)	Most sensitive test for primary hypothyroidism (i.e., TSH level is high before other tests show low T_4) Standard assay not reliable at low TSH levels; sensitive immunoradiometric and chemiluminescent assays improve detection of low levels

(continued)

▶ **TABLE 16.13** Tests Employed in the Evaluation of Patients with Thyroid Abnormalities (Continued)

Test	Purpose	Methodology	Comments
Thyroid scan	Functional status of nodular goiter	Radionuclide scanning	Often not needed in other types of thyroid pathology
Ultrasonography	Status of single nodules	Ultrasound scanning	Reliably discriminates between cystic and solid nodules in 90% of cases
Serum thyroid antimicrosomal antibodies	Distinguish between nodular goiter and thyroiditis	Tanned red blood cell agglutination test Complement fixation test Antimicrobial antibodies	High titers suggest Hashimoto's thyroiditis. Antibodies to thyroid microsomes are present in 70–90% of patients with chronic thyroiditis
Free thyroxine index (FT_4I)	Indirect correlation of free T_4	Calculation from results of T_3 resin uptake and total T_4 (serum $T_4 \times RT_3U$)	Good screening test since it is not affected by alterations in thyroxin-binding protein sites An index that generally correlates with free T4

	Hyperthyroidism	Hypothyroidism	Euthyroid with Increased TBG*	Euthyroid with Decreased TBG*
TOTAL T_4	Increased	Decreased	Increased	Decreased
T_3RU	Increased	Decreased	Decreased	Increased
FT_4I	Increased	Decreased	Normal	Normal
TSH	Decreased	Increased	Normal	Normal

*Thyroxin-binding globulins (TBGs)

TBGs may be increased in pregnancy, acute hepatitis, oral contraceptives, heroin abuse, or clofibrate use.

TBGs may be decreased in cirrhosis, nephrotic syndrome, androgens, and glucocorticoids.

Imaging

Noncontrast CT scanning (axial and coronal views to the orbital apex) is used to visualize the orbits, the EOMs, and the paranasal sinuses and to exclude retrobulbar tumors, orbital pseudotumors, or arteriovenous malformations as a cause of exophthalmos, particularly with unilateral involvement. Ultrasonography may be helpful in assessing anterior and midorbital disease. MRI may be useful in differentiating between EOMs that are actually inflamed and those that are fibrosed.

A careful eye examination should be performed on each patient. Depending on the stage of disease (see Table 16.12), any or all of the following procedures may be indicated: visual acuities, lid assessment, pupillary assessment, motility testing (including forced ductions), exophthalmometry, color vision perception, threshold perimetry, ophthalmoscopy, biomicroscopy, intraocular pressures (primary and upgaze), and/or visual-evoked potentials. External and fundus photography is a useful method of recording clinical status.

Note: Up to 50% of patients with optic nerve compression may have no fundus abnormalities.

The Treatment

The patient should be referred to a primary care physician or endocrinologist for management of systemic thyroid disorders. The patient with Graves' disease should be advised that the ophthalmopathy may progress even if euthyroidism is achieved and that smoking increases the risk of Graves' ophthalmopathy.

The choice of therapy for thyrotoxicosis is usually dictated by the etiology of the disorder, the patient's age, the size of the gland, the severity of disease, and in some cases, the desires of the patient. The ideal treatment for Graves' disease, which would correct the autoimmune responses in the thyroid and the orbits, is not available. Currently, there are three principal treatments—antithyroid drugs (methimazole and propylthiouracil), radioiodine (^{131}I), and total or subtotal thyroidectomy—all of which are effective. Unfortunately, no single treatment is guaranteed to result in permanent euthyroidism and each has certain advantages and adverse effects. ^{131}I, when compared to other forms of antithyroid therapy, is more likely to cause or exacerbate thyroid ophthalmopathy (particularly in cigarette smokers) unless low to moderate doses of oral prednisone are given for several weeks following radioiodine ablation.

Dysthyroid patients with eye signs should be evaluated and treated for the major complications of thyroid orbitopathy. The conditions include:

- Exposure keratopathy—the cornea should be protected with sunglasses, artificial tears, ointments, taping of the lids, tarsorrhaphy, or canthoplasty.
- Diplopia—small-angle tropias because of EOM entrapment can sometimes be managed with prism. Patients with large-angle deviations may benefit by recession of the restricted muscles. Surgery should typically be considered only after the eye signs have been stable for at least 6 months, unless the patient has a disabling head posture or disabling diplopia.
- Optic neuropathy—signs of optic nerve compression indicate a need for immediate treatment with high-dose steroids (prednisone 60 to 100 mg p.o. qd for 2 weeks), orbital radiotherapy, or graded surgical decompression of the orbit. While all three forms of therapy have been used, external beam orbital radiation may be of questionable value, as it appears to offer little in the way of long-term benefits. Because orbital radiotherapy is not innocuous, it should only be considered for patients with optic neuropathy but not for patients with mild to moderate ophthalmopathy.

Note: When optic neuropathy develops in thyroid disease, it will typically occur on the side of the less proptotic, more crowded orbit, which is also usually the "white" noncongested eye.

Several other forms of therapy have proven useful in certain cases.

- Cessation of smoking
- Moisture chambers or swimmers goggles to protect exposed corneas

- Elevation of the head and diuretics (HCTZ 50 mg p.o. qd) to help reduce eyelid and orbital edema
- Botulinum toxin injections for dysthyroid upper lid retraction and for selected cases of strabismus
- Other immunosuppressive agents (i.e., cyclosporine, azathioprine)

ACQUIRED IMMUNODEFICIENCY SYNDROME
Padhmalatha Segu

CMV RETINITIS, NONINFECTIOUS HIV RETINOPATHY

BACKGROUND INFORMATION

The human immunodeficiency virus (HIV) is a retrovirus from the lentiviridae family. Over time, HIV weakens the immune system by attacking T-cells, B-cells, macrophages, microglial cells, and monocytes. A patient infected with HIV is considered to have acquired immunodeficiency syndrome (AIDS) when their T-cell count (CD4 count) falls below 200 cells/mm^3(less than 14%) and/or they contract an AIDS-defining illness such as cytomegalovirus (CMV) retinitis or Kaposi's sarcoma.

In 2002, over 800,000 AIDS cases and 195,000 HIV cases were reported in the United States by the Centers for Disease Control (CDC). Worldwide, 40 million people are estimated to be living with HIV/AIDS, with southern Africa having the highest prevalence. The AIDS incidence and AIDS-related deaths in the United States have significantly decreased because of the advancements in anti-retroviral therapy.

Management of the HIV-positive patient includes monitoring the patient's CD4 count and viral load. The CD4 count monitors the status of the immune system and the viral load monitors the replication of the virus in the blood. A normal CD4 count in an immunocompetent patient is approximately 1000 cells/mm^3. HIV-positive patients with viral load levels greater then 100,000 copies/mL are considered to be at high risk for disease progression.

Several antiretroviral drugs have been approved by the Food and Drug Administration (FDA) for the treatment and management of HIV infection (Table 16.14). The antiretroviral medications are classified into three major categories: entry inhibitors (EI), reverse transcriptase inhibitors (RTI), and protease inhibitors (PI). Eyecare providers should be aware that in June 1997, the FDA published a warning that PIs may cause hyperglycemia and diabetes. Highly active antiretroviral therapy (HAART) is a combination of antiretroviral medications that often keeps the viral load at undetectable levels for several months and may include a PI.

CYTOMEGALOVIRUS (CMV) RETINITIS
ICD—9: 363.13

THE DISEASE

Pathophysiology

CMV may affect the lungs, brain, gastrointestinal tract, liver, spleen, and eyes, with chorioretinitis being the most frequent clinical manifestation. CMV causes a

▶ **TABLE 16.14 Antiretroviral Medications**

1. Reverse Transcriptase Inhibitors (RTI)	
a. Non-Nucleoside RTI	Rescriptor (delavirdine)
	Sustiva (efavirenz)
	Stocrin (efavirenz)
	Viramune (nevirapine)
b. Nucleoside RTI	Combivir (AZT and 3TC)
	Epivir (3TC, lamivudine)
	Emtriva (FTC, emtricitabine)
	Hivid (ddC, zalcitabine)
	Retrovir (AZT, zidovudine)
	Trizivir (AZT, 3TC, and abacavir)
	Videx (ddI, didanosine)
	Ziagen (abacavir)
	Zerit (d4T, stavudine)
c. Nucelotide RTI	Viread (tenofovir)
2. Protease Inhibitors	Agenerase (amprenavir)
	Crixivan (indinavir)
	Fortovase (saquinavir)
	Invirase (saquinavir)
	Norvir (ritonavir)
	Kaletra (lopinavir and ritonavir)
	Lexiva (fosamprenavir)
	Viracept (nelfinavir)
3. Entry Inhibitor	Fuzeon (enfuvirtide)

full-thickness retinal necrosis that will result in an absolute scotoma and irreversible blindness.

Etiology

Cytomegalovirus is a DNA virus of the herpes virus family. CMV is present in the general adult population and can be transmitted perinatally, through direct contact with infected secretions, sexual intercourse, blood transfusions, and/or organ transplants. In cases when the immune system is suppressed by disease or by medications, CMV may reactivate and can cause end-organ damage. CMV retinitis typically occurs when the immune system is severely suppressed and the CD4 count falls below 50 cells/mm^3.

The Patient

Clinical Symptoms
Most patients are asymptomatic unless the posterior pole is involved. Symptoms may include visual field loss, photophobia, photopsia, floaters, blurred vision, and/or metamorphopsia.

Clinical Signs
The diagnosis of CMV retinitis is based on clinical appearance and is often referred to as "cottage cheese and ketchup" or "pizza pie fundus." The fulminant form is associated

with dense confluent areas of hemorrhaging, exudates, retinal vascular sheathing, and necrotizing retinitis located in the posterior pole. The indolent form is "quieter" in appearance with less hemorrhaging and affects the peripheral fundus. Twenty percent of patients with CMV retinitis may develop a rhegmatogenous retinal detachment. Other clinical manifestations include cystoid macular edema, papillitis, cataract formation, and frosted branch angiitis.

Demographics

CMV is a ubiquitous organism, with 50 to 60% of the world's population testing seropositive for the virus; however, CMV is found in 90 to 100% of the homosexual population. CMV retinitis is considered to be the most common ocular opportunistic infection and leading cause of blindness in AIDS patients. Approximately 2% of patients with HIV have CMV retinitis as an AIDS-defining illness.

Significant History
- Ocular symptoms (see Clinical Symptoms)?
- Previous history of CMV retinitis?
- Weight loss, fever, pain with swallowing?
- Abdominal pain, blood in the stool, loss of appetite, diarrhea?
- Lowest and most recent CD4 count?
- Highest and most recent viral load?
- Adherence with antiretroviral therapy?

Ancillary Tests

Although, CMV can be cultured from blood, semen, urine, or tears, the diagnosis of CMV retinitis is primarily based on clinical presentation; therefore, diagnostic tests are usually not required. For patients unaware of their immune status, consider testing for HIV and obtaining a CD4 count.

The Treatment

The goal of therapy is to preserve vision and prevent further advancement of CMV retinitis. With the advent of new medications and formulations to treat HIV and CMV retinitis, life expectancy and maintenance of visual acuity has significantly improved. Treatment for CMV retinitis is based on the location of the retinitis *(posterior versus peripheral involvement)*, the patient's immune status, response to HARRT therapy *(patients with HIV)*, current medications, systemic health, and quality of life.

Traditionally, management consists of an induction phase and maintenance phase. The induction phase is the first stage of treatment in which the medication is administered frequently over a 2- to 3-week period or until there is a clinical response. The maintenance phase is the second stage of treatment in which the dosage of medication is reduced for the remainder of the patient's life in cases where the immune system remains compromised. Patients should be monitored closely for signs of reactivation of the retinitis during maintenance therapy.

▶ **TABLE 16.15 Treatment for CMV Retinitis**

Intravenous formulation	Cytovene (ganciclovir)
	Foscavir (foscarnet)
	Vistide (cidofovir)
Oral formulation	Cytovene (ganciclovir)
(after immune reconstitution)	Valcyte (valganciclovir)
Intraocular device	Vitrasert (ganciclovir)
Intravitreal injection	Cytovene (ganciclovir)
	Foscavir (foscarnet)
	Vitravene (fomivirsen)

Treatment for CMV retinitis includes the use of the antiviral agents (Table 16.15). Regression of CMV retinitis is usually apparent in 1 to 2 weeks, with resolution of the hemorrhages and fading of the opacified, necrotizing retinitis. The challenge with all available treatment modalities is progression and reactivation of CMV retinitis. Current treatment options are virostatic; therefore, the patient is required to maintain lifelong treatment and to be monitored for reactivation. In 1999, the CDC guidelines for prevention of opportunistic infections stated that chronic maintenance therapy for CMV retinitis could be discontinued if the patient's CD4 count remained above 100 to 150 cells/mm^3 each month for 3 to 6 consecutive months on HAART.

NONINFECTIOUS HIV RETINOPATHY
ICD—9: 362.84—Retinal ischemia
ICD—9: 362.81—Retinal hemorrhages
ICD—9: 362.83—Retinal edima

THE DISEASE
Pathophysiology

Noninfectious HIV retinopathy is the most common retinopathy seen in AIDS patients and is associated with a suppressed immune system. The presence of noninfectious HIV retinopathy indicates a breakdown in the blood retinal barrier, leading to retinal ischemia and ultimately increasing the risk for other infections such as CMV.

Etiology

The exact pathogenesis for HIV retinopathy is unknown. Postulated theories include immune complexes deposited within the retinal capillaries, direct endothelial cell damage by HIV, and/or increased levels of fibrinogen in the blood.

The Patient

Clinical Symptoms
The patient is typically asymptomatic.

Clinical Signs

The hallmark of noninfectious retinopathy is cotton wool spots (CWS). The presentation is often bilateral with multiple CWS distributed within the posterior pole. Other clinical manifestations include hemorrhages, capillary nonperfusion, microaneurysms, retinal vein sheathing, branch or central retinal vein occlusion, and branch retinal artery occlusion.

Demographics

Noninfectious retinopathy usually occurs in approximately 40 to 60% of AIDS patients. There is an associated risk for disease progression in patients with a CD4 count less than 50 to 100 cells/mm^3.

Significant History
- Lowest and most recent CD4 count
- Highest and most recent viral load

Ancillary Testing

The diagnosis of noninfectious HIV retinopathy is made based on clinical presentation; therefore, diagnostic tests are usually not required. For patients unaware of their immune status, consider testing for HIV and obtaining a CD4 count.

The Treatment

No specific treatment is indicated; however, it is important to monitor for the development of CMV retinitis. The differentiation between noninfectious HIV retinopathy and early CMV retinitis is extremely important for appropriate management. The initial presentation of CMV retinitis may be mistaken for HIV retinopathy in the early stages of the infection. In cases when uncertainty exists, fundus photographs are suggested, and the patient should be reexamined in 2 weeks. A patient with HIV retinopathy will show minimal change at the 2-week follow-up unlike CMV retinitis, which will typically show progressive changes.

LYME DISEASE
Nicky R. Holdeman

ICD—9: 088.81

THE DISEASE

Pathophysiology

Lyme disease, a tick-transmitted infection, is categorized into early disease (stages 1 and 2) and late disease (stage 3). In the early disseminated stage (stage 2) and chronic stage (stage 3), ocular involvement can occur.

After inoculation in the skin of a human host, the vector-borne spirochete *Borrelia burgdorferi* replicates and spreads within the dermis. The infection then disseminates to numerous organs by the hematogenous route but exhibits particular affinity for the heart, central nervous system, and joints.

Etiology

Lyme disease is caused by the spirochete *B. burgdorferi*. It is usually transmitted by the bite of an infected *Ixodes* tick. Ticks most commonly infected with *B. burgdorferi* usually feed and mate on the white-tailed deer and the white-footed mouse, which serve as reservoirs for the disease. Migratory birds disperse infected ticks over wide regions of North America and northern Europe.

The Patient

Clinical Symptoms
Stage 1 (Early Localized Disease; 1 to 4 Weeks After the Tick Bite)
- Expanding skin rash (occurs in 60 to 80% of patients)
- Constitutional flulike symptoms
  - headache
  - malaise
  - myalgias
  - fatigue
  - arthralgias
  - chills
- Some patients may be asymptomatic

Note: The classic skin rash usually begins 3 to 20 days after a tick bite, an incident recalled by only 20% of patients with Lyme disease.

Stage 2 (Early Disseminated Disease; Several Weeks to Months After Stage 1)
- Multiple or satellite skin lesions
- Stiff neck, headache
- Joint pain (particularly in the knee, elbow, and shoulder)
- Photophobia, inflamed eye, blurred vision, double vision

Stage 3 (Chronic or Late-Disseminated Disease; Several Months to Years After Stage 1)
- Joint pain (most often in the knees)
- Neuropsychiatric symptoms
  - memory loss
  - depression
  - dementia
  - sleep disorders
- Symptoms mimicking other CNS disorders
  - Multiple sclerosis (MS)–like syndromes
  - Strokelike symptoms
  - Parkinsonian symptoms

Clinical Signs

Stage 1

- Erythema migrans (EM) skin lesion. A red macule occurs at the location of the tick bite, expanding to become an annular rash with central clearing. The rash is painless and not infectious.
- Fever (100.4° to 103.1° F)
- Regional lymphadenopathy

Stage 2

- Multiple erythema migrans lesions
- Aseptic meningitis, encephalitis
- Cranial neuropathies (especially Bell's palsy)
- Heart block (varying degrees of A-V block)
- Pericarditis
- Orchitis, hepatitis, hematuria, proteinuria
- Iritis
- Arthritis (migratory arthropathy)
- Generalized lymphadenopathy

Stage 3

- Recurrent synovitis, tendonitis, bursitis, and/or arthritis
- Carpal tunnel syndrome
- Neuropathies (motor, sensory, or autonomic)
- Ophthalmic manifestations (see Table 16.16)

Demographics

Lyme disease is the most common vector-associated disease in the United States; 15,000 cases are reported each year. Prevalence increases with physician and patient awareness.

Risk of infection varies with region and time of year.

- Northeastern United States—May and June
- North central United States—May through August
- Western United States—January through May

Highest prevalence occurs in Connecticut, Rhode Island, New York, New Jersey, Pennsylvania, Wisconsin, Maryland, and Minnesota.

In endemic areas of Connecticut and New York, as many as 50 to 70% of *I. dammini* ticks are infected with *B. burgdorferi*. However, transmission of disease occurs in ≈10% of bites by infected ticks, and prompt removal of the tick decreases the risk of transmission.

Lyme disease can occur in all ages but is most common in children ages 5 to 9 and in adults 50 to 59 years of age living in heavily wooded areas.

Significant History

- Has the patient visited or lived in an endemic area for Lyme disease?
- Does the patient recall a tick bite? (Fewer than 20% of people remember having a tick bite.)

▶ **TABLE 16.16** Ophthalmic Manifestations of Lyme Disease

Lids
- Periorbital edema

Conjunctiva
- Conjunctivitis (with or without symblepharon)
- Injection without tearing

Cornea
- Interstitial keratitis (multifocal opacities with irregular borders throughout the stroma)

Uvea/Episclera/Sclera
- Uveitis (iritis; iridocyclitis, diffuse choroidal infiltration)
- Episcleritis
- Scleritis
- Panophthalmitis

Vitreous
- Pars planitis
- Vitreous clouding (vitreitis)

Retina
- Neuroretinitis
- Vasculitis
- Macular edema
- Exudative retinal detachments (may mimic V-K-H syndrome)

Optic Nerve
- Papilledema (associated with Lyme meningitis)
- Optic neuritis
- Optic perineuritis
- Ischemic optic neuropathy
- Optic atrophy
- Pseudotumor cerebri

Neuro-ophthalmologic
- Preganglionic Horner's syndrome
- Argyll Robertson pupils
- Bells palsy (may be recurring or bilateral)
- EOM palsies
- Orbital myositis
- Brainstem disorders
  - Skew deviation
  - Internuclear ophthalmoplegia
- Cortical blindness

Note: Because of the many potential conditions patient follow-up will depend on the type and severity of the ocular manifestations.

- If a tick bite occurred, how long was the tick attached to the skin? (Transmission of disease is extremely unlikely with less than 24 to 48 hours of tick attachment.)
- Hunters, campers, forest rangers, and the like may be at increased risk for Lyme disease.

Ancillary Tests

A clinical diagnosis of early Lyme disease in a patient with typical erythema migrans, in an endemic area, does not require laboratory confirmation.

Patients with nonspecific symptoms without objective signs of Lyme disease should not have serologic testing performed. Despite an enzyme-linked immunosorbent assay (ELISA) sensitivity of 89% and specificity of 72%, if the clinical suspicion is low, a positive test is more likely to be a false-positive than a true-positive.

The culture of *B. burgdorferi* from specimens on Barbour-Stoenner-Kelly medium permits a definitive diagnosis. However, positive cultures are usually obtained only early in the illness from biopsy samples of the EM lesions and generally have a fairly low yield. Laboratory confirmation typically requires detection of specific antibodies to *B. burgdorferi* (IgM and IgG) in serum by ELISA, followed by a Western blot test if the ELISA is positive.

Note: ELISA testing is frequently negative in stage 1 disease, which may then require acute and convalescent titers. A fourfold rise in antibody titer would be diagnostic of recent infection.

False-positive responses in the ELISA have been reported in Rocky Mountain spotted fever, Behçet's disease, syphilis, sarcoid, Vogt-Koyanagi-Harada (VKH) syndrome, systemic lupus erythematosus (SLE), juvenile rheumatoid arthritis (JRA), infectious mononucleosis, subacute infective endocarditis, leptospirosis, and viral illnesses, and in patients with gingival disease.

Later in the infection, polymerase chain reaction (PCR) testing is greatly superior to culture in the detection of *B. burgdorferi* in joint fluid. Up to 85% of synovial fluid samples are positive in active arthritis. It is questionable whether a positive PCR indicates active infection or is a marker for residual DNA indicative of an autoimmune arthritis.

The Treatment

Most features of Lyme disease respond to antibiotics, but the time to complete resolution may extend well beyond the treatment period. Despite the time lag, chronic antibiotic therapy is not indicated.

Treatment of early disease is most successful, leading to quicker and more complete recovery. Approximately 15% of patients who are untreated in stage 1 will develop stage 2 disease; however, up to 80% of patients not treated in stage 2 will ultimately develop stage 3 disease.

Stage 1 disease can usually be treated on an outpatient basis; stages 2 and 3 may require more intensive therapy based on symptoms (i.e., patients with objective neurologic findings such as meningitis require extended treatment with IV antibiotics). Prior treatment with systemic corticosteroids may make antibiotic therapy less effective.

For an early localized or early disseminated uncomplicated infection:

- Doxycycline, 100 mg p.o. bid for 10 to 14 days (do not use in children <12 or in pregnant women), or
- Amoxicillin, 500 mg p.o. tid for 10 to 14 days (pediatric dose 50 mg/kg/day in three divided doses), or

- Cefuroxime axetil, 500 mg p.o. bid for 10 to 14 days (pediatric dose 30 mg/kg/day in two divided doses), or
- Azithromycin, 500 mg p.o. qd for 7 to 10 days

Stage 2 and 3 disease often mandates treatment with IV antibiotics (i.e., ceftriaxone, cefotaxime, penicillin G) and requires careful monitoring over a period of months to years, based on severity of symptoms.

A Jarisch-Herxheimer–like reaction occurs in approximately 15% of patients within 24 hours of therapy.

Note: Prevention is the best way to avoid getting Lyme disease. Patients should be advised of the following:

- Avoid prime tick habitats.
- In tick-infested areas, wear a hat, long-sleeved shirts, and long pants with socks drawn up over the pants.
- Insect sprays that contain "deet" repel ticks. Use according to directions.
- Ticks prefer warm moist areas of the body, so thoroughly inspect the groin area, armpits, and scalp. If a tick is found, remove it immediately with tweezers.
- A vaccine for Lyme disease (LYMErix) is available in the United States and should be considered for individuals between the ages of 4 and 70 years who live in or visit high-risk areas and have frequent or prolonged exposure to *I. scapalaris* ticks. Three injections at 0, 1, and 12 months are recommended, but immunization only provides a 75% efficacy in preventing disease, and boosters are needed on a regular basis.

Because the vaccine is not always effective against Lyme disease, may be associated with minor adverse events, and does not protect against other tickborne infections, vigilance for tick bites must remain a priority.

Chapter 17

Glaucoma and Related Conditions

OCULAR HYPERTENSION (OHT)
G. Richard Bennett

ICD—9: 365.01

THE DISEASE
Pathophysiology

OHT is a condition in which elevated intraocular pressure is found in individuals without detectable glaucomatous damage on standard clinical tests such as automated perimetry and optic nerve head evaluation. Elevated intraocular pressure is generally defined as IOPs greater than 21 mm Hg or 22 mm Hg by Goldmann tonometry. An estimated three to six million people in the United States, including 4 to 7% of those older than 40 years, are at increased risk of developing primary open-angle glaucoma and subsequent visual loss. There is much evidence that substantial damage occurs to the optic nerve fibers before glaucomatous damage is detectable by current clinical methods. The Ocular Hypertensive Treatment Study (OHTS) found that 9.5% of ocular hypertensives suffered clearly detectable clinical damage to the visual field and/or the optic nerve in the first 60 months of that study. Prophylactic medical treatment reduced the risk of developing damage to the optic nerve and visual field by more than 50% during the first 60 months of the OHTS.

Etiology

The precise etiology for ocular hypertension has not yet been determined, but most authorities attribute the elevated intraocular pressure to a reduced aqueous outflow facility in patients at risk.

The Patient

Clinical Symptoms
OHT is a condition without symptoms, which sometimes leads to difficulty in educating the patient with respect to the importance of close observation and possibly treatment.

Clinical Signs

- Ocular hypertension is associated with elevated IOPs but normal optic nerve head appearance and normal threshold visual fields. Central corneal thickness (CCT), as measured by corneal pachymetry, is variable but may contribute valuable information with respect to risk of progression. The OHTS demonstrated a substantially higher risk to ocular hypertensives with large cup/disc ratios but relatively thin (below 555 microns) central corneal thicknesses. It is important NOT to apply this to other glaucoma suspects who do not show elevated IOPs, as OHT individuals have a considerably thicker average CCT (570 microns) than the general population.
- Gonioscopy will demonstrate normal anterior chamber depth and anatomy.
- Ophthalmoscopy will show a healthy optic nerve head with an intact neuroretinal rim 360°.

Demographics

Groups at higher risk include patients with very elevated intraocular pressures, African Americans, older patients, patients with large vertical cup/disc ratios (>0.5), and patients with thin CCTs (<555 microns).

Significant History

A family history of primary open-angle glaucoma (POAG) and a personal history of vascular disease are considered significant risk factors by many authorities.

Ancillary Tests

- Threshold visual fields
- Pachymetry
- Optic nerve photography (stereo)
- Imaging (HRT II, GDx, OCT)

The Treatment

The initial management is generally close observation. The OHTS demonstrated that patients with OHT are at risk for significant vision loss but that this is generally a slowly progressive condition and most patients will never require treatment. It is critical to identify those patients at greatest risk (high IOPs, thin CCTs, large cup/disc ratios) and treat those patients. Treatment is usually topical medical therapy. Laser (ALT/SLT) or surgical intervention would only be considered under extraordinary conditions without demonstrable visual field or optic nerve damage.

Initial Medical Therapy

The following medications are options for initial therapy:

- Topical prostaglandin analogs (latanoprost 0.005%, travoprost 0.004%, or bimatoprost 0.03%) at bedtime

- Topical β-blocker (timolol 0.25 to 0.5%, levobunolol 0.25 to 0.5%, betaxolol 0.25% or carteolol 1.0%) q AM or bid
- Topical brimonidine 0.15 or 0.2% three times a day
- Topical carbonic anhydrase inhibitors (dorzolamide 2% or brinzolamide 1%) three times a day

PRIMARY OPEN-ANGLE GLAUCOMA (POAG)
G. Richard Bennett and Michael B. Caplan

ICD—9: 365.11

THE DISEASE
Pathophysiology

POAG is a progressive optic neuropathy that is associated with an elevated intraocular pressure, progressive cupping of the optic nerve, and visual field loss. Intraocular pressure is thought to be elevated because of an obstruction to aqueous outflow through the trabecular meshwork.

Etiology

While the exact etiology is unclear, elevated intraocular pressure plays an important role in the development of POAG. Glaucoma probably has a polygenetic mode of inheritance.

The Patient

Clinical Symptoms
POAG is usually asymptomatic. In advanced stages, the patient may complain of decreased peripheral or central vision.

Clinical Signs
POAG is usually bilateral but can be asymmetric. The intraocular pressure is usually >21 mm Hg.; however, because intraocular pressure fluctuates, it does not have to be >21 mm Hg on every examination. As many as 25% of patients with open-angle glaucoma present initially with IOPs lower than 22 mm Hg. Gonioscopy demonstrates an open anterior chamber angle without anatomic abnormalities and should be considered an important procedure in the evaluation of a glaucoma suspect. There are no specific corneal or iris abnormalities. Fundus examination (best achieved by a binocular examination of the posterior pole with a 60, 78, or 90 diopter lens, or a fundus contact lens) can reveal increased or asymmetric cupping, as well as notching or thinning of the neuroretinal rim. Splinter disc hemorrhages are occasionally seen and suggest the glaucoma is not adequately controlled, especially in patients with relatively low pretreatment IOPs. Defects in the nerve fiber layer may precede progressive optic nerve cupping. Common visual field defects include nasal steps, arcuate defects, and

paracentral scotomas, often with significant asymmetry between the superior and inferior hemifields. The OHTS has demonstrated the importance of performing pachymetry to determine central corneal thickness in POAG and OHT (ocular hypertension) patients.

Demographics

The risk factors for developing POAG include an elevated intraocular pressure, increased age, family history of glaucoma in a first-degree relative, Hispanic or African American race, high myopia, thin central corneal thickness, and possibly vascular diseases. Ocular hypertension is a significant risk factor, but most people with ocular hypertension do not develop glaucoma (optic nerve changes and visual field defects).

Significant History

- History of risk factors (family history of POAG, age, race, diabetes mellitus, myopia >8D, systemic hypertension, and/or systemic hypotension)
- A history of pulmonary disease, heart disease, kidney stones, depression, and drug allergies is important in determining appropriate therapy for glaucoma

Ancillary Tests

- Threshold visual fields
- Pachymetry
- Optic nerve head photography (stereo)
- Imaging (HRT II, GDx, OCT)
- Color vision testing
- Diurnal IOPs

The Treatment

Topical medical treatment may include:

1. Prostaglandin Analogs
   Prostaglandin analogs have become a major first-line drug in the treatment of open-angle glaucoma because of superior efficacy, convenience, and safety.
   - Latanoprost (Xalatan 0.005%) at bedtime
   - Bimatoprost (Lumigan 0.03%) at bedtime
   - Travoprost (Travatan 0.004%) at bedtime
   - Unoprostone isopropyl (Rescula 0.15%) twice a day (actually a docosanoid and the least effective of this class of drugs)
2. Topical β-blockers
   Topical β-blockers were traditionally the first line of medical therapy unless contraindicated by medical conditions.
3. Selective β-blockers
   - β-1 selective: Betaxolol (Betoptic 0.5% twice a day, Betoptic-S 0.25% twice a day)
4. Nonselective β-blockers
   - Timolol maleate (Timoptic 0.25% twice a day, Timoptic 0.5% twice a day, Timoptic XE 0.25 or 0.5% qam every day)
   - Timolol hemihydrate (Betimol 0.25 or 0.5% twice a day)

- Levobunolol (Betagan 0.25% every day or twice a day, Betagan 0.5% every day or twice a day)
- Metipranolol (Optipranolol 0.3% twice a day)—may be associated with uveitis
- Nonselective with ISA (intrinsic sympathomimetic activity): Carteolol (Ocupress 1.0% twice a day)
- Combination with dorzolamide (Cosopt twice a day = 0.5% Timoptic + 2.0% Trusopt)

5. Topical Carbonic Anhydrase Inhibitors
   - Dorzolamide (Trusopt 2.0% three times a day)
   - Brinzolamide (Azopt 1.0% three times a day)
6. Miotics
   - Pilocarpine is started in low concentrations (0.5 to 1.0%) and increased (up to 2.0 to 6.0%) depending on the intraocular pressure and patient tolerance. Pilocarpine is frequently given four times a day; however, two or three times a day dosing may be sufficient in some cases.
   - Pilocarpine can also be prescribed as a gel (Pilopine gel 4% at bedtime) or as an implant (Ocusert pilo-20, which is replaced weekly).
   - Other miotics (carbachol 1.5 to 3.0% three times a day, phospholine iodide 0.06, 0.125, 0.25% twice a day) are occasionally used in pseudophakic or aphakic patients.

   Note: Miotics are not commonly used in the United States today because of newer, more effective medications with fewer side effects.

7. Epinephrine Compounds (not commonly used in the United States today)
   - Dipivefrin (Propine 0.1% twice a day)
   - Epinephrine 1 to 2% (Epifrin once or twice daily)
8. α-Agonists
   - Apraclonidine (Iopidine 0.5% three times a day)—not generally used as a maintenance drug because of significant tachyphalaxis. Very useful in short-term lowering of IOP.
   - Brimonidine 0.2% three times a day, 0.15% with purite preservative three times a day (Alphagan-P)

   Note: Oral medical treatment—used in urgent care for very elevated IOPs but used rarely today for treatment of POAG because of significant side effects.

9. Carbonic Anhydrase Inhibitors
   - Methazolamide (25-mg or 50-mg tablets) 25 to 100 mg orally two to three times a day
   - Acetazolamide (250 mg orally four times a day or 500-mg sequels orally twice a day)
10. Laser Surgery
    - Argon laser trabeculoplasty (ALT) is effective in reducing the intraocular pressure in approximately 80% of patients with POAG. The intraocular pressure frequently increases over time and the success rate drops to 40 to 50% after 5 years.
    - Selective laser trabeculoplasty (SLT) is as effective as ALT and may be repeatable after the treatment effect decreases over time.

11. Filtration Surgery
    ■ Trabeculectomy has an 80 to 90% success rate in lowering intraocular pressure to ≤21 mmHg in patients with POAG. Antimetabolites, such as 5-FU and Mitomycin-C, are useful in cases that are at an increased risk for failure.
12. Other Surgical Options
    ■ Shunt tubes (Molteno, Schocket, Baerveldt, Ahmed, etc.)
    ■ Cyclodestructive procedures (cyclocryotherapy or laser transscleral cyclophotocoagulation or endophotocoagulation of the ciliary processes)

There is not a "cookbook" for the treatment of POAG. Each patient must be considered individually to determine the appropriate treatment. Factors to consider include: age of the patient, medical history (avoid topical β-blockers in patients with emphysema, asthma, heart block, decompensated heart failure), ocular history (prostaglandin analogs may exacerbate epithelial HSV keratitis, CME, uveitis), drug allergies, comfort, convenience, and compliance. Lastly, each practitioner should consider the safety, cost, dosage frequency, side effects, and efficacy of all medications.

LOW/NORMAL-TENSION GLAUCOMA (NTG)
G. Richard Bennett and Michael B. Caplan

ICD—9: 365.12

THE DISEASE
Pathophysiology

Low-tension glaucoma (or normal-tension glaucoma) is present when there is optic nerve cupping, visual field defects consistent with glaucoma, and intraocular pressures <22 mm Hg without treatment. No other identifiable cause is present for the cupping and visual field changes. It is critical to exclude contributing systemic diseases (vascular occlusive disease, space-occupying lesions, etc.) before establishing a diagnosis of NTG.

Etiology

NTG has been shown to be a pressure-dependent disease, with IOP lowering of 30% or more often proving beneficial in slowing the rate of progression. Etiology is elusive with non-IOP–dependent risk factors such as hypotension, cardiovascular disease, atrial fibrillation, migraine syndrome, apoptosis, vasospasm, connective tissue disorders, anemia, sleep apnea, and hypothyroidism, potentially contributing to the disease process.

The Patient

Clinical Symptoms
Like many other types of glaucoma, patients are usually asymptomatic until the optic nerve damage is severe enough to cause visual loss.

Clinical Signs

Optic nerve cupping is present and can be asymmetric. Superficial disc hemorrhages and peripapillary atrophy appear to be more common in low-tension glaucoma compared to primary open-angle glaucoma and may have a greater significance with respect to progression. Visual field defects are frequently like those in primary open-angle glaucoma. Often the visual field defects are denser and steeper and involve the paracentral area with encroachment of fixation. Intraocular pressure is consistently <22 mm Hg. The angle is open by gonioscopy without peripheral anterior synechiae. Exclude other retinal and optic nerve anomalies (i.e., colobomas, optic pits, tilted disc, myopic discs, ischemic optic neuropathy, macular disease, retinal artery occlusion, drusen, etc.).

Demographics

Low-tension glaucoma is more common in elderly patients. It is unusual to diagnose low-tension glaucoma in patients less than 50 years of age.

Significant History

It is important to note other causes of glaucoma or other conditions that could produce similar optic nerve and visual field changes. Ask about previous ocular trauma, steroid use, uveitis (red eye and photophobia), hypotensive episodes, sleep-disordered breathing or sleep apnea, anemia, ischemic optic neuropathy, or angle-closure glaucoma.

Patients taking oral or topical β-blockers at nighttime may be at increased risk for progressive vision loss.

Ancillary Tests

Automated visual field testing and a stereoscopic evaluation of the optic nerve (with a slit lamp and a 60-, 78-, or 90-diopter lens, fundus contact lens, or Hruby lens) are performed. Diurnal IOP measurements can be helpful in identifying patients with intermittent pressure elevations >21 mm Hg.

Pachymetry is indicated as thin corneas can underestimate the true IOP.

Hematologic studies including a CBC (for anemia or polycythemia), RPR, FTA-ABS (for syphilis), and an ESR (for temporal arteritis) may be useful in some cases.

Blood pressure and pulse should be measured.

Multiple IOP measurements at different times of the day should be obtained prior to initiating therapy.

It may be appropriate to have the patient see an internist for a complete exam, emphasizing the need to investigate for cardiovascular disease and carotid occlusive disease.

In unusual cases (patients <60 years of age, visual fields that are rapidly progressive or show defects that respect the vertical midline, reduced central visual acuity, asymmetry of the cups or fields with symmetrical IOPs, or discs that show more pallor than cupping), consider neuroimaging (CT scan or MRI).

The Treatment

Treatment for low-tension glaucoma is similar to primary open-angle glaucoma. Attempt to lower the intraocular pressure by at least 30% below the level where damage has occurred. Reduction in pressure may be accomplished by medical therapy, laser trabeculoplasty, or filtration surgery.

Medical Therapy
- Brimonidine 0.15 or 0.2% three times a day
- β-blockers: Betaxolol 0.25 to 0.5% twice a day, carteolol 1.0% twice a day, and so on. Note that some authorities suggest that topical noncardioselective β-blockers may interfere with perfusion to the ONH and are not the ideal therapy in NTG.
- Topical carbonic anhydrase inhibitors: Dorzolamide 2% or brinzolamide 1% three times a day.
- Latanoprost (Xalatan 0.005%), travoprost (Travatan 0.004%), or brimatoprost (Lumigan 0.03%) once a day in the evening.

Argon laser trabeculoplasty (ALT) or selective laser trabeculoplasty (SLT) may be effective in some low-tension patients; however, the results have been inconsistent.

Filtration surgery is used when progressive optic nerve cupping and visual field loss occurs and there is significant danger of loss of quality of life and the intraocular pressure cannot be lowered with more conservative therapy. If a low target pressure is desired, consider trabeculectomy with early suture lysis and/or antimetabolites (such as Mitomycin-C or 5-FU) or full-thickness procedures.

Recent studies have advocated the use of oral calcium-channel blockers in patients with low-tension glaucoma who have progressive cupping or visual field loss. Proof of their efficacy awaits the results of future long-term studies. It is important for NTG patients to avoid taking these agents just prior to sleep with resultant lowering of blood pressure and perfusion to the optic nerve.

STEROID-INDUCED GLAUCOMA
G. Richard Bennett and Michael B. Caplan

ICD—9: 365.03

THE DISEASE

Pathophysiology

Steroid-induced elevations in intraocular pressure appear to be secondary to decreased facility of aqueous outflow. There are several proposed mechanisms, including an accumulation of glycosaminoglycans or aqueous debris in the trabecular meshwork because of inhibition of phagocytosis or inhibition of prostaglandin synthesis, or possibly a certain protein(s) may initiate the response.

Etiology

Elevated intraocular pressure has been associated most commonly with the use of topical steroid eyedrops or periocular repository steroid injections. The pressure response can occur within a week or may be delayed for months or years. Systemic steroids, steroid creams used on the skin near the eye or in areas away from the eye, inhaled steroids, injected steroids, implantable steroids, and nasal corticosteroids have all been associated with an increase in intraocular pressure.

The Patient

Clinical Symptoms

The patient is usually asymptomatic unless the intraocular pressure increases enough to cause corneal edema (decreased vision, halos, photophobia) or pain. The patient may have symptoms from the ocular disorder that is being treated with steroids (photophobia from iritis).

Clinical Signs

Prolonged elevations of intraocular pressure can cause optic nerve cupping and visual field defects similar to primary open-angle glaucoma. Clinical signs of the ocular disorder that is being treated with steroids can be seen (cells, flare, anterior or posterior synechiae, or engorged iris vessels from iritis), as can other ocular side effects of chronic ocular steroid use, such as posterior subcapsular cataracts or atrophy of the skin near the eyelids.

Demographics

Steroid-induced elevations in intraocular pressure are more common in patients with pre-existing glaucoma, high myopes (>5D), diabetics, and in those with a family history of glaucoma.

Approximately one-third of the normal population will develop a moderate increase in IOP following ocular, topical corticosteroid use; however, 5 to 6% will show a markedly elevated IOP response.

Significant History

Significant history includes the type of steroid and the duration of use, previous ocular disorders, a history of diabetes mellitus or myopia, or a family history of glaucoma.

Ancillary Tests

- Threshold visual fields
- Stereo disc photographs
- Gonioscopy
- Laser interferometry (if cataracts are present)

The Treatment

Steroid-induced intraocular pressure elevations almost always respond within days to weeks of stopping the steroids. It is not always possible to abruptly stop steroids because of the underlying ocular disorder being treated. In patients with iritis, it is often difficult to determine whether the increased intraocular pressure is because of steroids or inflammation. If iritis is still present, increase the steroid to treat the iritis and consider medical therapy to reduce the IOP. When the inflammation has decreased then taper the steroids.

Options for treatment include:

- Decreasing the effects of steroids by:
  - Stopping the steroid.
  - Decreasing the frequency or strength of the steroid being used.
  - Using a different type of steroid (fluorometholone, rimexolone, loteprednol, or medrysone are less prone to pressure elevations than prednisolone or dexamethasone).
  - Using nonsteroidal anti-inflammatory eyedrops (diclofenac 0.1%, ketorolac 0.5%) instead of steroids.
- Medications to decrease the intraocular pressure may be needed if the intraocular pressure is very high or if the elevated intraocular pressure persists after changing, reducing, or stopping the steroids.
  - β-blockers (timolol 0.25 to 0.5% twice a day, levobunolol 0.25 to 0.5% once or twice a day, Timoptic XE 0.25 to 0.5% once a day, carteolol 1.0% twice a day, betaxolol 0.25 to 0.5% twice a day)
  - Apraclonidine 0.5% three times a day or brimonidine 0.15 or 0.2% three times a day
  - Carbonic anhydrase inhibitors (dorzolamide 2% three times a day, brinzolamide 1% three times a day, methazolamide 25 to 50 mg one to two tablets orally two to three times a day, or acetazolamide 250 mg orally four times a day or 500-mg sequels orally twice a day)
  - Miotics and prostaglandin analogs should be avoided if the patient has recently had ocular inflammatory disease.
- Removal of an injected intraocular or periocular steroid may be required.
- Occasionally, glaucoma surgery is necessary if the intraocular pressure does not respond to discontinuing the steroid and/or medical therapy.

GLAUCOMA ASSOCIATED WITH INFLAMMATION

G. Richard Bennett and Michael B. Caplan

ICD—9: 365.62

THE DISEASE

Pathophysiology

Intraocular inflammation can cause an elevated intraocular pressure by several different mechanisms. Inflammation can increase resistance to aqueous outflow by causing dysfunction or swelling of trabecular sheets and endothelial cells or by causing a breakdown in the blood-aqueous barrier, which allows inflammatory cells or fibrin to accumulate in the trabecular meshwork. Prostaglandin production may produce elevated intraocular pressure by causing a breakdown in the blood-aqueous barrier. If posterior synechiae, secondary to inflammation, completely obstruct the flow of aqueous humour from the posterior to the anterior chamber, the peripheral iris will bow forward, causing iris bombe. This bowing can cause acute or chronic angle-closure glaucoma. Peripheral anterior synechiae formation may cause chronic angle-closure glaucoma. In many instances, multiple mechanisms occur simultaneously.

Etiology

There are many etiologies of intraocular inflammation (see sections on uveitis). Frequently the cause of iridocyclitis is never determined.

One must distinguish uveitic glaucoma from angle-closure glaucoma, which may produce a mild to moderate iritis.

The Patient

Clinical Symptoms
Photophobia, red eye, pain, and decreased vision may be present.

Clinical Signs
Elevated intraocular pressure, ciliary flush, flare and cells in the anterior chamber and anterior vitreous, miosis, keratic precipitates, and engorged iris vessels may be seen. Gonioscopy is important to determine whether the angle is open or whether peripheral anterior synechiae partially or completely close the angle. Chronically elevated IOP may cause optic nerve and visual field changes.

Demographics

The demographics of the group at risk will depend on the etiology of the intraocular inflammation.

Significant History
- Previous history of intraocular inflammation
- Duration of current symptoms
- Presence of systemic diseases associated with intraocular inflammation
  - Sarcoidosis
  - Ankylosing spondylitis
  - Juvenile rheumatoid arthritis
  - Behçet's disease, ulcerative colitis, Crohn's disease, and so on
- History of trauma

Ancillary Tests

See the section on uveitis for the approach to and laboratory tests for suspected etiologies of intraocular inflammation. Secondary glaucomas should specifically be excluded. Usual glaucoma testing (visual fields, gonioscopy, optic nerve photography, etc.) may be indicated in some patients.

The Treatment

- Topical steroids are titrated, depending on the severity of intraocular inflammation. The specific steroid used will depend on the amount of inflammation and how well the intraocular pressure can be controlled. Traumatic uveitis may not require aggressive therapy, while some inflammatory situations require frequent (every hour) instillation of steroids. Prednisolone acetate 1.0% and dexamethasone 0.1% are potent anti-inflammatory agents and are very useful in treating moderate to severe inflammatory disease. These agents show a higher incidence of steroid-induced elevated intraocular pressure than fluorometholone 0.1 or 0.5%. Rimexolone 1% or loteprednol 0.5% also offers potent anti-inflammatory properties with a lower incidence of intraocular pressure elevation than prednisolone acetate, prednisolone phosphate, or dexamethasone. Certain inflammatory conditions (epithelial herpes simplex keratitis, fungal infections, etc.) may preclude intervention with steroids.
- Periocular or systemic steroids are sometimes indicated for severe inflammation or inflammation that is not responsive to topical steroids.
- Cycloplegic eyedrops one to three times per day (scopolamine 0.25%, homatropine 5.0%, cyclopentolate 1.0%, or atropine 1.0%) are used to decrease pain from ciliary spasm and decrease the potential for posterior synechiae.
- Topical nonsteroidal anti-inflammatory drops (ketorolac 0.5%, diclofenac 0.1%) are sometimes helpful as an adjuvant to topical steroids. They are titrated according to the level of inflammation.
- Control the intraocular pressure.
  - Topical β-blockers (timolol 0.25 to 0.5% twice a day, levobunolol 0.25 to 0.5% twice a day, Timoptic XE 0.25 to 0.5% once a day, carteolol 1.0% twice a day, betaxolol 0.25 to 0.5% twice a day)
  - Carbonic anhydrase inhibitors (dorzolamide 2% or brinzolamide 1% drops three times a day, methazolamide 25 to 50 mg one to two tablets orally two to three times a day, acetazolamide 250 mg orally four times a day or 500-mg sequels twice a day)
  - Topical apraclonidine 0.5% three times a day or brimonidine 0.15 or 0.2% three times a day
  - Oral or intravenous osmotic agents if the initial pressure is very high (oral isosorbide 45% 1.0 to 1.5 g/kg, oral glycerol 50% 1.0 to 1.5 g/kg or IV mannitol 20% 1 to 2 g/kg over 45 to 60 minutes)
  - Occasionally glaucoma filtration surgery with local antimetabolite therapy (mitomycin-C or 5 FU) is indicated if the intraocular pressure cannot be controlled medically.

Note: Avoid miotics (pilocarpine), prostaglandin analogs, and laser trabeculoplasty while inflammation is present.
- Treat the underlying systemic disease if one is present.

GLAUCOMATOCYCLITIC CRISIS (POSNER-SCHLOSSMAN [P-S] SYNDROME)
Nicky R. Holdeman and Michael B. Caplan

ICD: 364.22

THE DISEASE
Pathophysiology

Glaucomatocyclitic crisis is an unusual type of acute, recurrent uveitis and secondary glaucoma.

The exact mechanism of this condition is unknown; however, trabeculitis may contribute to the pathogenesis, as tonographic studies indicate a reduction in outflow facility during an attack.

Etiology

While the exact etiology has yet to be defined, herpes simplex virus and prostaglandin E have both been implicated as possible causes.

Increased levels of prostaglandins in the anterior chamber may account for the decreased facility of outflow and breakdown of the blood aqueous barrier.

The Patient

Clinical Symptoms
In general, symptoms are remarkably mild and few in relation to the magnitude of the intraocular pressure.

The patient may be asymptomatic, or may report slight discomfort, blurred vision, and halos if the intraocular pressure is significantly elevated and corneal epithelial edema is present.

Clinical Signs
Glaucomatocyclitic crisis is generally unilateral and is associated with a significant increase in intraocular pressure (>30 mm Hg and often between 40 and 60 mm Hg). Inflammation is minimal. There are a few cells and mild flare in the anterior chamber. Keratic precipitates appear for a few days, are small, flat, and nonpigmented, and tend to appear in the lower third of the cornea. The conjunctiva has minimal injection. The angle is open, and there are no anterior or posterior synechiae. Occasionally there is heterochromia with slight pupillary constriction or pupillary enlargement of the affected eye.

Between attacks, all tests are within normal limits, including IOP and outflow facility.

Demographics

Usually occurs in patients between the ages of 20 to 50 years and is seldom seen after the age of 60.

Significant History

The patient may report intermittent episodes of unilateral blurred vision and ocular discomfort as recurrent attacks are common. Recurrences tend to occur at intervals of a few months to several years.

Ancillary Tests

There appears to be an association of glaucomatocyclitic crisis with primary open-angle glaucoma. Some patients can experience optic nerve cupping and visual field loss because of repeated attacks or because of underlying POAG. Consequently, patients with P-S syndrome should undergo a complete glaucoma evaluation (e.g., gonioscopy, pachymetry, stereo disc photos, and formal visual field testing).

The Treatment

Glaucomatocyclitic crisis is self-limited and will usually resolve with or without treatment. The episodes typically last from several hours to a few weeks. Between attacks, the patient is asymptomatic, the intraocular pressure is normal, and there is no intraocular inflammation.

The treatment of glaucomatocyclitic crisis is aimed at controlling the intraocular pressure, decreasing inflammation, and maintaining ocular comfort during an acute attack. Treatment is usually not required between episodes.

- Topical β-blocker (timolol 0.5% bid, levobunolol 0.5% bid, metipranolol 0.3% bid, carteolol 1.0% bid, betaxolol 0.25% bid)
- Topical α-agonist (apraclonidine 0.5% or brimonidine 0.15 or 0.20% bid-tid)
- Topical carbonic anhydrase inhibitors *or* oral CAI if necessary (dorzolamide 2% tid, brinzolamide 1% tid, methazolamide 25 to 50 mg one to two tablets p.o. bid-tid, acetazolamide 250-mg tablets p.o. qid or 500-mg sequels p.o. bid)
- Topical steroids (fluorometholone 0.1 or 0.25% qid, rimexolone 1% qid, or lotoprednol 0.5% qid)
- Cycloplegic agents for comfort if needed (cyclopentolate 1.0%, bid-tid, homatropine 5% bid-tid). Cycloplegics are seldom required, as there is little ciliary muscle spasm.
- Oral NSAIDs (indomethacin) and topical NSAIDs have been effective in reducing inflammation and in lowering the IOP in some patients.

Note: Patients with P-S syndrome have an increased incidence of elevated IOP in response to topical steroids. Prolonged treatment with corticosteroids should be avoided.

Laser trabeculoplasty (ALT/SLT) is generally not effective in controlling the elevations in IOP.

NEOVASCULAR GLAUCOMA
G. Richard Bennett and Michael B. Caplan

ICD—9: 365.63

THE DISEASE
Pathophysiology

Retinal hypoxia, caused by numerous etiologies, provides the stimulus for neovascularization of the iris and the anterior chamber angle. Neovascularization of the iris consists of a fibrovascular membrane that can obstruct outflow through the trabecular meshwork either by covering the anterior chamber angle or by contracting, which causes peripheral anterior synechiae formation.

Etiology

The most common causes of retinal hypoxia resulting in neovascular glaucoma are diabetic retinopathy, central retinal vein occlusion (CRVO), and ocular ischemic syndrome (carotid occlusive disease). Some of the other etiologies include branch retinal vein occlusion, central retinal artery occlusion, chronic retinal detachment, chronic uveitis, intraocular tumors, radiation therapy, and trauma.

The Patient
Clinical Symptoms
Occasionally neovascular glaucoma is asymptomatic. More often, symptoms include red eye, pain, decreased vision, and photophobia. Nausea and vomiting may be present if the intraocular pressure is very high.

Clinical Signs
Neovascularization of the iris can be confined to the pupillary margin or may extend into the angle. Conjunctival injection, corneal edema, iritis, significant elevations of intraocular pressure, hyphema, and ectropion uvea are frequently present. Gonioscopy may reveal an open angle with or without neovascularization, or may demonstrate partial or complete closure secondary to anterior synechiae. Retinal examination may reveal proliferative diabetic retinopathy, retinal hemorrhages or shunt vessels from previous vascular occlusions, or other retinal pathology that may help determine the cause of ocular ischemia.

Demographics

The demographics depend on the etiology of the retinal hypoxia. However, proliferative diabetic retinopathy (PDR) is the most common cause of neovascular glaucoma. About 33% of patients with proliferative diabetic retinopathy will develop rubeosis irides.

Significant History

The medical history is essential in determining the cause of neovascular glaucoma. Diabetics will usually have a long history of poorly controlled diabetes mellitus. Patients with CRVO are typically vasculopathic and will usually relate a sudden, unilateral, painless, visual loss within the past 6 months. In ocular ischemic syndrome, a history of stroke, amaurosis fugax, chronic ocular or periocular pain, and medical or surgical treatment for carotid occlusive disease may be elicited.

Ancillary Tests

Fluorescein angiography can help determine the etiology and extent of ocular ischemia. Patients suspected of having ocular ischemic syndrome will need noninvasive studies to assess the degree of carotid artery obstruction. A HbA1C should be obtained on all diabetic patients at least three times per year.

The Treatment

The goals of treatment are to identify and eliminate the hypoxic stimulus in order to promote regression of neovascularization, to reduce the intraocular pressure, and to control pain and ocular inflammation.

- If the retina can be visualized, prompt panretinal photocoagulation is the treatment of choice to eliminate the hypoxic stimulus. If the view to the retina is poor, retinal cryotherapy, transcleral retinopexy, or retinal endolaser may be used. If ocular ischemia is secondary to carotid occlusive disease, a carotid endarterectomy or stent may be indicated.
- To control intraocular pressure:
  - β-blockers (timolol 0.25 to 0.5% twice a day, levobunolol 0.25 to 0.5% twice a day, Timoptic XE 0.25 to 0.5% once a day, carteolol 1.0% twice a day, or betaxolol 0.25 to 0.5% twice a day).
  - Apraclonidine 0.5 to 1.0% two to three times a day or brimonidine 0.15 or 0.20% three times a day.
  - Oral carbonic anhydrase inhibitors (methazolamide 25- to 50-mg tablets one to two orally two to three times a day, acetazolamide 250 mg orally four times a day or 500-mg sequels orally twice a day).
  - Oral or intravenous osmotic agents: one of the following may be indicated—use with caution in diabetics: Oral glycerol 50% 1.0 to 1.5 g/kg, oral isosorbide 45% 1.0 to 1.5 g/kg, IV mannitol 20% 1 to 2 g/kg over 45 minutes.
  - Trabeculectomy is indicated if the intraocular pressure is not adequately controlled with medical therapy. Antimetabolites, such as mitomycin C or 5-FU, are frequently used. Preferably iris neovascularization will have time to regress after retinal ablation prior to performing a trabeculectomy.
  - Shunt tubes, cyclocryotherapy, and transcleral laser cyclophotocoagulation can also be used to lower the intraocular pressure.

- Goniophotocoagulation (the use of laser to directly treat neovascularization in the angle) may be useful in slowing the rate of angle closure while waiting for regression of neovascularization following panretinal photocoagulation or retinal cryotherapy.
- Topical steroids (prednisolone, rimexolone, dexamethasone) and/or cycloplegic drops (scopolamine 0.25%, cyclopentolate 1.0%, or homatropine 5% three times a day) can help reduce inflammation, congestion, and pain.
- As in other inflammatory diseases, miotics, epinephrine, prostaglandins, and laser trabeculoplasty is contraindicated.

PIGMENTARY GLAUCOMA
G. Richard Bennett and Michael B. Caplan

ICD—9: 365.13

THE DISEASE
Pathophysiology

It has long been theorized that deposition of pigment in the trabecular meshwork causes the intraocular pressure to increase by impeding outflow of aqueous. If pigment dispersion is noted without evidence of glaucoma, pigment dispersion syndrome is present. If evidence of glaucoma is detected (elevated intraocular pressure, visual field loss, or optic nerve cupping), then pigmentary glaucoma is present.

Etiology

The dispersion of pigment is secondary to contact between the lens zonules and the iris. As the pigment is rubbed off the iris pigment epithelium, it is deposited in various ocular structures including the trabecular meshwork.

The Patient

Clinical Symptoms
Patients are usually asymptomatic. Intermittent blurred vision and halos may be reported if a sudden liberation of pigment causes the intraocular pressure to elevate significantly and corneal edema develops. Symptoms may occur after exercise or pupillary dilation.

Clinical Signs
There are many clinical signs of pigment dispersion. Slit-lamp examination may demonstrate Krukenberg's spindles (vertical linear accumulations of pigment in corneal endothelial cells), iris pigment dusting (which may cause heterochromia), midperipheral spoke-like iris transillumination defects, and pigment deposition on the periphery of the lens (Zentmayer ring or Scheie line). Pigmented cells in the anterior chamber are sometimes seen, particularly after dilation or vigorous physical activity. Gonioscopy reveals an open angle with increased pigmentation of the trabecular meshwork and

Schwalbe's line (Sampaolesi's line). The midperipheral iris may have a concave configuration. There are often wide fluctuations in intraocular pressure. Pigment dispersion is usually bilateral but may be more evident in one eye versus the other.

Demographics

Pigment dispersion syndrome and pigmentary glaucoma occur most often in myopic males between 20 and 50 years old. Approximately one-third of patients with pigment dispersion syndrome will eventually develop pigmentary glaucoma. Pigment dispersion is less common among African Americans but may be associated with radial depositions of pigment on the anterior lens capsule.

Significant History
- Episodes of blurred vision or halos

Ancillary Tests
- Threshold visual fields
- Gonioscopy
- Stereo optic nerve photography
- Tonometry after aerobic exercise

The Treatment

Medical Treatment
- Pilocarpine helps reduce zonular/iris contact and, therefore, can decrease the dispersion of pigment and lower the intraocular pressure. It is, however, poorly tolerated in many young adults because of accommodative spasm. With many other therapeutic choices, pilocarpine has become infrequently used. The incidence of retinal detachment is also increased in myopes using pilocarpine.
- β-blockers (timolol 0.25 to 0.5% twice a day, levobunolol 0.25 to 0.5% every day, twice a day, Timoptic XE 0.25 to 0.5% once a day, carteolol 1.0% twice a day, metipranolol 0.3% twice a day, betaxolol 0.25 to 0.5% twice a day) are effective at lowering the intraocular pressure in pigmentary glaucoma but do not decrease the liberation of pigment.
- Carbonic anhydrase inhibitors (dorzolamide 2% or brinzolamide 1% drops three times a day, methazolamide 25- to 50-mg one to two tablets orally two to three times a day, acetazolamide 250 mg orally four times a day or 500-mg sequels orally twice a day) are occasionally used if other medical or laser procedures are ineffective in lowering intraocular pressure.
- α agonist (brimonidine 0.15 or 0.2% three times a day) is useful, particularly in patients who cannot tolerate β-blockers.
- Prostaglandin agonists: latanoprost (Xalatan 0.005%), travoprost (Travatan 0.004%), or bimatoprost (Lumigan 0.03%) at bedtime.

Note: Aqueous suppressants could potentially increase the viscosity of the aqueous, thus exacerbating the concentration of pigment cells in the trabecular meshwork.

Surgical Therapy

- Laser trabeculoplasty of only one-half of the angle is usually sufficient to lower the intraocular pressure dramatically. Lower energy settings can often be used because of heavy trabecular meshwork pigmentation. The pressure lowering effect of trabeculoplasty is frequently lost earlier in pigmentary glaucoma than in primary open-angle glaucoma.
- Some data suggests that a peripheral iridectomy may be effective in decreasing pigment dispersion by equalizing the pressure in the anterior and posterior chambers, thereby reducing concavity of the iris and decreasing contact between the lens zonules and peripheral iris.
- If medical and laser therapy is not effective, trabeculectomy is indicated. (Patients with pigment dispersion syndrome can be followed without treatment in most cases.)

EXFOLIATIVE GLAUCOMA (PEX)
G. Richard Bennett and Michael B. Caplan

ICD—9: 365.52

THE DISEASE

Pathophysiology

Exfoliative glaucoma is a type of open-angle glaucoma in which white fibrillar material gets deposited in various locations in the eye. Exfoliation syndrome has the same clinical presentation without evidence of glaucoma. The exact mechanism of obstruction to aqueous outflow in exfoliative glaucoma is uncertain. It could be a result of blockage of the trabecular meshwork by exfoliative material, dysfunction of trabecular endothelial cells, or from the deposition of pigment in the trabecular meshwork. There is also a high prevalence of primary open-angle glaucoma in the contralateral eye of unilateral cases of exfoliative glaucoma. This suggests that an underlying predisposition to glaucoma may exist in some patients with exfoliation syndrome who go on to develop glaucoma.

Etiology

The exfoliative material comes from many sources as part of a generalized basement membrane disorder.

The Patient

Clinical Symptoms

The patients are usually asymptomatic until the glaucoma is very advanced.

Clinical Signs

Exfoliative glaucoma may be unilateral or bilateral but marked asymmetry is usually present. Unilateral cases can become bilateral. The most striking clinical finding in exfoliative glaucoma usually involves the lens, which characteristically has several zones of involvement of the anterior capsule. There is a peripheral granular zone, a middle clear zone, and a central translucent zone. The middle clear zone is felt to be caused by the action of the iris removing the exfoliative material from that area of the lens. Additional areas where exfoliative material can be seen include the pupillary margin, the corneal endothelium, the anterior chamber angle, the lens zonules, and the ciliary processes. Frequently iris transillumination defects can be seen at the pupillary margin.

Gonioscopy may reveal exfoliative material in the angle or a patchy increase in trabecular meshwork pigment. A Sampaolesi's line (pigmentation along Schwalbe's line) is seen most often inferiorly. Higher mean IOPs, asymmetric disease, and more advanced optic nerve damage is found more typically than in POAG.

Demographics

The prevalence of exfoliation syndrome and exfoliative glaucoma varies significantly in different populations and increases markedly with age. It is very common in Scandinavian countries and rare in Eskimos. The prevalence of exfoliation in patients with glaucoma exceeds 50% in some Scandinavian countries. Approximately 5% of patients with exfoliation syndrome will develop glaucoma within 5 years, and approximately 15% by 10 years. Older Caucasian women are most likely to be affected.

Significant History

- Scandinavian ancestry
- No clear hereditary pattern

Ancillary Tests

- Threshold visual fields
- Gonioscopy
- Optic nerve head photography
- Optic nerve imaging (HRTII, GDx, OCT)

The Treatment

- Exfoliative glaucoma can be treated medically, essentially the same as primary open-angle glaucoma. However, patients with PEX are often more resistant to medical therapy. There is a high success rate with argon laser trabeculoplasty. Trabeculectomy is indicated when the intraocular pressure is not controlled medically or with trabeculoplasty.
- Extraction of the lens is not effective in treating the glaucoma.
- Patients with exfoliative glaucoma may have weakened zonules that may increase the complication rate during cataract surgery.

CONGENITAL GLAUCOMA

G. Richard Bennett and Michael B. Caplan

ICD—9: 743.20

THE DISEASE

Pathophysiology

Congenital glaucoma includes primary congenital glaucoma and congenital glaucoma associated with other ocular and systemic abnormalities. During development, the iris and ciliary body do not recede posteriorly, therefore, they insert anteriorly into the trabecular meshwork. The obstruction to aqueous outflow causes the intraocular pressure to increase. There are numerous types of infantile glaucoma associated with other ocular or systemic conditions. These include aniridia, goniodysgenesis (Axenfeld-Rieger syndrome, Peter's anomaly), congenital rubella, phakomatoses (Sturge-Weber syndrome, neurofibromatosis), persistent hyperplastic primary vitreous, homocystinuria, Marfan's syndrome, Pierre-Robin syndrome, Lowe's syndrome, microcornea, and microspherophakia.

Etiology

The vast majority of cases of primary congenital glaucoma are sporadic; however, a polygenetic inheritance pattern may be involved in approximately 10% of cases.

The Patient

Clinical Symptoms
See Clinical Signs.

Clinical Signs
Primary congenital glaucoma is bilateral in 70% of cases. Common signs include elevated intraocular pressure, increased corneal diameter (>12 mm), blepharospasm, photophobia, tearing, corneal edema and clouding, optic nerve cupping, and Haab's striae (horizontal tears in Descemet's membrane). Gonioscopy reveals a flat, high iris insertion, and peripheral iris hypoplasia.

An exam under anesthesia is sometimes required to confirm the diagnosis. It is important to note that the intraocular pressure will decrease with most general anesthetic agents; therefore, tonometry is performed as soon as the patient is asleep. Ketamine is frequently used since the intraocular pressure usually does not decrease immediately, and, in fact, it can increase.

Demographics

Primary congenital glaucoma occurs in about 1 in 30,000 live births and accounts for about one-half of glaucoma in children. Approximately 60% of cases are diagnosed by age 6 months and 80% are diagnosed by 1 year; 65% of the patients are male. Approximately 20% of patients are noted to have Wilms' tumors.

Significant History

The date of onset of clinical signs (patients diagnosed before 1 month old and after 24 months old have a worse prognosis), the presence of other systemic abnormalities, a history of forceps delivery (which can cause corneal edema secondary to a tear in Descemet's membrane), infections during pregnancy, and a family history of congenital glaucoma are important to elicit.

Ancillary Tests

Clinical evaluation allows diagnosis.

The Treatment

Primary congenital glaucoma is best treated surgically. Goniotomy or trabeculotomy are the initial procedures of choice. Medical therapy is usually not successful in controlling the intraocular pressure, but it may be useful while the patient is awaiting surgery or as an adjuvant to surgery if the intraocular pressure is not sufficiently lowered by surgery alone.

LENS-INDUCED SECONDARY OPEN-ANGLE GLAUCOMA
G. Richard Bennett and Michael B. Caplan
ICD—9: 365.51

THE DISEASE
Pathophysiology

Lens-induced secondary open-angle glaucoma is divided into three entities:

- Phacolytic (lens protein) glaucoma occurs when lens proteins leak from a mature or hypermature lens and obstruct outflow through the trabecular meshwork.
- Lens-particle glaucoma is induced by ocular surgery or trauma. Lens material is released and obstructs the trabecular meshwork.
- Phacoanaphylaxis occurs after penetrating trauma or surgery when a patient becomes sensitized to their lens protein, causing an autoimmune reaction. Glaucoma can develop when the inflammation affects the trabecular meshwork, or secondary angle closure can occur if extensive peripheral anterior synechiae form.

Etiology

See earlier.

The Patient

Clinical Symptoms

All three types of lens-induced secondary open-angle glaucoma may present with unilateral pain, red eye, decreased vision, photophobia, or tearing.

Clinical Signs

- Phacolytic (lens protein) glaucoma:
  - Mature or hypermature lens, cells and intense flare, corneal edema, significantly elevated intraocular pressure, conjunctival injection, and white material on the capsular surface or in the anterior chamber. The anterior chamber is open by gonioscopy. A hypopyon may be present.
- Lens-particle glaucoma:
  - Elevated intraocular pressure, cortical lens material in the anterior chamber, cells and flare, corneal edema, and occasionally a hypopyon is present. In traumatic cases, a tear in the capsule may be seen.
- Phacoanaphylaxis:
  - Keratic precipitates on the intraocular lens and cornea, residual lens material, intense cell and flare, and frequently a hypopyon. Progression may lead to posterior synechia, cyclitic membrane, and phthisis of the globe.

Demographics

Phacolytic (lens protein) glaucoma usually occurs in adults (because mature or hypermature cataracts are usually seen in adults). Lens-particle glaucoma and phacoanaphylaxis can occur at any age within hours or months after surgery or trauma.

Significant History

- Ocular trauma or cataract surgery
- History of previous episodes of uveitis

Ancillary Tests

If a diagnostic paracentesis is performed:

- Phacolytic (lens protein) glaucoma and phacoanaphylaxis will show macrophages that are swollen and filled with lens material.
- Lens-particle glaucoma will demonstrate macrophages and fragments of lens material.
- Gonioscopy typically reveals open angles that may later progress to secondary angle closure
- Optic nerve head assessment

The Treatment

1. Phacolytic (lens protein) glaucoma: The goal of treatment is to quickly control the intraocular pressure and inflammation and then remove the cataract.

- Lower the intraocular pressure
  - Topical β-blocker (timolol 0.25 to 0.5% twice a day or levobunolol 0.25 to 0.5% twice a day or Timoptic XE 0.25 to 0.5% once a day or carteolol 1.0% twice a day or betaxolol 0.25 to 0.5% twice a day)
  - Topical, oral, or intravenous carbonic anhydrase inhibitor (dorzolamide 2% or brinzolamide 1% drops three times a day, acetazolamide 500-mg IV, or acetazolamide 250 mg orally four times a day or 500-mg sequels orally twice a day)
  - Topical apraclonidine 0.5% three times a day or brimonidine 0.15 or 0.20% three times a day
  - Hyperosmotic agents (if needed): Oral glycerol 50% 1.0 to 1.5 g/kg, oral isosorbide 45% 1.0 to 1.5 g/kg, IV mannitol 20% 1 to 2 g/kg over 45 minutes
- Decrease the inflammation
  - Topical prednisolone acetate 1% or rimexolone 1% every hour
- Cycloplege the pupil
  - Cyclopentolate 1.0% or scopolamine 0.25% three times a day
- Cataract extraction is usually performed soon after the diagnosis is made and after initial attempts to control the intraocular pressure and inflammation
2. Lens-particle glaucoma
   - Medical therapy to lower the intraocular pressure (see earlier)
   - Topical prednisolone acetate 1% or rimexolone 1% four times a day (the goal is to prescribe enough topical steroid to reduce intraocular inflammation but not to suppress the absorption of lens material)
   - Topical cycloplegic (cyclopentolate 1.0% or scopolamine 0.25% three times a day)
   - If the intraocular pressure does not respond to medical therapy, consider surgery to remove the residual lens material
3. Phacoanaphylaxis
   - Medical treatment is used to lower the intraocular pressure and control the intraocular inflammation (see phacolytic glaucoma listed earlier). Subconjunctival steroids (methylprednisolone 40 mg) or a brief course of systemic steroids (oral prednisone approximately 60 to 80 mg every day) may be required to decrease inflammation.
   - Surgery is frequently needed to remove the lens material after initial attempts to decrease the intraocular inflammation.

ANGLE-RECESSION GLAUCOMA
G. Richard Bennett and Michael B. Caplan

ICD—9: 364.77

THE DISEASE

Pathophysiology

Blunt trauma can cause recession of the anterior chamber angle and eventual development of glaucoma. Angle recession is because of tearing between the circular and longitudinal fibers of the ciliary muscle. Intraocular pressure can become elevated months to years after the blunt injury, because of scarring of the trabecular meshwork. Patients with greater than 270° of angle recession are at greater risk for developing glaucoma.

Etiology
- Blunt ocular trauma

The Patient

Clinical Symptoms
Patients are usually asymptomatic but may complain of unilateral visual loss if glaucoma becomes advanced.

Clinical Signs
Gonioscopy reveals a broad ciliary body band, increased visibility of the scleral spur, torn iris processes, and a deepening of the iris recess. Gonioscopy is a critical procedure in the evaluation of the patient with suspected traumatic glaucoma. It is important to compare the angle anatomy with the contralateral eye, which should be examined first. Elevated intraocular pressure, cupping of the optic nerve, and visual field defects are usually unilateral or asymmetric. Other signs of trauma (iridodialysis, cyclodialysis, iris sphincter tears, Vossius ring, cataract, dislocated lens, vitreous changes, retinal breaks, or choroidal rupture) are sometimes present. In patients who develop glaucoma in an eye with angle recession, there is an increased incidence of open-angle glaucoma in the contralateral eye.

Demographics

Blunt trauma is most common in males <30 years old; however, it can occur at any age. The prevalence of angle recession is high (60 to 94%) if a hyphema occurs at the time of blunt trauma. Glaucoma develops in 2 to 10% of patients with angle recession.

Significant History

The patient can usually recall blunt trauma to the affected eye.

Ancillary Tests
- Gonioscopy
- Threshold visual fields
- Optic nerve head imaging (HRT II, GDx, OCT)
- Optic nerve head photography

The Treatment

Medical treatment of angle recession glaucoma includes:

- Topical β-blockers (timolol 0.25 to 0.5% twice a day, levobunolol 0.25 to 0.5% every day or twice a day, Timoptic XE 0.25 to 0.5% once a day, carteolol 1.0% twice a day, betaxolol 0.25 to 0.5% twice a day).

- Carbonic anhydrase inhibitors (dorzolamide 2% or brinzolamide 1% drops three times a day, methazolamide 25- to 50-mg one to two tablets orally two to three times a day, or acetazolamide 250 mg orally four times a day or 500-mg sequels orally twice a day).
- Brimonidine 0.15 to 0.20% two to three times a day.
- Miotics, such as pilocarpine, should not be used; they are frequently ineffective and may elevate intraocular pressure as a result of decreased uveoscleral outflow.
- Prostaglandin analogs (latanoprost 0.005%, travoprost 0.004%, bimatoprost 0.03%) at bedtime.

Laser trabeculoplasty can be attempted prior to filtration surgery if medical therapy does not adequately lower the intraocular pressure. The success rate is significantly lower than in primary open-angle glaucoma, especially if there is extensive angle recession.

Surgical treatment includes trabeculectomy, shunt tubes, or cyclodestructive procedures.

IRIDOCORNEAL ENDOTHELIAL (ICE) SYNDROME
G. Richard Bennett and Michael B. Caplan

ICD—9: 364.51

THE DISEASE
Pathophysiology

Iridocorneal endothelial syndrome is a spectrum of clinical entities in which there is a disorder of the corneal endothelium and endothelialization of the anterior chamber angle and iris surface. Glaucoma is a prominent feature of ICE syndrome and is caused by an obstruction to aqueous outflow as a result of anterior synechiae formation or by the cellular membrane that covers the angle. Contraction of the cellular membrane in the angle and on the iris surface is believed to contribute to the various anterior segment abnormalities seen in ICE syndrome.

Etiology

The exact etiology of iridocorneal endothelial syndrome is unknown. This condition appears to be acquired, not inherited. It has been suggested that herpes simplex virus infection may be related.

The Patient

Clinical Symptoms
Frequently ICE syndrome is asymptomatic. Symptoms may include decreased vision and pain either from corneal edema or glaucoma. Some patients may note displacement of the pupil or other iris abnormalities.

Clinical Signs

The full manifestations in ICE syndrome are almost always unilateral and are not associated with other systemic abnormalities. Subtle abnormalities of the corneal endothelium may be detected in the contralateral eye. The corneal endothelium has a fine-hammered, beaten, silver appearance and corneal edema may occur. Peripheral anterior synechiae, which extend past Schwalbe's line, are often present. Glaucoma is common. Iris and corneal abnormalities are the basis for distinguishing the various clinical entities:

- Progressive iris atrophy (essential iris atrophy):
  - Marked iris atrophy, corectopia, ectropion uvea, and iris hole formation.
- Chandler's syndrome:
  - Corneal endothelial changes and corneal edema are usually the prominent features of Chandler's syndrome. Mild iris atrophy and mild, if any, corectopia may be present.
- Cogan-Reese syndrome (iris nevus syndrome):
  - Iris atrophy is variable. Pedunculated, pigmented nodules of the surface of the iris, composed of iris stroma and surrounded by the cellular membrane, are present.

Demographics

- ICE syndrome usually manifests in early or middle adulthood and is more common in women.
- Whites are affected more often than Blacks.

Significant History

- It is rare to elicit a family history of similar ocular abnormalities
- Onset in adulthood, not congenital

Ancillary Tests

- Gonioscopy
- Threshold visual field testing
- Optic nerve head photography
- Optic nerve imaging (HRT II, GDx, OCT)
- Specular microscopy

The Treatment

Treatment is not indicated unless the patient develops glaucoma or corneal edema. Lowering the intraocular pressure may help improve the corneal edema in some cases.

Treatment of Glaucoma

- Medical treatment is used to decrease aqueous production or increase uveoscleral outflow:

- Topical β-blocker twice a day (timolol 0.25 to 0.5%, levobunolol 0.25 to 0.5%, carteolol 1.0%, betaxolol 0.25 to 0.5%, or Timoptic XE 0.25 to 0.5% once a day)
- Carbonic anhydrase inhibitors (dorzolamide 2% or brinzolamide 1% drops three times a day, methazolamide 25- to 50-mg one to two tablets orally two to three times a day, or acetazolamide 250 mg orally four times a day, or 500-mg sequels orally twice a day)
- Brimonidine 0.15 to 0.20% two or three times a day
- Prostaglandin analogs (latanoprost 0.005%, travoprost 0.004%, bimatoprost 0.03% at bedtime). This class of drugs is usually most efficacious in lowering the IOP in ICE syndrome patients.
- Surgical considerations include trabeculectomy, shunt tubes, or cyclodestructive procedures.
- Laser trabeculoplasty is not indicated because of the angle abnormalities.
- Miotics are not effective because of obstruction of the trabecular meshwork.

Treatment of Corneal Edema
- Hypertonic saline (NaCl 5% drops four times a day and NaCl 5% ointment at bedtime)
- Corneal transplant if indicated and if glaucoma is controlled

---

MALIGNANT GLAUCOMA (CILIARY BLOCK GLAUCOMA, AQUEOUS MISDIRECTION)
G. Richard Bennett and Michael B. Caplan

ICD—9: 365.83

THE DISEASE
Pathophysiology

Malignant glaucoma is felt to be caused by a posterior misdirection of aqueous into or behind the vitreous cavity. As aqueous accumulates in the vitreous, the anterior chamber becomes diffusely shallow or flat and the intraocular pressure increases.

Etiology

Malignant glaucoma occurs most often in phakic patients with angle-closure glaucoma who have undergone glaucoma filtration surgery. It can occur immediately after surgery or even months later. It may be related to the discontinuation of cycloplegics or the initiation of miotics. Malignant glaucoma is believed to be caused by a relative block to the anterior flow of aqueous where the ciliary processes, anterior hyaloid face, and lens meet (it can also occur in aphakic patients).

The Patient

Clinical Symptoms

Symptoms can include pain, loss of vision, photophobia, nausea, and vomiting; however, some patients may be asymptomatic.

Clinical Signs

The anterior chamber is diffusely shallow or flat despite a patent peripheral iridectomy. The intraocular pressure is elevated. Ciliary processes are rotated anteriorly and may be seen touching the lens through the peripheral iridectomy. Fundus examination shows no elevation of the choroid.

Demographics

Malignant glaucoma has been reported to occur in 0.6 to 4% of patients who have had surgery for angle-closure glaucoma.

Significant History

- Previous angle-closure glaucoma
- Previous ocular surgery
- Recent changes in topical ocular medications
- Malignant glaucoma in the fellow eye

Ancillary Tests

- Gonioscopy
- Indirect ophthalmoscopy
- B-scan ultrasonography to exclude a choroidal detachment

The Treatment

- If the diagnosis of malignant glaucoma is suspected, first ensure that a patent iridectomy is present. If it is not, revise or perform a peripheral iridectomy to rule out pupillary block.
- Medical treatment of malignant glaucoma involves decreasing the intraocular pressure and eliminating the ciliary block. Initial medical therapy includes:
  - Atropine 1% 1 drop four times a day
  - Phenylephrine 2.5% 1 drop four times a day
  - Acetazolamide 500 mg orally or IV, then 250 mg orally four times a day
  - Topical β-blocker twice a day (timolol 0.5%, levobunolol 0.5%, carteolol 1.0%, betaxolol 0.25 to 0.5%)
  - Apraclonidine 1.0% twice a day or brimonidine 0.15 or 0.20% twice a day
  - Hyperosmotic agents are given initially and can be repeated bid. Options include: Oral glycerol 50% 1.0 to 1.5 g/kg, oral isosorbide 45% 1.0 g/kg, IV mannitol 20% 1 to 2 g/kg given over 45 minutes.
- If medical treatment is not successful, consider the following laser therapies:
  - YAG laser disruption of the posterior capsule and anterior hyaloid face in pseudophakic or aphakic patients.

- Argon laser shrinkage of ciliary processes through a peripheral iridectomy (this may help break the ciliolenticular block). Settings are adjusted according to clinical response. Initial settings can be 100 to 300 mw, 0.1 to 0.2 seconds, 100 to 200 micron spot sizes.

  Note: Medical therapy should be continued after laser procedures and gradually tapered. Atropine is frequently required indefinitely.
- Surgical therapy (partial vitrectomy and reformation of the anterior chamber) is considered if other treatment modalities are unsuccessful.

PLATEAU IRIS
G. Richard Bennett and Michael B. Caplan

ICD—9: 365.02—Plateau iris configuration
ICD—9: 365.41—Plateau iris syndrome

THE DISEASE
Pathophysiology

Plateau iris is divided into plateau iris configuration and plateau iris syndrome. Plateau iris configuration is an anatomic variation of the anterior chamber angle that can predispose the patient to acute angle-closure glaucoma with a relatively small degree of pupillary block. Plateau iris syndrome refers to angle-closure glaucoma secondary to a plateau iris configuration, which is not responsive to peripheral iridectomy.

The iris plane is flat and the peripheral iris angles sharply posterior prior to insertion into the ciliary face. This anatomic structuring creates a narrow angle that is susceptible to closure if the peripheral iris rolls into the angle either spontaneously or after dilation.

Etiology

There is an abnormal configuration of the iris insertion into the anterior chamber angle (see earlier).

The Patient

Clinical Symptoms
Patients with plateau iris configuration are usually asymptomatic unless angle-closure glaucoma occurs. If angle-closure glaucoma develops, the patient can have decreased vision, pain, nausea, and vomiting.

Clinical Signs
Gonioscopy will reveal the aforementioned anatomic changes in the angle. In cases of acute angle-closure glaucoma secondary to plateau iris, the anterior chamber is deeper and the iris plane is flatter than acute angle-closure glaucoma secondary to a pure pupillary block mechanism. Look for a patent peripheral iridectomy in cases of acute angle-closure glaucoma to help diagnose plateau iris syndrome. If the intraocular pressure

is still significantly elevated after a peripheral iridectomy is performed for acute angle-closure glaucoma, one must also consider malignant glaucoma (diffusely shallow anterior chamber) and chronic angle closure secondary to anterior synechiae.

Demographics

Acute angle-closure glaucoma secondary to plateau iris tends to occur in younger patients than acute angle-closure glaucoma secondary to pupillary block. It should also be suspected in myopic patients who present with acute angle closure.

Significant History

- Recent dilation or acute angle-closure glaucoma not responding to a patent peripheral iridectomy

Ancillary Tests

- Gonioscopy
- Ultrasound biomicroscopy
- Optic nerve head assessment

The Treatment

- Initially treat acute angle closure medically followed by peripheral iridectomy (see treatment in Acute Angle-Closure Glaucoma section). If plateau iris configuration is present, the peripheral iridectomy will help resolve the attack.
- If angle-closure glaucoma occurs after obtaining a patent iridectomy, then plateau iris syndrome is present and should be treated chronically with miotics (pilocarpine 0.5 to 1.0% three to four times a day).
- Iridoplasty may be useful in alleviating the angle closure in plateau iris syndrome.
- Gonioplasty may be helpful in cases of iris plateau syndrome.
- In patients with plateau iris configuration who have not had an attack of acute angle closure, the angle is followed closely. Consider a peripheral iridectomy if there is evidence of progressive narrowing or peripheral anterior synechiae formation.

Chapter 18

Retina and Vitreal Disease

RETINAL TEARS AND RHEGMATOGENOUS DETACHMENT

W. Craig Lannin

ICD—9: 361.32—Horseshoe tear of retina without detachment
ICD—9: 361.0—Retinal detachment with retinal defect

THE DISEASE

Significant ocular morbidity is associated with retinal detachment, and to lesser extent retinal tears. As typical symptoms usually herald the possible development of a retinal tear, educating at-risk patients about the nature and significance of such symptoms is an important means of reducing the incidence of progression to rhegmatogenous detachment. Compared to retinal detachment surgery, the treatment of retinal tears is less expensive, requires less rehabilitation, is technically less demanding, results in fewer serious complications, and is much less likely to be associated with significant visual loss.

Pathophysiology

Retinal detachment can result from a variety of mechanisms. Rhegmatogenous retinal detachment results from the passage of fluid from the vitreous cavity through a hole or tears in the retina into the subretinal space. Although round atrophic holes may lead to retinal detachment, the majority of clinically significant retinal detachments result from retinal tears secondary to vitreoretinal traction. An important event in the genesis of such tears is posterior vitreous detachment.

Retinal tears often occur along the posterior border of the vitreous base or at other sites of vitreoretinal adhesion, following spontaneous or traumatic posterior vitreous detachment. After the vitreous has separated from its broad area of contact with the retina, which usually closely follows detachment at the optic disc, vitreoretinal traction is increased at sites of normal and abnormal adhesion. Vitreous movement initiated by rapid head turning or eye rotation is then translated through force vectors to these focal areas of residual vitreoretinal attachment, and may lead to the genesis of a retinal tear.

Unusually strong vitreoretinal adherence may be associated with developmental anomalies, including cystic retinal tufts and localized posterior extensions of the vitreous base. Exaggerated adherence is also often found along the course of retinal blood vessels and is reflected in the frequent association of vitreous hemorrhage with acute retinal tears. Finally, firm vitreoretinal adhesions are associated with obvious areas of retinal alteration, including retinal lattice degeneration and sites of previous inflammation.

In order for a rhegmatogenous retinal detachment to develop, there must be a break in the retina and liquefied vitreous overlying the break. Posterior vitreous detachment increases the probability of occurrence for both of these conditions. Initially, the sub-retinal fluid is composed of fluid originating in the vitreous cavity, but this is most likely augmented by serum derived from the choriocapillaris as time passes. Variables that influence whether fluid gains access to the subretinal space include the amount of traction being exerted on the edges of the break, the effects of gravity (location of the break above or below the horizontal midline), and the lifestyle and activities of the affected person.

Etiology

Risk factors for retinal tears and detachment include myopia, a history of cataract surgery, ocular trauma, lattice degeneration, a familial history of tears/detachment, and a history of either condition having occurred in the fellow eye. About half of all patients who have a retinal detachment are myopic, and about a third have had cataract surgery. YAG laser capsulotomy has also been identified as an independent risk factor. A history of posterior capsular rupture and vitreous loss increases the risk of subsequent detachment.

The Patient

Clinical Symptoms

Symptoms of an acute retinal tear may include a sudden onset of floaters and debris, photopsia, and blurred vision, but these same symptoms can also occur in uncomplicated posterior vitreous detachment. Photopsia associated with vitreoretinal traction is typically of very short duration, unlike the scintillations encountered with migraine or other vascular disturbances.

When a retinal detachment has occurred, patients may additionally become aware of visual field loss, with the perception of a mobile shadow or curtain obscuring their vision. If the macula is involved, there will usually be significant loss of central visual acuity as well. Patients with chronic, slowly progressive or demarcated detachments, usually in the inferior retina, may be asymptomatic.

Clinical Signs

Posterior vitreous detachment is often a precursor of retinal tears and detachment, and is evident clinically in most cases. Slit-lamp exam may reveal the presence of fine-pigment granules in the anterior vitreous (tobacco dust), which, in the absence of a history of prior intraocular surgery, is highly suggestive of a retinal break. When a vitreous hemorrhage occurs in association with posterior vitreous detachment, a retinal tear will be present about 70% of the time. Binocular indirect ophthalmoscopy with scleral depression or peripheral contact lens examination will, in most cases, demonstrate the attached flap of a retinal horseshoe tear under persistent vitreoretinal traction, or a free-floating operculum overlying a retinal hole indicates that traction has been released. The tear itself usually has a darker orange color than the surrounding retina because of the unimpeded illumination of the underlying choroid.

Horseshoe retinal tears occur with the greatest frequency in the superotemporal retina (60%), followed by the superonasal quadrant. Traumatic retinal dialyses have a propensity to occur in the inferotemporal retina, particularly in the young. Retinal breaks occur at or anterior to the equator in about 85% of cases.

The most obvious visible evidence of the presence of a detached retina is its elevation from the surface. The surface of the detached retina has a corrugated and often dimpled appearance and demonstrates movement with motion of the head and/or eye. Mobility may be significantly reduced in long-standing retinal detachments or in those complicated by proliferative vitreoretinopathy.

The differential diagnosis of rhegmatogenous retinal detachment includes exudative retinal detachment, traction retinal detachment, retinoschisis, retinal/choroidal tumor, and choroidal detachment. A thorough history and careful examination usually makes the distinguishing characteristics of these entities evident. Exudative detachment is characterized by shifting subretinal fluid, and the underlying inflammatory or other causative disorder is usually also apparent. Traction detachment is associated with a concave retinal configuration and lack of significant movement. Choroidal tumors and detachment can be distinguished from retinal detachment by their smooth contour and the presence of retinal pigment epithelium (RPE) and choroidal markings associated with the elevated retina.

The configuration of the detachment is an important clue to help pinpoint the location of the retinal break(s). With a superior detachment, the retinal break is usually at or near the 12 o'clock position. When a detachment of one inferior quadrant has occurred, a break will almost always be found superior to a line radially bisecting the area of detachment. In an inferior detachment, if the subretinal fluid extends higher on one side than the other, the break will be found on the higher side. About half of all retinal detachments are associated with a single break, but the possibility of multiple breaks must always be kept in mind.

Confrontation testing will often demonstrate a visual field defect, and Snellen acuity will be reduced if the macula is detached. Tonometry will usually reveal a relatively low intraocular pressure in an eye with a retinal detachment, although rarely the pressure may actually be higher than normal. Pupillary testing may demonstrate a relative afferent pupillary defect. Ultrasonography and occasionally electroretinography (ERG) may be helpful in cases where media opacity prevents adequate visualization of the retina.

Demographics

Approximately 1 out of every 15,000 individuals has a retinal detachment in any given year. The incidence of retinal breaks is significantly greater, about 6%, but the majority of these breaks are small atrophic holes with a low potential for progression to retinal detachment. Peak incidence of retinal detachment occurs between 50 and 70 years of age; the increased frequency in that age group largely reflects the incidence of both posterior vitreous detachment and of cataract surgery. Myopic detachments are most common between age 25 and 45. There is another smaller peak during the teenage years, and these detachments are frequently of traumatic origin. About 60% of retinal detachment patients are male, and trauma does not completely account for this propensity. Although familial patterns of retinal detachment are sometimes evident, most are sporadic. A large part of the familial risk profile is of an indirect nature, such as a genetic predisposition to myopia and/or lattice degeneration. Of all rhegmatogenous detachments, 50% have more than one break. The risk of retinal detachment in the second eye of an affected individual has been estimated to be about 10 to 15% in phakic individuals and 25 to 40% in aphakic or pseudophakic individuals.

The Treatment

Retinal Tear

Treatment for acute, symptomatic flap tears is justified as a means of reducing the risk of progression to retinal detachment. Such tears have been shown to progress to detachment in approximately one-third of cases. Treatment for symptomatic operculated holes is also justifiable, although the danger of progression is less than for a flap tear with persistent vitreoretinal traction. In asymptomatic patients, the decision whether or not to treat must be individualized, taking into account multiple factors. These include the location, type, and size of the break(s), with superior breaks, flap tears, and large breaks being considered for prophylaxis. If there is pigmentation around the break, it is not acute and treatment may not be indicated. If there is significant localized subretinal fluid around the break, treatment may be indicated. The presence of vitreous hemorrhage increases the risk associated with a retinal break. Other factors that must be weighed in the decision are the age and life expectancy of the patient; the patient's lifestyle; the status of the fellow eye, the refractive error; and, in particular, the degree of axial myopia; the presence of aphakia, pseudophakia, or anticipated cataract surgery; and the family history. The timing of treatment is dictated by the apparent degree of threat associated with a particular break.

Prophylactic treatment of retinal breaks is usually accomplished using either transconjunctival cryopexy or laser photocoagulation. The choice of technique is guided by the number, size, and position of the break(s), as well as by the preference of the patient and surgeon. There is some theoretical advantage of laser over cryotherapy because of the possibility of dispersing viable RPE cells with cryotherapy. Many surgeons feel that there is a greater risk for the subsequent development of an epiretinal membrane and macular pucker with cryotherapy. This has resulted in a trend toward increased utilization of laser for prophylactic treatment. However, there are some cases where cryotherapy still holds a distinct advantage, such as cases of very anterior breaks and when visualization is impaired because of the presence of significant cataract or vitreous hemorrhage. Other than in cases of giant tears or dialysis, scleral buckling is rarely utilized for prophylactic treatment.

Laser photocoagulation of retinal tears can usually be accomplished with only topical anesthesia, unless extensive treatment of multiple breaks and/or lattice degeneration is contemplated. Transconjunctival cryopexy is generally performed utilizing topical anesthesia augmented with a subconjunctival injection in the area overlying the break(s). Whichever modality is chosen, the goals of treatment are the same: to ensure an adequate width of treatment that completely surrounds the retinal break. The resultant scar will then isolate the break and prevent fluid from the vitreous cavity from gaining access to the subretinal space. Following surgery, the patient is instructed to restrict activity until an effective adhesion has developed, usually 7 to 10 days for cryopexy or a slightly shorter period of time for laser.

Prophylactic treatment of high-risk retinal breaks has been shown to be effective in significantly reducing the risk of subsequent retinal detachment. Serious complications are rare, with the most frequent visually significant adverse consequence being macular pucker. However, macular pucker also develops in association with retinal breaks that have not been treated.

Retinal Detachment

The decision to treat a retinal detachment must also be individualized, taking into account the likelihood of progression; the residual visual potential; the age, lifestyle, and life expectancy of the patient; the status of the fellow eye; and the patient's wishes. When an acute, macula-threatening or recent macula-off detachment is encountered, surgery is indicated as soon as possible. Appropriate bed rest and positioning instructions are given to reduce the possibility of extension of the detachment into the macula, if it is still attached. This may also allow for significant absorption of subretinal fluid prior to surgery. An inferior demarcated detachment may not require surgery. Likewise, the limited visual prognosis associated with a long-standing macula-off detachment may persuade the patient and surgeon not to pursue surgical intervention, particularly if there is excellent vision in the contralateral eye.

The surgical technique most commonly employed in the treatment of rhegmatogenous retinal detachment is scleral buckling (SB), in combination with retinopexy utilizing cryotherapy or laser photocoagulation. Cryotherapy or laser is necessary in order to produce a controlled inflammatory reaction that will result in a permanent adhesion of the retina once it is brought back into contact with the RPE. Laser cannot be effectively employed until after the retina has been brought back into close proximity with the pigment epithelium, whereas cryotherapy can be applied around the retinal breaks in the presence of subretinal fluid. The purpose of the buckle is to aid in bringing the treated breaks back into contact with the RPE and to relieve persistent vitreoretinal traction. The scleral buckle is created utilizing either solid silicone rubber elements or soft silicone sponges, which are permanently anchored to the sclera with sutures. Surgery is often performed under regional block anesthesia, although general anesthesia may be necessary if a lengthy procedure is a possibility.

Placement of the buckle can be segmental, with either radial or circumferential elements, or encircling, passing under the four rectus muscles. In some cases, a combination of an encircling band or tire is combined with a radial sponge. Drainage of subretinal fluid is often required in order to bring the retina into contact with the buckle and also to provide space to achieve an adequate buckle height without an excessive elevation of intraocular pressure. The need for drainage is influenced by several factors, including the amount of retinal elevation; the number, size, and position of retinal breaks; and the duration of the detachment, as long-standing subretinal fluid becomes highly viscous and resistant to reabsorption. A successful surgical outcome is dependent on finding and closing *all* the retinal breaks, not necessarily only the causative break.

Alternative methods of retinal reattachment surgery include pars plana vitrectomy (PPV), pneumatic retinopexy, and a temporary balloon buckle. Pars plana vitrectomy has become the method of choice for treating retinal detachments associated with giant retinal tears, and for dealing with other complicated scenarios. Vitrectomy is also necessary to repair recurrent retinal detachments associated with significant proliferative vitreoretinopathy (PVR). The vitrectomy is often supplemented with adjunctive techniques, including the use of membrane dissection, internal drainage of subretinal fluid, laser, fluid-gas exchange, intraocular silicone oil, and, particularly in the treatment of giant tears, liquid perfluorocarbon. In many cases, it is also necessary to employ a scleral buckle as well.

PPV has become increasingly popular, particularly in Europe, as a primary procedure for rhegmatogenous retinal detachment. In the United States, many surgeons employ primary PPV for pseudophakic detachments. Reported advantages of PPV over SB include better intraoperative control, the avoidance of a very soft eye during surgery, the avoidance of drainage complications, and a lower incidence of refractive change and diplopia. Disadvantages include the invasive nature of the surgery and the associated risk of endophthalmitis, cataractogenesis in phakic patients, the higher rate of iatrogenic and missed/new breaks, more frequent persistent postoperative intraocular pressure elevation, the more technologically demanding nature of the procedure requiring more skilled assistance and nursing, and probably its increased expense.

Pneumatic retinopexy is an effective method of repair, if cases are selected carefully. It can only be utilized for detachments with superior breaks and cases of single breaks or breaks separated by no more than 1 clock hour. The technique consists of a pars plana injection of perfluorocarbon gas, again combined with cryopexy and/or laser photocoagulation. The patient must be willing and able to sustain a strict postoperative positioning regimen, or the chances of success are dramatically reduced. The head is positioned so as to bring the position of the break to the 12 o'clock meridian, so that the gas bubble completely covers the break. This must be continued until the break has been brought back into contact with the RPE, and a good cryopexy or laser scar is forming. In general, better results have been obtained in phakic patients. Pneumatic retinopexy is contraindicated in the presence of extensive lattice degeneration or significant PVR. Gas injection may also be utilized in conjunction with scleral buckling, in order to facilitate the reabsorption of subretinal fluid.

Approximately 80 to 85% of primary retinal detachments can be successfully repaired utilizing a single SB operation, and approximately 92% of detachments overall can be successfully repaired, including those that require two or more procedures. The success rates for PPV are similar to those of SB in uncomplicated cases. The success rates for PPV in complicated cases of retinal detachment (RD) are significantly higher than with SB. The one-operation success rates with pneumatic retinopexy are somewhat less than with either SB or PPV, but failed attempts at this procedure do not seem to significantly jeopardize the final outcome. An important advantage of pneumatic retinopexy is its significantly lower overall costs relative to SB and vitrectomy, which must be performed in the operating room. There may also be faster rehabilitation with pneumatic retinopexy, at least in some cases.

Visual results following retinal detachment surgery are in large part determined by the preoperative visual acuity and the status of the macula. Overall, 55% of anatomic surgical successes will achieve at least 20/50 vision within 6 months of surgery, but about 15% will be left with 20/400 or worse. The average long-term visual result for a repaired macula-off detachment is about 20/70 acuity.

Patients with a retinal tear and/or a retinal detachment require careful follow-up to watch for the development of complications and to monitor the status of the fellow eye. The most common cause of failed surgery is the development of PVR. PVR is characterized by the development of epiretinal and/or subretinal membranes that distort the retinal surface into fixed folds and often reopen existing breaks or cause new ones to form. Its development portends a relatively poor prognosis, particularly in regard to the visual outcome. Other significant complications include intraoperative subretinal hemorrhage, retinal incarceration, new retinal break formation, postoperative choroidal detachment, diplopia, strabismus, cystoid macular edema, and macular pucker.

DEGENERATIVE RETINOSCHISIS
W. Craig Lannin

ICD—9: 361.10

THE DISEASE

Degenerative (age-related, senile) retinoschisis is a relatively rare precursor to clinically significant (progressive) retinal detachment (RD) but can sometimes be difficult to distinguish from a chronic detachment. This differentiation is one of the most clinically important aspects of retinoschisis. There is a congenital form of retinoschisis, but this discussion is limited to the more common degenerative form.

Pathophysiology

Degenerative retinoschisis represents a splitting of the retina, usually originating in the outer plexiform layer, and develops as a progression of peripheral cystoid degeneration. Cystoid degeneration is found in the vast majority of adult eyes, and begins with the development of tiny spaces within the outer plexiform layer. As the cysts enlarge, the spaces are bridged by glial cell fibers that extend from the external to the internal limiting membranes. This process begins near the ora serrata and extends circumferentially and posteriorly but usually not posterior to the equator. Based on pathologic and less distinctly clinical features, cystoid degeneration may be subdivided into typical and reticular forms. The much less common reticular form has a greater potential to spread more posteriorly, beyond the equator.

With further enlargement of the cysts, the stretched glial pillars may eventually rupture, resulting in the development of retinoschisis. The inner wall of the schisis cavity consists of the internal limiting membrane, the nerve fiber layer, the retinal vessels, and the inner plexiform layer. The outer wall is composed of degenerated elements of the inner nuclear, outer plexiform, and outer nuclear layers, with a relatively well-preserved photoreceptor layer. The cavity itself contains a hyaluronidase-sensitive mucopolysaccharide substance. The margins of the schisis are contiguous with areas of cystoid degeneration.

Degenerative retinoschisis may also be divided into typical and reticular forms. Both types are usually found in the temporal retina, particularly the inferotemporal quadrant. The reticular form is also seen in the nasal retina more frequently than is the typical form. Reticular retinoschisis is more often highly bullous and frequently has an extremely thin inner wall. Reticular schisis also usually extends posterior to the equator, unlike typical schisis, and may rarely even threaten the macula.

Etiology

Cystoid degeneration is almost universal in adult eyes, but retinoschisis is much less common. It is not certain why in some cases cystoid degeneration progresses to degenerative retinoschisis. There does not appear to be a genetic predisposition to this process. Bullous retinoschisis seems to be more common when zones of typical and reticular cystoid degeneration overlap.

Some authors contend that the precipitating factor is age-related degenerative change in the inner retinal layers related to vascular insufficiency and impaired cellular nutrition. This theory is supported by the increasing prevalence of retinoschisis with advancing age and by the association of vascular abnormalities seen with some cases of the condition.

Other authors believe that vitreoretinal traction plays a role in the development and progression of retinoschisis. However, studies have failed to demonstrate that vitreoretinal relationships play a significant role in these events, and posterior vitreous detachment in the presence of retinoschisis only rarely results in the development of a progressive, symptomatic RD.

The Patient

Clinical Symptoms

The vast majority of patients (99%) with retinoschisis are asymptomatic. Although retinoschisis causes an absolute visual field defect, most patients are unaware of these, except in those rare cases where the schisis extends posteriorly into the macular region. The reasons for the usual lack of recognition of the field cut include the typically very slow or lack of progression of the retinoschisis and the fact that nasal field loss associated with the usual temporally located schisis can be easily overlooked.

Complications of retinoschisis include retinal detachment and vitreous hemorrhage. The localized, nonprogressive type of retinal detachment does not usually cause symptoms, but progressive, clinically significant detachments do. Vitreous hemorrhage, causing an acute onset of floaters, or hemorrhage into the schisis cavity may rarely be associated with retinoschisis, but such hemorrhages are usually minor. Incidental posterior vitreous detachment is a more common source of both vitreous hemorrhage and floaters in general.

Clinical Signs

The inner layer of the retinoschisis is visible as a smooth-domed elevation containing the retinal vessels. The retinal vessels may appear white because of sheathing. Retinoschisis is found predominantly in the temporal retina and is usually bilateral, although it may be asymmetric in extent and elevation. The schisis cavity may increase or decrease in height over time, and complete disappearance has been noted in 2% of cases. Tiny glistening flecks are often seen on the inner layer, although these have little clinical significance. New areas of schisis may develop elsewhere in about 10% of cases. Posterior extension of the retinoschisis may occur, although involvement of the macula is rare. Most cases stop within 3-disc diameters (DD) of the macula. Fundus contact lens examination is useful in the recognition of outer and inner layer holes.

Holes may develop in either the inner, outer, or both of the walls of a retinoschisis cavity in about 15% of cases. Outer layer holes are much more common than inner layer holes. Clinically, what appears to be an inner layer hole may actually represent only an area of extreme thinning. When an inner layer hole does develop, it is usually quite small and difficult to appreciate clinically. Outer layer holes are usually much more obvious, as they tend to be large. They have a rounded contour, may be single or multiple, and are seen typically in association with reticular retinoschisis. Outer layer holes often have a posteriorly rolled edge.

Although progressive rhegmatogenous retinal detachment is the most important clinical complication of degenerative retinoschisis, this is actually rare, accounting for probably no more than 2.5% of all detachments. In about 6% of cases of retinoschisis, localized, asymptomatic, nonprogressive or very slowly progressive retinal detachments develop, and these do not extend much beyond the border of the area of schisis. There may be a fine demarcation line present if one of these localized subclinical retinal detachments is present. All schisis-related retinal detachments are associated with outer layer holes. The viscosity of the fluid within the retinoschisis cavity is probably an important factor in inhibiting the progression of schisis-related detachments with outer layer holes. Inner-layer holes or traction-related tears are also sometimes present, particularly with progressive, symptomatic retinal detachments.

The differential diagnosis of degenerative retinoschisis includes retinal detachment, choroidal detachment/tumors, and juvenile (X-linked) retinoschisis. The latter two groups are usually easily excluded with a thorough history and careful examination. In some cases, the differentiation of retinoschisis from a chronic retinal detachment can be challenging (Table 18.1).

▶ **TABLE 18.1 Clinical Signs: Retinoschisis Versus Retinal Detatchment**

	Retinoschisis	Retinal Detachment
Laterality	Usually bilateral	Usually unilateral
Surface contour	Smooth	Corrugated
Mobility with eye movement	Less mobile	More mobile
Vitreous cells	Absent, if schisis isolated	Often present
Vascular sheathing and flecks	Often present	Absent
Demarcation lines	Usually absent	Often present, if chronic
Underlying RPE degeneration	Usually minimal, if isolated	Significant, if chronic
Visual field defect	Absolute	Relative
Refractive error	More often hyperopic	More often myopic
Retinal break(s)	Outer/inner layer possible	Full thickness

Demographics

The prevalence of retinoschisis is 3 to 4% in patients over age 10, and 7% in patients over age 40. No significant differences in the incidence of degenerative retinoschisis based on racial, sexual, or geographic factors have been elucidated. Degenerative retinoschisis is more common in hyperopic eyes. Retinoschisis is bilateral in more than 80% of cases. The risk of progression to clinical RD is approximately 1 in 2,000.

The Treatment

Treatment is rarely required for degenerative retinoschisis. Only in those rare cases when progressive, clinically significant retinal detachment develops is surgery indicated. This usually entails cryotherapy and scleral buckling to close the outer wall breaks, most often with drainage of subretinal fluid. However, if the outer layer breaks are posterior, multiple, and/or large, cryotherapy with drainage and intraocular gas injection or vitrectomy techniques may be required. Patients with localized detachments, particularly those with demarcation lines, may be managed conservatively with periodic follow-up and education about the warning symptoms of progressive retinal detachment. Prophylactic treatment of outer layer holes is of dubious value, as progressive retinal detachment rarely occurs and treatment is not without risk. This may be justified in cases where there has been a schisis-related detachment in the opposite eye. Treatment of posterior extension of retinoschisis is rarely indicated, as the risk of macular involvement is quite small, and again treatment may be associated with complications. All patients with retinoschisis should be followed up at least every 6 to 12 months, depending on the duration and stability of the condition. They should be instructed to call promptly in the event of the development of symptoms suggestive of retinal tear or detachment.

POSTERIOR VITREOUS DETACHMENT (PVD)
Michael J. Trad

ICD—9: 379.21

THE DISEASE

Pathophysiology

Posterior vitreous detachment represents a cortical vitreous and hyaloid membrane detachment from the posterior retina. PVD occurs as a result of anterior contractional forces exerted by the overlying fibrous vitreous at the vitreous base, secondary to fibrillary degeneration and hyaloid membrane thinning. Fibrillary degeneration encompasses both syneresis (vitreal shrinkage) and liquefaction of vitreous. Gravitational forces also play a role in the inferior and anterior collapse of the vitreal body. However, PVD may also occur without collapse, although this is less common. PVD also is termed complete when it extends to the ora serrata or incomplete when involving only specific regional areas.

PVD is of greatest clinical concern as a result of its potential to cause retinal tears at pre-existing sites of increased vitreoretinal adherence (lattice degeneration, retinal tuft, etc.). This tractional influence may result in retinal hemorrhage and tear; vitreous hemorrhage (those associated with PVD are usually small and self-limiting); macular edema, hole, or epiretinal membrane; and retinal detachment (secondary to continuous flow of liquid vitreous through retinal breaks).

Etiology

PVD typically occurs as a normal consequence of aging but can also be associated or potentially linked to trauma, chorioretinitis, myopia, vigorous exercise or isolated head movement, heavy lifting, aphakia, and pseudophakia.

The Patient

Clinical Symptoms
- Floaters
- Transient photopsia
- Blurred vision
- Metamorphopsia

Clinical Signs
Prominent Signs
- Prepapillary floater in the shape of an annular ring, line, or other geometric form
- Occasionally, preretinal and vitreous hemorrhage, retinal hemorrhage, retinal tear, and retinal detachment

Subtle Signs
- Macular edema
- Macular hole
- Pseudo-operculum anterior to macula
- Epiretinal membrane
- Retinal striations
- White without pressure
- Schaffer's sign (tobacco dust)–pigmented particles in anterior vitreous
- Peripheral retinal operculum (if associated with a retinal break)

Demographics
- PVD rarely occurs in patients younger than 45 years of age unless associated with chorioretinitis or trauma.
- Vitreous detachment of the optic disc is present in approximately one-half of all patients older than 50 years of age.
- By age 65, approximately 31% of the population has experienced a complete PVD.
- Complete PVD is much more common than incomplete PVD.
- Up to 50% of PVDs are associated with photopsia.

- Approximately 90% of patients who report concurrent flashes and floaters have PVD, and 11% have retinal breaks.
- Retinal breaks occur in up to 15% of patients with symptomatic PVD.
- 7.5% of PVDs have an associated vitreous hemorrhage.
- Traction at the posterior pole resulting in macular edema occurs in about 2.5% of symptomatic PVDs.

Significant History
- Trauma
- Chorioretinitis
- May potentially be precipitated by aphakia, pseudophakia, myopia, heavy lifting, and vigorous exercise or isolated head movement

Ancillary Tests

Ocular assessment for PVD may include confrontation visual fields, Amsler grid, biomicroscopy, and dilated fundus evaluation (binocular indirect ophthalmoscopy with scleral depression, direct ophthalmoscopy, Goldmann three-mirror lens, and biomicroscopic indirect lenses).

The Treatment

No treatment for PVD is necessary, although retinal consultation may be warranted in cases of retinal tear and/or detachment, extensive vitreous hemorrhage (rare), macular edema or hole, and epiretinal membrane formation. Patients with no apparent retinal involvement at the time of initial presentation must be thoroughly educated as to the necessity to return immediately upon recognition of new floaters or flashes. It is this early stage in which symptomatology is detectable that is vital in providing a therapeutic window of opportunity for the prevention of retinal detachment. Differing opinions prevail as to both the usefulness and frequency of regular follow-up visits because retinal tears may occur anywhere from a few weeks to a decade after initial examination of uncomplicated PVD. Conservative follow-up typically involves monthly visits for the initial 3 months, followed by yearly examination.

IDIOPATHIC EPIRETINAL MEMBRANES (IERMs)
Michael J. Trad

ICD—9: 362.56

THE DISEASE
Pathophysiology

Idiopathic epiretinal membranes are nonvascular proliferative lesions of the macular or paramacular vitreoretinal interface and typically develop unilaterally in individuals 50 years of age and older. IERMs are believed to develop secondary- to venous-flow impedance at retinal arteriosclerotic arteriovenous crossings, posterior vitreous detachment, and/or subclinical focal retinal inflammation. These conditions may disrupt the retina's internal limiting membrane (ILM) at sites where it is thin and firmly adherent (blood vessels and optic disc), stimulating a reparative process in which Muller cell processes and astroglial cells migrate through ILM breaks to proliferate on the retinal surface (within the subhyaloid space). Other IERMs that are composed of collagen ("cortical vitreous preretinal membranes") or a combination of collagen and retinal glial cells may also occur.

IERMs typically display little or no progression. However, some may grow and contract enough to cause irregular folding of the retina's ILM and nerve fiber layer. In rare instances, significant vision loss can occur when further tractional forces result in cystoid macular edema (CME), macular holes, or retinal detachment.

Etiology

Epiretinal membranes (ERMs) have been described differently in the literature, depending upon their etiology, appearance, and/or clinical stage, and include idiopathic epiretinal membrane, preretinal membrane, preretinal gliosis, preretinal macular fibrosis, cellophane maculopathy/retinopathy, crinkled cellophane, star folds, surface-wrinkling retinopathy, macular pucker, pigmented macular pucker, pigmented preretinal membrane, primary retinal folds, and silent central retinal vein obstruction. Some ERMs may be associated with ocular and/or facial trauma, retinal vascular disorders (e.g., diabetes), vitreous hemorrhage, retinal breaks and detachment, intraocular inflammation (e.g., toxoplasmosis), photocoagulation, or previous anterior segment or vitreoretinal surgery. Most IERMs are idiopathic.

The Patient

Symptoms and signs of IERMs are dependent upon the extent of the disease process and the presence of secondary tractional sequelae, such as CME.

Clinical Symptoms
Typically, there are no subjective complaints, and IERMs are found on routine examination. However, patients may complain of blurred vision and/or metamorphopsia. Decreased depth perception, diplopia, and absolute scotoma are also infrequently observed.

Clinical Signs
Prominent Signs
- Decreased visual acuity (dependent upon the extent and location of membrane formation and presence of secondary sequelae)
- Amsler grid metamorphopsia
- Loss of foveal reflex
- Semitranslucent to opaque gathered-pleat or volcano pattern appearance of IERM with deviation of retinal vasculature and retinal folds

Subtle Signs
- Cellophane reflex of retinal surface (best observed with the binocular indirect ophthalmoscope, accessory biomicroscopic lenses, and/or red-free filter of the direct ophthalmoscope)
- Perimacular vasculature may be slightly tortuous, and vessels may appear to straighten toward the area of the IERM

Other signs include posterior vitreous detachment ("partial" versus "complete"), retinal thickening (suggesting macular edema), macular hole, and retinal break/detachment.

Demographics
- IERM is much more prevalent in patients over the age of 50 (6.4% of individuals within this age group are thought to have the condition).
- Unilateral IERM occurs in 70 to 90% of cases.
- Approximately 1 to 2% of unilateral cases eventually become bilateral.
- IERM affects both sexes equally.
- Posterior vitreous detachment occurs in 80 to 90% of cases.
- CME has been reported to occur in 16% of patients with IERM.
- In 77% of cases, vision is 20/60 or better, while 61% have acuity of 20/40 or better.

Significant History
- Usually none (possibly posterior vitreous detachment)

Ancillary Tests

Ocular assessment of IERM would include best corrected visual acuity, pupil assessment, Amsler grid, color vision, and dilated fundus examination.

Fluorescein angiography is usually not necessary but may be indicated when acuity is worse than 20/40 (especially when a partial posterior vitreous detachment is present), concurrent CME is suspected, or the condition occurs in younger individuals.

The Treatment

In most cases, surgical intervention is not warranted as IERMs are usually self-limiting with a final visual acuity of 20/40 or better. Patients are instructed on routine Amsler grid usage, and follow-up examinations are scheduled according to individual case severity.

Surgery may be indicated, however, if visual acuity is 20/60 or worse but is initiated only after contemplating pre-existing permanent macular damage as well as anticipated surgical trauma. When surgery is performed, a pars plana approach with a closed intraocular microsurgical technique (vitrectomy with membrane peeling) is employed. Stabilization of visual acuity typically occurs 1 to 3 months postoperatively, and in 83% of cases improves by at least two Snellen lines. Epiretinal membranes recur at an incidence of approximately 3 to 4%.

OCULAR HISTOPLASMOSIS SYNDROME (OHS)
Michael J. Trad

ICD—9: 115.02

THE DISEASE
Pathophysiology

Ocular histoplasmosis syndrome presents initially in the posterior pole, peripapillary area, and peripheral retina as a bilateral, multifocal choroiditis. Active "histo" lesions are comprised of lymphocytes, plasma cells, and macrophages and may disrupt Bruch's membrane and subsequently damage the RPE and outer retinal layers.

It is believed that 10 to 30 years after the initial infection in which inhaled particles of fungus enter the body, reactivation of the disease and subretinal neovascular membrane (SRNVM) progression may occur. A potential visually devastating maculopathy may ensue when SRNVM extension results in hemorrhagic RPE and/or neurosensory retinal detachment, and ultimately disciform scar formation.

Etiology

Systemic histoplasmosis is a fungal infection caused by the yeast *Histoplasma capsulatum*. *H. capsulatum* spores present in soil (in close proximity to the droppings from chickens, other birds, and bats) are inhaled into the pulmonary system and then travel via the bloodstream to the eye (choroid) and/or other organ systems.

Although cases of OHS may be found anywhere throughout the United States because of population migration, OHS typically affects individuals living in the so-called histo belt of the Ohio and middle Mississippi valleys, Alabama, Arkansas, Illinois, Indiana, Iowa, Kansas, Kentucky, Louisiana, Maryland, Mississippi, Missouri, Nebraska, Ohio, Oklahoma, Tennessee, Texas, West Virginia, and Virginia. OHS usually occurs in immunocompetent persons without overt systemic manifestations, but may present opportunistically in immunocompromised patients (e.g., AIDS).

The Patient

Patients are usually asymptomatic unless significant macular or peripapillary retinal involvement occurs. In these instances, blurred or distorted vision and field loss may be experienced.

Clinical Signs
Prominent Signs
- Classic triad of peripapillary atrophy, peripheral chorioretinal atrophic spots, and macular subretinal neovascularization
- Absence of anterior uveitis
- Disciform macular scar
- Metamorphopsia or relative scotoma on Amsler grid
- Hemorrhagic/serous retinal and RPE detachment

- Optic disc edema, choroidal hemorrhage
- Vitreous hemorrhage (infrequent)

Subtle Signs

- Absence of vitritis (vitritis concurrent with OHS-like signs may indicate an inflammatory disorder, such as pseudo-POHS, a subtype of acute zonal occult outer retinopathy)
- Gray-green area in macular or peripapillary area indicating the presence of an SRNVM
- Linear streak lesions at the equator, which run parallel to the oral serrata (infrequent)

Demographics

- OHS patients typically range in age from 20 to 50 years.
- OHS occurs six times more frequently in Whites than in Blacks.
- OHS occurs with equal frequency between the sexes.
- Bilateral macular involvement is more common in men than in women.
- Maculopathy presents in individuals between the ages of 20 to 40 years.
- Each year in the United States, at least 2,000 individuals experience significant visual loss because of OHS.

Significant History

Past or present residence in the histo belt; past exposure to chickens, pigeons, or parakeets; immunodeficiency states (e.g., AIDS may reactivate OHS); stress may precipitate macular involvement

Ancillary Tests

Ocular assessment for OHS may include visual acuity, color vision, Amsler grid, confrontation fields, pupils, biomicroscopy, tonometry, dilated funduscopy, and fundus photography.

Visual field testing, electroretinogram (ERG), and visual-evoked potentials (VEP) may be necessary in differentiating OHS from pseudo-OHS (a IIB subgroup of acute zonal occult outer retinopathy).

Laboratory studies are rarely necessary, as the diagnosis is usually made on fundus appearance alone. However, in rare instances chest x-ray, histoplasmin skin testing, and HLA gene typing (HLA DR-2 gene) may be utilized.

Fluorescein (FA) and indocyanine green (ICG) angiography may be useful in cases of presumed or active maculopathy.

The Treatment

Patients should undergo bilateral FA in a very timely manner when there is clinical suspicion of active macular involvement (unilateral or bilateral). The early phase of the FA displays SRNVMs as lacy fans of vessels, while later phases are characterized by hyperfluorescence.

The Verteporfin in Ocular Histoplasmosis (VOH) Study demonstrated efficacy for photodynamic therapy of SRNVMs. Most patients with SRNVMs within 1500 microns (1 disc diameter) of the fovea have a poor visual prognosis if left untreated. The Ocular Histoplasmosis Study (one part of the Macular Photocoagulation Study) demonstrated the efficacy of argon blue-green laser photocoagulation in treating SRNVMs 200 to 2500 microns from the foveal avascular zone (FAZ) center and krypton-red laser for lesions within 200 microns of the FAZ.

Although there is a generally poor visual prognosis for subfoveal neovascular membranes, surgery that separates the membrane from adjacent RPE and sensory retina may be utilized. In addition, subretinal hemorrhage may be removed by employing recombinant tissue plasminogen activator.

Recurrence of SRNVMs necessitates home Amsler grid testing, monitoring of systemic hypertension (which may exacerbate recurrences), and yearly ocular examination (or more frequently if necessary).

OCULAR TOXOPLASMOSIS
Nicky R. Holdeman

ICD—9: 771.2—Other congenital infections
ICD—9: 130.0—Meningoencephalitis due to toxoplasmosis

THE DISEASE
Pathophysiology

Toxoplasma gondii is the most common cause of infectious retinochoroiditis in the world, accounting for 30 to 50% of cases in otherwise healthy individuals. In addition to retinochoroiditis, the organism may also produce other functional changes including a dense vitritis, vitreous detachment, iridocyclitis, perivasculitis, retinal detachment, neovascularization, cataracts, and glaucoma. Because the organism is an intracellular parasite, the retina sustains the primary insult and the major damage.

Recurrent retinochoroiditis occurs when tissue cysts release parasites that invade and destroy retinal cells. As they proliferate, parasites stimulate inflammatory reactions, resulting in clinically apparent lesions. Factors related to reactivation of disease in otherwise healthy individuals are not known, and recurrences cannot be predicted.

Etiology

T. gondii is a small obligate intracellular protozoan parasite affecting humans and animals; nearly one-third of all humans have has been exposed to this parasite. Multiplication occurs in the intestines of cats, and the oocyst forms are shed in the stool. The most common routes of human transmission are by intrauterine infection, by ingestion of contaminated food or undercooked meat, or through inhalation of oocysts in cat litter. Cysts may remain viable in the soil for extended periods of time.

The Patient

Clinical Symptoms

The patient will generally not complain of pain, but rather of an increase in floaters and a reduction of vision in the affected eye.

Clinical Signs

The appearance of a toxoplasmosis lesion varies depending on whether the infection is in an active or inactive state, and on the immune status of the patient.

Active retinochoroiditis, in an immunocompetent patient, typically appears as a unilateral, creamy-white, fluffy, necrotic, retinal lesion with blurred margins. Recurrent disease often occurs next to an old scar to produce a "satellite lesion." Usually, a hazy vitreous overlies the lesion, giving a "headlight in the fog" appearance.

In immunocompromised patients, the active condition is bilateral in 20% of cases. The retinal lesions are often extensive and may consist of large areas of retinal necrosis or retinochoroiditis without adjacent pre existing retinal scars. These atypical retinal lesions may be associated with cerebral involvement, myocarditis, and pneumonitis.

The ocular complications of toxoplasmosis may include SRNVM, vessel occlusions, preretinal gliosis, retinal breaks, retinal detachments, macular edema, papillitis, optic nerve atrophy, synechia, cataract, and/or glaucoma. A mild anterior chamber reaction may be seen in some patients.

Inactive lesions produce a well-demarcated chorioretinal scar with bare sclera often surrounded by hypertrophic retinal pigment epithelium.

Demographics

The frequency of ocular involvement in postnatally acquired toxoplasmosis is not known, but the incidence of acquired infections is probably greater than originally suspected. There is clear evidence that acquired toxoplasmosis can induce ocular lesions.

It has long been believed that the vast majority of cases of ocular toxoplasmosis involving adults are late sequelae of a congenital infection with the mother acquiring a primary infection during pregnancy, then passing it to the fetus transplacentally. Congenital infection has been estimated to affect 3,000 infants born in the United States each year. When primary infection of the mother occurs during pregnancy, there is a 40% chance of fetal infection. Although congenital infection can affect any organ, ocular disease is the most common manifestation resulting in irreversible damage to the retina in utero. *Toxoplasma* organisms invade the retina of the fetus, where they may change into the cystic form. Most active cases are thought to represent a late manifestation of this intrauterine infection, where the cysts rupture and liberate parasites in surrounding cells.

Recurrences often manifest between ages 11 and 40, with the mean age of first presentation being approximately 29 years. The disease is rather uncommon in early childhood and after the age of 50, but severe or acquired cases of ocular toxoplasmosis have been reported in older patients without suspected or documented immunodeficiency. Recurrences have been observed in 49% of patients within 3 years.

Legal blindness (BCVA ≤20/200) in at least one eye may be expected in 24% of patients (i.e., macular involvement, vitreous hemorrhage, SRNVM, or retinal detachment).

Significant History

- Is the patient aware of having contracted any congenital infections?
- Does the patient eat raw or undercooked meat?
- Is there an exposure to cats or cat litter?
- Inquire about immunosuppression or risk factors for AIDS in patients with active bilateral, atypical, or multifocal lesions.

Ancillary Tests

The diagnosis of ocular toxoplasmosis is usually made by the classic fundus findings; however, several tests can be used to confirm clinical impressions or assist in atypical cases.

- Serology is supportive but not diagnostic in adults, as 20 to 70% of the general population will show positive titers.
- The most commonly used serologic tests are the IFA and ELISA for toxoplasmosis, which can be done on blood, CSF, and aqueous. These tests permit separation of IgM and IgG antibodies. The presence of IgM antitoxin titers indicates a recent acquisition of infection. Recurrent retinochoroiditis is usually associated with stable, low IgG titers and no IgM antibody. A positive test, even at a 1:1 dilution, corroborates the diagnosis.
- In difficult or atypical cases, anterior chamber paracentesis to detect local antibody production may be helpful. If IgG antibodies in the aqueous are higher than in the serum, the diagnosis is supported. In addition, polymerase chain reaction (PCR) tests to detect *T. gondii* DNA in the aqueous can help confirm the diagnosis and help differentiate ocular toxoplasmosis from similar retinal lesions caused by herpesvirus or other infectious agents.
- The Sabin-Feldman dye test, which was the original standard test for toxoplasmosis, requires working with live *Toxoplasma* organisms and is seldom used today.
- Fluorescein angiography may be useful in helping to identify sub-retinal neovascular membranes and/or macular edema.

The Treatment

The treatment for ocular toxoplasmosis is not uniform. Some lesions, if they are small and in the retinal periphery, are generally not a threat to vision, and if they occur in an immunocompetent host may simply be followed. Activity in the lesion may persist for up to 4 months, but will spontaneously resolve.

Large active lesions, or those that threaten the optic nerve or macula, are often treated with a combination of systemic steroids plus one to three antitoxoplasmic agents. It should be noted, however, that there is a lack of evidence to support routine antibiotic treatment for acute toxoplasmic retinochoroiditis and that treatment is often associated with adverse effects.

Corticosteroids are rarely employed in the treatment of immunocompromised patients and should never be used without antimicrobial therapy. Steroids are often given concurrently with antitoxoplasmic drugs to alleviate inflammation, especially when the lesions are located near or in the macula.

- Prednisone 40 to 80 mg p.o. daily is begun after the second or third day of antitoxoplasmic therapy until day 10, and then tapered gradually over a period of 4 to 5 weeks. Stop steroids before antitoxoplasma medications.

Antitoxoplasmic drugs include pyramethamine (which is probably the most effective drug against ocular toxoplasmosis), sulfadiazine, clindamycin, azithromycin, and tetracycline. Trimethoprim-sulfamethoxazole has been used with variable results.

- Pyrimethamine—loading dose of 75 to 150 mg p.o. the first day, then 25 mg p.o. bid for 3 to 6 weeks. Follow complete blood counts and give folinic acid (leucovorin) 3 to 5 mg p.o. two to four times weekly to minimize bone marrow depression (thrombocytopenia, leukopenia, megablastic anemia).
- Sulfadiazine—loading dose of 2 grams p.o. the first day, then 1 gram p.o. qid for 3 to 6 weeks depending on clinical response.
- Clindamycin—150 to 300 mg p.o. qid. Useful adjunct to above therapy or may be used with only sulfadiazine. Concentrates in the choriod, but is expensive. Monitor for pseudomembranous colitis. Limit treatment to 4 weeks.
- Azithromycin—500 mg on day 1 followed by 250 mg per day, alone or in combination with pyrimethamine, appears to be effective in treating sight-threatening lesions with fewer side effects than other antibiotics.
- Tetracycline—loading dose of 1 gram p.o. on the first day, then 500 mg p.o. qid for 3 to 6 weeks.
- Trimethoprim (160mg)/sulfamethoxazole (800 mg)—the use of this drug for the treatment of ocular toxoplasmosis in humans is limited, although many uveitis specialists concur that it is an effective therapy and is generally well tolerated. There is also evidence that long-term treatment (up to 20 months) with TMP/SMX significantly reduces the rate of recurrence of retinochoroiditis in patients with a history of multiple previous recurrences.

Because some of these drugs may have significant side effects, it is advisable to follow these patients with an internist.

Intravitreal injections of clindamycin and dexamethasone are generally well tolerated and may offer an additional treatment strategy in patients who are unable to afford or tolerate systemic therapy, or whose disease progresses despite systemic therapy.

There appears to be an increased risk of reactivations of ocular toxoplasmosis following cataract extraction. This finding would imply that prophylactic treatment with antitoxoplasmic agents prior to and after surgery might be prudent for patients at risk for visual loss.

Anterior segment inflammation varies from a minimal response to a severe granulomatous iritis and is treated with topical cycloplegics (e.g., homatropine 5% bid-tid) and/or topical steroids (e.g., prednisolone acetate 1% qid) as the need exists.

TOXOCARIASIS
Nicky R. Holdeman
ICD—9: 128.0

THE DISEASE
Pathophysiology

Toxocariasis is a clinical syndrome resulting from parasitic invasion of human viscera with subsequent migration of the larvae to various organs. Toxocara does not develop beyond the larval state in the incidental human host, thus eggs are not found in the stool of humans.

Etiology

Toxocariasis most commonly results from infections with larvae of the canine round-worm, *Toxocara canis*. The adult worms live in the intestinal tracts of their primary hosts and release large numbers of eggs in the stool. The eggs can remain active and infective in the soil for months to years.

Human infections are generally acquired by young children who ingest the ova from soil or sand contaminated with animal feces, most often puppies. The eggs hatch in the intestine, and liberated larvae then penetrate the mucosal wall and are disseminated by the systemic circulation to the liver, lung, brain, kidney, striated muscle, CNS, heart, and the eye where they may produce an eosinophilic granulomatous inflammation. Remains of larvae are found within the granulomas, which contain eosinophils and histiocytes.

The Patient

Clinical Symptoms
Symptoms will vary depending on the organ involved. Children, usually before the age of 3, may develop acute systemic disease (i.e., visceral larvae migrans [VLM]). If so, the migrating larvae may produce symptoms such as malaise, fever, cough, skin rash, and/or abdominal pain.

Patients with ocular toxocariasis may complain of visual impairment in one eye, or may be referred for evaluation of leukocoria or strabismus.

Eye pain is not typical in this condition.

Clinical Signs
Patients with VLM may demonstrate lymphadenopathy, hepatomegaly, fever, wheezing, or a variety of other findings with diverse organ invasion.

In the eye, toxocariasis can have three different presentations.

- Peripheral chorioretinal granuloma—usually associated with dense fibrous bands in the vitreous with dragging of the macula; may mimic pars planitis.

- Posterior pole chorioretinal granuloma—a white mass, 1 to 6 mm in diameter, is seen with an accompanying vitritis; usually located in the macula or in the papillo-macular bundle.
- Endophthalmitis—chronic, diffuse, painless uveitis with a cloudy vitreous. There may be a secondary cataract, cyclitic membrane, and/or retinal detachment.

It is rare to have VLM and ocular disease concurrently. Ocular toxocariasis is typically a unilateral disorder, but confirmed cases of bilateral panuveitis have been reported.

Demographics

- Visceral larva migrans usually presents around the age of 2 years.
- Most cases of ocular toxocariasis occur in children 5 to 10 years of age, with a range of 2 to 30 years. By the time the child seeks eye care, systemic manifestations have usually resolved.
- The largest numbers of cases of ocular toxocariasis have been reported in the United States; however, the disease has been seen in many countries worldwide.

Significant History

- Is there known exposure to puppies, especially 2 weeks to 6 months of age? (>50% of puppies and 20% of adult dogs harbor the parasite.)
- Is there a history of geophagia?
- Did the child play in a sandbox?
- Is there a history of ingesting uncooked foods?

Ancillary Tests

The diagnosis of both visceral larva migrans and ocular toxocariasis is typically made based on the appropriate signs and symptoms, together with a history of exposure to infected pets or pica. In atypical cases, the diagnosis can be aided by an ELISA titer of undiluted serum, which has a high sensitivity and specificity (90%) for toxocara antibodies.

Occasionally, in cases of ocular toxocariasis, the serum ELISA titers may be normal but antibody titers of intraocular fluids may be elevated which permits a diagnosis.

Visceral larva migrans is often associated with a marked leucocytosis, with 30 to 80% because of eosinophils. Ocular toxocariasis is usually not associated with a peripheral eosinophilia; however, eosinophils found in the vitreous can be helpful in the diagnosis.

Ultrasonography, to detect the intraocular calcifications of a retinoblastoma, can assist in the differential diagnosis.

The Treatment

The medical management of ocular toxocariasis is unclear, as no proven treatment is available. While the acute systemic infection is often treated with thiabendazole, mebendazole, albendazole, or diethylcarbamazine, the use of these antihelminthic agents is of questionable benefit in ocular toxocariasis as the disease is self-limiting, the amount of ocular absorption is unknown, and the reaction to a dead nematode can increase ocular inflammation. If oral antihelmenthics are employed, it is recommended that they be used in conjunction with steroids to decrease the inflammatory process.

Suggested regimens for ocular toxocariasis may include a combination of:

- Thiabendazole 25 mg/kg p.o. bid for 3 to 7 days. Maximum of 3 grams daily.
- Prednisone 40 mg p.o. daily for 5 to 10 days followed by taper to control the vitritis (in some cases, subconjunctival injections of steroids may be preferable to oral usage).

Anterior uveitis, if present, is typically mild and should be treated with topical steroids and cycloplegics as clinically indicated.

If subretinal larva is visualized outside the foveal area, photocoagulation or cryocoagulation may be used to destroy the organisms.

Surgery is sometimes required for complications such as tractional retinal detachments.

Note: Controlling toxocara infections in dogs and puppies is essential if there are children in the household.

AGE-RELATED MACULAR DEGENERATION (AMD)
Helmut Buettner

ICD—9: 362.50

THE DISEASE
Pathophysiology

The earliest ophthalmoscopically detectable change of age-related macular degeneration is the formation of "drusen," which are yellow-gray, slightly elevated round deposits under the RPE. They contain, among amorphous material, incompletely digested retinal photoreceptor and RPE-cell organelles, pointing toward a primary malfunction of the RPE. Thickening and accumulation of lipids in Bruch's membrane probably interferes further with the elimination of retinal (photoreceptor) break-down products and results in an increase in the number and size of drusen, which eventually may become confluent and form a serous detachment of the RPE. It is at this stage that blood vessels extending from the choriocapillaris are most likely to invade and penetrate the degenerated Bruch's membrane and grow under the RPE. Exudation and hemorrhage from these choroidal neovascularization are the main causes of sudden, profound loss of central vision in this "wet" form of AMD. Eventually, the exudative or hemorrhagic disciform detachment caused by the choroidal neovascularization transforms into a disciform scar, representing the end-stage of "wet" macular degeneration. Not all drusen become large and confluent and form a pigment epithelial detachment, often giving rise to choroidal neovascularization. Drusen may become dehydrated and calcified and the RPE may atrophy in a sharply outlined geographic pattern in the posterior pole. This gradually progressing atrophy results in profound visual loss when it extends into the center of the macula. Drusen, pigmentary abnormalities, and geographic atrophy of the RPE are the main ophthalmoscopic features of the "dry" form of macular degeneration.

Etiology

Age-related macular degeneration is a chronic degenerative disease of Bruch's membrane and the retinal pigment epithelium, resulting in damage to the macular photoreceptor cells. Age, heredity, and race are established etiologic factors of AMD. Other factors include hypertension, cardiovascular disease, smoking, and exposure to sunlight (ultraviolet light). Low antioxidant (carotenoids, vitamins C and E) blood levels appear to have either causative or exacerbating significance in the development of the disease.

The Patient

Clinical Symptoms
- Initially may be asymptomatic
- Blurred vision
- Metamorphopsia
- Central blind spot

Clinical Signs
The hallmark clinically detectable abnormality and earliest sign of AMD are round, slightly elevated yellowish-gray deposits under the RPE primarily in the posterior pole, called "drusen." Drusen, which are composed of eosinophilic material between the basement membrane of the RPE and Bruch's membrane, may become visible ophthalmoscopically as early as the fourth decade of life, generally grow in number, enlarge with progressing age, and may become confluent. Mottled pigment eventually accumulates around the drusen. Drusen and pigmentary changes, often arranged in a reticular pattern, may also be found in the midperipheral fundus. At this stage, visual acuity is usually normal, but symptoms of requiring more light to read or mild metamorphopsia may be noted. This manifestation of AMD is also referred to as the dry form of macular degeneration and is seen in about 90% of individuals with AMD. Atrophy of the retinal pigment epithelium may develop in a sharply outlined or geographic pattern (geographic atrophy) which, when involving the fovea, leads to severe loss of central vision.

The individual with large drusen surrounded by pigment proliferation is at greatest risk of developing the wet or exudative form of AMD encountered in about 10% of patients with the disease. The wet form of AMD is characterized by leakage of fluid alone, resulting in a pigment epithelial detachment and/or serous neurosensory retinal detachment, or leakage of fluid and blood from neovascularization arising from the choroidal circulation. The neovascularization eventually transform into scar tissue (disciform scar), which can extend under the entire posterior pole. The retinal photoreceptor cells overlying such a scar degenerate resulting in severe loss of central vision, also noted by the patient as a blurred spot or scotoma in the central visual field.

Demographics

Age-related macular degeneration is the most common cause of legal blindness in the United States and Western Europe. Ten percent of the population over age 65 in the United States exhibit fundus changes of AMD (large drusen and pigment mottling in the macula), and 1% will be legally blind (20/200 or less vision bilaterally) from the disorder. AMD affects primarily blue-eyed, White individuals, women more often than men. It rarely causes visual loss in Black persons. Many individuals with AMD have other family members affected by the disease.

Ancillary Tests

In addition to a detailed eye examination including biomicroscopy, a number of tests are extremely helpful in diagnosing and managing patients with AMD. The Amsler grid allows the detection and localization of changes in the central visual field caused by AMD. It also allows the patient with AMD to self-monitor the central visual field for the development of visual symptoms or their changes. Fluorescein and indocyanine green angiography are extremely helpful in the identification and classification of anatomic and functional abnormalities associated with AMD. These angiographic techniques are particularly useful in the exact localization of neovascularization, important for the planning and performance of their treatment. Optical coherence tomography (OCT) can provide cross-sectional high-resolution images of the retina, pigment epithelium, and inner choroid in the macular area, helpful in monitoring the disease or its response to treatment.

The Treatment

Population-based studies have shown that individuals who have consumed a diet rich in antioxidants (green leafy vegetables, red wine) throughout their lives have a lower risk of developing and losing vision from AMD. These studies led to a large, prospective randomized trial of the affect of high-dose vitamins and minerals on the progression of AMD in patients with large drusen in the macula. In the Age-Related Eye Disease Study (AREDS), individuals who received the vitamins and minerals had a lower risk of both progression of their AMD and visual loss from AMD as compared to individuals who received a placebo. Other measures aimed at preventing development or progression of AMD include cessation of smoking, optimal control of cardiovascular disease and risk factors, and minimizing exposure to ultraviolet light (UV) by wearing appropriate UV-blocking glasses.

For extrafoveal choroidal neovascular membranes, conventional thermal photocoagulation is the treatment of choice. For occult subfoveal neovascularization transpupillary thermo-therapy (TTT), using an infrared laser is being evaluated.

The growth of subfoveal choroidal neovascularization can also be stopped with photodynamic therapy (PDT), a combination of photosensitizing drugs and infrared laser irradiation. Specifically, a large randomized collaborative study, Treatment of Age-Related Macular Degeneration with Photodynamic Therapy (TAP), showed that 67% of eyes with predominantly classic subfoveal neovascularization treated with verteporfin had lost fewer than 15 letters of vision after 12 months as compared to only 39% of eyes treated with placebo. The verteporfin treatment benefit was still present after 2 years. Subsequent studies also demonstrated the benefit of verteporfin treatment of occult subfoveal choroidal neovascularization (CNV) in AMD.

TAP inclusion criteria specifies that patients should be ≥50 years of age, the CNV should be under the geometric center of the foveal avascular zone, fluorescein angiography should show evidence of a classic CNV, and the area of CNV should encompass at least 50% of the area of the total neovascular lesion, Snellen visual acuity should be approximately 20/40 through 20/200, and the greatest linear dimension of the lesion should be ≤5400 microns (not including any area of prior laser photocoagulation).

Macular translocation, a delicate surgical procedure that relocates the macular retina over healthier retinal pigment epithelium adjacent to the neovascularization, which are then destroyed with conventional photocoagulation, can in selected cases of AMD improve or preserve central vision.

The pharmacologic treatment of subfoveal choroidal neovascularization with various vascular growth factor inhibitors (rhuFab V2, Pegaptabnib sodium) and steroid derivatives (Anecortave acetate) is currently undergoing clinical trials and may soon add new treatment modalities for selected forms of AMD.

STARGARDT'S DISEASE
Jerome Sherman

ICD—9: 362.75

THE DISEASE

Stargardt's disease or dystrophy, occasionally termed *juvenile macular dystrophy*, is the most common form of inherited juvenile macular degeneration. It is characterized by progressive and symmetrical atrophy of the macula that affects individuals with previously normal vision. Stargardt's disease is often considered a form of fundus flavimaculatus, where macular atrophy predominates early in the disease progression. Perhaps the most accurate name is "Stargardt's Disease with Fundus Flavimaculatus" because most patients have both the macular atrophy and the characteristic flecks.

Pathophysiology

Although most eye clinicians regard Stargardt's disease and fundus flavimaculatus as different manifestations of the same disease, for classification purposes they are interchangeable. The term *fundus flavimaculatus* is applied when the characteristic subretinal flecks, which are fish-tail or pisciform in shape, are scattered throughout the fundus. When the flecks are very subtle, confined to the posterior pole or nonexistent, the macular atrophy is properly termed *Stargardt's dystrophy*. Although some patients present initially with only the macular atrophy while others present with only the flecks, long-term follow-up of either group reveals the eventual ophthalmoscopic finding of both the macular atrophy and the characteristic flecks.

Stargardt's disease has its onset within the first two decades of life. A patient initially presents with a decrease in visual acuity. Although visual acuity loss is often proportional to the degree of macular atrophy, it is not at all rare for a patient to present with reduced visual acuity but with a normal appearing fundus. Numerous patients with an eventual diagnosis of Stargardt's have been initially misdiagnosed as malingering. Macular lesions may precede the flecks. Thus, the diagnosis of Stargardt's disease is sometimes made before other signs of fundus flavimaculatus are evident.

Etiology

Stargardt's disease is most typically a result of an autosomal recessive gene. As with all autorecessive disorders, a high incidence of consanguinity can be established through the appropriate questions. A very small number of families have an autosomal dominant form. All autosomal recessive forms of Stargardt's and fundus flavimaculatus have been mapped to the short arm of chromosome 1. The autosomal dominant form of these disorders map to chromosome 13q34 and the long arm of chromosome 6. It has been found that the causal gene of Stargardt's disease, ABCA4 (located on the short arm of chromosome 1), is a mutated photoreceptor cell-specific adenosine triphosphate-binding transporter. It is expressed in rod but not cone photoreceptors. The variations in sequencing of the ABCA4 gene appear to be responsible for the varied clinical presentations observed in patients with Stargardt's dystrophy.

The Patient

Clinical Symptoms
The initial presenting symptom is always that of decreased central vision in an individual with prior normal vision. In the later stages of the disease, there may also be noticeable color vision defects. Night blindness is usually not a complaint. Photophobia is rare as an early complaint, but some patients report that they are bothered by glare.

Clinical Signs
The onset of Stargardt's disease is usually in the first or second decade of an individual's life. The most characteristic finding of Stargardt's dystrophy is a progressive and symmetrical atrophy of the macula with previously normal vision. Visual acuity initially varies from 20/25 to 20/60 and progresses to 20/200. Although the progression of visual loss is variable, it is generally found to be similar with members of the same pedigree.

The initial fundus exam may be unremarkable with perhaps only a loss of the foveal reflex. Through the course of disease progression, a number of discrete yellowish pisciform flecks are evident at the level of the retinal pigment epithelium (RPE) surrounding the macula or are scattered throughout the posterior pole. Vessels are not usually attenuated. Over time, the retinal pigment epithelium may take on a "bull's-eye pattern" of loss. In the later stages of disease, the macula is often described as having a "beaten bronze" appearance with a horizontal oval area (approximately 2 DD by 1.5 DD). As the macular atrophy continues to develop, the flecks extend to the midperiphery. There is an enlargement of the RPE cells that is thought to be secondary to excessive lipofuscin deposition in the zones of the flecks with a total disappearance of the cones, rods, and RPE cells in the circumfoveal zone. These small, deep flecks that appear around the lesion and in the periphery have the appearance of classic fundus flavimaculatus and thus are thought to be the same disease. It is when the macular lesions precede the flecks that the disorder may be diagnosed as Stargardt's disease.

A small number of patients (approximately 1%) who present with what appears to be Stargardt's disease progress to an overall retinal degeneration. Although very rare, even within the same family, one member may have Stargardt's but another member has retinitis pigmentosa.

Demographics

Stargardt's disease is the most common form of inherited juvenile macular degenerations and is often diagnosed within the first two decades of life. The prevalence of Stargardt's disease worldwide is estimated to be 1 in 8,000, whereas the incidence of fundus flavimaculatus is said to be 1 in 10,000. Patients initially present with reduced central vision. Once a visual acuity of 20/40 is reached, there is often a rapid progression of visual loss until acuity is reduced to 20/200. There is over 50% likelihood that an individual with Stargardt's may retain a visual acuity of 20/40 in at least one eye by age 20. The probability of maintaining 20/40 visual acuity is over 30% by age 30 and over 20% by age 40. By age 50, approximately half of patients have visual acuities of 20/200 or worse.

Ancillary Tests

Ocular assessment may include visual acuity, dilated fundus evaluation, standard visual field testing, color vision testing, fluorescein angiography, electroretinography (ERG), and electro-oculography (EOG). Fluorescein angiography enables the detection of the macular abnormality by depicting multiple, irregular hyperfluorescent spots. The flecks observed ophthalmoscopically can either be nonfluorescent or hyperfluorescent. Therefore, the spots may not correspond directly to the flecks. In the case of a bull's-eye lesion, the central area is normally surrounded by a hyperfluorescent area. In about 50% of Stargardt cases, there is a generalized dark "silent" choroid. Color defects are often mild red-green dyschromatopsia and gradually progress to achromatopsia in late macular atrophy. ERGs are found to be normal or slightly abnormal with reduced B-wave amplitudes. The result of the EOG is dependent on the extent of retinal pigment epithelium involved and is usually normal until later stages. Visual fields demonstrate initial central scotomas, which often progress to absolute scotomas. Peripheral vision is maintained even in late stages of the disease. A rare case may present with a normal ERG that progresses to a completely extinguished ERG. This suggests that retinitis pigmentosa on occasion can present initially as Stargardt's disease.

The Treatment

There is no treatment for Stargardt's disease. Vision loss is inevitable, so the best possible prescription should be provided with the recommendation of lenses to block short wavelength light. Individuals with the disorder often benefit from low vision rehabilitation including vision aids and orientation and mobility training. Genetic counseling and testing is fundamental. Psychological counseling may be needed to assist in coping with the trauma of rapid vision loss. No proven vitamin therapy exists. A few patients who present with Stargardt's later develop unrelated glaucoma, and hence procedures such as

IOP measurements, disc assessment, and retinal nerve fiber layer measurements should be considered. Although Stargardt's is not treatable, the unrelated glaucoma is treatable. Brimonidine lowers IOPs but may have neuroprotective qualities as well. Some nonhuman studies have concluded that brimonidine not only protects ganglion cells but also may protect photoreceptors. No proof exists in humans at the present time.

IDIOPATHIC CENTRAL SEROUS CHORIORETINOPATHY (ICSC)
Michael J. Trad

ICD—9: 362.41

THE DISEASE
Pathophysiology

Idiopathic central serous chorioretinopathy is a transient, unilateral serous detachment of neurosensory retina and retinal pigment epithelium (RPE). It occurs most frequently in young, White adult males and is not associated with any predisposing pathological alterations of the retina/RPE/choroid interface, such as drusen or choroidal neovascularization. Although the exact pathogenesis of ICSC is unknown, research suggests that an underlying dystrophic, inflammatory, or ischemic mechanism may cause either a focal or diffuse dysfunction of the RPE's tight junctions and/or choriocapillaris vascular network. This allows choriocapillary serous fluid access through Bruch's membrane (frequently causing an RPE detachment) and the RPE into the subretinal space. A localized retinal detachment results when subretinal fluid separates the RPE from the neurosensory retina.

Etiology

As its name implies, the cause of ICSC is unknown (idiopathic); however, many schools of thought exist as to its etiology. The most frequently advocated theory suggests that patients under high degrees of emotional and/or physical stress exhibit heightened sympathetic tone manifested by increased levels of circulating epinephrine or catecholamines. Thus, the classic patient profile is best exemplified by a young, compulsive, Type-A personality male. ICSC has also been reported in association with pregnancy, solid organ transplantation, and Cushing's syndrome.

The Patient

Symptoms and signs of ICSC are dependent upon the extent and duration of the disease process.

Clinical Symptoms
- Sudden onset of mild to moderate vision loss in one eye
- Distortion of vision

- Mild central loss of vision
- Image size difference between eyes (smaller image in the affected eye)
- Decreased depth perception
- Color vision disturbance

Clinical Signs
Prominent Signs
- Mild to moderate (20/20 to 20/80) unilateral decrease in visual acuity
- Amsler grid metamorphopsia
- Amsler grid relative central scotoma
- Color desaturation
- Increased photostress recovery time
- Decreased contrast sensitivity
- Delayed VEP latency
- Loss of foveal reflex

Subtle Signs
- Amsler grid micropsia
- Unilateral hyperopic shift
- Dome-shaped elevation of macula (and/or other posterior pole location), indicating a retinal detachment
- Light reflex ring around sensory detachment (dome)
- Lemon-drop nodule within sensory elevation (indicating an RPE serous detachment)
- Active peripheral ICSC lesions in the affected and/or opposite eye
- Yellow precipitates on the sensory detachment's undersurface or a gray, diffuse subretinal fibrin layer (indicating a later stage in the disease process)
- Teardrop-shaped areas of RPE dropout in the peripheral retina of either eye (indicating past bout of ICSC)

Demographics
- ICSC has been observed more frequently in Whites than in Blacks.
- Men have a higher incidence of the disease than women (depending on the study, the reported ratio of males to females ranges from 2:1 to 7:1).
- The age of onset is generally between 30 and 50 years, with a range from 27 to 60 years of age and older.
- There is an increased incidence of ICSC in women during pregnancy.
- ICSC may be of greater incidence in patients with Cushing's syndrome than in the general population.
- Up to 50% of ICSC cases recur.
- In approximately 10 to 25% of cases, the opposite eye will develop symptomatic ICSC after a delay of a number of weeks.
- Approximately 50 to 60% of patients recover visual acuity of 20/20, but 5 to 10% suffer a permanent loss of vision worse than 20/40. Up to 90% of patients experience a resolution of acuity to at least 20/40 within 1 to 6 months. Patients recover visual acuity within 3 months in 60% of cases, while in 20% it may take longer than

6 months. Most patients, however, will experience some degree of visual disturbance after resolution of ICSC.
- Patients undergoing laser treatment of ICSC experience resolution of vision within 5 weeks, while untreated patients recover in 23 weeks (median duration).
- Patients with ICSC who undergo laser photocoagulation develop choroidal neovascularization (CNV) approximately 2 to 5% of the time.

Significant History

Usually none but may be associated with stress, pregnancy, solid organ transplantation, or Cushing's syndrome.

Ancillary Tests

Ocular assessment of ICSC would include best-corrected visual acuity, pupil assessment, visual field testing, color vision, contrast sensitivity, photostress recovery time, and dilated fundus examination.

OCT and FA should be done to confirm the diagnosis. The angiographic appearance of ICSC is variable, but most leaks occur within one disc diameter of the fovea. Classically with FA, the disease demonstrates focal hyperfluorescence at a leakage site in the early phase, which progresses in time to form an inverted smokestack (10 to 23% of cases). However, the most frequently observed pattern (65%) is a point stain in the venous phase. These small leaks are associated with much less extensive retinal detachments than those displaying smokestack staining. The remaining two FA patterns observed in ICSC are diffuse (12%) and sub-RPE pooling with punctate leakage through the RPE into the subretinal space (4%). If no leaks are observed during the FA, the disease process may have resolved or the leakage is outside of the macula. In the latter instance, it is critical to rule out other causes of serous detachments, such as congenital optic disc pits, choroidal neoplasm, metastatic carcinoma, peripheral retinal holes/tears, and uveal effusion. Indocyanine green (ICG) angiography is also utilized to image the choroidal vasculature and may demonstrate multifocal areas of choroidal hyperpermeability.

The Treatment

No treatment is usually indicated, as ICSC generally resolves within a few weeks to months. However, if the patient has critical visual demands and/or the subretinal fluid fails to reabsorb after 4 to 6 months, laser photocoagulation may be considered.

In those cases when argon or krypton photocoagulation is contemplated, FA should be performed within at least 1 week of the laser treatment. Also, it is important to consider that while photocoagulation may initially hasten visual recovery, it typically does not influence the long-term visual prognosis, that is, whether treated or not vision will ultimately be the same. When laser treatment is performed, FA leakage points at least 200 microns outside of the FAZ are best treated with direct photocoagulation, while leaks within 200 microns of the FAZ fare better with indirect application of the krypton red laser. Burn spot size is typically 100 to 150 microns, and the lowest possible laser energy should be employed. As mentioned earlier, CNV may occur in approximately 2 to 5% of photocoagulated patients, and up to 50% of ICSC cases may recur. In addition, photo-dynamic therapy (PDT) with ICG guidance has recently been suggested as a potential treatment for ICSC.

ANGIOID STREAKS
Mohammad R. Rafieetary and Christopher Willingham

ICD—9: 363.43

THE DISEASE
Pathophysiology

Angioid streaks are sharply demarcated, irregular, tapering, linear cracks in Bruch's membrane. They are thought to occur as a primary abnormality of the fibers of Bruch's membrane and from an increased availability or pathologic deposition of metal salts. As a result, there is increased fragility of Bruch's membrane, which can secondarily lead to the development of a choroidal neovascular membrane (CNVM).

Etiology

Angioid streaks are found in association with a number of conditions, including pseu-doxanthoma elasticum (PXE) (Grönblad-Strandberg syndrome), osteitis deformans (Paget's disease), sickle cell hemoglobinopathies, senile elastosis of the skin, and hy-pertensive cardiovascular disorders. Other less frequent causes are fibrodysplasia hy-perelastica (Ehlers Danlos syndrome), senile actinic elastosis, retinal exsanguination, lead poisoning, hemochromatosis, acquired hemolytic anemia, hypercalcemia, hyper-phosphatemia, tuberous sclerosis, Sturge Weber syndrome, and neurofibromatosis.

Approximately 50% of angioid streaks are idiopathic.

By far, the most common cause of angioid streaks is PXE, which is characterized by wrinkled skin with loose folds, particularly in the neck, axillae, groin, and the flexor aspects of joints. Major complications of PXE include hypertension, myocardial infarc-tion, intermittent claudication, stroke, and recurrent gastrointestinal bleeding. When associated with PXE, angioid streaks may be seen at a young age. If present in Paget's disease, angioid streaks are usually a late finding. Sickle cell disease will most likely have already been diagnosed prior to this finding.

The Patient

Symptoms and signs correspond to the underlying systemic disease or the extent of macular involvement.

Clinical Symptoms
Most patients with angioid streaks are visually asymptomatic. Loss of vision, meta-morphopsia, and color vision changes occur particularly when there is leakage of fluid through a defect in Bruch's membrane in the posterior pole.

Clinical Signs

Prominent Signs

- Angioid streaks originate in the peripapillary region as grayish or dark-reddish lines. They extend radially and taper off as they reach posterior to the equator. Ophthalmoscopically, they are seen at the level of the RPE and thus are deeper than the retinal vessels. They have a crack-like or jigsaw-like appearance.
- Extensive subretinal hemorrhaging may occur, which may spontaneously resolve.
- Disciform scarring is common.

Subtle Signs

- Disappearance of angioid streaks with pressure on the globe
- Macular drusen
- Fibrous tissue cuffs bordering the wider proximal portions of angioid streaks
- Drusen of the optic nerve head
- Mottled-background fundus appearance
- Peripheral punched-out chorioretinal scars

Demographics

Angioid streaks are rarely noted in children. They develop in the second or third decade of life. They are usually bilateral with asymmetrical presentation. Angioid streaks occur in 87% of patients with PXE, 22% with sickle cell disease, and 15% with Paget's disease.

Significant History

Patients with one of the underlying disorders as discussed under etiology.

Ancillary Tests

Ocular assessment includes visual acuity, pupil testing, color vision, Amsler grid, intraocular pressure, slit-lamp examination, and dilated fundus evaluation. Other ancillary testing includes fluorescein angiography (in the presence of macular lesions, subretinal fluid or hemorrhage or reduced visual acuity), visual fields are usually normal, dark adaptation and electrophysiology.

Expected Findings

- Visual acuity: Normal, unless involvement of the posterior pole
- Visual fields: Normal or central scotomata with macular involvement
- Color vision: Normal, unless vision loss
- Fluorescein angiography: Hyperfluorescence is usually noted in early phase and persists through the recirculation. Dye leakage can be noted from some of the cracks and also from associated CNVMs
- Dark adaptation: Normal
- Electroretinography: Normal
- Electro-oculography: Normal, unless extensive disease in the macular region

■ Laboratory studies: Sickle cell testing, serum alkaline phosphatase, phosphorus, urine calcium levels in suspected PXE, skin biopsy, cardiovascular and gastrointestinal evaluation in suspected cases of PXE

The Treatment

Angioid streaks require no treatment. If there is an associated CNVM, the membrane should be treated. Current therapies include thermal photocoagulation and photodynamic therapy. Future studies may show some benefit in treating the CNVMs with intraocular antiangiogenic agents or periocular steroidal agents.

Any systemic disease should be referred for further evaluation by an internist or an appropriate subspecialist.

HIGH MYOPIA
Mohammad R. Rafieetary and Steve Charles
ICD—9: 360.21

THE DISEASE
Pathophysiology

High myopia is characterized by refractive error of ≥ -6.00 diopters and axial length >26.5 mm. If the axial length extends to 32.5 mm, then the patient is said to have "pathologic" myopia. Other terms have been used to recognize a spectrum of condition; these include *progressive myopia, degenerative myopia,* and *malignant myopia*. Use of these terms can unnecessarily alarm those highly myopic patients who may never experience any significant vision loss. For the sake of discussion and simplification, the term *high myopia* is used in this chapter to discuss all arrays of this condition.

The pathogenesis of retinal disease in high myopia is not clearly understood, although it is thought to be either because of biomechanical abnormalities and/or a heredodegenerative process.

Etiology

The exact etiology of high myopia is not known. Both dominant and recessive autosomal patterns of inheritance have been found, but many sporadic occurrences also exist. Pathologic findings associated with high myopia are believed by some to result from progressive elongation of the globe. This theory may be flawed, as patients with low to moderate degrees of myopia (<6 D) may present with retinal complications. Conversely, patients presenting with high degrees of myopia may have relatively normal funduscopic findings.

The Patient

Symptoms and signs depend on the extent of the myopic error and the extent of the retinal change.

Clinical Symptoms

The patient with high myopia often complains of poor distance vision and floaters at an early age. By middle age, disturbances of central vision including metamorphopsia and central vision loss may occur. Progressive central degeneration may lead to hemeralopia, where the patient experiences better vision in dim, as opposed to bright, illumination.

Clinical Signs

Prominent Signs

- Refractive error of ≥ -6.00 diopters
- Axial length >26.00 mm
- Peripapillary "myopic" or temporal crescent (hallmark)
- Macular degeneration–type findings
- Forster-Fuchs spot (circular macular dark spot)
- Lacquer crack (breaks in Bruch's membrane appearing as yellow streaks)

Subtle Signs

- Temporal optic-disc pallor
- Titled optic disc
- Geographic areas of RPE atrophy
- Posterior staphyloma
- Nuclear sclerosis and posterior subcapsular opacities
- Open-angle, pigmentary, and low-tension glaucoma
- Chorioretinal atrophy
- Macular hemorrhages (with or without choroidal neovascular membrane)
- Choroidal neovascular membrane (CNVM)
- Lattice degeneration
- Retinal detachment
- Vitreal condensation and floaters

Demographics

Myopia is one of the leading causes of blindness worldwide. The prevalence of high myopia varies among different ethnic groups. In the United States, the condition is reported in 2.1% of 17 year olds. The incidence usually peaks at 20 years of age. Of these myopes, only around one-third may have the pathologic findings.

Women are thought to be more likely to develop higher degrees of myopia.

Genetic factors also play a major role. Blacks are usually less myopic, while Asians, especially the Chinese, are affected at a much higher frequency.

Differential diagnosis for retinal findings associated with high myopia include macular degeneration, ocular histoplasmosis, tilted disc syndrome, gyrate atrophy, toxoplasmosis, and traumatic retinal scars.

Significant History
- Nearsightedness at a young age
- Family history of myopia

Ancillary Tests

Ocular assessment includes visual acuity, pupil testing, color vision, Amsler grid, intraocular pressure, slit-lamp examination, dilated fundus examination with scleral indentation, visual field examination, and fluorescein angiography. Consider doing axial length measurements and keratometry. Record both a manifest and cycloplegic refraction.

The Treatment
- Correct the refractive error with glasses, contact lenses, or refractive surgery.
- Retinal breaks should be prophylacticly treated with laser or cryotherapy. Any retinal detachment should be managed appropriately.
- Choroidal neovascular membranes are treated appropriately with respect to their size and location by focal photocoagulation, photodynamic therapy, or submacular surgery.

GYRATE ATROPHY
Mohammad R. Rafieetary and Christopher Willingham

ICD—9: 363.54—Central choroidal atrophy, total
ICD—9: 363.57—Other diffuse or generalized dystrophy, total

THE DISEASE
Pathophysiology

Gyrate atrophy is a progressive, bilateral, autosomal recessive condition. It is caused by a decrease in the activity of the mitochondrial enzyme, ornithine aminotransferase, which is responsible for the breakdown of ornithine to delta-pyrroline-5-carboxylic acid, which is then converted into proline. As a result, patients have abnormally high ornithine levels in all body fluids. These levels are usually 6 to 15 times higher than normal. The high ornithine levels are believed to cause most of the pathology in gyrate atrophy. Other abnormalities include lower than normal serum lysine levels and a deficiency of creatinine or phosphocreatinine.

Etiology

Gyrate atrophy is a genetic disorder, resulting in mutations of the ornithine aminotransferase gene found on chromosome 10. It is considered an inborn error of amino acid metabolism.

The Patient

Symptoms and signs are those of progressive night blindness (nyctalopia) and visual acuity loss that usually begins in the first decade of life. The course of the decline in visual function such as visual field and electrophysiologic findings are usually slow.

Clinical Symptoms
- History of seizures
- Progressive night blindness leading to complete blindness between the ages of 40 and 50, if untreated

Clinical Signs
Prominent Signs
- High myopia
- Astigmatism
- Posterior subcapsular cataracts
- Irregular, sharply defined areas of chorioretinal atrophy
- Scalloped borders between normal and abnormal retinal pigment epithelium

Subtle Signs
- Yellowish appearance of fundus and disc
- Retinal vessel attenuation
- Fine, sparse, straight scalp hair with areas of alopecia

Demographics

The highest incidence of gyrate atrophy is reported in Finland in approximately 1:50,000 of the population.

The classic clinical presentation is high myopia in the first decade, night blindness in the second decade, cataracts in the third decade, and progressive chorioretinal atrophy and macular involvement leading to blindness in the fourth decade.

Significant History
- Known family history of disease

Ancillary Tests

Ocular assessment includes visual acuity, correction of myopia and astigmatic refractive errors, fundus evaluation, and fluorescein angiography. Visual field testing as well as color vision should be monitored. Other testing could include electroretinography, electro-oculography, and dark adaptation studies.

Laboratory studies: Serum ornithine levels. Electroencephalography will show diffuse slow-wave activity and skeletal muscle biopsy will show ultrastructural abnormalities.

The Treatment

Treatment involves maintaining serum ornithine levels between 55 and 355 uM with arginine-deficient diet by restricting arginine-rich foods such as nuts and legumes. Oral pyridoxine (vitamin B_6) 15 to 20 mg daily may reduce serum ornithine, while massive doses (500 to 750 mg) may improve retinal function. Orally administered α-aminoisobutyric acid can also reduce serum ornithine. Genetic counseling should be offered. Oral lysine administration to a few sample sizes of patients with B_6-nonresponsive gyrate atrophy has been shown to reduce plasma ornithine concentrations by 21 to 31% within 1 to 2 days. Genetic counseling must be considered.

CHOROIDAL FOLDS
Mohammad R. Rafieetary and Steve Charles

ICD—9: 743.54

THE DISEASE

Pathophysiology

Choroidal folds are parallel furrows (striae) usually seen in the posterior pole. These inner choroidal folds may also involve the Bruch's membrane, RPE, and even the sensory retina.

Etiology

The possible cause for choroidal folds includes choroidal congestion, scleral folding, and contraction of the Bruch's membrane. The conditions that could arise to such findings include orbital disease such as orbital tumors or thyroid ophthalmopathy, choroidal tumors, ocular hypotony, and intracranial hypertension (with or without presence of papilledema). Other miscellaneous causes include posterior scleritis and scleral buckle surgery. Idiopathic choroidal folds may be seen in hyperopic eyes with short axial length and normal vision.

Recently, a syndrome of bilateral choroidal folds and optic neuropathy has been described in middle-aged patients with hyperopia and short axial length. It has been speculated that these patients have a constricted scleral canal, causing optic disc congestion and complicated nonarteritic anterior ischemic optic neuropathy as a variant of the crowded disc syndrome.

The Patient

Asymptomatic cases are not uncommon. However, metamorphopsia may be the initial presenting symptom. Visual acuity may be normal or reduced, depending on the etiology, duration, and the location of the folds.

Patients may also have symptoms relating to the primary disease. For example, a patient with thyroid eye disease may present with symptoms associated with this condition, while choroidal folds are simply an incidental finding.

Clinical Signs

Funduscopic presence of folds primarily in the posterior pole.

Prominent Signs

- Horizontal parallel folds
- Occasional vertical, oblique, or irregular orientation
- Pale color of the crest of the fold
- Hyperopia
- Papilledema (usually chronic)
- Choroidal tumors
- Hypotony (e.g., following filtration surgery)
- Scleral buckle
- Thyroid ophthalmopathy

Demographics

Other than the idiopathic cases seen in hyperopic eyes with short axial length and presence as a secondary sequela of the contributory conditions, there is no specific demographic distribution.

Significant History

History of attributing medical or ocular conditions including prior ocular trauma and surgeries must be thoroughly investigated.

Ancillary Tests

Fluorescein angiography is helpful, showing alternating streaks of hyper- and hypofluorescence at the level of the RPE. Radiologic studies of the head and the orbit are highly recommended when retrobulbar disease is suspected. Lumbar puncture must be considered in patients suspicious to have increased intracranial pressure (such as pseudotumor cerebri).

The Treatment

There is no specific treatment for choroidal folds. In the presence of an underlying cause, the treatment is tailored to the origin of the disease.

CHOROIDEREMIA

Mohammad R. Rafieetary and Christopher Willingham

ICD—9: 363.50

THE DISEASE

Pathophysiology

The pathophysiology of choroideremia is poorly understood. It is a bilateral, X-linked recessive disorder that is characterized by progressive degeneration of the retinal pigment epithelium, retina, and choroid. Clinically, this leads to a bared sclera. There is variable visual field and vision loss.

Etiology

Choroideremia is transmitted in an X-linked recessive manner, with males exhibiting the full extent of the disease and females usually being asymptomatic carriers. Less than 5% of carriers are afflicted with the severe form of the disease.

The gene responsible for choroideremia has been localized to Xq13-q22 by linkage analysis. The protein product of this gene plays a vital role in intracellular vesicular transport.

The Patient

Symptoms generally begin in the first and second decades of life. Initially, these include problems with dark adaptation and difficulty with night vision. The progression of the disease will lead to significant visual field constriction and severe central vision loss by the fifth to seventh decades of life. Loss of macular function usually occurs in the later stages of the disease.

Clinical Symptoms
Retinal findings may be detected as early as the first decade of life. Retinal changes may be present in both affected males and asymptomatic female carriers.

Clinical Signs
Prominent Signs
- Pigment stippling
- Focal atrophy of the RPE
- Regions of choroidal atrophy with exposed choroidal vessels
- Diffuse choroidal thinning and sclerosis of choroidal vessels
- Scattered areas of normal choroid in the macula and peripheral retina
- Baring of sclera
- Pale optic disc

Subtle Signs
- Fine fibrillar vitreal degeneration
- Posterior subcapsular opacities
- Myopia
- Small, glistening intraretinal flecks

Demographics

Because this disease is inherited in a recessive X-linked manner, half of the male offspring of female carriers will be affected, and all the daughters of affected males will be carriers.

Significant History

■ Known family history of disease

Ancillary Tests

A practical immunoblot assay has been developed to diagnose patients with choroideremia. Ocular assessment should place emphasis on funduscopic evaluation, visual field testing, and fluorescein angiography. Color vision remains normal initially. Abnormal ERG findings may present even in early disease.

The Treatment

There is no treatment for choroideremia. Some symptoms may be helped with sunglasses. Low vision aids and field expanders may be tried in early stages of the disease. Genetic counseling must be considered.

ARTERIAL OCCLUSIVE DISEASE

Mohammad R. Rafieetary and Steve Charles

ICD—9: 362.30—Retinal vascular occlusion, unspecified
ICD—9: 362.31—Central retinal artery occlusion
ICD—9: 362.32—Arterial branch occlusion
ICD—9: 362.33—Partial arterial occlusion
ICD—9: 362.34—Transient arterial occlusion

THE DISEASE

Pathophysiology

Arterial occlusive disease, especially when sudden, leads to retinal ischemia and, consequently, loss of sight. The pattern of neuroretinal damage corresponds to the involved arterial network. This may include the occlusion of the ophthalmic artery, the central retinal artery that leads to central retinal artery occlusion (CRAO), one of the branches, hence a branch retinal artery occlusion (BRAO), or cilioretinal artery occlusion (CIRAO).

There are some similarities as well as a few differences in these conditions. All result in some degree of vision loss varying from mild changes to no light perception. The latter is more common with acute ophthalmic artery occlusion (OAO).

Approximately 5 to 10% of patients presenting with a CRAO may in actuality be experiencing an acute OAO. The neuroretinal ischemia leads to opacification of the superficial retina presenting as areas of retinal whitening in the acute phase, and in CRAO, formation of the foveal cherry-red spot, which is classically only seen in 30% of OAO cases. The retinal whitening usually resolves within 4 to 6 weeks, leaving a pale optic disc and a normal-appearing but dysfunctional retina.

Approximately 57% of retinal arterial occlusions involve the central retinal artery, whereas branch retinal arteries account for 38%. The most frequently affected region of the retina in BRAO is the superior temporal area. CIRAO accounts for only 5% of retinal occlusions.

Etiology

There are over 60 conditions and etiologic factors that lead to arterial occlusion. These can be subclassified as conditions leading to embolus formation, traumatic and iatrogenic, coagulopathies, collagen vascular and inflammatory disorders, ocular conditions associated with retinal arterial obstruction (e.g., optic disc drusen), vasculitidies, and a number of miscellaneous conditions (e.g., Fabry's disease).

In 20% of cases, intra-arterial emboli can be identified. These include emboli from cardiac lesions, artificial cardiac valves, bacterial endocarditis, and mitral valve prolapse or from atherosclerotic deposits within the carotid arteries (Hollenhorst plaque). Other sources of emboli include intravenous drug abuse, lipid emboli (pancreatitis, Purtscher's retinopathy), radiologic studies, head and neck corticosteroid injection, trauma, coagulopathies, and thrombi secondary to giant cell arteritis.

In nonembolic episodes, the exact mechanism responsible for the occlusion may be difficult to determine. A consideration of the etiologies of arterial occlusive disease is related to the associated systemic abnormality. Patients with hypertension, diabetes, and migraine headaches, and women who take oral contraceptives and smoke are all at higher risk of developing occlusion.

The Patient

Most patients present with a sudden, painless loss of vision in one eye. An afferent pupillary defect can appear within seconds after occlusion of the retinal vascular system. Some patients may have a previous history of amaurosis fugax.

Clinical Symptoms

Unilateral, painless, sudden vision loss (CRAO, OAO) or loss of partial visual field (BRAO, CIRAO). In OAO, 90% of patients will have no light perception, while in CRAO, 90% of patients will have counting fingers to light-perception vision. About 80% of eyes with BRAO improve to 20/40 or better. About 90% of eyes with CIRAO improve to 20/40 or better vision, and 60% return to 20/20.

Clinical Signs
Prominent Signs
- Retinal whitening or opacification
- Cherry-red spot in CRAO (in OAO, 30% have definitively, 40% questionable, and 30% lack)
- Optic atrophy late in CRAO and OAO and segmental optic atrophy in BRAO
- Afferent pupillary defect

Subtle Signs
- Retinal arterial thinning, atherosclerosis, and occlusion
- Segmentation or "boxcarring" in both arteries and veins
- Intra-arterial emboli and plaques
- Retinal pigment epithelial changes in OAO
- Iris and disc neovascularization and arterial shunts as late sequelae
- Anterior ischemic optic neuropathy with CIRAO

Demographics

Most arterial vascular occlusions occur in older adults, with a mean age in the early 60s. Men are more frequently affected than women, and there is no predilection for either eye. Most cases are unilateral, with only 1 to 2% of cases being bilateral. Bilateral involvement could indicate giant cell arteritis or cardiac valvular disease. Arterial occlusion in a younger individual could indicate coagulopathy or trauma, or in females with a history of migraine and oral contraceptive use, vasospastic disease.

Significant History
- Hypertension
- Diabetes
- Cardiac valvular disease
- Carotid artery disease
- Giant cell arteritis or other vasculitides

Ancillary Tests

Ocular assessment includes visual acuity and ophthalmoscopic examination. Electroretinography shows reduced B-wave amplitude in CRAO and reduced or absent A- and B-waves in OAO.

Fluorescein angiography shows delay in retinal arterial filling and delay in arteriovenous transit time in CRAO. Delayed choroidal filling is absent in CRAO but present in OAO. Late staining of the retinal pigment epithelium is absent in CRAO but variably present in OAO.

Laboratory studies: CBC with differential; plasma glucose; ESR; C-reactive protein; platelet count; lipid profile; antinuclear antibody (ANA); rheumatoid factor; anticardiolipin; antiphospholipid antibody; lupus anticoagulant; hemoglobin electrophoresis; serum protein electrophoresis; and homocysteine level.

Noninvasive testing: Blood pressure; carotid auscultation; cardiac evaluation (electrocardiogram, Holter monitor, and echocardiogram); carotid duplex ultrasound; ophthalmodynamometry or oculoplethysmography is optional.

The Treatment

Treatment should be started as soon as possible, preferably within the first 2 hours. There are no effective treatments for cases presenting several hours or days after onset. Any underlying systemic disease should also be treated.

In acute presentation of occlusions from emboli, immediate ocular massage may dislodge the embolus. Also, inhalation of a mixture of 5% CO_2 combined with 95% O_2 for 15 minutes (this can be accomplished by breathing in a paper bag), followed by breathing room air for 15 minutes over 6 to 12 hours may help. If not contraindicated, two adult-size aspirin should be given immediately, followed by a once-a-day daily dose. Paracentesis of the anterior chamber with a 30-gauge short needle on a tuberculin syringe will quickly lower intraocular pressure and may dislodge an embolus. The intraocular pressure (IOP) should be maintained at a low level with oral acetazolamide, 250 mg (when it is not contraindicated) every 6 hours for several days. Topical IOP-lowering medications may be as effective; avoid β-blockers and miotics.

Approximately one-third of patients may have improvement in their vision after anterior chamber paracentesis and inhalation of a 95% oxygen and 5% carbon dioxide mixture.

RETINAL VENOUS OCCLUSIVE DISEASE
Michael J. Trad

ICD—9: 362.35—Central retinal vein occlusion
ICD—9: 362.36—Venous tributary (branch) occlusion
ICD—9: 362.83—Retinal edema

THE DISEASE
Pathophysiology

Central Retinal Vein Occlusion (CRVO)
- CRVO: Thrombosis of the central retinal vein (CRV) in the area of the lamina cribrosa causes increased venous resistance.
- Type II papillophlebitis: Inflammatory occlusion of the CRV occurs in young adults.
- Hemicentral retinal vein occlusion (hemi-CRVO): Occlusion of one of the two main branches of the CRV occurs anterior to the retrolaminar area, where the two branches ultimately become the single vessel of the CRV.

Branch Retinal Vein Occlusion (BRVO)
- BRVO: An underlying tributary of a primary retinal venule at an arteriovenous (AV) crossing is compressed by a sclerosed arteriole. In time, the venule lumen becomes further stenotic, occlusion occurs, and the branch vein and its capillary bed are damaged. BRVO occurs most frequently in the superotemporal retina because this is the site of the most AV crossings. Additionally, BRVO may occur at or distal to the disc margin.
- Macular BRVO (MBRVO): A small tributary branch near the macula occludes.
- Peripheral BRVO (PBRVO): Also known as Twig BRVO, venous occlusion occurs beyond the second venous bifurcation.

Etiology

CRVO in adults younger than 40 to 50 years of age is termed *papillophlebitis* and is subclassified into two types: Type I (exemplified by disc edema and a paucity of additional retinal pathology), and Type II, which resembles CRVO. The cause of papillophlebitis is undetermined in the vast majority of cases, but occasionally it may be associated with systemic hypertension, heart disease, pulmonary disease, gastrointestinal disease, hyperlipidemia, renal disease, arthritis, migraine, anemia, viral infection, collagen vascular disease, hyperviscosity states, acquired immunodeficiency syndrome (AIDS), pregnancy, carotid artery disease, drugs (e.g., oral contraceptives), glaucoma, cilioretinal artery occlusion, or optic disc drusen.

In individuals over 50 years of age, systemic hypertension, hyperlipidemia, hypercholesterolemia, hypertriglyceridemia, and diabetes are the most common etiologies of CRVO. Other causes in this age group may include cardiovascular disease, chronic pulmonary disease, vasculitis, drugs (e.g., oral contraceptives), hemodialysis, hypercoagulable states, platelet abnormalities, trauma, AIDS, thyroid disease, migraine, orbital tumor, glaucoma, and disc drusen.

The most common etiologies of BRVO are systemic hypertension, arteriosclerosis, diabetes, hypercholesterolemia, and hyperlipidemia. Other etiologies may include arteritis; carotid artery disease; cavernous sinus thrombosis; cystic fibrosis; diseases of red blood cells, white blood cells, platelets, and plasma constituents; superior vena cava syndrome; lateral sinus thrombosis; orbital vein thrombosis; Coats's disease; von Hippel-Lindau disease; glaucoma; retinal phlebitis; Eale's disease; and disc drusen.

The Patient

Symptoms and signs vary according to the site and extent of retinal venous occlusion.

Clinical Symptoms
Most venous occlusions usually produce painless unilateral vision loss or blind spots (the exception is PBRVO, where patients are typically asymptomatic).

Clinical Signs
See Table 18.2.

Demographics
- 90% of all venous occlusions are unilateral. However, the fellow eye may eventually become occluded in 10% of cases.
- 55% of patients with CRVO are male.
- CRVO usually occurs after the age of 50.
- Papillophlebitis occurs most commonly in males.
- Papillophlebitis occurs in patients from 12 to 49 years of age, with the mean age being 35.8 years.
- 85% of patients with BRVO are between 50 and 80 years of age.
- BRVO occurs in individuals from 30 to 90 years of age, with an average age of 62.6 years.

TABLE 18.2 Clinical Signs of Retinal Venous Occlusive Disease

	CRVO	BRVO
Prominent signs:		
Visual acuity	Often 20/200 in ischemic CRVO while better than 20/200 in nonischemic CRVO (unless significant macular edema) Typically 20/40 or better in papillophlebitis	Typically 20/20 to 20/30 unless partial or full macular edema is present (may decline to 20/100 or worse) Compromised in 85% of MBRVO
Retinal hemorrhages	Present in all quadrants in CRVC Present in both quadrants of either the superior or inferior retina (hemi-CRVO) Greater in number and extend into the periphery (in ischemic CRVO and ischemic hemi-CRVO) when compared with nonischemic counterparts Greater in number and extend over the entire posterior pole (in type II papillophlebitis) when compared to type I papillophlebitis	Present as a wedge-shaped area whose apex points to the site of occlusion (hemorrhage usually doesn't cross the horizontal raphé (BRVO)) BRVO most commonly occurs in the superotemporal retina (more AV crossings) BRVO may occur coincident with or distal to the disc margin Present in close proximity to a venous macular tributary branch (MERVO) Present in one quadrant after the second venous bifurcation (PBRVO)
Disc edema	Present in CRVO, hemi-CRVO, and papillophlebitis	Not present
Cotton wool spots (CWS)	Multiple number in ischemic CRVO and ischemic hemi-CRVO but rare in nonischemic counterparts	Greater number in ischemic BRVO
Macular edema	Greater degree in ischemic CRVO and ischemic hemi-CRVO	Present in 48–58% of BRVO Present in 85% of MBRVO
Dilated, tortuous venules	Present	Present
Neovascular glaucoma	Present in 10–20% of CRVO Present in 60% of ischemic CRVO May be present in ischemic hemi-CRVO	Rare
Subtle signs:		
Relative afferent pupillary defect (RAPD)	Often present in ischemic CRVO	Absent
Collateral vessels	Present on disc in nonischemic CRVO	May cross the horizontal raphé in BRVO
Neovascularization of the iris (NVI)	Present in 20% of CRVO	May occur in BRVO (rare)
Neovascularization of the disc (NVD) or elsewhere in the retina (NVE)	Present in 40–60% of ischemic CRVO Higher risk of development in ischemic CRVO or ischemic hemi-CRVO	May occur infrequently in BRVO (25–30%)
Decreased intraocular pressure	Greater decrease in ischemic CRVO Greater decrease in CRVO than BRVO	Not affected in MBRVO nor PBRVO

Other signs that may present in CRVO and/or BRVO include microaneurysms, exudates, intraretinal microvascular abnormalities (IRMA), retinal edema, epiretinal membrane, arteriolar sheathing, vitreous hemorrhage, and retinal detachment.

- BRVO occurs more frequently in males and hyperopes and has a strong association with systemic disease (57%).
- 4 to 5% of BRVOs are bilateral.
- BRVO is second to diabetic retinopathy as the most common retinal vascular disease.

Significant History

See Etiology.

Ancillary Tests

Ocular assessment includes best-corrected visual acuity, color vision, confrontation fields, Amsler grid, ocular motilities, pupillary testing, slit-lamp exam, applanation tonometry, gonioscopy, and dilated retinal examination. Fundus photography and automated visual field examination may also be utilized. Additionally, an ERG is recommended in cases of CRVO.

Laboratory studies include CBC with differential and platelets, PT, PTT, lipid profile, fasting blood sugar, erythrocyte sedimentation rate, C-reactive protein, antinuclear antibodies, FTA-ABS, and serum protein electrophoresis.

Other laboratory tests may include antiphospholipid antibodies, hemoglobin electrophoresis, cryoglobulins, VDRL, and HIV.

Other testing includes blood pressure measurement, chest x-ray, cardiovascular evaluation (electrocardiogram, echocardiography), carotid auscultation, ophthalmodynamometry, oculopneumoplethysmography, carotid duplex ultrasonography, and orbital-brain MRI may be indicated in some instances.

FA is done later in the disease process when hemorrhaging clears adequately. When hemorrhaging clears sufficiently, FA is used to assess unresolved macular edema or suspected retinal neovascularization.

The Treatment

Medical Evaluation (All Venous Occlusions)
- Control any underlying medical condition(s).
- Recommend cessation of smoking.
- Address present systemic medication(s) that may potentially play a contributory role (oral contraceptives, diuretics, etc.).

Medical Treatment
1. CRVO (and hemi-CRVO)
   - Consider anticoagulation therapy (questionable efficacy) with monitoring of blood levels.
2. Papillophlebitis
   - Generally none, although steroid therapy early in the disease process may be beneficial in some cases.

3. BRVO
   - No treatment indicated.

Ophthalmic Treatment and Follow-Up

1. CRVO (and hemi-CRVO)
   - Decrease intraocular pressure in either eye if elevated.
   - Monthly follow-ups for the first 6 months and then in accordance with clinical findings over the 2-year follow-up period.
   - Neovascular glaucoma is most likely to occur in the first 2 to 5 months (100-day glaucoma) after initial presentation but may occur anytime over the 2-year follow-up period. Therefore, follow-up visits should include slit-lamp biomicroscopy to rule out rubeosis as well as gonioscopy to assess for angle neovascularization (NVI). Panretinal photocoagulation (PRP) should be initiated if either iris or angle neovascularization is present.
   - Consider ERG (if ischemic CRVO is suggested by diminished B-wave on 30-Hz Flicker ERG, consider panretinal photocoagulation when appropriate).
   - Perform FA when hemorrhaging is sufficiently cleared. Consider panretinal photocoagulation (PRP) if CRVO is ischemic (defined as $\geq$10 disc diameters of nonperfusion). If ischemic, follow up every 2 to 3 weeks after PRP (observing for NVI) for the first 6 months; if nonischemic, observe for conversion to ischemic CRVO (most likely during the first 4 months) on monthly basis for the first 6 months.
   - The Collaborative Central Vein Occlusion Study (CVOS) demonstrated that grid laser photocoagulation is not visually beneficial in treating macular edema, and in fact actually tended to worsen vision in patients older than 65 years of age.
   - Follow up on yearly basis for the development of chronic open-angle glaucoma.
   - Other potential treatments described include intravitreal tissue plasminogen activator (t-PA), intravitreal triamcinolone acetonide, retinochoroidal anastomoses, and radial optic neurotomy.
2. Papillophlebitis
   - Typically is self-limiting over a 6- to 18-month period. Follow up every month for the first 4 months and then every 2 months until resolution.
3. BRVO
   - Follow up every month for the first 4 months and then every 2 months until resolution. Assess for retinal and iris neovascularization (NVI rarely occurs).
   - If retinal neovascularization occurs and/or is suspected, perform FA. If capillary nonperfusion is confirmed, perform sector PRP to ischemic area.
   - When chronic (3 to 6 months) macular edema persists in conjunction with visual acuity less than 20/40, consider FA. If macular perfusion is evident on FA, consider macular grid laser treatment. Follow up on a yearly basis for the development of chronic open-angle glaucoma.
   - Another potential treatment described is adventitial sheathotomy/arteriovenous crossing dissection.

OCULAR ISCHEMIC SYNDROME (OIS)

Mohammad R. Rafieetary

ICD—9: 362.84

THE DISEASE

Pathophysiology

Ocular ischemic syndrome was initially termed *venous stasis retinopathy* and is a condition typically caused by severe carotid artery obstruction. However, at times chronic ophthalmic artery and rarely central retinal artery occlusion can result in a similar presentation.

Etiology

Atherosclerotic stenosis is the most common etiology. However, giant cell arteritis and other vaso-inflammatory conditions can also be responsible.

Hemodynamic flow is usually not significantly affected until at least 70% stenosis. Most OIS patients have at least 90%, and in one-half of patients, there is 100% occlusion of the carotid artery on the same side.

The Patient

Vision loss is noted by approximately 90% of patients with OIS. In others, the diagnosis is made by clinical observation of the posterior and anterior segment findings.

Clinical Symptoms

In addition to vision loss, other symptoms include visual disturbance (e.g., afterimages); alteration of light to dark adaptation; ocular or periorbital pain (40%), which may be related to increased intraocular pressure; and transient monocular vision loss (amaurosis fugax) in 10% of cases.

Differential diagnosis of OIS includes diabetic retinopathy and central retinal vein occlusion.

Clinical Signs
Prominent Signs
- Distended veins with irregular caliber (typically not tortuous)
- Attenuation of retinal arteries
- Microaneurysms
- Midperipheral retinal hemorrhages (80%)
- Iris neovascularization (65%)
- Posterior segment neovascularization (NVD 35%, NVE 8%)
- Macular edema (15%)
- Neovascular glaucoma
- Episcleral injection

- Corneal edema
- Mild anterior uveitis (20%)

Subtle Signs
- Iris atrophy
- Iris neovascularization with normal intraocular pressure
- Central retinal artery occlusion
- Cherry-red spot
- Flare response greater than cellular response in patients with iritis
- Keratic precipitates
- Cataract (hypermature, in end stages of disease)
- Spontaneous pulsations of the central retinal artery (4%)
- Cotton wool spots (4%)
- Hollenhorst plaques

Demographics

Ocular ischemic syndrome usually occurs in persons over 50 to 80 years of age, with a mean age of 65. A definitive incidence rate has not yet been established and will be difficult to establish because of the large number of misdiagnosed cases. Men comprise two-thirds of the cases. There is no racial predilection. The condition affects the left and right eyes with equal frequency. The disease is unilateral 80% of the time; however, there may be a higher incidence of mild involvement of the fellow eye.

Significant History
- Hypertension
- Diabetes
- Hyperlipidemia
- Ischemic heart disease
- Previous cerebrovascular accident or transient ischemic attack
- Peripheral vascular disease (cold hands, spasm of arm muscles with exercise)

Ancillary Tests

Careful examination of the iris under slit lamp as well as gonioscopy prior to pupil dilation should be done. Fluorescein angiography may show delayed choroidal filling as well as prolonged arm-to-retina circulation time, increased retinal arteriovenous transit time, late-phase staining of the retinal vessels, macular edema, microaneurysms, and retinal capillary nonperfusion. ERG shows decreased (and extinguished in severe cases) amplitude of both the A- and B-waves.

Carotid artery evaluation should include ophthalmodynamometry, oculoplethysmography, and Doppler ultrasound. Arm pulses, cardiac, and carotid auscultation should be performed. Invasive testing including carotid angiography may be considered.

Medical evaluation should also include CBC with differential, ESR, C-reactive protein, ANA, blood chemistry with complete lipid profile, and an echocardiogram in the presence of retinal arterial plaques.

The Treatment

If the carotid artery is not 100% obstructed, carotid endarterectomy surgery can reverse the syndrome if the disease is detected before iris neovascularization develops. Anticoagulation (e.g., warfarin) or antiplatelet (e.g., aspirin) may be helpful and is necessary to prevent other complication such as cerebrovascular accidents. Extracranial-intracranial bypass surgery has been found to be useless in reducing stroke risk.

Panretinal photocoagulation (PRP) is considered in the presence of neovascularization. This is effective in about one-third of cases. Any neovascular glaucoma should be managed medically or surgically.

DIABETIC RETINOPATHY

Michael J. Trad

ICD—9: 250.50—Diabetes with ophthalmic manifestations
ICD—9: 250.51—Type 1 (juvenile type), not stated as uncontrolled
ICD—9: 250.52—Type 2 or unspecified type, uncontrolled
ICD—9: 250.53—Type 1 (juvenile type), uncontrolled
ICD—9: 362.01—Background diabetic retinopathy
ICD—9: 362.02—Proliferative diabetic retinopathy
ICD—9: 362.83—Retinal edema

THE DISEASE

Pathophysiology

Hyperglycemia-induced biochemical changes, alterations in vascular flow, and platelet aggregation caused by endocrine factors are thought to represent the primary mechanisms responsible for diabetic microvascular disease (retinopathy).

- Background Diabetic Retinopathy (BDR)/Mild Nonproliferative Diabetic Retinopathy (Mild NPDR). The earliest histological alteration in retinal capillaries appears to be a selective loss of intramural pericytes as a result of hypoxia. With the disappearance of pericytes, small focal outpouchings (microaneurysms) form throughout the venous (and secondarily arteriolar) side of the capillary network. In time, proliferating endothelial cells thicken microaneurysmal walls and form additional basement membrane, eventually resulting in endothelial dropout and microaneurysmal occlusion and/or leakage (hemorrhage).
- Preproliferative Diabetic Retinopathy (PPDR)/NPDR. Capillary degeneration causes further retinal hypoxia, which in turn leads to capillary circulatory closure, cotton wool spots, venous caliber irregularities, and formation of intraretinal microvascular abnormalities (IRMAs) from shunt vessels on closure margins.
- Proliferative Diabetic Retinopathy (PDR). Retinal hypoxia causes the release of vascular endothelial growth factor (VEGF), which provides the angiogenic stimulus for new blood vessel formation (neovascularization) from IRMAs and/or other ischemic foci. Neovascularization may occur at the disc (NVD) or elsewhere in the retina (NVE).

In time, NVE perforates the retinal internal limiting membrane (ILM), proliferates along the ILM surface, and adheres to the posterior hyaloid face (NVD has greater initial access to the vitreous because of the physiological absence of an ILM overlying the disc). Proliferating retinal glial cells, in turn, provide the fibrotic scaffold for further neovascular expansion and vitreal attachment. It is this resultant fibroglial vitreoretinal adhesion that provides the tractional impetus for the development of vitreous hemorrhage and retinal detachment.

- Diabetic Macular Edema (DME). Diseased capillaries leak because of damage to the blood-retinal barrier and the tight junctions between endothelial cells. Capillary exudation results in retinal edema and lipid (hard exudate) accumulation. DME may occur at any stage of retinopathy.

Etiology

Diabetic retinopathy (DR) occurs in both insulin-dependent (IDDM) and noninsulin dependent (NIDDM) diabetics. Diabetes mellitus (DM) is a metabolic disorder of carbohydrate (glucose) metabolism that involves insulin resistance, relative or absolute insulin deficiency, or both. Hyperglycemia is the hallmark of this chronic disease that results in both long-term macro- and microvascular (retinal) complications. The exact process by which diabetes causes retinopathy is not fully understood but may involve hypercoagulation and increased protein glycosylation. Diabetes has recently been reclassified into four subtypes: prediabetes, type 1, type 1.5, and type 2.

The Patient

Symptomatology varies depending upon the stability of glucose levels, degree of retinopathy, and presence of macular edema. Patients may experience blurred, distorted, and/or fluctuating vision; color vision disturbance; and flashes and floaters.

Clinical Signs (vary depending upon the stage of retinopathy)
Prominent Signs
- Decreased acuity (unilateral or bilateral)
- Color vision abnormalities
- Amsler grid metamorphopsia and/or scotomas
- Confrontation field defects
- Dot hemorrhages and microaneurysms (indistinguishable ophthalmoscopically but differentiated by fluorescein angiography)
- Blot hemorrhages
- Nerve fiber layer (flame-shaped) hemorrhages
- Arteriolar narrowing
- Hard exudates (often in a complete or semicircinate pattern)
- Cotton wool spots
- Venous caliber irregularities (tortuosity, beading)
- IRMA

- NVD*
- NVE*
- Preretinal fibrosis* (fibrotic proliferation)
- Preretinal hemorrhage*
- Vitreous hemorrhage*
- Retinal detachment*

Subtle Signs
- Increased hyperopia secondary to macular edema
- Rubeosis iridis (rule out retinal neovascularization)
- Macular epiretinal membrane*
- Macular hole* (full or partial thickness)
- Retinal edema/thickening (nonexudative)

Demographics
- Diabetes mellitus is the leading cause of blindness in the United States for persons aged 20 to 74 years. Fifty percent of all blindness related to diabetic retinopathy can be prevented by early diagnosis and proper management.
- Insulin-dependent diabetics typically do not demonstrate retinopathy until at least 5 years after diagnosis of diabetes. Only 11 to 17% of type 1 diabetics demonstrate retinopathy during the first 5 years. However, nearly all insulin-dependent diabetics display retinopathy after 15 years of the disease.
- Twenty percent of noninsulin-dependent diabetics display retinopathy at the time of initial diagnosis, while 60 to 80% will have some degree of retinopathy after having the disease for 15 or more years.
- Patients with retinal neovascularization have an approximate average life expectancy of 6 years.
- Twenty-five percent of type 1 diabetics will develop PDR after 15 years, and half will demonstrate such changes after 20 or more years.
- After 15 years, 5 to 20% of NIDDM patients will have PDR.
- Within 5 years of onset of PDR, one-half of all diabetics experience a reduction in visual acuity to 20/200 or less.
- Within 10 years, all patients with NVD and three-fourths with NVE are blind in at least one eye.
- Diabetic maculopathy represents the most common cause of visual loss in diabetics. Approximately 3% of all diabetics would currently be expected to have DME.

Significant History
- Pertinent symptomatology (polydipsia, polyuria, polyphagia, etc.), which may suggest DM
- Family history of DM

---

*Denotes association with PDR.
*Denotes macular pathological changes secondary to diabetic retinopathy (signs are not diagnostic of diabetic retinopathy itself).

- Ethnic background (Hispanic, Black, or Native American)
- Previous report of gestational diabetes or delivery of babies larger than 9 lbs
- Pregnancy
- Obesity
- Drug-induced hyperglycemia (glucocorticoids, β-blockers, etc.)
- Hypertension
- Hyperlipidemia
- Duration and type of DM
- Stability, frequency of monitoring, and most recent measurement of blood glucose level

Ancillary Tests

Ocular assessment for diabetic retinopathy may include visual acuity, pupil assessment, extraocular motilities, Amsler grid, color vision, biomicroscopy, tonometry, gonioscopy, contrast sensitivity, dilated stereoscopic fundus examination, and fundus photography.

Laboratory studies: fasting blood glucose, glycosylated hemoglobin, glucose tolerance, and lipid profile.

Other testing includes blood pressure, B-scan ultrasonography (when indicated), retinal fluorescein angiography.

The Treatment

Management of Systemic Disease

Patients suspected of having diabetes should be referred to a physician for a fasting blood glucose (pregnant women should be tested for glucose intolerance and managed in conjunction with their obstetrician), lipid profile, and blood pressure assessment. Elevated glucose level, hyperlipidemia, and hypertension are risk factors for the development and progression of hard exudates and generalized diabetic retinopathy. Therefore, it is also prudent to ensure that all known diabetics achieve and maintain appropriate blood glucose, serum lipids, and systemic blood pressure control.

Management of Diabetic Retinopathy

- Diagnostic Staging of Disease (Table 18.3A). The Diabetic Retinopathy Study (DRS), Early Treatment of Diabetic Retinopathy Study (ETDRS), and the Diabetic Retinopathy Vitrectomy Study (DRVS) provide the basis for management and treatment protocols regarding diabetic retinopathy. Nonproliferative diabetic retinopathy (NPDR), proliferative diabetic retinopathy (PDR), and diabetic macular edema (DME) represent the three basic classifications/entities of diabetic retinopathy.

  NPDR encompasses both the traditional background (BDR) and preproliferative diabetic retinopathy (PPDR) stages. Characteristic finding of NPDR include microaneurysms, intraretinal hemorrhages (dot, blot, or flame-shaped), hard exudates, cotton wool spots, IRMA, and venous irregularities (tortuosity, beading). NPDR may be further subclassified into mild, moderate, severe, or very severe levels based upon the presence of characteristic retinal findings and comparison to modified Airlie House retinal photographic standards.

▶ **TABLE 18.3A** Guidelines for Staging of Diabetic Retinopathy

Category	Characteristics
Normal	No diabetic retinopathy
Mild nonproliferative diabetic retinopathy (no CSME)	At least 1 microaneurysm H/Ma <Standard Photograph 2A[†]
Moderate nonproliferative diabetic retinopathy (no CSME)	H/Ma ≥Standard Photograph 2A[†] and/or soft exudates, VB, IRMA to mild degree
Severe nonproliferative diabetic retinopathy (preproliferative diabetic retinopathy) (no CSME)	IRMAs present in 1 or more quadrants ≥Standard Photograph 8A[†] VB ≥Standard Photograph 6B[†] in 2 or more quadrants H/Ma ≥Standard Photograph 2A[†] in 4 or more quadrants
Early proliferative diabetic retinopathy (no CSME)	Neovascularization of the disc or elsewhere, which does not meet the DRS's high-risk characteristics
High-risk proliferative diabetic retinopathy	Moderate or severe neovascularization on or within 1 DD of the optic disc (NVD) >1/4 to 1/3 disc area (Standard Photograph 10A[†]) with/without vitreous or preretinal hemorrhage. -OR- Mild new neovascularization on or within 2 DD of optic disc (NVD) if fresh vitreous or preretinal hemorrhage. -OR- Moderate or severe new neovascularization elsewhere (NVE) if fresh vitreous or preretinal hemorrhage (Standard Photograph 7[†])
Preretinal and/or vitreous hemorrhage	Vitreous or preretinal hemorrhage presumed to be from either ruptured NVD or NVE or possibly retinal tear
Tractional retinal detachment	Retinal detachment associated with fibrotic proliferation
Neovascularization of iris	Any new vessel growth at the iris sphincter, iris surface, or anterior chamber angle Indicative of severe ocular hypoxia
Macular edema *May occur at any stage of diabetic retinopathy*	Thickening of retina within 1 DD of center of macula. -OR- Hard exudates within 1 DD of center of macula with associated retinal thickening -OR- Signs <definition of clinically significant macular edema (CSME)
Clinically significant macular edema (CSME) *May occur at any stage of diabetic retinopathy*	Retinal thickening at or within 500 μm (1/3 DD) of center of macula. -OR- Hard exudates at or within 500 μm of center of macula if associated with thickening of adjacent retina. -OR- Zone(s) of retinal thickening 1 DD area in size, at least part of which was within 1 DD of center of macula

H/Ma, hemorrhages and/or microaneurysms; IRMAs, intraretinal microvascular abnormalities; VB, venous beading; ETDRS, early treatment diabetic retinopathy study; DRS, diabetic retinopathy study.
[†] Photo references are to the Airlie House Classification System.
Developed by the National Systemic Disease Committee of the American Optometric Association, St. Louis, MO. Reprinted with permission.

PDR may include neovascularization of the disc (NVD), neovascularization elsewhere in the retina (NVE), preretinal fibrosis, preretinal hemorrhage, vitreous hemorrhage, and tractional retinal detachment. PDR is further subclassified into mild, moderate, or high-risk levels.

DME is categorized as either clinically insignificant or significant (CSME). CSME is defined as retinal thickening or hard exudate formation at or within one-third DD

▶ TABLE 18.3B   General Guidelines for the Management of Diabetic Retinopathy

Category	Management*
Normal	Document and educate the patient.
	Communicate/send letter to patient's physician.
	Follow up with dilated fundus exam in 1 y.
Mild nonproliferative diabetic retinopathy (no CSME)	Document and educate the patient.
	Communicate/send letter to patient's physician.
	Follow up in 12 mo depending on extent of lesions.
Moderate nonproliferative diabetic relinopathy (no CSME)	Document and educate the patient.
	Communicate/send letter to patient's physician.
	Follow up in 6–12 mo.
	Note. Underestimating the level of retinopathy will grossly underestimate the risk of progression to proliferative retinopathy.
Severe nonproliferative diabetic retinopathy (preproliferative diabetic retinopathy) (no CSME)	Document and educate the patient.
	Communicate/send letter to patient's physician.
	Obtain retinal consult within 2-4 weeks; follow up in 2–3 mo.
	Note. Very strong risk for progression to proliferative diabetic retinopathy.
Early proliferative diabetic retinopathy (no CSME)	Document and educate the patient.
	Communicate/send letter to patient's physician.
	Obtain a retinal consult within a 2 week period.
	Note. Panretinal photocoagulation may be indicated in some patients at this stage. Very high risk of progression to severe proliferative diabetic retinopathy (high-risk characteristics).
High-risk proliferative diabetic retinopathy	Document and educate the patient.
	Communicate/send letter to patient's physician.
	Obtain a retinal consult ASAP (within 24–48 h).
	Note. Very high risk of severe vitreous hemorrhage and/or vision loses over 2 y period. DRS and ETDRS proved benefit of panretinal photocoagulation intervention.
Preretinal and/or vitreous hemorrhage	Document and educate the patient.
	Communicate/send letter to patient's physician.
	Obtain retinal consult ASAP (within 24–48 h).
	Note. Treat as high-risk proliferative diabetic retinopathy. DRS and Diabetic Retinopathy Vitrectomy Study proved that panretinal photocoagulation treatment or early vitrectomy may improve visual outcome.
Tractional retinal detachment	Document and educate the patient.
	Communicate/send letter to patient's physician.
	Obtain retinal consult within 1 week; vitrectomy may be indicated as it may improve vision.
Neovascularization of iris	Document and educate the patient.
	Communicate/send letter to patient's physician.
	Obtain retinal consult ASAP (within 24 48 h).
	Note. Panretinal photocoagulation may prevent the development of neovascular glaucoma.
Macular edema	Document and educate the patient.
May occur at any stage of diabetic retinopathy	Communicate/send letter to patient's physician.
	Obtain retinal consult within a 2-week period.
	Note. Focal laser treatment may be indicated in some patients.
Clinically significant macular edema (CSME)	Document and educate the patient.
May occur at any stage of diabetic retinopathy	Communicate/send letter to patient's physician.
	Obtain retinal consult within 2-week period.
	Note. ETDRS proved benefit of focal laser treatment in improving visual outcome.

H/Ma, hemorrhages and/or microaneurysms; IRMAs, intraretinal microvascular abnormalities; VB, venous beading; ETDRS, early treatment diabetic retinopathy study; DRS, diabetic retinopathy study.

*Coexisting medical conditions (i.e., hypertension, renal disease, hyperlipidemia, pregnancy) may indicate the need for more frequent evaluation.

from the center of the macula or retinal thickening of at least one disc area (DA) in size that intrudes in part within one DD of the fovea. As mentioned earlier, DME may occur at any stage of DR.

- Management and Treatment. Patients without severe nonproliferative diabetic retinopathy (PPDR) may be followed by their eyecare practitioner according to the guidelines set forth in Table 18.3B. Patients with macular edema, severe NPDR, or early PDR should be scheduled for consultation with a retinal specialist within a 2- to 4-week period. Focal laser treatment benefits those with CSME and may also be necessary in some patients with non-CSME. Panretinal photocoagulation (PRP) may be beneficial in some patients with early PDR.

    Patients with neovascularization of the iris (NVI/rubeosis), high-risk PDR, and preretinal and/or vitreous hemorrhage should be examined by a retinal specialist within 24 to 48 hours. PRP or early vitrectomy may be indicated to prevent neovascular glaucoma and/or deleterious vitreoretinal sequelae. When tractional retinal detachment is observed, vitrectomy may improve visual outcome, and thus retinal consultation should be obtained within 7 days.

    Lastly, it is important to not overlook the necessity for low-vision rehabilitation and/or psychosocial counseling referral for both those who have suffered profound visual loss or are very fearful of potential future visual compromise or blindness.

HYPERTENSIVE RETINOPATHY
Michael J. Trad

ICD—9: 362.11

THE DISEASE
Pathophysiology

The severity and duration of systemic hypertension (HTN) affects the retinal arterioles in different manners. The initial neuroretinopathic response is one of arteriolar vasoconstriction, with the degree of such corresponding to the severity of systemic HTN (this relationship is less direct in the elderly population, however, as pre-existing arteriolosclerosis limits the extent of arteriolar attenuation). Long-standing HTN ultimately results in disruption of the blood-retinal barrier through degeneration of circumcapillary pericytes and muscle cells. Sustained HTN also is related to arteriolosclerosis of vessel walls, as demonstrated by endothelial and medial hypertrophy, as well as intimal hyalinization. Subsequent retinal venous nicking at arteriovenous (AV) crossing sites may occur because of compression by an arteriole's thickened wall.

Etiology

- Essential HTN (Primary HTN, Idiopathic HTN). No known underlying etiology is known to cause this type of HTN. However, factors such as obesity, smoking, and so on may play a role. More than 95% of all cases of HTN are classified as essential.

- Secondary HTN. An underlying cause for HTN is identified and may include oral contraceptive use, preeclampsial/eclampsia, renal disease, adrenal disease (including pheochromocytoma), hyper- or hypothyroidism, coarctation of the aorta, and vasculitis.

The Patient

Symptoms and signs vary depending upon the severity and duration of systemic HTN, as well as the timeliness and success of medical intervention.

Clinical Symptoms

Usually patients are asymptomatic, although some may present with decreased vision.

Clinical Signs

Prominent Signs

- Grade I hypertensive retinopathy (HR): Mild, generalized bilateral attenuation of arterioles beyond the second bifurcation.
- Grade II HR: Greater generalized arteriolar attenuation than grade I with the addition of focal attenuation.
- Grade III HR: Grade II changes with the addition of cotton wool spots (CWS). Nerve fiber layer (NFL) hemorrhages and exudates frequently are present.
- Grade IV HR: Grade III changes plus bilateral disc edema (disc pallor and optic atrophy may ultimately occur). A macular star is also often present.

Subtle Signs

- Grade I HR: Early arteriolosclerosis as manifested by an abnormally bright arteriolar light reflex.
- Grade II HR: Exudates (if occurring in the macula, they may take on a star appearance), NFL hemorrhages and dot/blot hemorrhages may be present. AV crossing changes such as Salus's sign (nicking), Bonnet's sign (venule banking), and Gunn's sign (right-angle deflected venules) may also be present.
- Grade III HR: Grade II subtle signs with advanced arteriolosclerotic copper-silver wire light reflex.
- Grade IV HR: Choroidal infarcts in the peripheral retina may be present: Elschnig's spots (black pigment flecks surrounded by a bright yellow or red halo) and Sieger's streaks (chains of pigmented spots/clumps that follow the course of sclerosed choroidal vessels).

Other signs may include branch retinal vein occlusion, central retinal vein occlusion, branch retinal artery occlusion, central retinal artery occlusion, vitreous hemorrhage, arterial microaneurysm, retinal neovascularization, retinal detachment, and ischemic optic neuropathy. Also, unilateral HR may be indicative of contralateral carotid occlusive disease.

Demographics

More than 25% of the U.S. population has systemic HTN. The incidence of HTN is greater in Blacks than in Whites. The 3-year survival rate is 22% for patients with grade III HR and 6% for those with grade IV HR.

Significant History
- Known HTN
- Diabetes
- Pregnancy
- Obesity
- Smoking
- Cardiac disease
- Hyperlipidemia
- Oral medications (contraceptives, steroids)
- Renal disease

Ancillary Tests

Ocular assessment includes best-corrected visual acuity, color vision, confrontation fields, Amsler grid, pupillary testing, slit-lamp exam, applanation tonometry, and dilated retinal examination. Fundus photography and automated visual field examination may also be utilized.

Laboratory studies: Typically none, although specific blood testing may be indicated in some instances.

Noninvasive testing: Blood pressure. The Seventh Report of the Joint National Committee on Prevention, Detection, Evaluation and Treatment of High Blood Pressure (JNC7) was released on May 14th, 2003. New guidelines in categorizing hypertension are as follows:

- Normal: <120/<80 mm Hg
- Prehypertension: 120–139/80–89
- Stage 1 hypertension: 140–159/90–99
- Stage 2 hypertension: > or = 160/> or = 100

Invasive testing: Usually none, although intravenous fluorescein angiography of the retina may be performed in some cases.

The Treatment

All patients presenting with elevated blood pressure measurements should be referred to their primary care practitioner, medical internist, or a hospital emergency room if necessary according to the conservative guidelines in Table 10.4.

Follow-up for HR varies according to the stage of severity but typically is performed every 3 to 12 months.

▶ TABLE 18.4 Medical Management of Hypertensive Retinopathy

Signs/Symptoms	Medical Consultation within . . .
Systolic blood pressure (BP) of 140–159 mm Hg and/or diastolic BP of 90–99 mm Hg	1 mo
Systolic BP 160–179 mm Hg and/or diastolic BP 100–109 mm Hg	2 weeks
One or more of the following: systolic BP 180 mm Hg, diastolic BP 110 mm Hg, grade IV HR, breathing difficulties, and chest pain	Immediate

SICKLE CELL HEMOGLOBINOPATHIES
Mohammad Rafieetary and Steve Charles

ICD—9: 362.10—Background retinopathy, unspecified
ICD—9: 362.13—Changes in vascular appearance
ICD—9: 362.15—Retinal telangiectasia
ICD—9: 362.16—Retinal neovascularization NOS
ICD—9: 362.29—Other nondiabetic proliferative retinopathy

THE DISEASE

Pathophysiology

Sickle cell diseases are genetic abnormalities involving the production of hemoglobin. The abnormal globin chains cause distortion of the erythrocyte (sickling), which in turn causes hemolysis and intermittent vascular obstruction. The intravascular sickling causes sludging of blood flow with reduction in red cell survival, leading to chronic anemia.

The intensity of the disease state corresponds to the amount of sickle hemoglobin and its disposition to sickle in the presence of hypoxia and acidosis.

Etiology

Sickle cell can be divided into SS or sickle cell anemia (homozygous: both parents with the disease); AS for sickle cell trait, AC (heterozygous with 50% hemoglobin S or C); and SC, SThal (double heterozygous) genotypes.

The Patient

Patients with sickle cell anemia (SS) exhibit severe systemic morbidity including bone marrow infarcts, bone trabeculation and sclerosis, aseptic necrosis, joint pain, abdominal pain, dyspnea, stroke, and seizures. Orbital involvement of a sickle crisis may include proptosis and pain. Patients with sickle cell trait (AS, AC) usually do not have any significant systemic or ocular manifestations.

Patients who are double heterozygous (SC, SThal) have a relatively unremarkable systemic course yet exhibit the most severity when it comes to ocular changes.

Clinical Symptoms
Most patients will have few if any ocular symptoms. Some may complain of floaters and flashes of light. In advanced disease, significant vision loss can occur.

Clinical Signs
Sickle cell retinopathy can be staged as follows:

- Stage 1: Background (nonproliferative): venous tortuosity, vascular loops, peripheral occluded vessels, "salmon patch" hemorrhages, schisis cavity with overlying "iridescent spots," black sunbursts, cotton wool patches, angioid streaks, comma-shaped conjunctival vessels
- Stage 2: Arteriolar-venule anastomoses: Peripheral "silver wire" vessels
- Stage 3: Neovascular changes (proliferative): so-called sea-fan peripheral neovascularization (autoinfarcted in 60% of cases)
- Stage 4: Vitreous hemorrhage and vitreous traction (most common is SC)
- Stage 5: Retinal detachment: both tractional and rhegmatogenous retinal detachments are possible

Prominent Signs
- Salmon patches—pink color intraretinal and subretinal hemorrhages
- Black sunbursts—black midperipheral chorioretinal scars with spiculated borders
- Iridescent spots—refractile deposits over schisis cavities
- Sea fans—peripheral retinal neovascularization, these grow on the retinal surface in a circumferential pattern
- Sclerosed peripheral retinal vessels
- Vitreous hemorrhage
- Retinal detachment

Subtle Signs
- Schisis cavities
- Areas of white without pressure
- Angioid streaks
- Mottled brown areas
- Comma-shaped capillaries of the conjunctiva and on the optic nerve head
- Macular arteriolar occlusions
- Iris atrophy

Demographics

Originally, sickle cell hemoglobinopathies were noted in some areas of Africa; now these are the most common hemoglobin diseases affecting man throughout the world.

The genes predisposing to these conditions are found primarily, but not exclusively, among certain ethnic populations. Individuals of African, Saudi Arabian, Asian, or Mediterranean lineage are at greater risk for these hemoglobinopathies.

In North America, the incidence of any sickle hemoglobin is approximately 10%. The sickle cell trait (AS) is estimated to occur in 8% and hemoglobin C trait in 2% of Blacks in the United States. Proliferative retinopathy is uncommon in these groups.

Americans also suffer sickle cell homozygote (SS) at 0.4%, with approximately 3% incidence of proliferative retinopathy, SC 0.2% and 33%, and SThal 0.03% and 14% respectively.

Significant History
- African, Saudi Arabian, Asian, or Mediterranean heritage
- Known history of sickle cell hemoglobinopathy

Ancillary Tests

Examination of the anterior segment concentrating on conjunctival blood vessels and iris integrity and fundus evaluation with special emphasis on the peripheral retina. Fluorescein angiography to identify capillary dropout and leakage.

Laboratory Tests: Sickle cell prep and hemoglobin electrophoresis.

The Treatment
- Ablative treatments to eliminate neovascular tissue, such as laser photocoagulation, cryotherapy, and diathermy, have been tried. Laser photocoagulation appears to be the most promising, with the fewest side effects. Laser should be applied in a peripheral scatter or PRP-like pattern, not directly to the neovascular or feeder vessels.
- Vitreous hemorrhage may be monitored with B-scan ultrasound. In the absence of retinal detachment and anterior segment neovascularization, vitreous hemorrhages may be monitored for several weeks to a few months for spontaneous clearing of blood and vitrectomy performed for nonclearing hemorrhages.
- Retinal detachment repair with vitrectomy, if indicated. Preoperative exchange transfusion may be utilized in select cases. The patients should be kept well hydrated and well oxygenated in the perioperative period.

ACUTE RETINAL NECROSIS (ARN)
Mohammad R. Rafieetary

ICD—9: 363.08

THE DISEASE
Pathophysiology

Acute retinal necrosis, also known as acute necrotizing herpetic retinitis, is a fulminant infectious chorioretinal disease. Although, ARN usually occurs in otherwise healthy individuals, it can be seen in immunocompromised patients. Clinically, ARN is characterized by peripheral necrotizing retinitis, occlusive retinal arteritis, and vitritis. Approximately one-third of cases are bilateral (BARN).

Etiology

Varicella zoster virus (HZV) usually seen in older patients, herpes simplex virus (HSV) usually seen in younger patients, and rarely cytomegalovirus (CMV) have been identified as underlying pathogens. In cases of herpes, the condition most likely begins as a latent neural infection. A few cases have also been reported following epidural corticosteroid injections for back pain.

The Patient

Symptoms and signs usually begin suddenly and progress quickly.

Clinical Symptoms

The patient with ARN complains of blurred vision, often with floaters, ocular pain, and photophobia. Further loss of visual function may be noted with the progression or late sequelae of the condition.

Clinical Signs

Prominent Signs

- Multiple white or yellowish opaque patches of thickened retina (usually in the periphery)
- Posterior pole may be unaffected until later
- Sharp demarcation line between normal and abnormal retina
- Retinal vasculitis and vascular sheathing
- Severe anterior chamber reaction
- Vitritis (may be severe)
- Anterior uveitis (may be granulomatous)
- Episcleral injection
- Regional periarteritis with sheathing
- Peripheral intraretinal hemorrhages
- Rhegmatogenous retinal detachment
- Exudative retinal detachments

Subtle Signs

- Increased intraocular pressure
- Optic neuropathy (disc edema, pallor and relative afferent pupillary defect)
- Decreased color vision
- Retinal neovascularization
- Iris neovascularization

Demographics

Acute retinal necrosis occurs equally in both males and females and at almost any age. The disease is unilateral in two-thirds of cases. If the second eye is involved, it is usually affected in a matter of days or weeks. Rhegmatogenous retinal detachments with multiple retinal breaks occur in up to 70 to 85% of patients within 2 to 3 months. Tears are usually located at the margin between the normal and the affected retina.

Significant History

- Sudden, painful vision loss in an otherwise healthy or immunocompromised patient.

Ancillary Tests

Ocular assessment includes visual acuity, intraocular pressure, pupil testing, slit-lamp examination, and careful dilated fundus evaluation. Fluorescein angiography may be helpful.

Laboratory studies: CBC with differential, ESR, RPR, FTA-ABS, HIV, PPD, toxoplasmosis titers, chest x-ray, urine for cytomegalovirus. HZV and HSV (type 1 and 2) IgG and IgM titers.

The Treatment

The patient should be promptly started on intravenous acyclovir (5 to 10 mg/kg or 1500 mg/m^2 of body surface area/day divided in 3 doses for 10 to 14 days. This is followed by 4 to 8 weeks of oral acyclovir (400 to 800 mg 5 times daily). The antiviral therapy can reduce the chance of the fellow eye involvement in unilateral cases. Treat anterior segment involvement with topical steroid (prednisolone 1% q2 to 6 hours) and cycloplegic (homatropine 5% tid). Oral steroid treatment is controversial; however, prednisone may be given to reduce inflammation after the first 48 hours. Anticoagulation with heparin and Coumadin for 2 or 3 weeks or antiplatelet such as aspirin can be tried to treat potential arterial occlusive changes. Prophylactic retinal laser photocoagulation may prevent rhegmatogenous retinal detachments. Vitrectomy with long-acting gas or silicone oil or scleral buckling can also be tried to manage rhegmatogenous retinal detachments.

RETINITIS PIGMENTOSA (RP)
Jerome Sherman

ICD—9: 362.74

THE DISEASE

Although much has been learned about the myriad progressive retinal degenerations, the term *retinitis pigmentosa* is still commonly used even though the disorder is not typically an inflammation and is sometimes present without retinal pigmentary proliferation. At the present time, RP is best regarded as a phenotypic description of a group of related retinal dystrophies regardless of which of the nearly 100 genetic defects is implicated. When genetic testing of RP patients becomes widespread, the entire present classification will likely be altered.

Pathophysiology

RP is a retinal disorder with primary involvement of both the retinal pigment epithelium and the photoreceptors. Historically, typical retinitis pigmentosa referred to the form of RP affecting the rods to a greater extent than the cones. Hence, the presenting symptom would be reduced side vision and difficulty seeing at night. A smaller number of patients were classified as having inverse retinitis pigmentosa with cone involvement greater than rod involvement. In these patients, the presenting complaint would relate to poor central vision and sometimes reduction of color vision discrimination. Some clinicians advocate a simplistic but accurate classification of rod-cone vs. cone-rod degeneration.

RP is generally classified as a progressive disorder although the rate of degeneration is often very slow and not obvious to the patient from year to year. Whenever possible, RP should be differentiated from the various congenital stationary night blindness (CSNB) disorders that, unlike RP, demonstrate no field or ERG progression on serial analysis.

Although most cases of RP occur in patients without associated systemic conditions, a minority present with a retinal degeneration as part of a syndrome. These include Lawrence-Moon, Bardet-Biedl, Usher, Alport, Refsum, Kearns-Sayre, Alstrom, and Zellweger.

Etiology

Various mutations or alterations in the RDS/peripheren gene, which is found on chromosome arm 6p, or in the protein rhodopsin, which has been mapped to chromosome arm 3q, result in various retinal degenerations. Other forms of RP have been mapped to chromosomes 1, 7, 17, and 19. Retinal degeneration with hearing loss, specifically Usher's syndrome, has been mapped to chromosome arm 11q in about three-fourths of studied cases. In Kearns-Sayre syndrome (KS), mitochondrial mutations and deletions have been identified. In KS, progressive external ophthalmoplegia presents with a retinal degeneration. In total, nearly 100 mutations associated with the various retinal degenerations have been identified.

The Patient

Clinical Symptoms

Most patients with rod-cone degeneration present with nyctalopia (loss of night vision) and sometimes report difficulty with night driving and problems with entering a dimly lit movie theater or a dark stairwell. Loss of peripheral vision may result in a history of tripping over unseen objects and bumping into furniture or doorframes, and difficulty in playing games such as baseball, tennis, and basketball.

In contrast, patients with cone-rod degeneration present with difficulty in seeing the blackboard at school, reading street signs, and recognizing faces. Reduced color vision is reported somewhat less frequently.

Clinical Signs

The most characteristic and diagnostic finding is diffuse arteriolar attenuation. Pigmentary changes include pigment loss, pigment clumping, and pigment migration. The common appearance of "bone spicules" represents pigment migration from the retinal pigment epithelium to the retinal nerve fiber layer (RNFL), with pigment clumping on retinal vessels within the RNFL. Some cases present with arteriolar attenuation without pigmentary changes, a disorder sometimes termed *retinitis pigmentosa sine pigmento*. Although the disc has been classically described as pale and waxy, disc changes are generally mild and not diagnostic. Bull's-eye maculopathy is not a rare observation, especially in cone-rod degenerations. Posterior subcapsular cataracts (PSC) occur in about one-third of cases. Disc drusen and drusen around the disc occurs in less than 5% of cases. White to yellow flecks or spots are occasionally seen in RP. Retinitis pigmentosa albescens (RP with white dots) demonstrates a much-reduced ERG, whereas fundus al bipuntatus (a form of CSNB) has normal or near normal ERGs following several hours of dark adaptation. A form of cystoid macular edema occurs in a small percentage of RP patients.

The full-field ERG is the single-most diagnostic test in the evaluation of a patient suspected of having a retinal degeneration. In a patient with one of the many pseudoretinitis pigmentosa etiologies, the ERG is often normal or near normal. In RP, the ERG is typically very reduced in amplitude or even extinguished under both photopic and scotopic conditions. In very early RP, the ERG is somewhat reduced in amplitude and delayed. In rod-cone degeneration, the ERG abnormality is greater under scotopic conditions (dark adapted with a dim white or blue stimulus) than under photopic conditions (light adapted and 30 Hz flicker). In cone-rod degeneration, the opposite ERG profile is encountered. Serial ERGs are helpful to document progression. Note that the ERG is often markedly reduced in a patient with a well-documented family history of RP but with no symptoms of nyctalopia. Hence, the ERG is diagnostic of RP in a patient with preclinical disease. A normal ERG in another family member in the same pedigree represents nearly conclusive evidence that RP is not present. In general, the ERG deficits occur prior to symptoms, and a flat ERG does indicate that the patient is blind. However, a flat ERG confirms advanced degeneration and a very poor prognosis even if the patient has only mild symptoms.

Demographics

The incidence of RP in the United States and worldwide is approximately 1 in 4,000. Autosomal dominant, autosomal recessive, and X-linked pedigrees have been reported. Autosomal dominant RP, the mildest form, accounts for nearly one-fourth of total cases. The other two forms of inheritance account for somewhat fewer cases. About half of patients with RP have no identifiable inheritance pattern and are termed *primary* or *simplex.* In contrast to the classical nuclear inheritance patterns above, cytoplasmic DNA mutations are the culprits in the mitochondrial syndrome, Kearns-Sayre.

Males and females are affected equally except for the X-linked pedigrees. The age of onset is highly variable and ranges from infancy to as late as beyond age 50. The so-called early onset cone-rod degeneration appears to occur in the first several years of life, and patients with mild autosomal dominant RP may present in their 50s with initial symptoms. Patients with cone-rod degeneration often become legally blind at a young age, but patients with typical rod-cone degeneration often retain good central visual acuity until the fifth or sixth decade of life.

Significant History

In addition to documenting the symptomatology, a detailed family history with pedigree should be sought. With documented genetic transmission, the diagnosis is better supported. However, a drug history that excludes the phenothiazines and the chloroquines is still essential to rule retinal toxicity. In addition to drug toxicity, certain other disorders, which result in a pigmentary retinopathy, should be considered and eliminated. The diagnosis of these pseudoretinitis pigmentosas is often aided by laboratory tests.

Ancillary Tests

Syphilis, the great masquerader, can mimic virtually all ocular conditions, including RP. When indicated, obtain a Venereal Disease Research Laboratory (VDRL) test and a fluorescent treponemal antibody (FTA-ABS).

If the fundus exam reveals scalloped areas of pigment changes, consider ornithine levels to confirm or deny a diagnosis of gyrate atrophy.

If other neurological abnormalities are present, consider serum phytanic acid levels. Consider an electrocardiogram to rule out heart block in a patient with both progressive external ophthalmoplegia and retinal degeneration because of probable Kearns-Sayre syndrome.

The Treatment

There is no agreed upon, proven treatment for RP. Sunglasses to avoid unnecessary light exposure are recommended by most clinicians for such activities as skiing and sunbathing. Antioxidants may be useful, but no evidence in favor of supplementation exists at present. Vitamin A palmitate (15,000 international units [IU] a day) appears to slow the progression by about 2% per year. But vitamin A intake at this level for many years has potential risks that need to be considered. High doses of vitamin E (400 IU a day) may decrease the beneficial affect of vitamin A. No evidence exists for lutein and bilberry to slow the degeneration.

If cystoid macular edema is confirmed with fluorescein angiography, oral carbonic anhydrase inhibitors (CAIs), such as acetazolamide, may prove helpful. Topical CAIs have not been studied. In about one-third of RP patients, early PSC cataracts will be present and cataract extraction should be considered. The surgery will hopefully improve central visual acuity, but will have little beneficial effect on visual fields.

MACULAR HOLE
Helmut Buettner

ICD—9: 362.54

THE DISEASE
Pathophysiology

An idiopathic age-related macular hole typically begins to develop in the presence of liquefied empty vitreous in the premacular area in the absence of a posterior vitreous detachment. The cortical vitreous, adherent to the surface of the retina and probably invaded by contracting retinal glial cells, exerts tangential traction leading to a foveolar (stage 1 A–impending macular hole) and foveal (stage 1 B–impending macular hole) detachment. In about 50% of these eyes, a spontaneous detachment of the cortical vitreous occurs in the foveal area, relieving the tangential traction and resulting in cessation of progression in the process of macular hole formation and resolution of the foveolar or foveal detachment. In the other 50% of eyes, a small oval or horseshoe-shaped retinal defect develops centrally or eccentrically within several months, called a stage 2 hole. Separation of the cortical vitreous often occurs at this stage, giving rise to a semitranslucent operculum-like structure in front of the macular hole on the surface of the posterior hyaloid face. The foveolar retinal receptor cells retract centrifugally until the retinal defect has reached 400 to 700 microns in diameter in most cases of what is now termed a stage 3 macular hole. The cortical vitreous, however, remains attached at the optic nerve head. Once the cortical vitreous has separated from the entire posterior pole including the optic nerve head, often evidenced by the presence of a Weiss' ring, the defect is designated a stage 4 macular hole.

The process of macular hole formation from stage 1 to stage 4 takes in general about 6 months, but may be completed in a few weeks in some eyes. While abortion of the hole formation process at an early stage (stage 1 A and B) is common with the development of a vitreous separation, closure of a fully developed macular hole (stage 3 and stage 4) occurs spontaneously in only rare cases. Spontaneous closure is usually associated with the formation of an epiretinal membrane.

The chance of developing a macular hole in the fellow eye is estimated at 10 to 15% and about 5% in the presence of a posterior vitreous detachment.

Etiology

A macular hole, a retinal defect in the center of the macula, may develop in association with trauma, inflammation, retinal vascular disease, or vitreoretinal interface changes such as epiretinal membranes and vitreoretinal traction. However, the vast majority of macular holes encountered are idiopathic and age-related in nature.

The Patient

Clinical Symptoms
The patient with an impending macular hole usually mentions metamorphopsia and slight decrease of central vision as the initial symptoms.

Clinical Signs

Biomicroscopy shows a yellow spot 100 to 200 microns in diameter (stage 1 A–impending macular hole) or yellow ring 200 to 300 microns in diameter (stage 1 B–impending macular hole) in the center of the macula. The foveal depression is generally less obvious or absent, and the overlying, attached vitreous appears optically empty. If the process of macular hole formation is not aborted at this stage with the development of a posterior vitreous detachment, a small centrally or eccentrically located full-thickness retinal defect develops (stage 2 macular hole). While some of these stage 2 macular holes remain unchanged in appearance with stable visual function, the majority will, usually over weeks or months, enlarge and develop a partial detachment of the cortical vitreous often with the appearance of an operculum-like opacity in front of the hole. As the retinal defect enlarges, a detachment of the neurosensory retina surrounding the macular hole develops. Once the hole has reached 400 microns in diameter, it is called a stage 3 hole. In most eyes, vision has dropped to about 20/80 to 20/200 by this time. While in a stage 3 hole, vitreofoveal separation has usually occurred, a complete posterior vitreous separation including the optic nerve head with the appearance of a Weiss' ring is the hallmark of a stage 4 macular hole. The operculum-like prefoveal opacity is now visible as a focal opacity in the posterior hyaloid face, which is no longer attached. A stage 4 macular hole most commonly measures 400 to 700 microns in diameter, with the vision ranging from 20/200 to 20/400 in the majority of cases. The surrounding neurosensory retinal detachment becomes quite obvious. Especially with longer-standing macular holes, rarefaction of the retinal pigment epithelium and often gray-yellow drusen-like nodules of thickened retinal pigment epithelium develop in the center of the hole. These changes are well visible on fluorescein angiography as a window-type defect.

Solitary drusen, cystoid macular edema, serous macular detachment in central serous retinopathy or age-related macular degeneration, epiretinal membranes, and a lamellar macular hole may at times be mistaken for an impending or full-thickness macular hole.

Demographics

Idiopathic age-related macular holes have their peak incidence in the seventh decade of life and are encountered more often in women than men at a ratio of 2:1 or 3:1.

Ancillary Tests

With the development of a macular hole, both distance and near visual acuity are found to be diminished, often associated with metamorphopsia. Evaluation of the central visual field with the Amsler grid shows in the early stages of macular hole formation often only distortion of the lines of the grid, while in the later stages, a distinct scotoma corresponding to the macular defect is often identified by the patient. At this stage, the patient may also see a central gap in a streak of light projected onto the macula (positive Watzke-Allen sign). Microperimetry of the central visual field using a scanning laser ophthalmoscope allows a sophisticated analysis of scotomata while observing the macula. The value of focal electroretinography in the functional evaluation of eyes with macular holes remains uncertain.

Color and red-free light fundus photography may aid in the recognition of retinal surface changes associated with a macular hole. Fluorescein angiography may be of equivocal diagnostic value in the early stages but clearly show a window-type defect in the later stages of a macular hole. Fluorescein angiography is also of value in differentiating the various stages of a macular hole.

Biomicroscopy, using a posterior pole contact lens, is the gold standard for the clinical examination of the posterior pole and macula. High-magnification stereopsis and slit-beam illumination with different wavelength light (white, blue, red-free light) allow for the most detailed visual evaluation not only of the retina but also of the vitreoretinal interface changes associated with macular hole formation.

The more advanced vitreoretinal interface changes may also be demonstrable with ultrasonography. However, the newest and most valuable imaging technique is optical coherence tomography (OCT). Using the principle of interferometry, the vitreoretinal changes associated with the various stages of a macular hole are shown in high-resolution cross-sectional images.

OCT allows the clinician to differentiate a pseudomacular hole (defect in an epiretinal membrane simulating a macular hole) from a true macular hole. A true macular hole in its earliest stage (stage 1) presents as yellow foveal dot clinically and as a separation of the photoreceptor outer segments from the retinal pigment epithelium with blunting of the foveal depression but no retinal defect on OCT. The process progresses with the formation of a small central or eccentric full-thickness retinal defect (stage 2), which enlarges (stage 3) and evolves into a mature stage 4 macular hole with the development of a complete posterior vitreous detachment. Referral for surgery to close a stage 2, 3, or 4 macular hole should be considered because it has a good chance of improving visual function. A stage 1 macular hole, however, is not a candidate for surgery because of generally minor visual loss and more importantly the high rate of spontaneous abortion of the process with recovery of vision.

The Treatment

Before the recognition of tangential vitreoretinal traction as the main mechanism in the pathogenesis of an idiopathic age-related macular hole, laser photocoagulation was used with rather limited success to treat the neurosensory detachment surrounding the macular hole. With the refinement of vitrectomy techniques in the late 1980s, the first surgical attempts to manage macular holes were directed at aborting the process of hole formation by removing the cortical vitreous in eyes with stage 1 incipient holes. This procedure, however, was shown to be ineffective in preventing the progression to a full-thickness macular hole. However, performing a vitrectomy with peeling of the cortical vitreous, filling the vitreous cavity with a slowly disappearing gas, and placing the patient in a face-down position for 1 to 2 weeks proved effective in closing a full-thickness macular hole in 90 to 95% of the cases with significant improvement of vision to the 20/40 or better level in about 50% of eyes. In the few cases where histopathologic examination of an eye after successful surgical closure of a macular hole was possible, the mechanism of hole closure appeared to be the proliferation of glial cells closing the retinal defect with centripetal pulling of retinal photoreceptors.

Complications of macular hole surgery include retinal detachment occurring in about 5 to 8% of the eyes and the formation or progression of a cataract occurring in all eyes. Other significantly less common complications are peripheral visual field defects, intraocular pressure elevations and glaucoma, proliferative vitreoretinopathy, and endophthalmitis.

Chapter 19

Neuro-ophthalmic Disease

PUPIL ABNORMALITIES

Leonid Skorin Jr. and Bruce G. Muchnick

ICD—9: 379.40

THE DISEASE

Pathophysiology

Pupil size reflects the neural input of both the sympathetic and parasympathetic systems on the dilator and sphincter muscles, respectively, of the iris. Normal pupils are 3 mm to 4 mm in diameter in ambient light and are relatively equal in size. This equality in pupil size is a result of the bilateral symmetrical afferent input to the Edinger-Westphal complex in the midbrain and because of the symmetrical output of the paired sympathetic nuclei in the hypothalamus. Any disruption of the neural pathway or iris architecture will lead to abnormalities of the pupillary state.

Etiology

A relative afferent pupillary deficit (RAPD) or Marcus Gunn pupil will result from a significant unilateral or asymmetric visual deficit caused by retinal or optic nerve disease (optic neuropathy).

Anisocoria is the state where the two pupils are unequal in size. The etiology depends on whether the abnormal pupil is the dilated or constricted pupil.

Dilated pupils can occur from iris sphincter trauma, Adie's tonic pupil, third-nerve palsy, or pharmacologic blockade. Constricted pupils can occur with iritis, pharmacologic blockade, Horner's syndrome, Argyll Robertson pupil, or long-standing Adie's pupil. Physiologic anisocoria is present when the pupil size difference remains the same in both bright light and in darkness.

The Patient

Symptoms and signs will vary according to the underlying etiology.

Clinical Symptoms

Patients with a RAPD will complain of vision and color loss in the affected eye.

Patients with anisocoria are often asymptomatic or may complain of other symptoms, such as droopy eyelid, blurred vision, focusing problems, or diplopia, depending on any accompanying symptoms.

Clinical Signs
Prominent Signs
- With RAPD, there will be a positive swinging flashlight test (see Fig. 19.1).
- Anisocoria—Pupillary size difference that may vary between light and dark.
- Adie's tonic pupil—The affected pupil is larger and reacts poorly to light or near stimuli.
- Argyll Robertson pupil—The miotic pupils are irregular and do not respond to light with poor dilation in the dark yet good near response.
- Pharmacologic pupil—Either miotic or dilated pupil that does not respond to any pharmacologic testing.
- Horner's syndrome—Miotic pupil accompanied by ptosis and possibly anhidrosis. Anhidrosis will be present if the lesion involves the sympathetic pathway proximal to the bifurcation of the common carotid artery.
- Third-nerve palsy—Dilated pupil accompanied by ptosis and extraocular muscle palsies.
- In light-near dissociation of pupils, there is better pupillary response to near stimuli than to light stimuli. This is found in optic neuropathy, retinopathy, Adie's tonic pupil,

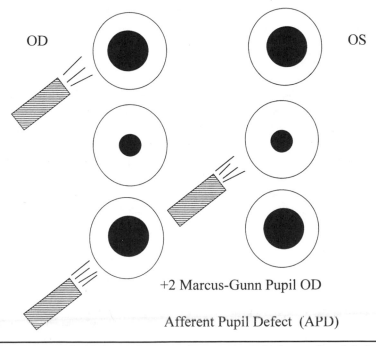

OD   OS

+2 Marcus-Gunn Pupil OD

Afferent Pupil Defect (APD)

FIGURE 19.1. Swinging flashlight test (examiner facing patient). Right eye affected; Left eye normal. Illustration courtesy of Kathleen A. Skorin, C.O.A.

Argyll Robertson pupil, Parinaud's dorsal midbrain syndrome, aberrant regeneration of the third nerve, and diabetes.

Demographics

Physiologic anisocoria is usually <1.0 mm and can change from day to day.

It is as common in men as in women, in the morning as in the afternoon, in the young as in the aged. The prevalence of physiologic anisocoria is approximately 20%.

Significant History

- History of optic nerve disease or retinopathy
- Recent changes in pupil size

Ancillary Tests

Swinging flashlight test. In this test, light is directed first into one pupil, then moved over quickly to the other pupil, and repeated several times while both pupils' response is observed. The test is done in a dimly lit room, with the patient gazing at a distant target and not at the light source. Allow just 3 to 5 seconds of illumination on each side.

When both afferent pathways are normal, the pupils remain essentially the same size no matter which side is illuminated. When an afferent defect is present, the pupils become larger when the light is directed to the involved side (see Fig. 19.1).

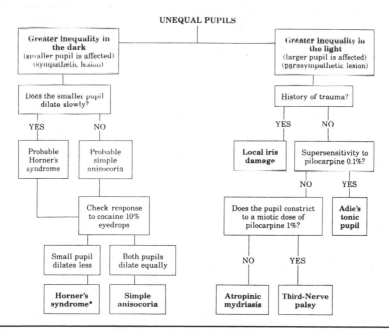

FIGURE 19.2. Flow chart for evaluation of anisocoria. (From Multack RF, Lannin WC, Olbum JR. Improving diagnostic acumen in pupillary evaluation: A review for the primary care physician. *J Am Osteopath Assoc* 1989;89:917–924. Reprinted with permission.)

The RAPD can be measured subjectively or objectively with neutral density filters.

To measure an RAPD objectively, a neutral density filter is held in front of the un-involved eye as the swinging flashlight test is performed. The filter density is increased until the pupil reactions on the swing test are equal.

Anisocoria is evaluated by determining whether pupillary inequality is caused by a defect in sympathetic or parasympathetic innervation, or is because of a structural disorder of the iris. Therefore, a comparison of pupil size by measurement should be done in bright and dim ambient illuminations (Fig. 19.2).

The Treatment

The treatment of pupillary abnormalities is directed to the underlying cause. (See specific sections on optic neuropathies, retinopathy, Horner's syndrome, Adie's tonic pupil, Argyll Robertson pupil, third-nerve palsy).

ADIE'S TONIC PUPIL

Leonid Skorin Jr. and Bruce G. Muchnick

ICD—9: 379.46

THE DISEASE

Pathophysiology

Tonic pupils occur from damage to the ciliary or the postganglionic short ciliary nerves that innervate the pupillary sphincter and ciliary muscles.

Selective damage causes areas of the iris to contract, with adjacent areas experiencing sector paralysis.

Etiology

Most cases of tonic pupil are idiopathic, although some follow a mild upper respiratory infection or other viral illness. Ocular and orbital trauma or surgery can also cause a tonic pupil.

If the tonic pupil is accompanied by diminished deep tendon reflexes, it is known as Holmes-Adie syndrome. This can be explained by concurrent involvement of the ciliary ganglion (tonic pupil) and dorsal root ganglion (areflexia).

Other causes of tonic pupil, especially if bilateral, include orthostatic hypotension, diabetes mellitus, Guillain-Barré syndrome, dysautonomias (such as Riley-Day syndrome), and acute ophthalmologic polyneuritis (Fisher syndrome). Other causes include infections, uveitis, sarcoidosis, orbital and intraorbital surgery, laser therapy, and trauma.

Bilateral tonic pupils that are mid-dilated and react poorly to light are also found in Parinaud's dorsal midbrain syndrome. Unlike true Adie's tonic pupils, these pupils constrict normally to convergence. Other signs of Parinaud's syndrome include supranu-clear paresis of vertical gaze, eyelid retraction, impaired vergence eye movements, convergence-retraction nystagmus, and skew deviation. These signs are not found in Adie's tonic pupil.

The Patient

The patient is often asymptomatic or will have accommodative difficulties with anisocoria.

Clinical Symptoms

The patient with tonic pupil may complain of pupil size difference, photophobia, or blurred near vision with difficulty focusing.

Clinical Signs
Prominent Signs

- Unilateral irregularly dilated pupil with poor to no response to light and shows a slow constriction to near stimulus with slow redilation

Subtle Signs

- Sectoral iris paralysis
- Irregular (vermiform) movements of the iris sphincter
- Defective accommodation

Demographics

Up to 80% of tonic pupils are unilateral initially, and after 1 or 2 months, a tonic pupil may become miotic and smaller than the fellow pupil. Of the unilateral cases, approximately 4% become bilateral each year.

Tonic pupils occur in younger individuals (20 to 40 years of age), and there is a female predilection, with up to 70% of cases occurring in young women.

From 50 to 90% of patients with tonic pupil will also have diminished deep tendon reflexes.

Significant History

- Recent viral illness
- Ocular or orbital trauma
- Hypotension
- Diabetes

Ancillary Tests

Ocular assessment includes visual acuity, extraocular muscle testing, accommodation testing, slit-lamp evaluation of the iris, and fundus evaluation.

Pupil testing should be performed for light and near. To test for cholinergic supersensitivity, have the patient look at a distant target and administer pilocarpine 0.125%

in each eye. Remeasure the pupil size after 15 minutes, making sure the patient does not do any near work.

The tonic pupil will constrict significantly as compared with the normal pupil.

Occasionally, an acute tonic pupil will not show cholinergic supersensitivity until several months later. No neuroimaging studies are necessary once the Adie's tonic pupil is pharmacologically confirmed. All patients with bilateral tonic pupils, whether dilated or miotic, should have serological testing for syphilis (FTA-ABS). Neurosyphilis may cause bilateral tonic pupil confirmed on cholinergic supersensitivity testing.

The Treatment

No treatment is necessary in an asymptomatic patient. If the patient is photophobic, dilute pilocarpine or tinted lenses can be helpful. Reading difficulties can be corrected with appropriate refractive correction for near work, often requiring unequal near adds. Consider colored contact lenses to hide any anisocoria.

ARGYLL ROBERTSON PUPIL

Leonid Skorin Jr. and Bruce G. Muchnick

ICD—9: 379.45

THE DISEASE

Pathophysiology

The lesion responsible for pupillary abnormality is uncertain but may originate in the region of the Sylvian aqueduct in the rostral midbrain interfering with the light reflex fibers and supranuclear inhibitory fibers as they approach the Edinger-Westphal nuclei. The more ventrally located fibers for near response are not affected. In addition, the miosis found in classic Argyll Robertson syndrome can be explained by a lesion rostral to the oculomotor nuclei for pupillary constriction. This would interrupt the supranuclear inhibitory pathways from the higher brain centers thus producing a spastic paralysis in the oculomotor nuclei yielding a miotic pupil.

Etiology

The Argyll Robertson pupil has been recognized as the hallmark of late central nervous system syphilis. Other possible causes include tabes diabetica, multiple sclerosis, encephalitis, sarcoidosis, chronic alcoholism, trauma, neoplasm, and diabetes mellitus.

The Patient

The patient will present with abnormal pupils characterized by miosis, unresponsiveness to light stimulus, and contraction on near effort in eyes with intact visual function.

Clinical Symptoms
The patient with Argyll Robertson pupils is often asymptomatic. The condition is typically bilateral and may be either symmetric or asymmetric. With few exceptions, it is permanent and usually stable but may deteriorate toward total pupil immobility. It develops over months to years.

If because of neurosyphilis, any signs that are present may include mixed neurologic features. These include meningeal syphilis (headache, nausea, vomiting, neck stiffness), microvascular syphilis (stroke), and parenchymal syphilis (paresthesias).

Clinical Signs
Prominent Signs
- Miotic, irregular pupils that do not react to light but react briskly to a near stimulus

Subtle Signs
- Pupils dilate poorly in the dark
- Pupils dilate poorly to mydriatic agents
- Usually bilateral but asymmetric
- Iris atrophy

Demographics

Up to 80% of patients with neurosyphilis will have Argyll Robertson pupils.

Significant History
- Tertiary syphilis
- Diabetes mellitus
- Demyelinating disease
- Trauma
- Neoplasm

Ancillary Tests

Ocular assessment includes visual acuity, extraocular muscle testing, testing pupillary reaction to light and near, slit-lamp evaluation for iris atrophy or interstitial keratitis, and fundus evaluation. Argyll Robertson pupils dilate poorly if the iris atrophy is extensive. The less the atrophy, the better the dilation. Likewise, miotics work poorly in the highly atrophied iris and well in the uninvolved iris. Iris atrophy may be visualized by transillumination of the globe.

Laboratory studies: VDRL, RPR, FTA-ABS, MHA-TP.

The Treatment

Treatment is indicated if there is active disease, and the patient should have an internal medicine evaluation.

CAT SCRATCH DISEASE (CSD)

Joseph W. Sowka and Leonid Skorin Jr.

ICD—9: 078.3

THE DISEASE

Pathophysiology

Cat scratch disease is an infection caused by a fastidious gram-negative bacillus from exposure to an infected cat or kitten. The most common manifestation of CSD in humans is regional lymphadenitis. Other systemic manifestations include Parinaud's oculoglandular syndrome (conjunctivitis, retrotarsal conjunctival granulations, regional preauricular and cervical lymphadenitis, and fever), hepatosplenic infection, encephalopathy, osteomyelitis, and endocarditis. In immunocompetent individuals, the disease is typically self-limiting over the course of 3 to 6 weeks.

Beyond Parinaud's oculoglandular syndrome, the ocular manifestation most associated with CSD is neuroretinitis, a combination of disc edema with stellate macular star of exudates. Cat scratch disease appears to be the most common cause of neuroretinitis. In cases of neuroretinitis, vision is often affected, but to a variable degree. Vision may range from 20/20 to count fingers. Dyschromatopsia and a relative afferent pupil defect may be present to variable degrees. Other posterior segment findings include peripapillary serous macular detachment, discrete foci of retinitis manifested as white retinal or choroidal lesions, vitritis, and submacular exudates. Anterior uveitis may also occur.

Etiology

The causative organism of CSD is the gram-negative rod, *Bartonella henselae*. However, other strains of the organism, notably *Bartonella quintana*, have been implicated in the disease as well. The disease is transmitted by the scratch or bite of an infected cat or kitten, which are natural hosts for these organisms. About 10% of pet cats and 33% of feral cats are bacteremic with these organisms. Arthropod vectors exist as well, but transmission through fleas is questionable. There may or may not be a history of a scratch or bite, but contact with felines is invariably present.

After an incubation period of several days to weeks, the patient develops a self-limiting regional lymphadenopathy with a small cutaneous lesion at the site of inoculation. The patient will demonstrate fever and flu-like symptoms, which will typically resolve over 3 to 6 weeks.

The Patient

The patient is typically younger and has had exposure to cats or kittens. Often there will be a history of a bite or scratch, but this history is not always present. The patient will manifest a flu-like illness with lymphadenopathy and fever.

Clinical Symptoms

- Regional lymphadenopathy
- Fever
- Small cutaneous lesion at site of inoculation
- Parinaud's oculoglandular syndrome
- Painless vision loss (typically unilateral)
  - May be asymptomatic
  - May diminish to count fingers
- Dyschromatopsia

Clinical Signs

- Conjunctivitis
- Retrotarsal conjunctival granulations
- Regional preauricular and cervical lymphadenitis
- Stellate neuroretinitis (disc edema with macular star of exudates): Macular star may develop late in the disease
- Vision ranging from 20/20 to count fingers
- Relative afferent pupil defect (+/−)
- Anterior uveitis
- Focal retinochoroiditis
- Submacular exudates with overlying serous retinal detachment
- Disc edema
- Disc edema with associated peripapillary or macular serous retinal detachment

Demographics

CSD typically afflicts young, otherwise healthy adults. It occurs commonly in children. Higher incidence is reported in fall and winter, attributed to seasonal breeding of cats.

Significant History

Despite the name, a scratch or bite from a cat is not always present. However, contact or exposure to cats or kittens is invariably reported. Patients may not remember a scratch or bite, but the disease is suspected in patients developing painless vision loss or disc edema following a febrile illness.

Ancillary Tests

The definitive test for CSD is the ELISA *Bartonella henselae* titer. In that there are other species that can cause CSD, it is appropriate to obtain titers for *Bartonella quintana* as well. Sera from 95% of patients with clinically defined CSD show IgG titers of 1:64 and above. Early in the disease process, IgG may be absent, but IgM may be positive. In some cases, there will be a false-negative ELISA despite clinical signs and symptoms of CSD. An alternate diagnostic modality is a polymerase chain reaction analysis of lymphadenopathy aspirate and should be considered in the clinical situation where CSD is strongly suspected and ELISA titers are either negative or borderline.

The Treatment

In immunocompetent individuals, CSD is generally a benign self-limiting disease with an excellent prognosis with little chance for morbidity. Medical treatment is generally unnecessary. The organism is quite susceptible to a number of antibiotics, such as penicillin, cephalosporins, aminoglycosides, tetracyclines, macrolides, fluoroquinolones, and rifamicin. While the benefit of therapy in immunocompetent patients is unknown, cases complicated by ocular involvement are recommended for therapy. Azithromycin is the drug of choice if treatment is initiated. For pediatric patients, an initial dose of 10 mg/kg on the first day, followed by 5 g/kg/day for the following 4 days is the recommended regimen. For older children and adults, the recommended regimen is 500 mg on the first treatment day, followed by 250 mg per day for the next 4 days. This is most often used when there is vision loss from neuroretinitis. Whether oral prednisone has a role in the management of this disease is unknown.

Long-term prognosis for patients with ocular involvement is good, but some individuals may acquire a mild postinfectious optic neuropathy.

HORNER'S SYNDROME

Leonid Skorin Jr. and Alan G. Kabat

ICD—9: 337.9—Unspecified disorder of autonomic nervous system
ICD—9: 954.0—Injury to cervical sympathetic

THE DISEASE

Pathophysiology

Partial or complete interruption of the oculosympathetic pathway results in Horner's syndrome. The oculosympathetic pathway is composed of three neurons:

- First-order neuron—This central neuron arises from the posterior hypothalamus, traveling through the brainstem and cervical cord, and synapsing at the ciliospinal center of Budge at C8-T2.
- Second-order neuron—These preganglionic neuron fibers exit the spinal cord primarily with the first ventral thoracic root and continue through the stellate ganglion at the pulmonary apex to the superior cervical ganglion at the bifurcation of the internal and external carotid arteries (C3-C4).
- Third-order neuron—This postganglionic neuron originates from the superior cervical ganglion and travels along the internal carotid artery, penetrating the base of the skull and continuing through the cavernous sinus. The fibers that will innervate the eye and Muller's muscles of the eyelids then enter the orbit via the superior orbital fissure. Fibers destined for the dilator muscle enter the eye via the long posterior ciliary nerves.

Etiology

- First-order neuron—Cerebrovascular disease (Wallenberg's lateral medullary plate infarction syndrome), cervical trauma, Arnold-Chiari malformation, demyelinating disease (e.g., multiple sclerosis), syringomyelia, tumors of the pons, third ventricle, cervical cord or pituitary, osteoarthritis of the neck with bony spurs.
- Second-order neuron—Tumors of the chest apex (Pancoast's tumor) or superior mediastinum, lymphadenopathy, aortic aneurysm, thyroid enlargement, surgical intervention (thyroidectomy, radical neck surgery, carotid angiography).
- Third-order neuron—Vascular headache syndromes (migraine, cluster, Raeder's paratrigeminal neuralgia), cavernous sinus or middle cranial fossa lesions, basal skull fracture, carotid-cavernous fistula, nasopharyngeal carcinoma, otitis media, sinusitis, trigeminal herpes zoster, Tolosa-Hunt syndrome, carotid artery occlusion or dissection.
- Congenital—Birth trauma sustained during labor or delivery, cervical and mediastinal neuroblastoma.

The Patient

The classic Horner's syndrome triad consists of unilateral ptosis, miosis, and anhidrosis.

Clinical Symptoms

A patient with a recent onset Horner's syndrome will complain of a droopy eyelid and the inability to sweat on one side of the face, provided the lesion occurs distal to the carotid bifurcation, since most of the sudomotor sympathetic fibers to the face travel with the external carotid artery.

Clinical Signs

Prominent Signs

- Anisocoria, which is greater in dim illumination
- Upper eyelid ptosis
- Diminished iris pigment in the affected eye (heterochromia irides), if congenital

Subtle Signs

- Upside-down ptosis or elevation of the lower eyelid
- Apparent enophthalmos from a narrowed palpebral fissure
- Dilated conjunctival and facial vessels
- Decreased intraocular pressure
- Increased accommodative amplitude
- Absence of dilation to psychosensory stimuli

Demographics

Horner's syndrome can occur at any age, and there is no sex predilection. From birth to age 20 years, trauma is the most significant cause. From 21 to 50 years, almost half the cases result from tumors. In patients over 50 years of age, neoplasia is the most important cause. Horner's syndrome is the initial sign of malignancy in 35% of patients. Overall, the cause of Horner's syndrome can be identified in only 60% of patients.

Significant History
- New onset of headache
- Trauma
- Recent cardiac, neck, thoracic surgery
- Recent stroke

Ancillary Tests

Ocular assessment includes visual acuity, extraocular muscle testing, pupil testing, levator function testing, visual fields, slit-lamp examination, and fundus evaluation. Evaluate old photographs. Definitive diagnosis is based on the results of pharmacologic testing of pupillary response, first to cocaine and then to hydroxyamphetamine.

- Cocaine test. Cocaine produces dilation of the pupil by preventing reuptake of norepinephrine. If the sympathetic innervation to the eye is interrupted at any level (central, preganglionic, or postganglionic), cocaine will have no dilation effect. Cocaine helps confirm the presence or absence of oculosympathetic palsy by increasing pupillary inequality. This test does not indicate the location of the lesion. (The patient may test positive on drug testing for 48 hours following the cocaine test.)

   Cocaine (4 to 10%), one drop is placed in each eye and then repeated in several minutes. The pupils should be evaluated after 50 to 60 minutes. A Horner's pupil does not dilate as well as the normal pupil.
- Hydroxyamphetamine test. Hydroxyamphetamine (Paredrine) 1% causes a release of norepinephrine from the nerve endings at the myoneural junction, stimulating the dilator muscle. This helps distinguish a third-order neuron from a first-order neuron and second-order neuron. Third-order neuron lesions are considered to be "benign" while first- and second-order lesions are potentially life threatening.

   Hydroxyamphetamine testing should not be performed for 48 hours following the cocaine test.

   Hydroxyamphetamine 1% is placed in each eye, repeating one drop 1 minute later. The pupils are evaluated in 30 minutes. The normal pupil will dilate, while a third-order neuron lesion pupil will show no dilation. Pupillary dilation will be normal if the Horner's syndrome is a result of lesions of the first-order or second-order neurons.
- Laboratory studies. Lab studies are not diagnostic of Horner's syndrome; however, they may aid in identifying the underlying etiology, particularly in cases of acquired disease. Some tests that may be considered include CBC with differential, serology testing for syphilis (FTA-ABS and RPR), and purified protein derivative for tuberculosis. Imaging studies may include chest x-ray with lordotic view to image the lung apex, CT scan or MRI of the brain, and x-rays of the cervical spine.

   A neurology consult should be ordered if a central lesion is suspected. If a malignancy is suspected, referral to an internist or oncologist is indicated.

   Vascular lesions require consultation with a vascular or thoracic surgeon.

The Treatment

Postganglionic lesions usually do not need treatment. Central or preganglionic lesions need to be addressed with appropriate consultation. Neurosurgical intervention may be required for potentially life-threatening situations.

Vascular headache syndromes (e.g., migraine, cluster) should be treated to minimize recurrence.

OCULOMOTOR-NERVE PALSY

Leonid Skorin Jr. and Joseph W. Sowka

ICD—9: 378.52

THE DISEASE

Pathophysiology

The oculomotor (third) cranial nerve innervates five extraocular muscles (the levator, superior, inferior and medial recti, and the inferior oblique) and carries the parasympathetic outflow to the ciliary ganglion, controlling pupillary constriction and accommodation. Any mechanism that disrupts this outflow will cause a partial or complete oculomotor-nerve palsy.

Etiology

Causes of nuclear oculomotor-nerve palsy include multiple sclerosis, vascular accidents, tumors, and infections. Midbrain vascular accidents account for the majority of fascicular palsies, involving both the oculomotor nucleus as well as the nerve's fascicles as they course through the parenchyma of the midbrain. After exiting the brainstem in the interpeduncular fossa, the oculomotor nerve passes inferolateral to the posterior communicating artery (PCA) and medial to the edge of the tentorium. In this region, it is vulnerable to damage from transtentorial herniation also known as uncal syndrome. Compression from an aneurysm of the PCA can also cause pupil-involving oculomotor palsy. Nerve damage can also result from subarachnoid hemorrhage and meningitis.

The disease processes within the cavernous sinus usually involve more than one nerve and include neoplasm, aneurysm, thrombosis, fistula, inflammation, and ischemia.

The oculomotor nerve divides into superior and inferior divisions at the level of the anterior cavernous sinus or superior orbital fissure. Superior-division palsies, involving the superior rectus and levator, may result from aneurysm, viral infection, diabetes, and enlargement of the third ventricle. Inferior-division palsies, involving the inferior rectus, inferior oblique, medial rectus, and ciliary sphincter, result from trauma, viral infections, local orbital disease, and brainstem vascular malformations. Orbital involvement, such as trauma, tumor, aneurysm, and infection from a tooth abscess, can damage the oculomotor nerve.

Aberrant regeneration or oculomotor synkinesis occurs only with mechanical disruption of fibers following an acute palsy such as from trauma or aneurysmal rupture and never from vasculopathic palsies. This type of misdirection can also be found in congenital oculomotor-nerve palsy and ophthalmoplegic migraine. Patients with ophthalmoplegic migraine are children and young adults who have a strong family history of migraine.

The Patient

Symptoms and signs depend on the location of the lesion that is disrupting the oculomotor nerve. Identifying pupil involvement is critical to diagnosis and management.

Clinical Symptoms

The patient with oculomotor-nerve palsy will complain of diplopia, droopy eyelid, difficulty focusing or reading, and possible eye or hemicranial pain.

Clinical Signs
Prominent Signs

- Complete palsy, which includes ptosis and restriction of ocular movement except for abduction and intorsion. The pupil may also be fixed and dilated.
- Superior-division palsy includes ptosis with a restriction in upgaze.
- Inferior-division palsy includes restriction in downgaze, restricted adduction, and pupil dilation.
- Nuclear-fascicular palsies may also involve contralateral hemiplegia, intention tremor, and ataxic gait, depending upon the location of the damage within the midbrain.

Subtle Signs

- Aberrant regeneration or oculomotor synkinesis
- Loss of accommodation
- Loss of near light reflex

Demographics

Approximately 20% of oculomotor third-nerve palsies are a result of expansion or hemorrhage of an aneurysm, and vasculopathic causes, such as diabetes, account for another 20%. Patients who have an underlying vasculopathic etiology are usually older than 45 years of age, and 60% or more are diabetic. Only 15% of oculomotor palsies are because of neoplasm. In children, 40% of oculomotor palsies are congenital, and 20% are because of trauma.

The pupil is spared in 80% of vasculopathic oculomotor nerve palsies and involved in 95% of aneurysmal palsies. Lesions in the cavernous sinus also may spare the pupil or present with a concurrent Horner's syndrome.

Significant History

- Diabetes
- Hypertension

- Hyperlipidemia
- Herpes zoster
- Leukemia
- New onset headache

Ancillary Tests

Ocular assessment includes visual acuity, extraocular muscle testing, visual field, exophthalmometry, levator function, and pupil assessment. If the pupil is dilated, then 0.125% pilocarpine should be instilled to assess for cholinergic suprasensitivity (Adie's pupil). If there is no response (constriction), then pilocarpine 1% should subsequently be instilled. With an oculomotor-nerve palsy there will be constriction of the affected pupil.

When the pupil is not involved, then a edrophonium test, evaluation of orbicularis strength, and evaluation of ptosis after sustained upgaze should be performed to rule out myasthenia gravis mimicking oculomotor palsy.

Neuroimaging with a CT scan or magnetic resonance imaging and magnetic resonance angiography, lumbar puncture, or cerebral angiography is indicated for all pupil-involved oculomotor palsies or pupil-sparing palsies if the patient is less than 45 years old with no vasculopathic history, has incomplete palsy, has a palsy that has not shown any improvement over 3 months time, or has more than just an isolated oculomotor deficit. Any patient who develops aberrant regeneration should also have neuroimaging.

Laboratory studies: CBC with differential, glucose tolerance test, ESR, RPR, antinuclear antibody. A blood pressure measurement should also be done.

The Treatment

Most patients with ischemic oculomotor-nerve palsies show improvement within 1 to 2 months and maximally by 6 months. While waiting for improvement to occur, the underlying vasculopathic abnormality should be corrected, and the patient may wear a temporary eye patch for any disturbing diplopic symptoms. Patients who have pupil-involving oculomotor palsies will need emergent evaluation and testing with possible hospitalization. If an intracranial aneurysm is the suspected cause of the oculomotor palsy, then the patient should be sent emergently to the hospital, as 20% of these patients die within 48 hours because of aneurysm rupture and subsequent subarachnoid hemorrhage.

Children with chronic oculomotor palsies may need Fresnel prism correction or botulinum toxin injection to the lateral rectus to prevent contracture of the muscle. Surgery should be delayed until 6 months from the time improvement has ceased. Ipsilateral horizontal recess-resect procedures work well if there is at least 50% medial rectus function. If the palsy is complete, large horizontal recess-resect procedures are combined with contralateral lateral rectus weakening and/or ipsilateral superior oblique transposition. Contralateral vertical muscle surgery may also need to be performed.

TROCHLEAR-NERVE PALSY
Leonid Skorin Jr. and Joseph W. Sowka

ICD—9: 378.53

THE DISEASE
Pathophysiology

The trochlear (fourth) cranial nerve is the only cranial nerve that exits at the dorsal aspect of the brainstem. The nerve fibers then cross and follow a long and circuitous course from the brainstem to the superior oblique muscles. This makes the nerve vulnerable to injury at many locations.

Etiology

Causes of nuclear-fascicular trochlear-nerve palsy include ischemia from infarction, hemorrhage, demyelination, and trauma. Bilateral trochlear-nerve palsies are often seen following blows to the head. Bilateral, and occasionally unilateral, trochlear-nerve palsies can be associated with a tumor of the pineal gland compressing the posterior midbrain in the dorsal midbrain syndrome. Loss of upward saccades and a light-near dissociated pupil accompany the trochlear palsy in dorsal midbrain syndrome. Distention of the fourth ventricle or contracoup forces transmitted to the brainstem by the free tentorial edge may injure the nerves. As the nerve courses through the cavernous sinus and orbit, it can be affected by inflammation, tumor, aneurysm, fistula, or trauma. Isolated trochlear-nerve palsies may be congenital and appear in late childhood to mid-adult life as a result of decompensation. Otherwise, most isolated acquired trochlear-nerve palsies are because of trauma, hypertension, atherosclerosis, and diabetes. More rare causes of palsy include herpes zoster ophthalmicus, collagen vascular disease, aneurysm, hydrocephalus, and encephalitis.

The Patient

Most patients with trochlear-nerve palsy will complain of vertical diplopia that is eliminated when one eye is closed.

Clinical Symptoms
- Vertical diplopia that is worse in the field of action of the involved superior oblique muscle
- Difficulty with near tasks or downgaze

Clinical Signs
Prominent Signs
- Positive Parks "three-step test"
  Step 1: Vertical deviation on the side of the lesion
  Step 2: Vertical deviation worsens on gaze away from the involved nerve

Step 3: On Bielschowsky head-tilt testing, the deviation is greater on head tilt toward the involved trochlear nerve

Subtle Signs
- Assumed or habitual head tilt toward the contralateral shoulder
- Large vertical fusional amplitudes
- Excyclotorsion as measured by double-Maddox rod test
- Hyperdeviation greater on downgaze

Demographics

The most common cause of trochlear-nerve palsy is trauma, which constitutes approximately 40% of the cases. In spite of the availability of improved diagnostic techniques, the number of cases remaining without a specific diagnosis is still approximately 30%. Ischemia causes 20% and tumors constitute 10% of acquired, isolated trochlear palsies.

Congenital trochlear palsies are also very common and can present in later life after decompensation. Approximately 30% of all trochlear palsies are bilateral, and the prevalence increases to 40% in those secondary to trauma.

Significant History
- Head trauma, especially blows to the vertex
- Hypertension
- Diabetes

Ancillary Tests

Ocular assessment includes visual acuity, extraocular muscle testing including the Parks three-step test and Bielschowsky's head-tilt testing. Measurement for excyclotorsion can be done with a double Maddox rod in a trial frame or phoropter, Maddox wing, or Lancaster red/green test. Cyclotorsion can also be evaluated with fundus examination or photography. Normally, the optic nerve is just slightly higher than the foveal area. In trochlear-nerve palsy, the optic disc is significantly higher than the fovea on fundus photography and lower on indirect ophthalmoscopy.

If congenital trochlear-nerve palsy is suspected, then measurement of the amplitude of vertical vergence should be done. In most patients, the normal value of vertical fusional amplitude is from 3 to 6 prism diopters. Patients with congenital trochlear palsy may be able to fuse anywhere from 10 to 30 prism diopters of deviation (using vertical prism bars). Evaluate possible long-standing palsy by reviewing old photographs, looking for the presence of head-tilting.

Laboratory studies: Glucose tolerance test, ESR, blood pressure measurement, edrophonium test if myasthenia gravis is suspected.

If the palsy has not resolved or improved in 4 months, or if any other neurologic signs are present, then the patient will also need neuroimaging, lumbar puncture, and cerebral angiography.

The Treatment

Because many acquired trochlear-nerve palsies spontaneously recover in 4 to 6 months, observation with patching for symptomatic diplopia is sufficient. If the deviation remains stable, prisms incorporated into glasses may be of benefit. Surgical correction has a high success rate. Surgery is undertaken when the deviation has been stable for at least 6 months.

ABDUCENS-NERVE PALSY
Leonid Skorin Jr. and Joseph Sowka

ICD—9: 378.54

THE DISEASE
Pathophysiology

The abducens (sixth) cranial nerve originates in the dorsal midpons with its nucleus being surrounded by the seventh nerve fascicle. This complex anatomic relationship helps determine the presence of associated findings. The abducens nerve fascicle travels anteriorly through the pons, lateral to the parapontine reticular formation, and through the pyramidal tract to exit the brainstem into the subarachnoid space. The subarachnoid space is the most common locus of an isolated, unilateral abducens-nerve palsy. The abducens nerve then continues up the clivus, over the petrous ridge along the base of the skull, entering the cavernous sinus and the orbit to innervate the lateral rectus muscle.

Etiology

Causes of nuclear-fascicular abducens-nerve palsies include tumors, demyelination, and vascular disease. The abducens nerve is vulnerable in the subarachnoid space from trauma and tumors. It is here that the nerve is affected by elevated intracranial pressure by downward displacement of the brainstem and secondary stretching of the nerve. Inflammation of the petrous bone and its dura may occur secondary to middle-ear infections, known as Gradenigo's syndrome. Traumatic abducens-nerve palsies may result from basilar skull fractures. Masses invading the base of the skull from the nasopharynx or at the cerebellopontine angle may cause abducens-nerve pareses.

Cavernous sinus and orbital etiologies include trauma, diabetes, hypertension, tumor, aneurysm, fistula, inflammation, and cellulitis. Isolated abducens-nerve palsy is seen in young patients with postviral syndrome and in adults with hypertension or diabetes with ischemic mononeuropathy.

The Patient

Most patients with isolated abducens-nerve palsy will complain of horizontal diplopia, which is greater at distance and is eliminated when one eye is closed.

Clinical Symptoms
Horizontal diplopia, worse at distance than near and exaggerated when the patient looks in the direction of the affected lateral rectus muscle.

Clinical Signs
Prominent Signs
- Abduction deficit
- Esotropia greater with paretic eye fixing a distant target, compared with unaffected eye fixing target
- No restriction on forced duction testing

Associated Syndromes
- Millard-Gubler—Ipsilateral abducens, and facial-cranial–nerve palsy with contralateral hemiparesis
- Raymond-Cestan—Ipsilateral abducens palsy with contralateral hemiparesis
- Foville's—Ipsilateral gaze palsy; ipsilateral trigeminal and facial-cranial–nerve palsy with ipsilateral Horner's syndrome
- Gradenigo's—Ipsilateral trigeminal pain, abducens, facial-cranial–nerve palsy, and hearing loss
- Pseudo-Gradenigo's—Ipsilateral abducens palsy, ipsilateral trigeminal pain, ipsilateral ocular irritation, and hearing loss
- One-and-a-half—Ipsilateral conjugate gaze palsy, internuclear ophthalmoplegia on gaze to contralateral side

Demographics

Abducens-nerve palsies occur more frequently than do palsies of the oculomotor or trochlear cranial nerve. Up to 30% of the time, the exact cause of abducens palsy remains unknown, while the rest of the time there appears to be an even distribution between tumor, vasculopathic causes, and trauma. Bilateral abducens-nerve palsies rarely result from vascular disease and are more common in children than in adults. Bilateral abducens palsies, especially with concurrent optic disc edema, strongly suggest increased intracranial pressure.

Significant History
- Head trauma
- Diabetes
- Hypertension
- New onset of headache, tinnitus, transient visual obscurations, nausea if increased intracranial pressure is suspected

Ancillary Tests

Ocular assessment includes visual acuity, extraocular muscle testing, forced duction testing, corneal sensitivity with cotton wisp, orbicularis strength, slit-lamp exam, and funduscopic evaluation for papilledema.

Laboratory studies: CBC with differential, glucose tolerance test, ESR, RPR, antinuclear antibody, and blood pressure measurement.

Neuroimaging with magnetic resonance imaging if a lesion of the brainstem or posterior fossa is suspected. CT scanning is preferred if sinus or mastoid disease is suspected. Lumbar puncture and cerebral angiography may also be necessary.

Edrophonium testing is indicated if myasthenia is a concern.

The Treatment

In an acute phase of an abducens cranial nerve palsy, simple occlusion with patching or temporary prisms if the deviation is small and not greatly noncomitant may be all that is necessary. Botulinum toxin injections into the ipsilateral medial rectus muscle may be necessary if the recovery is prolonged or the deviation is too large for prism correction or to prevent secondary contracture of the medial rectus. Surgical correction can be done after measurements have been stable for at least 6 months. An ipsilateral recess-resect procedure combined with a contralateral medial rectus recession may be indicated.

Any underlying medical problem must be identified and treated.

FACIAL-NERVE PALSY
Leonid Skorin Jr.

ICD—9: 351.0

THE DISEASE
Pathophysiology

Facial palsy is the most common of the cranial neuropathies. Bell's palsy is a facial palsy of no obvious cause whose presumed mechanism is swelling of the peripheral portion of the facial or seventh cranial nerve because of immune or infectious disease. The nerve becomes compressed and ischemic in its narrow course through the temporal bone. This mechanical compression causes interruption of the nerve's transmission, resulting in a conduction block and nerve degeneration. Additional immunological response may result in fragmentation and demyelination of the nerve sheath, causing loss of function. Because this condition is temporary, remyelination occurs after the inflammation resolves.

Etiology

True Bell's palsy or idiopathic facial palsy has no known underlying cause. Recent findings now strongly point to herpes simplex virus type I as the most likely cause of Bell's palsy. Other viral infections such as varicella-zoster, Epstein-Barr (infectious mononucleosis), measles, rubella, rabies, mumps, cytomegalovirus, infectious hepatitis, and human immunodeficiency are also known to cause facial palsy.

Herpes zoster can cause up to 13% of facial palsies. Herpes zoster infection of the geniculate ganglion with typical herpetic vesicular eruptions is known as Ramsay Hunt syndrome (herpes zoster oticus).

Bacterial infection is the cause of facial palsy up to 4% of the time. Tetanus, brucellosis, typhoid fever, leptospirosis, and diphtheria are rare examples. In endemic areas, up to 25% of acute facial palsies may be caused by Lyme disease. Lyme disease is a systemic spirochetal infection with *Borrelia burgdorferi* that follows the bite of the deer tick.

Facial palsy can be the result of middle-ear disease (otitis media with or without mastoiditis); malignancies of the parotid gland because the facial nerve runs through the gland; and neoplasms, both primary, such as schwannomas, or secondary, such as acoustic neuromas, which cause compression at the cerebellopontine angle. Up to 21% of the time, trauma is the cause. Primary neurologic disorders, such as Guillain-Barré and Melkersson's syndrome, may also cause facial palsy.

The Patient

Symptoms and signs may range from subtle weakness and facial muscle paresis to complete unilateral paralysis.

Clinical Symptoms

The patient with Bell's palsy complains of sudden unilateral facial weakness. There may be drooling after brushing the teeth or when drinking, an asymmetric appearance of the mouth, an inability to whistle, and excessive epiphora. The patient may describe a deadness, loss of feeling, or numbness. Up to 50% of patients experience pain behind the ear, sometimes even preceding physical changes. Hyperacusis (painful response to sound) and dysgeusia (distorted taste) are also common.

Clinical Signs
Prominent Signs
- Complete unilateral facial paresis or paralysis involving the forehead, orbicularis oculi, facial muscles of expression, and mouth

Subtle Signs
- Loss of facial creases and folds
- Widening of the palpebral aperture
- Lower lid ectropion
- Inability to blink
- Downturning of one side of mouth
- Corneal irritation from dry eye and exposure

Demographics

Bell's palsy is the most common peripheral facial palsy, occurring in 20 per 100,000 to 40 per 100,000 persons annually. Men and women of all ages are equally affected, with the majority of patients between the ages of 20 and 40. The condition affects the left and right sides of the face with equal frequency. It is bilateral at onset in about 0.3% of cases and recurrent in up to 11%. Up to 31% of patients with recurrent Bell's palsy are diabetics. A family history can be obtained in 2% of patients. The disease is 3.3 times more common in pregnant women and is especially prevalent in the third trimester or within the first week postpartum.

Significant History

- Prior exposure to stress, upper respiratory infection, cold, fever, dental extraction, menstruation, or driving with cold air blowing on the face
- Pregnancy
- Diabetes
- Hypertension
- Exposure to tick bite and skin rash (erythema chronicum migrans)
- Medical history of Guillain-Barré, Lyme disease, sarcoidosis, carcinomatous, treponemal, mycobacterial or cryptococcal meningitis, multiple sclerosis, if bilateral palsy is present

Ancillary Tests

Ocular assessment includes visual acuity, extraocular muscle testing, noting any muscle imbalance or nystagmus, corneal sensitivity with cotton wisp, slit-lamp exam with fluorescein, and rose bengal staining, Shirmer basal secretion test, orbicularis strength, and Bell's phenomenon. Otologic evaluation of the ear canal and tympanic membrane, looking behind the ear, hearing test in suspected cases of Ramsay Hunt syndrome.

Ancillary studies: CBC with differential, urinalysis, plasma glucose, ESR, chest x-ray, Lyme titer. In patients with complete paralysis, assessment of neural status by electrical tests is useful. These include maximal nerve stimulation, nerve conduction, electromyography (EMG), electroneuronography (ENOG). Imaging studies (MRI, CT) are indicated when the history or physical examination turns up suspicious findings or when facial movement does not recover within 6 months.

The Treatment

The one essential intervention in any facial palsy is corneal protection. Nonpreserved artificial tears during the day and bland ointment at night are mandatory. The patient may also physically close his or her eyelids when the eye is irritated. Moisture chambers, eyelid taping, external eyelid prosthesis, punctal plugs, botulinum toxin injection to induce upper eyelid ptosis, surgical placement of a stainless steel spring or gold weight to reanimate the upper eyelid, or partial tarsorrhaphy should be considered in cases of corneal compromise.

If the patient is seen within 2 weeks of onset of symptoms, oral prednisone 1 mg/kg of body weight daily (60 mg/day maximum) for 7 days, split into twice-daily dosing, then tapered over a subsequent 3 days can be started. Oral prednisone is most beneficial in patients with pain and complete paralysis. If seen within the first 3 days of symptom onset, oral antiviral agents (acyclovir 400 mg five times daily for 10 days, valacyclovir 500 mg three times daily for 7 days, or famciclovir 500 mg three times daily for 7 days) may be added to suspected herpes simplex palsies. The Quality Standards Subcommittee of the American Academy of Neurology recommends that the use of steroids is *probably* effective and under most circumstances should be considered but that antiviral agents should only *possibly* be considered.

Oral antiviral agents should be used in all cases of Ramsay Hunt syndrome. Lyme facial palsy is treated with amoxicillin, 500 mg four times a day for 3 to 4 weeks, or doxycycline, 100 mg two or three times a day for 3 to 4 weeks. Ceftriaxone, a third-generation cephalosporin, is used in amoxicillin and doxycycline failures.

Middle cranial fossa surgical decompression is of benefit in cases of complete acute paralysis between 3 and 14 days after onset, ENOG with >90% degeneration, and voluntary EMG with no motor-unit potentials.

CEREBRAL VENOUS THROMBOSIS
Bruce G. Muchnick

ICD—9: 325

THE DISEASE
Pathophysiology

Cerebral venous thrombosis describes the presence of a blood clot, or thrombus, within the venous system of the brain. This may lead to partial or complete occlusion of a cerebral vein, resulting in neurologic and visual dysfunction.

The blocking of a cerebral vein or dural sinus causes blood to be forced retrograde into the capillaries. This blocks oxygenated blood to the cerebral tissues, leading to ischemia, edema, and hemorrhagic infarction.

Etiology

A thrombus is an insoluble mass formed in the vascular system and composed of constituents of the blood. It forms on and is attached to the endothelium of the blood vessel. It may partially or completely occlude the lumen of the vessel.

The thrombus is composed primarily of platelets and fibrin. There may be an inflammatory response in the vessel wall accompanying the blood clot.

Cerebral venous thrombosis is caused by infectious or noninfectious processes. Acute inflammation can reach the cerebral veins and arise from infections of the mastoid air cells and paranasal sinuses. Infectious sources include fungi, virus (HIV), parasites (Trichinosis), and bacteria (syphilis).

Aseptic occlusion of the intracerebral venous structures can be caused by trauma, tumors, systemic diseases (Lupus), hypoperfusion (heart failure), and most commonly hypercoagulability.

No matter what the cause, cerebral venous occlusion results in hemorrhagic infarction of brain tissue and cerebral and subarachnoid hemorrhage.

The Patient

Clinical Symptoms
A low grade venous sinus thrombosis may be so mild as to produce only an increase in intracranial venous pressure, resulting in a mild headache. Focal seizures may occur if there is partial ischemia to the cerebral cortex. These seizures are sometimes preceded by a prodrome of numbness, weakness, behavioral changes, and headache.

A variety of visual field defects, both permanent or transient, may result from venous sinus thrombosis.

Clinical Signs

Depending on the location of the thrombosis, a wide range of neurological deficits may accompany cerebral venous thrombosis, including aphasia, memory loss, chills, sweats, and tachycardia. Ocular manifestations include pain around the eyes, orbital congestion, lid swelling, proptosis, and ophthalmoplegia.

An increase in cerebral spinal fluid level may result in papilledema.

Demographics

Because of the introduction of antibiotics, septic thrombosis has become relatively rare and accounts for about 10% of all cases of cerebral venous thrombosis in the Western world. In developing countries, the rate is higher (25%). The most common cause of aseptic venous thrombosis is hypercoagulability. One study showed that in cases of cerebral venous thrombosis, 12% were deceased within 3 years, 12% had seizures, 10% had motor deficits, 8% had visual field defects, 45% had headaches, and 83% were living independent lifestyles.

Significant History

- Inquire about the sudden onset of neurological deficits.
- Is the patient taking medications that may contribute to hypercoagulability states (birth control pills)?
- Is there any genetic disorder in the family or patient that may lead to a hypercoagulability state?
- Has there been any blunt injury to the head?
- Did the patient receive electroconvulsive treatment?
- Does the patient have any known systemic disorders?
- Does the patient have any signs of infection of the head or neck?

Ancillary Tests

The primary method of diagnosing cerebral venous thrombosis is noninvasive neuroimaging. This includes CT scanning and MR imaging. CT scanning may be performed unenhanced or with injection of iodinated contrast material. T1-weighted and T2-weighted MR images in patients with venous thrombosis reveal abnormalities in the veins and sinuses.

MR angiography (3D MR flow imaging) can reveal abnormalities in the intracranial and extracranial vasculature. Conventional (invasive) angiography can then confirm the diagnosis of thrombosis.

Laboratory tests (CBC with differential, blood cultures) should be utilized to rule out sepsis. Blood tests are helpful to detect a hypercoagulability state. These include CBC, erythrocyte sedimentation rate, C-reactive protein, prothrombin time, partial thromboplastin time, protein S deficiency, protein C deficiency, antithrombin III, factor

V Leiden (activated protein C resistance), anticardiolipin profile, lupus anticoagulant, homocysteine.

The Treatment

Treatment depends on the underlying cause of the thrombosis and location and severity of the neurological deficit.

- Septic thrombosis requires antimicrobial treatment and possible surgery
- Blood thinners (Heparin) are used in many cases to treat aseptic thrombosis
- Urokinase (thrombolysis) can be used in aseptic thrombosis
- Surgical removal of the thrombus
- Stent placement
- Treatment of elevated ICP (acetazolamide), lumbar punctures, or shunt procedures
- Long-term blood-thinner therapy (Warfarin)

CAVERNOUS SINUS SYNDROME

Leonid Skorin Jr. and Bruce G. Muchnick

ICD—9: 437.6—Nonpyogenic thrombosis of intracranial venous sinus
ICD—9: 325—Phlebitis and thrombophlebitis of intracranial venous sinuse

THE DISEASE

Pathophysiology

The cavernous sinuses are triangular interconnecting structures, the walls of each sinus extending from the superior orbital fissure to the posterior wall of the sella and created by dura mater. Each sinus contains the oculomotor, trochlear, abducens, and trigeminal cranial nerves. Other important structures include the sympathetic carotid plexus and the intracavernous carotid artery.

Etiology

The causes of cavernous sinus syndrome are varied. They include trauma; carotid-cavernous fistula; dural-cavernous fistula; pituitary adenoma or other neoplasm, either primary or metastatic, such as lymphoma or leukemia; inflammation from bacterial cause, such as sinusitis, viral, such as herpes zoster, fungal, such as mucormycosis, or idiopathic, such as Tolosa-Hunt syndrome.

The Patient

Symptoms and signs are those of multiple cranial-nerve palsies with pain and possible pupil involvement.

Clinical Symptoms

The patient may complain of double vision, pain that may be referred to the orbit or supraorbital region, photophobia, anisocoria, and eyelid drooping.

Clinical Signs

Prominent Signs

- Painful ophthalmoplegia
- Dilated pupil
- Horner's syndrome
- Exophthalmos
- Conjunctival chemosis
- Dilated episcleral and conjunctival blood vessels
- Ocular and cranial bruit

Subtle Signs

- Fever
- Nausea and vomiting
- Abnormal pulsations of the globe
- Nasal discharge of blood

Demographics

Septic thrombosis of the cavernous sinus is a potentially lethal disorder that often spreads from an infection of the face, mouth, throat, sinus, or orbit. Staphylococcal and streptococcal organisms are the most frequent cause. Most patients will have an elevated white blood count, and up to 70% will have positive blood cultures. Cerebrospinal fluid will indicate meningitis in 35%.

Mucormycosis is more rare and is seen in diabetic patients with ketoacidosis or in those with lymphoma or leukemia. Mortality may be as high as 90%.

Low-flow dural fistulas are usually spontaneous while high-flow are frequently caused by trauma. Dural fistulas close spontaneously or after carotid angiography nearly 50% of the time. High-flow fistulas rarely close spontaneously.

The frequency of Tolosa-Hunt syndrome is around 3% of all parasellar syndromes. It can range in patients from 3-1/2 years to 75 years, and there is no sex predilection, with the disease occurring more commonly in Whites. Pain is a uniform finding.

About 2% of pituitary adenomas compress the intrinsic structures within the cavernous sinus. About 20% of nasopharyngeal tumors present as a cavernous sinus syndrome, and up to 20% of cavernous sinus syndromes are a result of malignant nasopharyngeal tumors. Up to 23% of tumors found in the cavernous sinus are metastatic.

Significant History

- Recent facial infection
- Sinusitis
- Diabetes
- Debilitated state

- Past history of cancer
- New onset facial or orbital pain

Ancillary Tests

Ocular assessment includes visual acuity, extraocular muscle testing, corneal sensitivity with cotton wisp, pupil evaluation, exophthalmometry, testing for any resistance to retropulsion, slit-lamp evaluation for arterialization of episcleral or conjunctival vessels, orbicularis muscle strength, and ocular, orbital, temple, and carotid auscultation. The patient's temperature, nasal examination, and indirect pharyngoscopy and biopsies may be indicated.

Laboratory studies: CBC with differential, plasma glucose, ESR, antinuclear antibody, rheumatoid factor, chest x-ray, and neuroimaging of the sinuses, orbits, and brain. If infection is suspected, obtain blood cultures, cultures from the presumed primary source of infection, and lumbar puncture with cerebrospinal fluid analysis. If lymphadenopathy is present, a lymph node biopsy should be obtained. Magnetic resonance angiography or arteriography should be obtained in cases of suspected arteriovenous fistula.

The Treatment

Treatment depends on the source of the cavernous sinus syndrome. Infection will require hospitalization and intravenous antibiotics. Aseptic thrombosis may require systemic anticoagulation. Mucormycosis treatment includes amphotericin B and surgical debridement of necrotic tissue with stabilization of the metabolic state.

Treatment of a fistula is indicated for visual loss, intolerable pain, annoying tinnitus, or cosmesis. For fistulas of carotid origin, balloon embolization is used, while those of dural origin require particle embolization.

Intracavernous aneurysms are treated with balloon occlusion or surgical trapping.

Tolosa-Hunt syndrome responds quickly to oral prednisone, 80 to 100 mg once a day and is then tapered slowly as the pain subsides. Sometimes tapering may take months and recurrence is not uncommon.

CAROTID ARTERY DISSECTION
Bruce G. Muchnick

ICD—9: 443.21

THE DISEASE

Pathophysiology

Dissection represents a separation of the component layers of the carotid arterial wall because of the entrance and accumulation of intraluminal blood. Blood enters the vessel wall as a result of a breach in the endothelial layer. The resulting aneurysm may compromise the luminal diameter or cause an external diameter expansion. In either case, a second, false lumen is created of varying length. This second lumen may be stable, resolve, or occlude the true lumen, or burst through the entire wall and cause a severe hemorrhage.

Etiology

Dissecting carotid aneurysms may occur as a result of blunt trauma or penetrating injury of the head or neck. This includes head or neck surgery. Dissection of the carotid (CAD) may also arise spontaneously. Artery dissections are more common in individuals with predisposing systemic conditions such as connective tissue disease, Marfan's syndrome, syphilis, atherosclerosis, migraine, temporal arteritis, and systemic hypertension.

The Patient

Clinical Symptoms

Symptoms of dissection of carotid artery aneurysms are dependent on several factors, including the cause of the dissection, the site of the lesion, how the blood flow is affected, and whether aneurysmal rupture has occurred.

Minimally, and most commonly, there is headache and facial or neck pain. If progressive thrombosis (occlusion) occurs, or distal embolization, then more complicated symptoms may occur because of cerebral or retinal infarcts. Neurological symptoms may include hemiparesis, aphasia, tinnitus, subjective bruit, transient ischemic attacks (TIA), monocular blindness, and diplopia.

Clinical Signs

The clinical signs of carotid artery dissection typically include neurological and visual deficits. These include the neurological signs of a stroke (including hemiparesis, tongue deviation, and declining consciousness), ocular or visual signs (including visual loss, scintillating scotoma, and Horner's syndrome), and death.

Demographics

The incidence of artery dissection is unknown. In patients with completed stroke, the incidence of any artery dissection is 2.5%. In young individuals under 30 years of age with ischemic strokes, dissection is the cause in 22% of cases. About 1 in 3 patients with a dissecting artery have more than one involved vessel. The incidence of dissecting aneurysms is higher in men, most likely because of a higher rate of head or neck injury.

The peak age for a spontaneous carotid dissection is about 50 years of age. Atherosclerosis associated dissections average about age 59.

Half of patients with spontaneous carotid dissections have systemic hypertension. Ninety percent of patients with spontaneous carotid dissection present with a headache. Only 10% of patients with carotid dissection have eye, facial, or ear pain without headache.

Most patients who survive a spontaneous CAD do quite well, though about half report some residual neurological deficit. Traumatic CAD has a worse prognosis, often because of associated intracranial injury.

Significant History

- Any sudden headache?
- History of any head or neck trauma (no matter how trivial)?
- History of any head or neck surgery?
- History of TIAs?
- History of neurological deficits?
- Any sports-related head or neck injury?
- Any history of systemic conditions that may contribute to the formation of CAD?

Ancillary Tests

Neuroimaging is used to confirm the presence of CAD in suspected patients. These include:

- MR angiography
- Spinal CT angiography
- Conventional angiography
- Ultrasound (continuous wave Doppler ultrasound)
- Color Doppler flow imaging ultrasound
- Standard duplex ultrasound scanning

The Treatment

To treat the progressive thrombosis or distal embolization associated with CAD, medical treatment is directed at preventing further blood clotting. Immediate anticoagulation therapy is recommended in all patients with spontaneous dissection of the cervical portion of the internal carotid artery.

Standard anticoagulation, utilizing at first Heparin and later oral Coumadin, can reduce the risk of embolization, but may cause sudden, acute intracranial hemorrhaging. Rupture of a dissecting aneurysm remains a rare outcome of anticoagulation therapy.

The surgical approach to dissecting aneurysms depends on the location and extent of the lesion. Such surgical approaches manipulate the artery by either ligation, wrapping, resecting, reconstruction, or bypassing of the involved area.

TENSION-TYPE HEADACHE

Leonid Skorin Jr. and Lawrence D. Robbins

ICD—9: 307.81

THE DISEASE

Pathophysiology

The pain involved in tension-type headaches is best explained by the myofacial-central-vascular model. Input from the supraspinal control areas for muscle contraction is mediated by the central nervous system, specifically cortical, subcortical, and limbic mechanisms that cause the muscle to spasm. With prolonged periods of time of muscle contraction, tissue hypoxia results from small blood vessel compression. With tissue ischemia, there results the release of bradykinin, lactic acid, serotonin, and prostaglandins. This further results in muscle contraction and pain.

Etiology

Tension-type headache is thought to be partly caused by voluntary contraction of musculature, at times precipitated by stress and poor sleep that leads to inflammation and pain. Tension-type headache is a physical medical condition involving brain chemistry, as well as involving the cervical spine, the craniocervical junction, and the temporomandibular joint. Certain individuals do have a definite predisposition to these headaches. Approximately 50% of headache patients have an anxiety disorder, and 20% have either recurrent major depression or dysthymia. Bipolar illness is seen in 4 to 6% of headache patients.

Most patients with chronic tension-type headache have what is termed *transformed migraine*. They have a history of episodic migraine initially that has progressed to a chronic daily headache (CDH) over the years. CDH is seen in about 4% of the population and is defined as at least 15 headache days per month for at least 6 months. In 80% of cases, this process is associated with medication overuse and the development of rebound headaches. Episodic tension headaches are recurrent episodes of tension headache lasting minutes to days, but fewer than 15 per month or 180 days per year.

The Patient

Tension-type headaches are bilateral headaches with a pressing or tightening quality with usually no ocular symptoms or signs.

Clinical Symptoms

The patient with tension-type headache will complain of a constant aching, pressure, or tightness that is felt in a band around the head (i.e., the "hatband" area) and down the back of the neck. Occasionally, the patient may complain of soreness, cramping, or a feeling like a vise around the head or a weight on the head. Pain is usually bilateral but is sometimes worse on one side. The patient may also complain of dizziness, nausea, photophobia, or phonophobia. CDH patients awaken with their headache and go to sleep with it.

Clinical Signs
Prominent Signs
- Tender spots along cranial and neck musculature
- Sharply localized nodules in the cervical or pericranial muscles

Demographics

Tension-type headache is the most common type of headache, with a lifetime incidence of 69% in men and 88% in women. Tension headaches account for 47% of the headaches treated in a primary care practice. These headaches may begin at any age, but in 40% of patients they begin in childhood or adolescence. It is bilateral 90% of the time and strictly unilateral 10% of the time. The majority of patients with tension headache also experience periodic migraine headaches.

Significant History
- Myofascial pain syndrome
- Fibromyalgia

Ancillary Tests

A thorough headache history and complete ocular examination is necessary. Also, a complete neurologic evaluation should be performed. Muscles of the scalp and neck including the paraspinal and trapezius muscles should be palpated for tenderness. The temporomandibular area should be palpated to rule out dental occlusion problems. The temporal artery area should also be palpated to rule out temporal arteritis. With an unusual presentation or in those with new onset CDH, neuroimaging may be obtained.

The Treatment

Patients should be instructed to reduce precipitating factors and avoid stressful factors. Lifestyle changes should be reviewed. For selected patients, self-help books, relaxation exercises, or biofeedback are effective. Application of cold brings symptomatic relief in up to 70% of patients. Massage, physical therapy, and osteopathic manipulation can also be of benefit. Psychotherapy improves coping and is worthwhile even if it does not directly decrease head pain.

Symptomatic treatment consists of simple analgesics, such as acetaminophen, aspirin, or other nonsteroidals. Ibuprofen, 400 mg or 800 mg, or naproxen sodium, 275 mg to 550 mg, have been found to be very effective. Combination analgesic-sedative medications should be used cautiously because they have the potential to cause dependence. Midrin consists of a vasoconstrictor, isometheptane, combined with dichloraphenazone, a nonaddicting sedative, and 250 mg of acetaminophen. Midrin is primarily a migraine abortive agent, but it is effective for many patients with tension headache.

A realistic goal in using preventive medication is to improve the headache situation by 50 to 90%, while attempting to minimize medicine use. Prophylactic treatment includes the use of tricyclic antidepressants, such as amitriptyline hydrochloride. Doses should be started low and increased slowly every 3 to 7 days until the maintenance dose is reached. Alternative antidepressants such as the selective serotonin reuptake inhibitors (fluoxetine, sertraline) and the antiseizure medications sodium valproate or topiramate are highly beneficial in CDH.

MIGRAINE HEADACHE

Leonid Skorin Jr. and Lawrence D. Robbins

ICD—9: 346.0—Classical migraine
ICD—9: 368.12—Transient visual loss
ICD—9: 346.1—Common migraine
ICD—9: 346.2—Variants of migraine
ICD—9: 346.8—Other forms of migraine

THE DISEASE

Pathophysiology

The patient with migraine has an inherited susceptibility to headache. The expression of an altered migrainous threshold in headache-prone persons may depend on the balance between inhibitory and excitatory neurocircuits that are influenced by a complex interplay of exogenous and endogenous factors.

Migraine pain usually develops at a time when regional cerebral blood flow is reduced. In patients who have migraine with aura, there appears to be an initial decrease in volume of blood (oligemia) that originates from the occipital region and spreads anteriorly. This spreading oligemia may also relate to the spreading depression, which is a neurophysiological phenomena that represents a front of intense neural activity followed by neural silence. This spreading depression may also trigger a response of the trigeminovascular sensory fibers, resulting in neurogenic inflammation. This process consists of vascular dilation, enhanced leakage, or extravasation of plasma proteins across the endothelium with subsequent edema formation in vessel walls and a complex chain of chemical and physiologic events that excites, sensitizes, and lowers the threshold of the trigeminal nociceptive terminals. With the stimulation of these sensory fibers, substance P, bradykinin, calcitonin gene-related peptide, and serotonin are released, with serotonin being a key neurotransmitter in migraine.

Etiology

Various exogenous and endogenous triggers can help precipitate a migraine attack. Dietary factors appear to play a role in as many as 25% of migraineurs. The direct-acting vasoactive substances that can cause diet-precipitated migraine include amines (tyramine, phenylethylamine), nitrates (food coloring and preservative), monosodium glutamate (food additive), and alcohol. Indirect-acting vasoactive substances include caffeine and nicotine. Just as certain foods and other substances can trigger a headache, hunger, and its resultant hypoglycemia from missed meals, eating inadequate meals, dieting, or fasting can all cause headaches.

Prescription drugs can also induce a migraine attack. These include nitroglycerin, reserpine, nonsteroidal anti-inflammatory agents such as indomethacin, H2-receptor antagonists such as cimetidine and ranitidine, antibiotics such as griseofulvin and trimethoprim-sulfamethoxazole, and hormonal preparations such as oral contraceptives and estrogens.

Various physical and environmental factors, such as bright lights, sunshine, glare, strong odors, loud sounds, and weather or altitude changes, can all cause migraine headache. Stressful events, changes in routine, fatigue, excessive sleep, and physical activity can all trigger a migraine attack.

The Patient

Migraine is an episodic headache syndrome lasting 4 to 72 hours and is characterized by recurrent attacks that vary widely in intensity, frequency, and duration. Status migrainosis applies to migraine headaches that exceed 72 hours in length. Symptoms and signs depend on migraine type.

Migraine without Aura (Common Migraine)
Clinical Symptoms
- Unilateral, pulsing, throbbing, or pounding headache of moderate to severe intensity
- Can be aggravated by physical activity
- Accompanied by nausea and/or vomiting and photophobia or phonophobia

Clinical Signs
- Normal physical and neurologic exam
- Pallor of the face
- In women, there is often a positive relationship with menses

Migraine with Aura (Classical Migraine)
Clinical Symptoms
Approximately 20% of migraineurs experience an aura that lasts 10 to 20 minutes. The most common aura is visual and includes teichopsia, fortification spectrum, scintillating scotomas, and photopsias. Other aura include tingling (paresthesias) or numbness, motor disturbances such as monoparesis or hemiparesis, and cognitive or language disorders. Headache follows the aura. Vertigo or ataxia may occur.

Clinical Signs
- Normal physical and neurologic exam except for transient neuroparesis or hemiparesis

Migraine Aura without Headache (Acephalgic Migraine)
Clinical Symptoms
- Same as migraine with aura but no headache

Clinical Signs
- Same as migraine with aura

Complicated Migraine
Prodromal neurologic manifestations last for the entire headache attack or may even leave a permanent defect.

- Ophthalmoplegic migraine—The third cranial nerve is affected most often in children.
- Basilar migraine—Visual symptoms are similar to those of migraine with aura but affect both visual fields. Also will see vertigo, diplopia, disturbed consciousness, tinnitus, and ataxia.

- Hemiplegic migraine—Characterized by both motor and sensory symptoms occurring in a unilateral distribution.
- Retinal migraine—Fully reversible monocular scotoma or blindness lasting <60 minutes.

Demographics

Migraine is a common condition with a prevalence of 18% in females and 7% in males. Migraine without aura accounts for 80 to 85% of all vascular headaches. The peak ages are between 20 and 35 years old. Twenty-five percent to 40% of women with migraine suffer one to four or more severe, disabling attacks per month. Up to 75% of migraine patients report a first-degree relative having had migraine.

Significant History

Specific pattern of headache and the presence or absence of certain associated signs and symptoms.

Ancillary Tests

Ocular assessment includes visual acuity, extraocular muscle testing, pupil testing, intraocular pressure, fundus evaluation, and visual fields. A complete physical and neurologic examination is also necessary. Additional tests that are generally useful for diagnosis of headache are MRI of the brain, magnetic resonance angiography (MRA) to rule out intracranial aneurysms, lumbar puncture, and CT scan of the sinuses. Whether to do any additional testing at all depends upon the clinician's suspicion of organic pathology. Situations that raise the concern about organic pathology include:

1. Progressive headaches over days or weeks, increasing in intensity
2. New onset headaches, particularly in patients who never have headaches
3. New onset headaches with exertion
4. Neurologic symptoms or signs, stiff neck, papilledema, and changes in level of consciousness
5. Fever that is not explained
6. Radical increase or change in a pre-existing headache pattern

The Treatment

Nonpharmacologic treatment includes avoiding potential triggering factors, stress control, biofeedback, relaxation techniques, and cold application. Maintaining a headache calendar to better understand one's new onset headache is often helpful (Table 19.1). Symptomatic treatment includes simple analgesics such as aspirin or acetaminophen or nonsteroidal anti-inflammatory agents, such as ibuprofen or naproxen sodium, for mild to moderate headaches and combination analgesics, such as isometheptene with acetaminophen and dichloralphenazone (Midrin). Stronger symptomatic medications include corticosteroids, dihydroergotamine (available in IV, IM, and nasal spray), opioid analgesics, such as butorphanol nasal spray, or serotonin agonists such as sumatriptan. The serotonin agonists (triptans) are available in subcutaneous injection, tablet, nasal

▶ **TABLE 19.1   Headache Calendar for Patients**

At times, charting the headaches and trigger factors may help the patient and physician. The headache calendar is particularly useful in new onset headaches. The following is a sample headache calendar for patients.

Name _____

Headache Trigger Factors: (a) Stress, (b) after stress is over, (c) foods, such as chocolate or wine, (d) weather changes, (e) missing a meal, (f) (in women) menstrual or premenstrual days or hormone changes, such as with the birth control pill or during menopause, (g) bright lights or sunlight, (h) perfumes or other odors, (i) undersleeping, (j) oversleeping, (k) exercise or exertion, (l) cigarette smoke, (m) traveling, such as flying or car rides.

Overall Severity of the Headache That Day
Severity Scale

1	5	10
none	mild	moderate	severe

In the Overall Severity # column in the following chart, put one number down for how the whole day was overall.

Date	Trigger Factor #	Overall Severity #	"As Needed" Medicine & Did It Help?

Appendix C. Headache Calendar for Patients. (Adapted from Robbins LD. *Management of Headache and Headache Medications*. 2nd ed. Springer-Verlag, 2000, pp. 263–264. With permission.)

spray, and dissolving sublingual tablet form. Triptans have become the preferred first-line treatment of choice.

Prophylactic therapy is indicated when patients experience more than three headaches per month, attacks last more than 48 hours, attacks are severe, the patient is unable to cope with the attacks, treatment of an acute attack provides inadequate relief or therapy produces serious side effects, or attacks occur after prolonged aura. The patient's comorbidities (psychiatric, medical, gastrointestinal) determine which way to proceed with prophylactic therapy. β-adrenergic blocking agents, such as propranolol or atenolol, remain a good choice for prophylaxis of migraine. Other prophylactic medication include calcium channel blockers, such as verapamil, tricyclic antidepressants, such as amitriptyline and nortriptyline, and anticonvulsants, such as sodium valproate. Monoamine oxidase inhibitors, such as phenelzine, are stronger third-line considerations. Feverfew, a natural herb with its active ingredient parthenolide, can be taken as two or four tablets or capsules per day. Several vitamins and minerals have been found to be useful. These include magnesium oxide 250 mg or 500 mg once per day, riboflavin (vitamin B_2) 400 mg per day, pyridoxine (vitamin B_6) 50 mg or 100 mg per day, flaxseed oil 1,000-mg capsules one or two per day. Botulinum toxin injections are also being utilized as prophylactic headache therapy.

CLUSTER HEADACHE
Leonid Skorin Jr. and Lawrence D. Robbins

ICD—9: 346.2

THE DISEASE

Pathophysiology

There are three major clinicopathologic processes in the cluster headache syndrome: the cluster period, attack provocation, and pain production.

Cluster period occurrence appears to be related to seasonal photoperiod changes, with the greatest incidence of cluster headaches occurring in January and July, two weeks following the shortest and longest day of the year. Cluster headache patients appear to be unable to synchronize their hypothalamic suprachiasmatic nuclei, which are involved in coordinating the circadian rhythm with the photoperiods. As a consequence of these physiologic changes, chemoreceptor responses to hypoxemia may be diminished, resulting in impaired autoregulation of arterial oxygen concentration inducing a cluster attack. Distal pathways, such as the seventh cranial nerve, have been considered a potential major pain pathway. The trigeminovascular system and the release of substance P and other vasoactive substances in the sensory ganglia may also account for pain and autoimmune symptoms of cluster headaches.

Approximately 90% of all cluster headache sufferers have the episodic type. This condition is defined by periods of attack susceptibility (cluster period) followed by periods of nonattack (remissions). Cluster periods are most often found to recur cyclically, each lasting a mean of 2 months, followed by 1-year remissions. Ten percent of cluster patients have chronic clusters, where there is no break of at least 6 months between attacks. The mean frequency of cluster attacks during active periods is one to three per day for episodic cluster headache and two to four per day in the chronic type. Attacks last an average of 45 minutes, ranging from 15 minutes to 3 hours.

Etiology

Conditions that can cause hypoxemia and secondarily induce a cluster headache attack include REM sleep, periods of relaxation or exertion, high altitude, and vasodilators, such as nicotine, histamine, alcohol, nitroglycerin, and nifedipine. A substantial shift in the sleep–wake cycle may provoke a cluster period during periods of remission.

The Patient

Cluster headaches are usually stereotypical painful unilateral attacks with associated autonomic symptoms and signs.

Clinical Symptoms

The patient with cluster headaches will complain of severe, unilateral pain of sudden onset, and the pain is typically burning, stabbing, or a boring sensation in the eye, temple, forehead, jaw, or teeth with occasional radiation to the ear or neck. These attacks often occur in the evening or within 2 hours of the patient falling asleep, and the pain awakens the patient.

Cluster headache patients are rarely quiescent but are more often pacing, rocking, or moving about, and they may display odd behaviors such as violence, fugues, or trance-like states. At the end of an attack, the patient may be drained of all energy yet feel euphoric.

Clinical Signs
- Ipsilateral lacrimation
- Rhinorrhea and/or nasal stuffiness
- Conjunctival injection
- Complete or partial Horner's syndrome

Subtle Signs
- "Leonine" appearance
- Masculine body habitus
- Thick skin folds
- Coarse facial skin with telangiectasias
- Broad chin
- Well-chiseled lower lip
- Hazel eyes

Demographics

Cluster headache occurs mostly in White men with a male to female ratio of 4:1. The average age of onset is in the late 20s to 40s. The mean age of onset for women and chronic patients is older. The incidence of cluster headache is 0.4% in males and 0.08% in females. Approximately 10% of cluster patients give a positive family history for one or more relatives. Many patients "lose" their clusters in the late 40s or 50s, particularly if they have had them for many years.

Significant History

Typical cluster headache attack after exposure to alcohol, vasodilating drugs, high altitude, or strenuous exercise.

A rare unilateral headache that is related to cluster headache is SUNCT syndrome (short-lasting unilateral neuralgiform headache with conjunctival injection and tearing). Patients experience 5 to 7 attacks, lasting 5 seconds to 4 minutes in a typical hour. Twenty to 30 attacks per day are common. Pain occurs about the eye or temple and is stabbing or throbbing. The male to female ratio is 17:2. Conjunctival injection is very prominent, and other autonomic signs, such as forehead sweating, rhinorrhea, and tearing may be present.

Ancillary Tests

A thorough headache history and complete ocular examination is necessary. Also, a complete neurologic evaluation should be performed. If Horner's syndrome is also present, appropriate testing is indicated. In first episodes or unusual presentation, neuroimaging can be obtained.

The Treatment

Patients should be instructed to avoid any precipitating factors (alcohol, vasodilating drugs, etc.). Deep-breathing techniques or relaxation methods help some patients. Other techniques include application of ice or heat and pressing over the temple area.

An effective abortive treatment with a 60% success rate is oxygen inhalation, 8 liters per minute for 15 to 30 minutes utilizing a mask. The triptans, particularly sumatriptan injection (or the nasal spray), have become the treatment of choice.

Prophylactic treatment for episodic cluster: This regimen consists of oral prednisone, 20 mg per day for 3 days, then 10 mg once per day for 7 to 10 days, then stop. Prednisone can be used with calcium channel blockers. These agents can also be used alone if prednisone is of no relief. Verapamil, one 240-mg ER tablet, is taken once or twice a day. Prophylactic treatment for chronic cluster: Lithium carbonate, 300 mg two to four times a day, can be used with or without verapamil, one 240-mg ER tablet taken once or twice daily. Sodium valproate is also effective. Topiramate or indomethacin are also used prophylactically, for episodic or chronic cluster headaches.

NONPRIMARY HEADACHE
Leonid Skorin Jr.

ICD—9: 784.0

THE DISEASE
Pathophysiology

About 10% of headaches seen in emergency departments are because of secondary or morbid causes. Depending on the underlying cause, the pathophysiology will vary.

Etiology

Potentially dangerous causes of headache include subarachnoid hemorrhage, subdural or epidural hematoma, intracranial hemorrhage, stroke, dissection of carotid or vertebral artery, hypertensive encephalopathy, brain tumor, temporal arteritis, vasculitis, central nervous system infections, cavernous sinus disease, pseudotumor cerebri, and dural vein thrombosis.

The Patient

Symptoms and signs depend on the underlying cause of the headache.

Clinical Symptoms

- Subarachnoid hemorrhage (ICD—9: 430)—Sudden, severe, bilateral "thunderclap" headache with nausea, neck pain, or rigidity and loss of consciousness.
- Subdural or epidural hemorrhage (ICD—9: 432.1)—History of trauma with persistent headache, drowsiness, confusion, loss of consciousness.
- Intracranial hemorrhage (ICD—9: 431 or 432.9)—Unilateral, focal headache of mild to moderate severity. Headache occurs in up to 65% of patients.
- Stroke (ICD—9: 436)—Ischemic disease in the carotid circulation causes a frontal headache, usually in the eye or temple or the ipsilateral side 30% of the time, and disease in the vertebrobasilar system causes a posterior headache 59% of the time.
- Dissection of the carotid artery (ICD—9: 443.21) or vertebral artery (ICD—9: 443.24)—Carotid artery dissection causes sudden, nonthrobbing pain around the eye, frontal or temporal regions, angle of the mandible, or upper neck. Vertebral artery dissection manifestations can range from occipital or neck pain to coma.
- Hypertensive encephalopathy (ICD—9: 437.2)—Symptoms include headache, nausea, vomiting, visual disturbance, seizures, confusion, and coma.
- Brain tumor (ICD—9: 191.9)—Headache occurs in up to 60% of patients with brain tumor. It may be mild or severe, throbbing or steady, localized or generalized. It is worse in the morning and exacerbated by stooping, coughing, physical activity, or moving the head suddenly.
- Temporal arteritis (ICD—9: 446.5)—Headache accompanied by scalp tenderness, myalgias, malaise, jaw claudication, vision loss (which may be bilateral), and weight loss.
- Vasculitis (ICD—9: 710.0)—Headache with changes in mental state and coma.
- Central nervous system infections (ICD—9: 322.9)—A patient with meningitis will present with fever and headache and findings of stiffness when moving the neck anteriorly and posteriorly (meningismus).
- Cavernous sinus disease (ICD—9: 437.6 or 325)—Retro-orbital headache, diplopia, eyelid droop, facial pain, or numbness.
- Pseudotumor cerebri (ICD—9: 348.2)—Vascular-like headache of a chronic nature exacerbated by eye movements or Valsalva maneuver. Less frequent symptoms include transient blurred vision, diplopia, tinnitus, dizziness, or facial numbness.
- Dural vein thrombosis (ICD—9: 325)—Headache accompanying seizures and coma.

Clinical Signs

- Subarachnoid hemorrhage—Up to 78% of patients will present with nuchal rigidity. Ocular findings may include papilledema and retinal, preretinal, or even subconjunctival hemorrhages. Hypertension may also be present.
- Subdural and epidural hematomas—Focal neurologic signs are often absent. Occasionally, anisocoria may be seen.
- Intracranial hemorrhage—Signs of increased intracranial pressure or other neurologic signs.
- Stroke—Paralysis or paresis with occasional sensory deficits.
- Dissection of the carotid artery—Neurologic deficit contralateral to head or neck pain. About half the patients will have Horner's syndrome. A cranial or cervical bruit may be present.
- Hypertensive encephalopathy—Focal neurologic deficits, papilledema, retinal cotton wool spots, retinal hemorrhages in the presence of marked elevated blood pressure.
- Brain tumor—Papilledema and ataxia or hemiparesis may be present in long-standing cases.
- Temporal arteritis—Painful or pulseless temporal arteries with ischemic optic neuropathy, central retinal artery occlusion, or diplopia.
- Vasculitis—Hemiparesis, iritis or vitritis, accompanying polyarteritis nodosa, hypersensitivity vasculitis, Wegener's granulomatosis, or Behçet's disease.
- Central nervous system infection—Meningismus and fever.
- Cavernous sinus disease—Painful ophthalmoplegia, proptosis, and chemosis.
- Pseudotumor cerebri—Papilledema with occasional sixth-nerve palsy in young, obese female.
- Dural vein thrombosis—Papilledema with hemiplegia, paralysis of a leg, or convulsions and coma.

Demographics

Subarachnoid hemorrhage usually occurs in individuals over 30 years of age, with one-third occurring during strenuous activity, one-third during sleep, and one-third during random activity. If untreated, 50% of patients who survive the first 24 hours die within 2 weeks. The annual incidence of subarachnoid hemorrhage is 28/100,000.

Subdural and epidural hematomas usually result from trauma and account for 1 to 3% of major head injuries. The male to female ratio is as high as 4 to 1.

Stroke is the most frequent life-threatening disease of the nervous system and ranks third as a leading cause of death in the United States. The frequency of headaches in stroke can be as high as 38% and is seen more frequently in women and declines with increasing age. From 0.4 to 25% of all strokes are secondary to arterial dissection, with the highest incidence among young adults and middle-aged persons.

Hypertensive encephalopathy occurs both in chronically hypertensive patients with an abrupt rise in an already increased blood pressure and in previously normotensive patients, such as young women with toxemia of pregnancy.

The incidence of both primary and metastatic brain tumors is 8/100,000 each. Approximately 50% of the primary tumors are gliomas. The incidence of temporal arteritis can range from 3 to 174 per 100,000 in persons aged 50 years or older. Headache occurs in 70 to 90% of patients. Other vasculitidies have differing incidence and headache occurrence.

Bacterial meningitis can occur at any age and throughout the year. Viral meningitis occurs before age 40 and has the lowest incidence from January to June. The incidence of pseudotumor cerebri is 0.9/100,000 in the general population but 19/100,000 in obese young women. The incidence of dural vein thrombosis is increased in women between 20 and 35 years of age, possibly owing to the hypercoagulable states occurring with pregnancy and oral contraceptive use.

Significant History

Symptoms suggestive of secondary cause of headache include acute onset; progressive worsening of a subacute headache; headache accompanied by fever, nausea, and vomiting; and headache accompanied by new neurologic symptoms.

Ancillary Tests

- Subarachnoid hemorrhage—Unenhanced CT scans detect acute hemorrhage in about 90% of cases; however, sensitivity drops to 74% after 3 days. Most cases not detected on CT scan are found on lumbar puncture by red blood cells that do not clear in three samples of cerebrospinal fluid.
- Subdural and epidural hematomas—Both types of acute hematomas are hyperintense when diagnosed by CT scan.
- Intracranial hemorrhage and stroke—Both are identified on neuroimaging.
- Dissection of the carotid artery—The diagnostic "gold standard" is arteriography. Also consider magnetic resonance angiography.
- Hypertensive encephalopathy—Measure blood pressure, and evaluate urine for proteinuria. Neuroimaging may identify intracranial hemorrhage.
- Brain tumor—Contrast-enhanced neuroimaging.
- Temporal arteritis—Elevated ESR and C-reactive protein with a positive temporal artery biopsy.
- Vasculitis—Various serologic tests depending on suspected etiology.
- Meningitis—Neuroimaging followed by lumbar puncture to evaluate cerebrospinal fluid. CBC will have elevated white count.
- Cavernous sinus disease—Contrast-enhanced neuroimaging with magnetic resonance imaging being the diagnostic test of choice. Ophthalmic examination with attention to pupils, extraocular motility, Hertel exophthalmometry, and resistance to retropulsion.
- Pseudotumor cerebri—Normal neuroimaging with elevated cerebrospinal fluid level on lumbar puncture.
- Dural vein thrombosis—Magnetic resonance angiography with evaluation for inflammation or hypercoagulable states.

The Treatment

- Subarachnoid hemorrhage—Treatment options include bed rest, surgery to clip the aneurysm, management of hypertension, nimodipine therapy, and volume expansion.

- Subdural and epidural hematomas—Evacuation of blood and relieve intracranial pressure.
- Intracranial hemorrhage—Control hypertension and neurosurgical consultation.
- Stroke—Depending on time, antifibrinolytic agents may be initiated with a neurologic consultation.
- Dissection of the carotid artery—Use platelet antiaggregates or anticoagulation agents with surgical repair.
- Hypertensive encephalopathy—Blood pressure reduction and diuresis.
- Brain tumor—Neurosurgical consultation with corticosteroid therapy or diuresis to lower intracranial pressure.
- Temporal arteritis—Intravenous or high-dose oral corticosteroids.
- Vasculitis—Immunosuppression with corticosteroids or other immunosuppressive agents.
- Meningitis—Empirical therapy (antibiotics) can be initiated before return of culture results.
- Cavernous sinus disease—Treatment is specific to the underlying cause.
- Pseudotumor cerebri—Weight loss, acetazolamide, or furosemide to lower cerebrospinal fluid production, lumboperitoneal shunting, or optic nerve sheath decompression.
- Dural vein thrombosis—Anticoagulation with heparin sodium followed by warfarin sodium for 3 to 6 months.

MYASTHENIA GRAVIS (MG)
Leonid Skorin Jr. and Bruce Muchnick

ICD—9: 358.0

THE DISEASE
Pathophysiology

Myasthenia gravis is a disorder of neuromuscular transmission. A number of antibodies interact with the acetylcholine receptors located on the postsynaptic folds of the neuromuscular junction. The antibodies block the binding sites and accelerate receptor degradation, resulting in primary damage to the receptors themselves. In addition, there is widening of the synaptic cleft, allowing more time for acetylcholine esterase molecules to degrade the acetylcholine as it passively diffuses across the cleft.

Etiology

MG is an acquired autoimmune disease of the postsynaptic membrane. Circulating antibodies to acetylcholine receptors are detectable in the serum of around 90% of individuals with generalized myasthenia and from 50 to 70% of those with only ocular symptoms.

There are several illnesses associated with myasthenia, and all may play an enhancing effect. Encapsulated thymomas occur in 10% of myasthenics, almost all of them after age 30. Sixty-five percent of myasthenics will have thymic hyperplasia and 25% a normal or involuted thymus.

Elevated rheumatoid factors are found in 5% of myasthenics. Antinuclear antibody is elevated in 37%, and antithyroglobulin antibodies are elevated in 35% of myasthenics.

The Patient

Symptoms and signs may be isolated to ocular findings or more generalized fluctuating weakness and easy fatigability of certain skeletal muscles.

Clinical Symptoms

More than half of patients initially present with ocular symptoms that are exacerbated by use of muscles and improved by rest. These include diplopia, blurry vision, and eyelid drooping. In 14% of all patients with MG, the disease remains localized to the extraocular and orbicularis oculi muscles for the entire course of the disease. If the facial muscles are involved, the patient will have difficulty chewing or an abnormal smile or nasal speech. Dysphagia is caused by weakness of the tongue and palatal muscles. Difficulty in breathing results from weakness of the respiratory muscles. Limb weakness results in difficulty with gripping, brushing hair, dressing, or walking.

Clinical Signs

Prominent Signs
- Ptosis—Unilateral or bilateral and often asymmetric
- Simpson test—Extended upward gaze results in gradual lowering of eyelids
- Enhanced ptosis—Elevating the ptotic eyelid causes the opposite eyelid to close
- Ophthalmoparesis with the medial rectus, inferior rectus, and superior oblique most often involved

Subtle Signs
- Cogan lid-twitch sign
- Lid retraction from frontalis muscle strain
- Eyebrow thickening
- Peek sign from orbicularis oculi fatigue
- Reduced accommodation
- Mild pupil dilation or sluggish response to light
- Abnormal saccades
- Nystagmus

Demographics

MG is one of several disorders of the neuromuscular junction whose prevalence has been on the rise and is currently estimated to be 1 case in 10,000 to 20,000 people. Distribution is bimodal, affecting more women in their 20s and 30s and men in their 50s and 60s. The mean age of onset of ocular myasthenia is 38, and men are more often affected than women. No significant ethnic variability or strong genetic component has been noted.

Significant History

- Exacerbation of symptoms and signs by temperature extremes, infection, stress, malnutrition, pain, and certain drugs, such as aminoglycoside antibiotics, tetracyclines, and class I antiarrhythmics
- Thymoma
- Thyroid disease
- Rheumatoid arthritis
- Systemic lupus erythematosis

Ancillary Tests

Ocular assessment includes visual acuity, extraocular muscle testing, pupil testing, testing for accommodation, Simpson test, orbicularis function, and ice-pack test or sleep test.

An ice pack is applied to the affected eye for 2 minutes, and the eyelid is observed to see whether ptosis improves.

The patient sleeps or rests with his or her eyes closed for 30 minutes. Should have resolution of ptosis or ophthalmoparesis, with reappearance of either sign, 30 seconds to 5 minutes after opening his or her eyes.

The Tensilon (now available as Enlon) test employs edrophonium, an acetylcholinesterase inhibitor. The time of onset of edrophonium is 30 seconds, and the duration is 5 minutes.

A mixture of 10 mg per 1 cc is used. A test dose of 0.2 mL or 2 mg is given intravenously, and after 60 seconds, another 0.4 mL or 4 mg is again administered. If there is no definite clinical improvement then the remaining 0.4 mL or 4 mg is administered until a total of 1.0 mL or 10 mg has been given. A negative test does not exclude MG, and occasionally there is paradoxical worsening or false-positives. Because hypotension, bradycardia, or cardiac arrest can be seen with the use of edrophonium, appropriate life-support equipment should be available, including intravenous atropine 0.5 mg.

The neostigmine test is similar to the edrophonium test. Onset of action is 30 minutes after neostigmine, 1.5 mg, is given intramuscularly, 20 minutes after giving 0.6 mg of atropine. This test is particularly useful in testing children who tend to cry during the intravenous edrophonium test.

Laboratory studies: Acetylcholine receptor antibodies, antistriated muscle antibodies, thyroid function tests (T3, T4, TSH), antinuclear antibody, rheumatoid factor. Neurologic testing includes repetitive nerve stimulation, single-fiber electromyogram, and swallow function testing. A CT scan of the chest should be performed to identify any underlying thymoma.

The Treatment

- Occlusion of involved eye or Fresnel prisms.
- Treatment could be coordinated with a neurologist. The most commonly used anti-acetylcholinesterase medication is pyridostigmine bromide, 60 mg two or three times a day, and the dose is advanced until 120 mg every 3 hours or significant side effects occur.

- Other acetylcholinesterase inhibitors include neostigmine and ambenonium.
- Thymectomy is indicated in patients with generalized MG and who are between the ages of puberty and 60.
- Other immunosuppressives such as corticosteroids, azathioprine, cyclophosphamide, and cyclosporine can be tried. Corticosteroids, especially prednisone, is now standard drug therapy for MG refractory to antiacetylcholinesterase medications.

Plasmapheresis or plasma exchange is an effective short-term option for patients who have had a sudden exacerbation of their disease. This should be accompanied by hospitalization and ventilatory support. Another short-term option is intravenous immunoglobulin. It appears to have an equal efficacy to that of plasmapheresis.

BLEPHAROSPASM AND HEMIFACIAL SPASM
Leonid Skorin Jr.

ICD—9: 333.81—Blepharospasm
ICD—9: 351.8—Other facial nerve disorders

THE DISEASE
Pathophysiology

Both benign essential blepharospasm (BEB) and hemifacial spasm are dystonias dominated by involuntary sustained (tonic) or spasmodic (rapid or clonic), patterned, repetitive muscle contractions. The orbicularis oculi, procerus, and corrugator muscles are involved in BEB, and the facial muscles of expression are affected by hemifacial spasm.

Etiology

The exact etiology of BEB is unknown, but it is currently regarded as a dysfunction in the blinking reflex control center. Hemifacial spasm results from microvascular compression or irritation of the facial nerve by an aberrant artery, abnormal vasculature in the posterior fossa, or a cerebellopontine tumor.

The Patient

Symptoms and signs may initially be those of increased blinking that can lead to functional blindness from involuntary spasms of eyelid closure.

Clinical Symptoms

Patients with BEB initially complain of increased blinking lasting from seconds to minutes, ocular irritation, and photophobia that may affect only one side but eventually becomes bilateral.

Patients with hemifacial spasm will complain of similar symptoms, which are unilateral and extend to involve the facial muscles of expression and neck.

Clinical Signs

- BEB—Bilateral involuntary spasms of the orbicularis oculi, procerus, and corrugator musculature. Relieved by sleep.
- Meige's syndrome—Idiopathic orofacial dystonia with intermittent midfacial and lower facial movements accompanying BEB. Patients exhibit lip pursing, tongue protrusion, trismus (lockjaw), and speech difficulty.
- Breughel's syndrome—Oromandibular dystonia when the mandible is also involved. Contraction of the jaw and a widely open mouth with BEB.
- Segmental cranial dystonia—Includes involvement of muscles innervated by other cranial nerves with BEB.
- Apraxia of lid opening—Difficulty in initiating opening of eyelids in the absence of spasm. Seven percent of patients with BEB have apraxia of lid opening.
- Hemifacial spasm—Unilateral, involuntary, episodic bursts of tonic or clonic activity in the muscles of facial expression lasting from seconds to minutes. Not relieved by sleep.

Demographics

Prevalence of BEB is estimated at 133 per million. BEB usually begins in individuals aged 50 to 70 with a mean age of onset of 56 years. Almost two-thirds are female. Hemifacial spasm also occurs in middle-aged individuals and is more common in women. BEB and hemifacial spasm may occasionally be familial.

Significant History

- Dry eye syndrome
- Blepharitis
- Family history of tremor
- Prior head or facial trauma

Ancillary Tests

Ocular assessment includes visual acuity, biomicroscopy to identify any trichiasis, ectropion, entropion, uveitis, dry eye or blepharitis, tonometry to rule out glaucoma, and neuroophthalmic evaluation. Magnetic resonance imaging should be done in hemifacial spasm cases.

The Treatment

Patients often use various maneuvers such as singing, coughing, yawning, humming, doing mathematical calculations in their head, or applying pressure or tapping their temples to alleviate the spasms. Any underlying ocular (dry eye, blepharitis) or eyelid disorder (entropion, trichiasis) must be treated since it can aggravate the spasming. Conservative treatment includes sunglasses to relieve photophobia and ptosis crutches. Various medications have been tried for BEB with occasional success. These include clonazepam, carbidopa with levodopa, trihexypenidyl, carbamazepine, baclofen, haloperidol, and lithium.

The most effective nonsurgical treatment for BEB and hemifacial spasm is botulinum toxin injections. Botulinum toxin inhibits presynaptic release of acetylcholine at the neuromuscular junction, leading to muscle paralysis. Muscle paralysis is not permanent, and repeat injections are required every 3 to 6 months. Treatment with botulinum toxin results in 70% improvement in symptoms with a 90% patient acceptance rate. Doxorubicin can be used for injection chemomyectomy but with less predictable results and permanent muscle loss. Surgical treatment for BEB includes selective facial myectomy and for hemifacial spasm the Jannetta procedure, which involves microvascular decompression of the facial nerve.

TRIGEMINAL NEURALGIA
Bruce G. Muchnick

ICD—9: 350.1

THE DISEASE
Pathophysiology

Patients with trigeminal neuralgia, or Tic Douloreux, experience daily episodes of brief, sharp pain along the distribution of the trigeminal nerve. The pain usually lasts for only seconds and is most commonly distributed along the second and third divisions of the trigeminal nerve.

The painful episode may be triggered by speaking, chewing, touching the affected area, or shaving.

Etiology

Though the cause remains largely unknown, an irritation of the trigeminal nerve is believed to be a result, in some cases, of a compression by surrounding blood vessels, mass lesions, demyelination, and dental disease. These structural etiologies often have an area of associated numbness along the trigeminal distribution. Idiopathic causes tend not to have associated numbness.

The Patient

Clinical Symptoms
The pain is often described as a sharp, cutting, or tearing pain along one or more of the divisions of the trigeminal nerve. Though brief, the attacks of stabbing pain can be excruciating. Most commonly, the mandibular and maxillary divisions are involved. The pain is often described as episodes of unilateral electric shock-like facial pains separated by significant pain-free intervals.

Clinical Signs
Objective signs of sensory loss cannot be demonstrated. The diagnosis is usually based on history and clinical examination. Paroxysms of pain to the eye are very rare.

Demographics

It is the most frequent of all of the cranial neuralgias. The incidence of Tic Douleroux is believed to be one per one million persons per year. It occurs most commonly in middle-aged to elderly individuals.

Significant History
- History of episodes of stabbing, hemispheric facial pain lasting seconds.
- Age of patient significant.
- Any demyelinating-type symptoms?
- Any recent dental pain or dental work?

Ancillary Tests

Neuroimaging can rule out posterior fossa mass lesions, vascular compression at the base of the brain, and demyelinating disease.

Three-dimensional (3D) Constructive Interference in Steady-State (CISS) Magnetic Resonance (MR) imaging is useful in the detection of neurovascular compression compared with MR angiography.

The Treatment

Though trigeminal neuralgia may spontaneously remit, a plethora of traditional and alternative medical, as well as surgical, treatments may allow for pain reduction.

Pharmacotherapy includes the use of carbamazepine, still the first-line treatment, as well as gabapentin, phenytoin, baclofen, and tricyclic antidepressants. Alternatively, acupuncture therapy may help in those whose pain does not remit.

In cases that do not respond to medical treatment, percutaneous methods of trigeminal nerve root or ganglion destruction include glycerol injection, radiofrequency thermocoagulation, and balloon occlusion.

Immediate pain relief is obtained in 80 to 90% of cases surgically treated with microvascular decompression of the trigeminal nerve, and 70% of patients remain pain-free 10 years later. Gamma-knife radiosurgery is also showing excellent short-term results. In addition, dedicated linear accelerator radiosurgery is a precise and effective treatment for trigeminal neuralgia.

TRAUMATIC OPTIC NEUROPATHY
Alan G. Kabat and Leonid Skorin Jr.

ICD—9: 950.0

THE DISEASE
Pathophysiology

Optic nerve injury is a possible, though uncommon, sequelae of head or facial trauma. In the United States, traumatic optic neuropathy occurs in 0.5 to 5% of patients with closed head trauma and in approximately 2.5% of patients with midfacial fracture.

The exact pathophysiology is not thoroughly understood and is likely multifactorial. Several forms of optic nerve injury are known to occur, including optic nerve avulsion, neurotmesis (tearing of the optic nerve), optic nerve sheath hematoma, and optic nerve compression secondary to bony fracture of the orbital apex. Most commonly, however, concussive shock waves are implicated; transmission of these forces to the orbital bones and meninges results in contusion of the intracanalicular optic nerve. Subsequently, the nerve axons and microvasculature are compromised by ischemia and reactive edema, as well as generalized compressive forces. Occasionally, the neuropathy may develop some time after the initial trauma, a consequence of scarring within the optic canal that leads to secondary nerve compression.

Etiology

Traumatic optic neuropathy should be suspected in patients with vision loss who have sustained closed head or maxillofacial trauma. Trauma to the prechiasmal optic nerve may be classified as either posterior indirect, direct, or anterior indirect. *Posterior indirect* injuries are most common and typically result from frontal or midfacial blows as might occur in bicycle, motorcycle, or automobile accidents. *Direct* trauma occurs when an object or objects penetrates into the orbit and directly injures the optic nerve. Finally, *anterior indirect* describes an injury of the intraocular portion of the optic nerve, resulting from sudden rotation or anterior displacement of the eye by a finger or similar object.

The Patient

The typical patient will experience sudden loss of vision immediately or soon after trauma. Occasionally, the vision loss may be insidious, and in some cases, the patient may be unaware of any visual deficit until it is detected by routine examination. Ophthalmoscopy may not demonstrate significant evidence of injury at the time of the initial examination, particularly in cases of posterior indirect injury.

Clinical Symptoms
- Sudden, severe vision loss immediately or soon after blunt injury to the head

Clinical Signs
Prominent Signs
- Vision loss without external or ophthalmoscopic evidence of injury (with posterior indirect injury)
- Afferent pupillary defect
- Orbital compartment syndrome, if retrobulbar hemorrhage present in direct injury
- Vitreous hemorrhage, optic disc edema, venous congestion, central retinal artery occlusion, retinal edema (in anterior indirect injury)

Subtle Signs
- Color vision abnormality in affected eye
- Paracentral, arcuate, or altitudinal visual field defects
- Initial variable level of vision followed by deterioration

Demographics

Traumatic optic neuropathy most often affects males in their second decade. Various blunt and penetrating injuries have been shown to cause optic nerve injury. The most common causes are bicycle, motor vehicle, and sporting accidents and physical assaults.

Significant History

- Blunt injury to head or orbit
- Loss of consciousness
- Midfacial fractures
- Penetrating injury with entrance wound

Ancillary Tests

Ocular assessment includes visual acuity, extraocular motility testing, pupil testing, color vision, fundus examination, and visual field testing.

A complete neurologic assessment is indicated, especially if there was loss of consciousness. High resolution CT imaging of the orbital apex, optic canal, and cavernous sinus is essential; computed tomography is preferable to MRI when evaluating for bony fractures.

The Treatment

The appropriate treatment of traumatic optic neuropathy is the subject of significant debate. There are presently three options: (a) careful observation only; (b) systemic corticosteroid therapy; or (c) optic nerve decompression surgery.

While a significant number (15 to 33%) of patients with posterior indirect traumatic optic neuropathy experience spontaneous improvement of vision, there is great variability in outcome. Negative prognostic factors include blood in the posterior ethmoid cells, loss of consciousness, older age (i.e. >40), and no light perception vision at the initial presentation. During the 1980s and 1990s, it was considered standard practice to initiate megadose systemic corticosteroids therapy on virtually all patients with traumatic optic neuropathy within 8 hours of injury. This treatment modality was based upon findings from the Second National Acute Spinal Cord Injury Study. Those patients not responding to systemic corticosteroids therapy after several days or those with poorer visual acuity (i.e., count fingers or worse) at initial presentation were considered candidates for optic canal decompression surgery.

More recent studies, including the International Optic Nerve Trauma Study, have concluded that medical and/or surgical intervention might be of questionable value in some cases. These studies suggest that in patients without poor prognostic indicators, simply monitoring may be sufficient management. Furthermore, research has not conclusively shown any significant difference in final visual acuity related to dose (low vs. high vs. mega) or timing of corticosteroid therapy, nor is there a significantly different outcome between patients treated with steroids or surgical decompression of the optic canal. Patients with traumatic optic neuropathy should, therefore, be addressed and managed via one or more of the earlier-outlined options on an individual basis, following proper assessment and consultation.

In those cases that involve penetrating orbital injury or fracture of the sinus walls, systemic antibiotic therapy is mandatory to prevent secondary cellulitis.

OPTIC PITS
Joseph W. Sowka

ICD—9: 377.2

THE DISEASE
Pathophysiology

Optic pits are small, typically less than one-third disc diameter, excavations of the optic disc. They are considered atypical colobomas in that they can appear anywhere on the disc, whereas typical colobomas only appear inferiorly on the disc. Most often, they appear in the inferior to inferior-temporal part of the optic disc, though up to one-third will appear centrally on the disc. In approximately 85% of cases, pits occur unilaterally. While field and acuity loss may be present, the majority of patients are unaware of the presence of an optic pit.

Etiology

Optic pits are thought to occur from faulty closure of the embryonic fetal fissure during gestation. It has also been suggested that they occur from abnormal differentiation of primitive epithelia papilla. Arcuate visual field defects are the result of corresponding loss of retinal ganglion cells or secondary atrophy of attenuated nerve fibers. Depending upon the depth of the pit, paracentral visual field defects occur as well.

A significant number of patients with optic pits develop nonrhegmatogenous serous detachments of the macula. Patients with temporally located pits are more prone to this complication with resultant metamorphopsia and vision loss. The origin of the serous fluid is not well explained. The serous fluid may represent liquefied vitreous penetration and leaking vessels within the pit. New findings strongly suggest that serous macular detachments secondary to optic pits develop because of pre-existing schisis-like lesions, which connect the macula to the optic disc. Tangential traction by the vitreous may play a role in development of macular detachments.

The Patient

Patients with optic pits are typically asymptomatic unless there has been an associated serous macular detachment. However, the majority will manifest visual field defects with threshold testing. There is no racial or gender predilection. In that this is a congenital malformation of the disc, it is present at birth though often is not discovered until later in life.

Clinical Symptoms
- Often asymptomatic
- Visual field defects in arcuate bundles

- Paracentral scotomas
- Visual acuity reduction with macular detachment

Clinical Signs
- Discrete, round excavation of the optic disc
- Possible epiretinal membrane
- Possible serous elevation of the macula
- Possible macular hole
- Possible vision loss with maculopathy

Demographics

Patients with optic pits are often younger, as the pit is typically discovered at the patient's first dilated eye examination.

Significant History

Occasionally, patients with optic pits are mistakenly treated for normal tension glaucoma, as an optic pit may be confused with a focal rim defect that occurs in glaucoma. In that the field defect is in the arcuate bundle zone, a misdiagnosis of glaucoma is common.

Ancillary Tests
- There are no specific laboratory tests for patients with optic pits
- Visual fields should be done to assess any damage already present
- Amsler grid monitoring is advocated to identify early macular involvement

The Treatment

There is no direct treatment for optic pits. Concurrent maculopathy is all that needs to be addressed. Periodic monitoring, prophylactic laser photocoagulation, therapeutic laser photocoagulation after maculopathy has formed, oral steroids, and vitrectomy have all been tried. Macular detachments have recently been treated with vitrectomy and gas bubble tamponade. Vitrectomy with peeling of any epiretinal membrane as well as the internal limiting membrane is advocated in cases of optic pit–induced maculopathy.

LEBER'S HEREDITARY OPTIC NEUROPATHY (LHON)
Jerome Sherman

ICD—9: 377.16

THE DISEASE

Leber's hereditary optic neuropathy is a rare optic nerve disorder that results in profound bilateral loss of visual acuity, reduced color vision, and central-cecal visual field defects. Although the exclusive maternal inheritance pattern was noted nearly 150 years ago by Theodore Leber, specifics of the mode of transmission and pathophysiology of this intriguing disorder have only been identified within the past 15 years. Although LHON has always been classified as an acute onset disorder, careful follow-up studies of a large Brazilian pedigree have recently revealed that LHON is a chronic disease prior to and following the rapid stage of vision loss.

Pathophysiology

LHON is the paradigm of mitochondrial optic neuropathies. Mitochondria are increasingly recognized as central players in the life and death of cells and especially of neurons. The marked energy dependence of retinal ganglion cells (RGC) and their axons, which form the optic nerve, explain why the optic nerve is preferentially affected in LHON even though the causative mitochondrial mutation typically affects every cell in the body. Mitochondrial biogenesis occurs within the cellular somata of RGC in the retina. It needs the coordinated interaction of nuclear and mitochondrial genomes. Mitochondria are then transported down the axons and distributed where they are needed. These locations are along the unmyelinated portion of the nerve, under the nodes of Ranvier in the retrobulbar nerve, and at the synaptic terminals. Efficient transportation of mitochondria depends on multiple factors, including their own energy production, the integrity of the cytoskeleton and its protein components, and adequate myelination of the axons. Any dysfunction of these systems may be of pathological relevance for optic neuropathies with primary or secondary involvement of mitochondria. Clinical phenocopies of this pathology are represented by the wide array of optic neuropathies associated with vitamin depletion, toxic exposures, alcohol and tobacco abuse, and use of certain drugs.

All optic neuropathies result in loss of ganglion cells and their axons. In LHON, the initial loss is in the papillo-macular bundle. Recent histopathology demonstrates a marked loss of ganglion cells and their axons spreading to nearly the entire retina.

Etiology

The etiology of LHON is a point mutation in the mitochondrial genome. Sequencing studies of the genome from a large number of LHON patients have led to more than a dozen candidate mutations. Three of this group are considered primary mutations in that a single mutation can lead to the clinical disease. These mutations, which occur at nucleotide sites 3460, 11778, and 14484, result in amino acid substitutions in the ND1, ND4, and ND6 subunits, respectively, of respiratory chain complex 1. Because mitochondria are always found in the cytoplasm of cells and never in the nucleus, the DNA mitochondrial mutations are transmitted with the cytoplasm. Sperm cells, at the time of combination with the egg, shed all cytoplasm, and only the nucleus of the sperm cell enters to form the fertilized egg. Because all of the cytoplasm in the fertilized egg is derived from the egg, mitochondrial mutations are maternally inherited.

The Patient

Epidemiology

The average age of onset is within the third decade of life, although occasional cases as young as 4 and as old as 60 have been reported. Males are affected approximately four to five times as often as females for unknown reasons. Only females transmit the risk of optic neuropathy to their children. Because mitochondria are almost exclusively inherited from the mother, affected males never pass on the genetic mutation to their offspring. The true incidence of LHON is not known.

Clinical Symptoms
The typical patient is asymptomatic until sudden painless loss of central vision occurs in one eye, followed by a similar reduction in the fellow eye weeks to months later. Visual acuity often decreases to well below 20/400 in both eyes. Loss of color vision occurs early in the disease process. Problems with night vision and peripheral vision are not reported. Vision loss can progress to near total blindness, and eventual vision of "light perception only" is not rare.

Clinical Signs
When Theodore Leber first recognized the disorder in the 1860s, he described an unusual disc appearance at the time of onset: a hyperemic, blurred disc with numerous corkscrew-type vessels on the disc and immediately surrounding it as well as relative opacity of the retinal nerve fiber layer. This clinical appearance, termed *peripapillary telangiectatic microangiopathy*, is transient. Within several months after visual acuity loss, the disc becomes pale (especially temporally and corresponding to the papillomacula bundle), the retinal nerve fiber layer disappears, and the resultant disc appearance is indistinguishable from other etiologies of optic atrophy.

Significant History

In addition to the maternally inherited genetic defect that can be determined by obtaining a pedigree, recent evidence points to select environmental triggers that are often identified. These epigenetic triggers include smoking and alcohol consumption and at least partially explain why males in their 20s represent the largest group of those acutely affected.

Ancillary Tests

Although Leber reported that the transmission was exclusively through affected or unaffected mothers, it was not until about 130 years later that researchers proved that the maternal inheritance was because of specific point mutations on the mitochondrial DNA. Hence, genetic analysis is indicated in patients with an acute onset of optic neuropathy with questionable etiology. Several labs across the country have the expertise to identify the major point mutations responsible for LHON from a blood sample.

Fluorescein angiography in the acute phase reveals pseudodisc edema and telangiectatic vessels around the disc. Visual-evoked potentials may demonstrate abnormalities prior to visual acuity loss. GDx nerve fiber analysis (NFL) reveals profound and progressive loss of the NFL months to years after the acute onset of vision loss.

The Treatment

No therapeutic intervention has been proven effective, but avoidance of the identified epigenetic triggers (smoking, alcohol) is highly recommended in those at risk. Low-vision aids are sometimes helpful. Scant recent evidence exists that bromonidine may have neuroprotective qualities in LHON patients early in the disease course, and hence prior to widespread loss of ganglion cells and axons.

OPTIC NEURITIS

Alan G. Kabat and Leonid Skorin Jr.

ICD—9: 377.30—Optic neuritis unspecified
ICD—9: 377.31—Optic papillitis
ICD—9: 377.32—Retrobulbar neuritis (acute)

THE DISEASE

Pathophysiology

Optic neuritis refers to an inflammation of the optic nerve. When the anterior portion of the nerve including the optic disc is involved, the condition may be referred to as papillitis. If the posterior portion of the nerve behind the globe along is affected, the condition is known as retrobulbar optic neuritis. Patients with retrobulbar neuritis typically present with a normal-looking nerve head, as compared to the disc edema that is associated with papillitis.

Etiology

Demyelinating disease is the primary cause of optic neuritis in adults, and multiple sclerosis (MS) is by far the most frequent cause of demyelination. Optic neuritis is the initial manifestation of MS in about 20% of patients, though it occurs at some point in approximately 70% of all MS patients.

In children and immunocompromised adults, cases of optic neuritis are likely a result of an immune-mediated process. Etiologies may include viral infection (mumps, measles, chicken pox), bacterial infection (syphilis, Lyme disease, tuberculosis), fungal infection (cryptococcus, histoplasmosis), and systemic inflammation (sarcoidosis, lupus, Reiter syndrome, Crohn's disease, Behçet's disease).

The Patient

In a typical monosymptomatic event, there is progressive, painful, unilateral vision loss. Most patients with the demyelinating form of the disease are young, White females.

Clinical Symptoms

The patient with optic neuritis will complain of progressive vision loss in one eye, although bilateral vision loss, especially in children, can occur. Approximately one-third of patients maintain good vision (20/40 or better), one-third develop moderate vision loss (20/50 to 20/190), and one-third have severe vision loss (20/200 or worse). Patients may complain of other associated visual aberrations, including Riddoch phenomenon (the ability to see moving objects better than static objects) and Uhthoff's phenomenon (worsening of vision with increased body temperature).

Up to 90% of patients complain of periocular, retrobulbar, or eye pain. Pain is aggravated by eye movements.

Clinical Signs
Prominent Signs
- Variable monocular decrease in visual acuity
- Afferent pupillary defect
- Diffuse optic disc edema without associated hemorrhage
- Visual field changes (central, cecocentral, and altitudinal scotomas)

Subtle Signs
- Color vision loss
- Impaired contrast sensitivity
- Cells in vitreous with disc edema
- Cotton wool spots
- Decreased visual function in opposite eye

Demographics

Optic neuritis involves young adults most frequently between the ages of 20 and 45. Women are affected twice as often as men, and Whites are affected eight times more often than any other racial group. Within 15 years of onset of optic neuritis, about 60% of patients will manifest clinically definite MS.

Significant History
- Prior history of demyelinating symptoms, such as paresthesias, clumsiness of limbs, ataxia, diplopia, or urinary incontinence
- Recent history of viral or bacterial infection

Ancillary Tests

Ocular assessment includes visual acuity, extraocular motility testing to identify diplopia or elicit pain with movement, pupil testing, color vision, contrast sensitivity testing, red and brightness saturation testing, threshold visual fields, and visually evoked potential. Funduscopic evaluation, with emphasis on optic disc and vitreous, should also be conducted.

Laboratory studies: CBC with differential, ESR, antinuclear antibody, RPR, Lyme titer. In typical optic neuritis cases, these tests may not be needed.

Lumbar puncture may show evidence of a specific infection. Cerebrospinal fluid analysis in demyelinating disease can show oligoclonal bands, and immunoglobulin G may be elevated.

Imaging studies: MRI appears to be a good predictor for MS, demonstrating paraventricular white matter lesions sometimes called "unidentified bright objects" or "UBOs." MRI should be considered in all patients with optic neuritis, as the early detection of MS may facilitate treatment and remission.

The Treatment

Because up to 95% of patients' vision improves to 20/40 or better within 1 year after optic neuritis, regardless of the extent of vision loss or types of treatment, no intervention may be required. If an underlying immune-mediated condition is identified, however, systemic therapy is indicated.

The Optic Neuritis Treatment Trial addressed the issue of therapy for optic neuritis secondary to demyelinating disease. It concluded that oral prednisone alone actually increased the rate of new demyelinating events and should not be used. Intravenous methylprednisolone 250 mg, four times daily for 3 days, followed by 11 days of oral prednisone (1 mg per kg body weight per day) accelerated the rate of recovery during the first 2 weeks of treatment. In this same group of patients who had two or more typical demyelinating white matter lesions on MRI, there was a significantly lower rate of developing MS within 2 years; however, this benefit was no longer measurable after 3 years.

DOMINANT OPTIC NERVE ATROPHY
Bruce G. Muchnick

ICD—9: 377.16

THE DISEASE
Pathophysiology

This genetic optic neuropathy is characterized by a diffuse loss of retinal ganglion cells and their axons within the papillomacular bundle. The mechanism of the disease appears to be primary ganglion cell death.

Etiology

This form of optic neuropathy has a dominant inheritance pattern. The genetic defect has been identified on the chromosome 3q region.

The Patient

Clinical Symptoms
Symptoms are variable and range from none to profound visual impact. Visual acuity loss ranges from 20/25 to 20/400 (median 20/80). Color vision problems may be noticed

by the patient. The patients may complain of visual field constriction. There may be associated mental abnormalities or hearing loss.

Most typically patients are affected before the end of the first decade of life with a slowly progressive, painless, bilateral but symmetric visual loss. The onset is insidious.

Clinical Signs

Nystagmus may occur in early onset cases. Color vision testing may reveal tritanopia or dyschromatopsia. Visual field testing may reveal central, paracentral, or cecocentral scotomas. The optic nerve atrophy appears as a temporal wedge of pallor of the nerve head. Retinal findings may include peripapillary atrophy, loss of the foveal reflex, macular pigmentary changes, and arterial attenuation.

Demographics

This is the most common of the hereditary optic neuropathies. Fifty-eight percent of patients are 4 to 6 years old at onset. About one in five patients are never aware of any symptoms. Forty percent end up with visual acuity of 20/20 to 20/60. Forty-six percent end up with visual acuity of 20/60 to 20/100. Seventeen percent end up with visual acuity below 20/200. The visual acuity loss stabilizes in the second decade of life.

Significant History

- Reduced vision noticed in a preschooler?
- Optic nerve head pallor in a relative?
- Any unexplained visual loss in a relative?
- Any visual problems in a blood relative?

Ancillary Tests

- Visual acuity testing
- Visual field testing (if possible in a young person)
- Color vision testing (Farnsworth-Munsell 100-Hues test)
- Optic nerve photos
- Audiology testing
- IQ testing
- VEP (reduced amplitude and delayed)
- Test family members for evidence of linkage to chromosomes 3q and 18q
- Genetic testing
- Pedigree analysis
- In all cases of optic pallor in a child without affected family members, screen patient for compressive intracranial lesions

The Treatment

There is no known effective treatment for dominant optic atrophy. Low-vision referral should be made if the vision loss is significant. Genetic counseling must be offered.

PSEUDOTUMOR CEREBRI
Alan G. Kabat and Leonid Skorin Jr.

ICD—9: 348.2

THE DISEASE
Pathophysiology

Pseudotumor cerebri (idiopathic intracranial hypertension) is a disorder of intracranial pressure regulation, resulting in a syndrome of elevated intracranial pressure with normal cerebral anatomy and cerebrospinal fluid composition. While the precise etiology is unknown, suggested mechanisms include increased rate of cerebrospinal fluid production, reduced absorption of cerebrospinal fluid by the meninges surrounding the brain and spinal cord, sustained increase in intracranial venous pressure, and possible increased cerebral blood volume or extravascular fluid volume, simulating brain edema. That brain edema exists in pseudotumor cerebri has been partially substantiated by MRI studies, which show an increase in white matter signal, indicating an increase in overall water content. It is likely that pseudotumor cerebri is in fact a multifactorial disorder.

Etiology

Pseudotumor cerebri has no singularly recognized underlying cause. Numerous conditions have been associated with the disease. The most common ones are listed in Table 19.2.

The Patient

Symptoms and signs are those of increased intracranial pressure. The diagnosis is based on four key criteria (the Modified Dandy Criteria):

1. Intracranial pressure >200 mm H_2O (>250 mm H_2O in the clinically obese patient).
2. Normal cerebrospinal fluid composition (because of dilutional effect, a lower than normal protein value is acceptable).
3. Normal neuroimaging studies (notable exceptions include small or "slit-like" cerebral ventricles, as well as "empty sella syndrome").
4. Symptoms and signs indicative solely of elevated intracranial pressure.

Clinical Symptoms
The patient with pseudotumor cerebri will complain of headache (92%), transient visual obscurations (72%), pulsatile intracranial noises or tinnitus (58%), diplopia (35%), dizziness, nausea, or vomiting (21%), paresthesias, and photopsia.

Clinical Signs
Prominent Signs
- Papilledema (variable)
- Unilateral or bilateral abduction deficit (usually intermittent or transient) causing diplopia
- Visual field defects, such as enlarged blindspot and/or inferior-nasal steps

▶ TABLE 19.2 Causes of Pseudotumor Cerebri

Endocrine and metabolic

Menarche	Addison's disease
Menstruation	Hypoparathyroidism
Pregnancy	Hyperthyroidism
Oral contraceptive agents	Steroid use/withdrawal
Obesity	

Drugs and vitamins

Lithium	Danazol
Nalidixic acid	Keptone insecticide
Tetracycline	Hypervitaminosis A
Nitrofurantoin	Hypovitaminosis A
Amiodarone	Penicillin

Systemic diseases

Hypertension	Guillian-Barré
Systemic lupus erythematosus	Encephalitis
Sarcoidosis	Meningitis
Lyme disease	Post-status epilepticus
Anemias	Emphysema
Blood dyscrasias	Obstructive sleep apnea

Head trauma

Subtle Signs
- Paton's lines, which are circumferential retinal microfolds consistent with papilledema
- Choroidal folds
- Opticociliary shunt vessels

Demographics

Most patients with pseudotumor cerebri are female and between 20 and 45 years of age. Adult men are far less commonly affected; the female to male ratio is reported to be approximately 8:1. This sex predilection is not seen to exist in prepubescent children. The annual incidence in the general population of the United States is 0.9/100,000. However, in women aged 20 to 44 years, and those who are at least 20% over their ideal body weight, the annual incidence is as high as 19.3/100,000.

Significant History
- Obesity
- Endocrine and metabolic dysfunction
- Head trauma
- Hypertension
- Exposure to certain drugs or vitamins

Ancillary Tests

Ocular assessment includes visual acuity, visual field testing, extraocular motility evaluation, color vision, pupillary assessment, and fundus examination focusing on the optic nerves and posterior pole.

Neurologic evaluation should include blood pressure, neuroimaging (MRI) with and without contrast, and lumbar puncture.

The Treatment

- Although pseudotumor cerebri is sometimes described as a "benign, self-limiting disorder," severe vision loss and chronic physical impairment may occur.
- If visual function is normal and the patient is asymptomatic, treatment is unnecessary. If headache is the only symptom, it usually can be managed with prophylactic vascular headache remedies.
- If the patient is obese, weight loss should be strongly encouraged. Studies have shown dramatic improvement in some patients with as little as 6% reduction in body mass.
- Any potentially inciting vitamins or drugs should be discontinued.
- In the case of severe or intractable headaches, and/or persistent vision or visual field defects, medical therapy is typically initiated. The initial treatment of choice is oral acetazolamide 500 mg bid; furosemide or thiazide diuretics may be used in patients who are intolerant to carbonic anhydrase inhibitors. Corticosteroids may be less useful.
- If vision continues to deteriorate even on maximum medical therapy, then lumboperitoneal shunting or optic nerve sheath decompression (ONSD) should be performed. The success rate for ONSD ranges from 70 to 100%, depending upon the study. Up to 35% of initially successful ONSD surgeries may fail. Recently, however, mitomycin-C has been shown to safely and effectively increase the patency and hence the overall success rate of ONSD surgery.
- Gastric bypass surgery is a newly proposed treatment option for pseudotumor cerebri. Recent studies have reported significant intracranial pressure reduction following this procedure, as well as resolved or diminished symptoms in over 95% of patients.

OPTIC NERVE HEAD DRUSEN
Alan G. Kabat

ICD—9: 377.21

THE DISEASE

Pathophysiology

This condition involves the presence of retained hyaline bodies in the papilla anterior to the lamina cribrosa. In the majority of cases, there is little to no pathological impact; however, in rare instances, drusen can compress and compromise the nerve fibers and vascular supply, leading to visual field defects and disc hemorrhages, as well as slowly progressive optic atrophy in extreme cases. Disruption of the juxtapapillary tissue can also result in choroidal neovascular membrane formation, leading to subretinal hemorrhage and disciform retinal scarring.

Etiology

Optic nerve head drusen represent acellular laminated concretions within and between the nerve fibers of the papilla, composed primarily of mucopolysaccharides and proteinaceous material. In many cases, they are partially calcified, possibly as a result of accumulated axoplasmic derivatives from degenerating retinal nerve fibers; this is less common in children and more common in older individuals. Despite the similar nomenclature, there is no histopathological correlation between drusen of the nerve head and retinal drusen, the latter representing accumulated waste material of photoreceptor metabolism and composed of complex lipids.

The Patient

Optic nerve head drusen may be seen in patients of any race, age, or sex. A familial history is possible and likely. Also, the condition may be seen in association with other ocular disorders, including retinitis pigmentosa, angioid streaks, and X-linked retinoschisis.

Optic nerve head drusen tend to remain "buried" in children, but slowly become visible as they enlarge toward the disc surface and as the overlying retinal nerve fiber layer progressively thins. They are usually ophthalmoscopically detectable by the early to mid-teens.

Clinical Symptoms

Typically, patients with disc drusen remain asymptomatic, the finding discovered only upon routine ocular evaluation. Some cases may, however, present with mildly decreased visual acuity and visual field defects. Reports of recurrent, transient visual obscurations associated with disc drusen have also been documented.

Clinical Signs
Prominent Signs
- Bilaterally elevated optic discs with irregular or "scalloped" margins, and a small or nonexistent cup
- Refractile bodies on the surface of the disc, which may autofluoresce with red-free light

Subtle Signs
- Unusual vascular branching patterns that arise from a central vessel core within the nerve head
- An afferent pupillary defect may be noted if the condition is both significant and asymmetric
- Visual acuity and visual fields may be compromised in a small percentage of patients. Visual fields unfortunately are neither uniform nor diagnostic; patients may display nasal step defects, blindspot enlargement, arcuate scotomas, sectoral field loss, or altitudinal defects

Demographics

Optic nerve head drusen is encountered in approximately 2 to 5% of the general population and is bilateral in 70% of cases. It occurs primarily in Whites and is less common in patients of African descent. The condition may occur at any age, but because disc drusen tends to enlarge and become more prominent over time, it is more easily and commonly noted in older adults. An autosomal dominant inheritance pattern with incomplete penetrance has been identified.

Significant History
- Family history of optic nerve head drusen
- Associated ocular conditions: retinitis pigmentosa, angioid streaks, X-linked retinoschisis

Ancillary Tests

Ocular assessment includes visual acuity, pupil testing, contrast sensitivity, color vision testing, and threshold visual fields. Funduscopic evaluation, with emphasis on optic disc and peripapillary retina, is the primary means of diagnosis. Stereo disc photography is a helpful technique to monitor for progressive changes.

Imaging studies: Ultrasonography is extremely beneficial in confirming the diagnosis. The high reflectivity of calcified hyaline bodies is evident on B-scan ultrasonography, at low gain levels. CT scan of the nerve head can also reveal optic disc drusen. Should neovascular membranes be noted or suspected, intravenous fluorescein angiography is recommended. Calcified drusen may be seen to autofluoresce with the application of red-free light.

The Treatment

Optic nerve head drusen represent a normal physiologic variation, and hence most patients require only periodic evaluation every 6 to 12 months.

It is important for patients to self-monitor their vision, particularly because of the risk of choroidal neovascular membrane formation. Suspicion of membranes should prompt immediate fluorescein studies, followed by laser photocoagulation as indicated.

Unfortunately, for those who encounter progressive vision loss from optic nerve head drusen, no effective medical or surgical treatment has been identified to reverse the process.

TEMPORAL ARTERITIS
James A. Goodwin

ICD—9: 446.5

THE DISEASE
Pathophysiology

Temporal arteritis is an inflammatory disease of medium and large arteries that can be complicated by vision loss from arteritic ischemic optic neuropathy or less frequently from central retinal artery occlusion. On pathologic examination, the arterial wall is thickened by a granulomatous inflammatory process that is most intense at the level of the internal elastic lamina. The lumen of the artery is narrowed, and the internal elastic lamina becomes thickened and fragmented. The arterial wall is infiltrated with lymphocytes, plasma cells, and multinucleated giant cells.

Etiology

Temporal arteritis is an occlusive inflammatory process involving the ciliary arteries, ophthalmic arteries, extracranial arteries, the aorta, subclavian arteries, and occasionally the coronary arteries. The ocular complications result from involvement of the ciliary arteries and the ophthalmic artery. Intracranial vessels lack an internal elastic lamina and are rarely if ever the site of granulomatous inflammation. Stroke can complicate temporal arteritis, usually via artery to artery embolization from inflamed extracranial portions of the vertebral arteries and less commonly the external carotid arteries.

Polymyalgia rheumatica may be a prodromal symptom complex or may accompany temporal arteritis. Polymyalgia rheumatica is characterized by pain and stiffness of the neck and shoulder or pelvic girdles with extremely high erythrocyte sedimentation rate. The etiology of polymyalgia rheumatica is still enigmatic though it has been suggested to result from inflammation in the aortic arch causing referred pain in the neck and shoulders. Polymyalgia rheumatica has a very low incidence of ischemic visual or other neurologic complications and is generally treated with low-dose corticosteroids.

The Patient

Most patients are elderly with severe vision loss, headache, and malaise. The disease is almost never encountered in persons younger than 55 years, and most patients are in their 70s or 80s at presentation.

Clinical Symptoms

The patient with temporal arteritis may present with severe, sudden unilateral or bilateral vision loss or much less commonly with diplopia. Accompanying systemic symptoms include headache, which is found in up to 80% of patients; diffuse pain and tenderness of the scalp, face, or oral mucosa; pain in the temporomandibular joints or masseter areas brought on by chewing and relieved specifically by cessation of the muscle activity involved in chewing; depression; fatigue; general listlessness; migratory polyarthralgias; weakness; and loss of appetite.

Clinical Signs

Prominent Signs

- Anterior ischemic optic neuropathy, central retinal artery occlusion, or branch retinal artery occlusion
- Pallid disc edema with anterior ischemic optic neuropathy
- Retinal whitening (edema) with relative cherry-red spot at the macula in central retinal artery occlusion

- Retinal whitening in the involved territory of a branch retinal artery occlusion (upper or lower half of the retina)
- Tenderness to palpation of cranial arteries and focal skin erythema or even swelling overlying inflamed segments of cranial arteries

Subtle or Less Common Signs
- Weight loss
- Nerve fiber layer hemorrhages
- Narrowed arterioles
- Cotton wool spots
- Choroidal infarction
- Ocular ischemic syndrome
- Ulceration of scalp, tongue, oral mucosa
- Low grade fever
- Palpable indurated but often nonpulsatile temporal artery

Demographics

Temporal arteritis is a disease of the elderly, with few patients found under age 50 years. Women get the disease two to three times more often than men. In one study, the mean age at diagnosis was nearly 72 years with a range of 50 to 97. Studies from both the Mayo Clinic and Sweden have shown an increase in the incidence of the disease in the last 25 to 50 years, possibly from increased awareness, but a biologic cause is also suspected, possibly some form of infection.

Systemic signs and symptoms have been found to exist up to 9 months before the disease is confirmed.

Involvement of the second eye can occur in up to 75% of untreated cases. One-third will have vision changes in the second eye within the first 24 hours of the first eye being affected. One-third will have vision loss in the second eye within the first week and one-third between 1 to 4 weeks.

Significant History
- Elderly patient with typical symptoms or signs
- Amaurosis fugax

Ancillary Tests

Ocular assessment includes visual acuity, extraocular muscle testing, pupil testing, red saturation and light brightness testing, visual fields testing, and funduscopic examination.

Laboratory studies: ESR (top normal values: male = age/2, female = (age + 10)/2); quantitative C-reactive protein; CBC with differential; serum electrophoresis; fibrinogen level.

Definitive diagnosis is obtained with a temporal artery biopsy.

The Treatment

Treatment should be started immediately and should not be withheld until results of a temporal artery biopsy are available. Biopsy results may be positive for weeks, and the biopsy is more likely to be positive if the specimen is obtained within 7 to 10 days of the initiation of treatment. The rate of positive results is often quite high in clinical series published by centers specializing in rheumatology, but the overall positive rate in most series is around 20%. This means that if the clinical findings are strongly indicative of temporal arteritis, the corticosteroid treatment should be continued even if the biopsy is normal. Biopsy of the opposite temporal artery may increase the yield of positive results. Some reports indicate that external carotid angiography can identify involved segments in the superficial temporal artery to guide the surgeon where to take the biopsy and increase the positive yield. This can be accomplished now using selective magnetic resonance angiography of the external carotid artery with digital subtraction of the intracranial vessels.

Most patients can be treated with high dose oral prednisone (80 to 120 mg daily). It has also been advocated to initiate treatment with intravenous methylprednisolone 1 gram daily for 3 to 5 days and then treat with high-dose oral prednisone. This recommendation was prompted by the occasional onset of blindness in the second eye during the first few days on conventional high dose oral prednisone.

Before corticosteroid therapy is started, a chest x-ray, anergy panel, CBC, and stool guaiac test should be performed. Monitor blood tests (ESR, C-reactive protein) every 2 to 3 weeks. Treatment may be required for 3 months to several years but almost always for nearly a year. The patient should be seen every 3 to 4 weeks, with repeat erythrocyte sedimentation rate and C-reactive protein to decide on dosage reduction. More important than the laboratory values, however, is the need to keep the patient free of arteritic symptoms—mainly headache and jaw pain while the prednisone dosage is gradually reduced.

NONARTERITIC ISCHEMIC OPTIC NEUROPATHY

Alan G. Kabat and Leonid Skorin Jr.

ICD—9: 377.41

THE DISEASE

Pathophysiology

Ischemic optic neuropathy results from acute deprivation of blood to the optic nerve head, whose main vascular supply is derived from the posterior ciliary arteries and branches of the peripapillary choroidal arterial system. This results in infarction of the retinal nerve fiber bundles in the disc substance anterior to the lamina cribrosa. The term *nonarteritic* denotes that the etiology in these cases is not vascular inflammation.

Etiology

Nonarteritic ischemic optic neuropathy may occur as a result of arteriosclerotic or embolic lesions or from an acute alteration of the pressure-perfusion ratio at the nerve head. A decline in perfusion pressure below the critical level in the capillaries of the optic nerve head may be caused either by a marked fall in the mean blood pressure (e.g., shock, nocturnal hypotension, internal carotid artery or ophthalmic artery stenosis or occlusion) or a rise in intraocular pressure. Each patient with nonarteritic ischemic optic neuropathy may have a unique combination of systemic and local factors that together produce optic nerve head ischemic damage.

The Patient

Patients with nonarteric ischemic optic neuropathy are generally over 50 years of age. Whites appear to have a much higher incidence than other races; however, men and women are affected at virtually the same rate. Most patients report a sudden onset of variable vision loss noted upon awakening.

Clinical Symptoms

There is a rapid, painless unilateral loss of vision that is greatest at onset but may progress over the course of several weeks in up to 45% of cases. Typically, there are no antecedent ocular or systemic symptoms.

Clinical Signs

Prominent Signs

- Visual acuity is variable, ranging from 20/20 to no light perception. About 50% of cases are 20/60 or better, while about one-third of all cases are 20/200 or worse.
- Inferior altitudinal, inferior nasal, or cecocentral visual field defect.
- Afferent pupillary defect.
- Optic disc edema, usually in a sector with small flame-shaped hemorrhages and juxtapapillary arteriolar attenuation.

Subtle Signs

- Small or nonexistent physiologic cup in fellow eye know as "the disc at risk"
- Dyschromatopsia in the affected eye
- Filling defects in the optic disc, peripapillary choroid, or choroidal watershed zones on fluorescein angiography

Demographics

The age range of patients affected by nonarteritic ischemic optic neuropathy is from 40 to 80 years, but only about 5% of patients are older than 70 years. The disease occurs most often in the 56- to 70-year-old age group, though it has been noted in much younger patients with hypertension.

Up to 43% of patients will experience spontaneous recovery of vision by three or more lines of Snellen acuity at 6 months.

The risk of second-eye involvement is relatively small in nonarteritic ischemic optic neuropathy. In patients studied, less than 15% experienced fellow-eye involvement after 5 years. Of these patients, the greatest incidence was noted in those with diabetes and poorer baseline visual acuity in the initially affected eye. Age, sex, and smoking do not appear to be significant factors for fellow-eye involvement; by the same token, the use of aspirin has not been shown to offer any protective influence.

Significant History

- Hypertension
- Diabetes
- Hypercholesterolemia
- Cerebrovascular disease
- Transient nocturnal arterial hypotension
- Migraine or other vasospastic disorders
- Increased blood viscosity (e.g., polycythemia, thrombocytopenia, sickle cell anemia)
- Sleep apnea syndrome

Ancillary Tests

Ocular assessment includes visual acuity, pupil testing, color testing, red and brightness saturation testing, threshold visual fields, fundus examination, and fluorescein angiography.

Noninvasive testing includes measuring blood pressure.

Laboratory studies: CBC with differential; plasma glucose; serum lipid profile; ESR and C-reactive protein (to rule out temporal arteritis).

Imaging studies: Magnetic resonance imaging may be helpful in younger patients to differentiate between ischemic and demyelinating neuropathy (optic neuritis).

The Treatment

There is currently no effective treatment for nonarteritic ischemic optic neuropathy. The use of systemic corticosteroids is not supported by the literature. Some continue to advocate prophylactic aspirin therapy to protect against fellow-eye involvement, though prospective studies have shown no conclusive benefit. Aspirin is best used only in those patients with known thrombotic risk factors.

Patients with hypertension, diabetes, and hypercholesterolemia should address these significant risk factors by means of interventional therapy. Those suspected of having nocturnal hypotension should also seek care and/or consultation.

Surgical intervention, while widely advocated in the early 1990s, is no longer considered an appropriate form of therapy. The Ischemic Optic Neuropathy Decompression Trial demonstrated that optic nerve sheath decompression does not improve the course or outcome of the disease in most cases and may even be detrimental.

VISUAL HALLUCINATIONS
Leonid Skorin Jr.

ICD—9: 368.16

THE DISEASE

Pathophysiology

A visual hallucination is a visual experience that is based on endogenous neural activity rather than on exogenous, viewed objects. It is the subjective experience of a visual phenomenon without objective stimuli present in the environment. A similar term, *pseudohallucination,* can be used for the phenomenon where the subject is aware of the unreality of the sensory experience. If this pseudohallucination occurs in a visually impaired individual, it is known as Charles Bonnet syndrome (CBS).

There are two different types of visual hallucinations: elementary and complex. Elementary, or unformed visual hallucinations, are also called photopsias and consist of colored or colorless bright lights, flashes, spots, or streaks. Complex, or formed visual hallucinations, consist of formed images of objects or persons.

Visual hallucinations must be distinguished from visual illusions, which are altered perceptions of a viewed object, or palinopsia (visual perseveration), which is a persistent or recurrent perception of visual images after they have been removed from view and usually occur in a blind field of vision.

Etiology

CBS occurs more frequently in patients with a significant degree of visual loss and with bilateral as opposed to unilateral pathology. The most common pathology to cause CBS is age-related macular degeneration, but it has been associated with pathology at any level of the visual system.

CBS is thought to occur because of sensory deprivation. This theory has also been called the phantom-vision theory and compared with the phantom-limb syndrome. When the visual sensory cortex is deprived of normal afferent input, it exhibits spontaneous independent activity with resultant conscious imagery (release phenomenon). Beyond the vision loss, it is now felt that these individuals must also experience an overall reduction in their sensory stimulation. Social isolation such as living alone may create reduced levels of sensory stimulation conducive to forming such visual hallucinations in these visually impaired individuals.

The Patient

A typical CBS patient is elderly with significant bilateral visual impairment. He or she is often reluctant to admit to experiencing such hallucinations for fear of being labeled as crazy or insane.

Clinical Symptoms
- Visual hallucinations in a patient with normal mental health who has insight into his or her unreality
- Visual hallucinations are detailed, clearly focused images that may be static or dynamic, with or without color
- No evidence of delirium, dementia, impaired intellectual capacity, affective syndromes, paranoia, psychosis, intoxication, or neurological disease
- There should be no other delusions or hallucinations of the other senses

Clinical Signs
- Underlying severe bilateral vision loss
- Visual acuity in the better eye of 20/60 or worse

Demographics

Most patients with CBS are elderly, with a mean age of incidence around 75 to 80 years old. CBS has been reported in children who have experienced rapid visual loss.

If the patient is elderly, often he or she lives alone and because of his or her significant visual impairment is usually socially isolated.

Significant History

- Visual hallucinations
- Bilateral severe vision loss

Ancillary Tests

A complete eye examination should be performed to identify any possible correctable ocular pathology. Meticulous refraction and low-vision examination should be performed on all these patients.

The Treatment

Although anticonvulsants and neuroleptics have been tried, pharmacotherapy is rarely useful. Patients should be kept socially involved and busy with hobbies and other activities, which may help decrease symptoms.

Maximizing the patient's visual acuity with optical correction or surgery (as in the case of cataract extraction) may help to decrease the frequency or stop the hallucinations.

For most patients, the visual hallucinations disappear spontaneously. The majority of these patients are not disturbed by their hallucinations, once they know the reason for their occurrence. Patients usually feel great relief when told that their hallucinatory experiences are normal and do not signify any psychiatric disorder or dementia.

Chapter 20

Oculoplastics

ENTROPION
Shoib Myint

ICD—9: 374.00

THE DISEASE
Pathophysiology

Entropion, or inversion of the eyelid margin, can potentially lead to corneal opacification and subsequent damage leading to severe visual loss. It is one of the most common eyelid malpositions seen in clinical practice. The clinician must become familiar with the different etiologies of this condition so that the proper treatment option can be selected. Although involutional entropion is the type most frequently seen in clinical practice, other etiologies include congenital, acute spastic, and cicatricial. Involutional entropion is more common in the lower eyelid, while cicatricial is more common in the upper eyelid.

Etiology

Congenital entropion has been known to result from retractor dysgenesis, structural defects in the tarsal plate, and sometimes a shortening of the posterior lamella. Congenital entropion of the upper lid is composed of a horizontal tarsal kink. Congenital entropion should not be confused with epiblepharon in which the pretarsal muscle and skin override the eyelid margin and can potentially cause ocular irritation. The cilia in this case remain vertical.

Involutional entropion is the most common form of entropion and occurs in the lower eyelid. It has been postulated that increased horizontal eyelid laxity, disinsertion or attenuation of the eyelid retractor muscles and capsulopalpebral fascia, overriding of the preseptal orbicularis muscle, and involutional enophthalmos can all cause this type of entropion. Some believe that every involutional entropion has some horizontal eyelid structure component to it. Clinically, the disinsertion of the fascia can be seen as a white line below the inferior tarsal border, indicating the leading edge of the detached capsulopalpebral fascia. Other clinical clues include a deep inferior fornix, reverse ptosis of the lower eyelid (higher than normal), and minimal movement of the lower eyelid on downward gaze.

Cicatricial entropion results in vertical contracture of the posterior lamella of the eyelid. It most commonly occurs in the upper eyelid and can result in irritation of the globe from cilia or a keratinized lid margin. A number of factors can predispose one to this condition, including autoimmune (cicatricial pemphigoid), inflammatory (Stevens Johnson syndrome), infectious (trachoma, herpes zoster), surgical (posterior ptosis procedure, enucleation), and traumatic (chemical and thermal burns). Certain glaucoma medications such as miotics have been known to cause cicatricial entropion. This type of entropion can be differentiated from involutional entropion by the digital eversion test. An abnormal lid margin position will be corrected to its normal anatomic position with a digital traction of the involutional eyelid but not the cicatricial eyelid.

Spastic entropion occurs when the preseptal orbicularis muscle becomes overactive and hypertrophic because of inflammation, irritation, or surgery. This can be cyclic in nature. Acute spastic entropion can be induced clinically by asking the patient to tightly close their eyes.

The Patient

Clinical Symptoms

All forms of entropion can result in corneal irritation. If severe enough, it must be corrected surgically to prevent potential visual loss. Patients will most frequently complain of persistent tearing, foreign body sensation, and blurred vision. In acute spastic entropion, the symptoms may be periodic.

Clinical Signs
- Inward turning of eyelid and eyelashes
- Horizontal lid laxity
- Overriding preseptal orbicularis
- Enophthalmos
- Conjunctival injection
- Keratopathy

Physical testing for horizontal eyelid laxity includes the eyelid distraction test and the snap-back test. To perform the eyelid distraction test, grasp the lower eyelid and pull away from the globe. If the distance between the globe and the eyelid is 10 mm or greater, significant eyelid laxity is present.

The patient should not blink during the snap-back test. The eyelid is pulled downward and released. If it takes more than 10 seconds for the eyelid to reapproximate to the globe, laxity is present.

The orbicularis override test is positive if there is superior migration of the preseptal orbicularis as the patient squeezes his or her eyes closed.

The Treatment

Surgery is the best way to achieve long-lasting correction. While awaiting surgical repair, temporizing methods include lubricating ointments, soft bandage contact lenses, taping the lower eyelid away from the globe, and epilation.

Congenital entropion does not improve spontaneously and must be corrected surgically by reattaching the capsulopalpebral fascia to the inferior border of the tarsus on the lower lid.

Treatment of involutional entropion is directed toward correcting the underlying three pathophysiologic factors (disinsertion of the capsulopalpebral fascia, overriding of the preseptal over pretarsal components of the orbicularis muscle, and increased horizontal lid laxity). Some of the treatment measures include full-thickness marginal rotation sutures, tightening of the horizontal lid, and reattachment of the capsulopalpebral fascia. The three-suture technique (Quickert) is a useful in-office procedure that can correct the problem temporarily, and in some patients, on a long-term basis. The horizontal tightening procedure can be performed via the lateral tarsal strip or lateral canthal tendon plication.

One basic procedure to correct cicatricial entropion is the transverse blepharotomy described by Wies. This results in fracturing the tarsus with eversion of the margin. Overcorrection is achieved with slight ectropion to prevent inversion of the margin in the future.

Treatment options for acute spastic entropion include taping of the eyelid, cautery, botulinum toxin injection to the orbicularis oculi muscle, and various temporary suture techniques. However, because it is thought that an involutional component is present, a more permanent solution is surgery.

TRICHIASIS AND DISTICHIASIS
Geoffrey J. Gladstone

ICD—9: 374.05

THE DISEASE
Pathophysiology

Trichiasis is eyelashes that grow inward toward the eye. There is no actual entropion of the eyelid margin, and the eyelashes originate from a normal position. Distichiasis is inward-growing eyelashes that originate from a position posterior to the normal lashes. Typically, these originate from the meibomian gland orifices. Once again, the eyelid margin is not entropic. When subjected to chronic inflammation, a lash will grow from the meibomian gland orifice, producing distichiasis.

Etiology

Trichiasis can occur after eyelid trauma. It can be seen after surgical resection of eyelid margin tumors. Chronic inflammatory conditions such as ocular cicatricial pemphigoid, chronic blepharoconjunctivitis, and trachoma can also cause trichiasis. Trichiasis can occur with no apparent etiology.

Distichiasis can be congenital or acquired. Chronic blepharoconjunctivitis and other chronic inflammatory conditions can cause distichiasis. Distichiasis and trichiasis may be seen when eyelid tumors are present.

The Patient

Clinical Symptoms

The patient will usually complain of pain, irritation, and foreign body sensation. Epiphora will usually be present, and vision may be impaired.

Clinical Signs

On slit-lamp examination, misdirected lashes are visible. With distichiasis, the lashes can be seen emanating from the meibomian gland orifices, while with trichiasis, the lashes originate from a normal location.

The most significant signs are secondary to corneal and conjunctival abrasion from the misdirected lashes. A punctate or linear vertical keratopathy will usually be present. The distribution of the keratopathy will correspond to the location of the aberrant lashes.

Corneal ulceration can also occur. When present, this must be treated promptly and aggressively to prevent permanent vision loss.

A mucoid discharge is common, while a true infection is somewhat rare.

On eyelid eversion, a horizontal band of scar tissue known as Arlt's line can be present if the trichiasis is secondary to trachoma.

The lower eyelid should be pulled downward and the patient asked to look upward. Horizontal banding within the conjunctiva is known as a symblepharon. This is indicative of ocular cicatricial pemphigoid until proven otherwise.

The number of misdirected lashes as well as their distribution is important when trying to determine the proper treatment for trichiasis or distichiasis. A diagram can be drawn showing the areas of misdirected lashes on each eyelid.

Demographics

Areas of southeast Asia and the Middle East have a significant incidence of trachoma. Patients from these areas should be evaluated for trachomatous eyelid changes.

Significant History

- What country is the patient from?
- Did the patient have any prolonged eye infection?

Ancillary Tests

Whenever symblepharon is present, a biopsy should be considered to rule out the possibility of ocular cicatricial pemphigoid. This is important because prior to any surgical intervention in patients with ocular cicatricial pemphigoid, treatment with steroids or immunosuppressive agents should be considered.

The Treatment

Treatment of trichiasis and distichiasis depends on the extent and distribution of the aberrant lashes. If the abnormal lashes are in an isolated area, certain treatments are reasonable, while different procedures are indicated when the condition involves large areas of the eyelid.

Epilation of abnormal lashes is a simple but temporary solution to the problem. Almost always the lashes will regrow. Early in their growth, the lashes will be short and stubby. These lashes will often cause more irritation than longer more flexible ones.

Cryoablation is another option when a limited distribution of abnormal lashes is present. With this technique, a double freeze, thaw cycle is applied to the involved area. Several treatments may be necessary to achieve complete removal of the lashes. When treating distichiasis, the normal, anteriorly placed lashes will be destroyed along with the abnormal ones. If large areas of the eyelid are involved, cryoablation should be avoided as it can cause scarring and an abnormally displaced eyelid margin.

If abnormal lashes are present in a small area, consideration should be given to excising the area as a pentagonal wedge. The defect is then closed with standard techniques as for eyelid margin lacerations. The amount of eyelid that can be removed and closed in this fashion is directly related to the amount of eyelid laxity that is present. With this or other surgical techniques, it is important to rule out or treat ocular cicatricial pemphigoid prior to surgical intervention.

When a more diffuse trichiasis is present, consideration should be given to performing a Wies procedure. With this technique, a full thickness, horizontal incision is made 3.5 millimeters from the eyelid margin. The incision extends several millimeters medial and lateral to the area of abnormal lashes. Sutures are placed to rotate the eyelid margin away from the globe. An overcorrection of the margin is desired because the eyelid will rotate inward as it heals. The amount of overcorrection can be controlled by the suture placement. The more cicatrizing the condition, the more initial overcorrection is necessary.

With distichiasis, an almost unlimited number of surgical procedures have been described. This is the result of the extreme difficulty in successfully treating this condition. This limited prognosis should be communicated to the patient preoperatively. One useful technique involves the excision of the portion of the tarsus that contains the abnormal lash follicles. Using a posterior approach, the tarsus is excised from 0.5 to 2.5 millimeters from the eyelid margin. The area of excision encompasses the entire area of abnormal lashes. The abnormal follicles are completely removed. This leaves a defect in the tarsus that is filled by advancing the remaining tarsus into the defect. Even though the lash follicles have been removed, new lashes can grow from the remaining portions of the meibomian glands, leading to incomplete resolution of the problem. When effective, this procedure has the advantage of leaving the normal lashes in a normal position.

When the tarsal excision procedure has been ineffective, a Wies procedure should be considered. Although it is often efficacious, it has the disadvantage of bringing the normal lashes into an overrotated position. With this procedure, the distichiatic lashes must be brought into an overrotated position initially, but this overcorrection will generally resolve with time.

ECTROPION
Geoffrey J. Gladstone

ICD—9: 374.10

THE DISEASE
Pathophysiology

Ectropion is an outward turning of the eyelid. It can have a variety of etiologies. These include involutional, cicatricial, mechanical, and tarsal. It is crucial to determine the actual etiology, as this will guide the treatment.

Etiology

Involutional ectropion is the most common condition encountered. A progressive laxity of the lateral and or medial canthal tendon occurs. This leads to a horizontal eyelid laxity. Commonly, epiphora will commence, leading to rubbing of the eyelid and further weakening of the canthal tendons.

Cicatricial ectropion is secondary to a vertical skin shortage. This can occur after excessive skin removal. Lower eyelid blepharoplasty, eyelid reconstruction after tumor removal, and other types of surgery can cause a vertical skin deficiency. Thermal and chemical burns as well as cicatrizing dermatological diseases such as herpes zoster and acne rosacea can also be causative. Excessive exposure to the sun is another important predisposing factor. Chronic inflammation such as seen with blepharitis is occasionally implicated. Cicatricial ectropion can occur whether horizontal eyelid laxity is present or not.

Mechanical ectropion is somewhat rare and is seen when a mass is present on the eyelid. The weight of the mass pulls the eyelid away from the globe, causing the ectropion. This can be seen in neurofibromatosis and with other lesions that are allowed to get unusually large. The greater the horizontal eyelid laxity, the more easily the mass will pull the lid outward.

Tarsal ectropion is a distinct type of ectropion where little horizontal eyelid laxity exists and the eyelid turns outward by being hinged at the inferior tarsal border. Detachment of the eyelid retractors and conjunctival inflammation is thought to play a role in causing this condition.

The Patient

Clinical Symptoms
The patient will typically complain of epiphora, ocular irritation, a foreign body sensation, pain, and possibly decreased vision.

Clinical Signs
An outward turning of the eyelid is always present. This can vary from a very mild medial ectropion to a frank, diffuse ectropion. At times, the ectropion is only present in up gaze.

The ectropion will typically involve the entire eyelid. In cases of tarsal ectropion, the lid will hug the globe up to the inferior tarsal border. At this point, the lid turns outward.

The conjunctiva will often be hyperemic and thickened. A mucoid discharge is frequently seen. In long-standing cases, keratinization of the conjunctiva can be present.

Keratopathy will often be present. In severe cases, corneal ulceration is seen and must be treated promptly.

Laxity of the medial and or lateral canthal tendon will often be present. Medial canthal tendon laxity is often overlooked, leading to unsuccessful surgery or recurrence of the ectropion. The lateral canthal angle is usually several millimeters medial to the lateral orbital rim. In many cases of ectropion, the angle will be medially displaced, indicating laxity of the lateral canthal tendon. A displacement of 10 millimeters is not uncommon when significant laxity is present. The medial canthal tendon can be evaluated by grasping the medial eyelid and pulling it laterally. Normally, the punctum will move two or three millimeters. If the punctum moves to the medial limbus of the eye or further laterally (when the eye is gazing directly ahead), significant laxity is present. In these cases, the medial canthal tendon should be surgically tightened.

Other indicators of eyelid laxity include the eyelid distraction test and the snap-back test. To perform the eyelid distraction test, grasp the lower eyelid and pull it away from the globe. If the distance between the globe and the eyelid is 10 millimeters or greater, significant eyelid laxity is present. Another excellent test is the snap-back test. The patient must not blink during this test. The eyelid is pulled downward and released. If it takes more than 10 seconds for the eyelid to reapproximate to the globe, laxity is present.

In tarsal ectropion, eyelid laxity is absent while a severe ectropion is often seen. Conjunctival hyperemia and thickening are present.

A taut, wrinkle-free appearance to the lower eyelid skin can indicate solar damage and cicatricial change. Scar tissue from burns or previous surgery should be readily apparent.

Demographics

Demographics play a role in ectropion only with regard to sun exposure and surgery for skin carcinomas. Areas of the world with more sunshine and warmer climates will have an increased incidence of cicatricial ectropion secondary to solar damage and complications of reconstructive surgery for malignant skin carcinomas.

Significant History

- Does the patient have a history of work- or recreation-associated excessive exposure to the sun?
- Has there been previous cosmetic or reconstructive eyelid or facial surgery?
- Is there a history of dermatological conditions that affected the eyelids?

The Treatment

The treatment of ectropion is very dependent on the etiology. If the treatment is not directed at the underlying cause, it will not be successful.

Involutional ectropion is repaired surgically by tightening the medial and or lateral canthal tendons. When both are repaired, the medial canthal tendon should be repaired first, as a much smaller tissue excision will be needed laterally.

When repairing the medial canthal tendon, it is important to tighten the posterior and not the anterior limb of the tendon. Tightening the anterior limb will correct the laxity of the eyelid but will produce a gap between the eyelid and the globe medially. When the posterior limb is tightened, the eyelid is pulled posteriorly as well as tightened horizontally, keeping the medial lid in contact with the globe. A small portion of conjunctiva is removed just inferior and medial to the punctum. A 6-0 permanent, monofilament suture is placed between the medial-most tarsus and the remnant of the posterior limb of the medial canthal tendon. The conjunctiva is closed with a 6-0 plain suture.

The lateral canthal tendon is repaired with a lateral tarsal strip procedure. With this surgery, the eyelid is shortened horizontally and its attachment to the lateral rim strengthened. A lateral canthotomy and inferior cantholysis are made. The lower eyelid is pulled laterally, and its point of overlap with the lateral rim is noted. Lateral to this, all the eyelid tissue is removed (including the eyelid margin) except for the tarsus. This lateral tarsal strip is shortened and a permanent 5-0 suture used to attach the tarsal strip to the periosteum of the lateral orbital rim.

Cicatricial ectropion is repaired in several ways. In many cases, a full-thickness skin graft is utilized to replace the vertical skin deficiency. The skin can be harvested from the upper eyelids, retro- or preauricular, supraclavicular, and other areas. The retroauricular area has many advantages. Incision placement will vary depending on the etiology of the condition. It all cases, an incision is made and the scarred skin widely undermined. Any subcutaneous scar tissue is excised. The eyelid must rest without tension in a normal position. A horizontal tightening is performed if significant laxity is present. A full-thickness skin graft is placed on the defect. This is sewn in place and covered with a cotton-Telfa bolster. Often, a Frost suture is used to hold the eyelid in a slightly elevated position for the first week. The bolster is removed after one week.

In certain cases, a mid–face lift will be sufficient to recruit skin and allow the eyelid to assume a normal position. This has the advantage of not requiring a skin graft and potentially giving a better cosmetic result.

Repair of mechanical ectropion involves removing the mass that is pulling the eyelid downward. This can be relatively simple or involve resection of a portion of the eyelid. Skin grafting, as was described for repair of cicatricial ectropion, may be necessary. Simple or complex eyelid reconstruction may be indicated as well.

Tarsal ectropion is a unique condition and can be difficult to repair. The eye should be treated with an antibiotic steroid ointment for a week prior to and after surgery. This will decrease the conjunctival inflammation that contributes to the outward rotation. An incision is made at the inferior tarsal border and carried through the lower eyelid retractors. Chromic mattress sutures are then used to grasp the conjunctiva and eyelid retractors, closing the internal incision and exiting on the skin surface inferior to the conjunctival incision. These sutures place the retractors in proper position and pull the skin superiorly. The sutures are not removed and form a scar barrier to rotation within the eyelid.

FLOPPY EYELID SYNDROME (FES)

John D. Siddens

ICD—9: 374.50—Degenerative disorder of eyelid, unspecified
ICD—9: 728.4—Laxity of ligament
ICD—9: 374.9—Unspecified disorder of eyelid

THE DISEASE

Floppy eyelid syndrome is a clinical condition in which the eyelid has severe laxity. In the majority of cases, the patients are obese males. The upper eyelid is the primary lid involved and is rubbery, floppy, and easily everted. The majority of patients with FES have an associated chronic papillary conjunctivitis. Because the clinical condition is often unrecognized, the patient may have been treated unsuccessfully with artificial tears, topical antibiotics, steroids, or vasoconstrictive agents.

Pathophysiology

The pathophysiology is unclear, but it is believed that FES results from a decrease in tarsal elastin. Histologic evaluations with special stains, immunochemical studies, and electron microscopy have demonstrated this decrease in elastin.

Etiology

In one study, light microscopy of surgical specimens has demonstrated infestation by the mite *Demodex brevis*. The mite can damage the meibomian gland, with tear film and tarsal gland abnormality, increasing the clinical symptoms of FES. Patients with obstructive sleep apnea (OSA) often have hypoxia, which results from snoring and obstruction of the upper airway when they sleep on their back. These patients often sleep on their side to decrease the symptoms of OSA. While sleeping on one side, the face presses into the pillow, and the upper eyelid everts, causing mechanical inflammation and irritation to the conjunctival surface. It has been suggested that poor eyelid apposition to the globe may decrease proper lubrication to the eyelid, with resultant chronic papillary conjunctivitis. Some patients with FES present with keratoconus, which is thought to be a result of mechanical irritation to the cornea.

The Patient

Clinical Symptoms
Symptoms are usually worse in the morning, and as the day progresses, the inflammation does not resolve because of the associated corneal irritation.

Clinical Signs
The patient usually has bilateral chronic conjunctivitis, characterized by incessant irritation, tearing, and a thick ropy discharge.

The patient will often sleep poorly because of the OSA and may wake frequently as a result of snoring, apneic episodes, and ocular irritation. In more severe cases, the frequent lid eversion can result in keratopathy, which progresses to corneal ulceration and scarring with neovascularization and decreased vision. OSA may lead to systemic and pulmonary hypertension. Ultimately, congestive heart failure and cardiomyopathy can occur, thus the patient with FES should be referred to an appropriate internal medicine or pulmonary medicine specialist for further evaluation.

Demographics

FES is usually found in obese middle-aged Caucasian males, although the disease has been found in all races and both sexes.

Ancillary Tests

Examination of the patient will usually reveal excessive laxity in the eyelid. The lid can be easily everted and will feel rubbery and soft. The palpebral surface is inflamed and rubbery and may often appear atrophic. There is almost always a stringy, mucoid discharge, and the cornea may demonstrate a punctate keratopathy. Eyelash ptosis is a finding that is almost pathognomonic, a finding that is often accompanied by dermatochalasis, eyelid or brow ptosis. The lateral and medial canthal tendons may be loose or even disinserted. In more pronounced cases, slit-lamp examination will reveal rose bengal staining of the punctate corneal changes, as well as peripheral pannus or corneal thinning associated with keratoconus. Tear break-up time (TBUT) is usually reduced.

Histologic findings are not consistent, but light microscopy may demonstrate chronic conjunctival inflammation with increased polymorphonuclear leukocytes, eosinophils, and granulocytes; loss of meibomian glands; and granuloma formation. Immunohistological staining and electron microscopy can reveal a decrease in tarsal elastin.

The Treatment

Conservative treatment is optimal for mild or moderate cases. Intensive ocular lubrication will lessen the corneal and conjunctival symptoms. Erythromycin ophthalmic ointment may be combined with doxycycline if corneal or meibomian gland changes become significant. Taping the eyelids closed at night or having the patient wear a shield during sleep will prevent the eyelid from everting and help reduce symptoms. Treatment of OSA is imperative to reduce the sleep abnormalities and resultant ocular findings. OSA treatment may involve using nighttime continuous positive airway pressure (CPAP), weight reduction, and changing sleep habits. Surgical intervention for OSA may involve modification of the pharyngeal tissues, soft palate tissues, or skeletal abnormalities. The patient is encouraged to begin a weight-loss program supervised by a dietician.

If conservative treatment fails to resolve the symptoms, or the findings worsen, ophthalmic surgical intervention is mandated. Horizontal shortening of the eyelid is the primary treatment. In milder cases, a lateral canthal tendon plication or a tarsal strip procedure will resolve the symptoms. However, surgical removal of up to one-fourth to one-half of the eyelid may be necessary to correct more severe FES. Any associated periocular abnormalities, such as dermatochalasis or brow ptosis, may be corrected at the same time.

EYELID PTOSIS
John D. Siddens and Leonid Skorin Jr.

ICD—9: 374.30

THE DISEASE
Pathophysiology

Ptosis is a unilateral or bilateral droop of the upper eyelid, which occurs with the patient's head in an upright position and the eyes in primary gaze. The condition results in obstruction of primary vision or peripheral visual fields, with reduction of overall visual function.

Congenital ptosis results from a dystrophic levator muscle that is fibrotic and deficient in striated muscle fibers. The majority of all acquired ptosis cases are the result of levator disinsertion. The disinsertion of the levator has been shown to occur primarily as a result of microinfarction of the collagen bundles and other tissues within the levator aponeurosis. In some patients, the muscular fibers will be replaced with bundles of adipose tissue. When the levator aponeurosis begins to stretch or disinsert from the tarsal plate, the eyelid begins to fall, resulting in eyelid ptosis. If ptosis results from another cause, such as a neurogenic or myogenic etiology, the primary cause must be treated first, and then the lid position may be addressed.

Etiology

Ptosis may be classified into two overall types: congenital and acquired. Acquired ptosis may be further subdivided into aponeurotic, neurogenic, myogenic, mechanical, pseudoptosis, traumatic, or miscellaneous.

Congenital
This disorder is unilateral in up to 70% of patients and may be associated with strabismus, amblyopia, or anisometropic refractive error. Other related anomalies include double elevator palsy, jaw-winking phenomenon, and blepharophimosis (ptosis, epicanthus inversus and telecanthus), which is an autosomal dominant inherited syndrome.

Aponeurotic
This is the most frequent form of ptosis in the adult. It usually occurs as a result of the levator aponeurosis disinserting from, or separating from, the tarsal plate.

Neurogenic
Neurogenic ptosis may result from a variety of neurologic diseases, including multiple sclerosis, Guillain-Barré, third-nerve palsy, Horner's syndrome, and ophthalmoplegic migraine.

Myogenic
Myogenic ptosis may overlap with neurogenic causes but may result from myasthenia gravis, chronic progressive external ophthalmoplegia, and myotonic dystrophy.

Mechanical
Mechanical causes of ptosis include tumors involving the eyelid, scarring, or severe excess skin (dermatochalasis) weighing down the eyelid.

Pseudoptosis
This form of ptosis is not an actual eyelid droop at all. It is an apparent ptosis caused by insufficient posterior support of the eyelid, as seen in phthisis bulbi, microphthalmos, anophthalmos, and enucleation; hysterical ptosis; excessive skin on the brow and dermatochalasis; contralateral lid retraction such as occurs in thyroid disease; apraxia of lid opening and blepharospasm; and ipsilateral hypotropia.

Traumatic
Trauma may indirectly (blunt trauma) or directly (penetrating trauma) cause the levator aponeurosis to disinsert from the tarsal plate, resulting in eyelid ptosis.

Miscellaneous
A few causes of ptosis do not fit in any one category. These include ptosis during pregnancy and ptosis from contact lens or ocular prosthesis wear.

The Patient

The patient with ptosis will complain of having one or both eyelids obstructing their vision and of having heavy or sleepy lids.

Clinical Symptoms
- Obstructed superior vision
- Ocular fatigue

Clinical Signs
- Droopy upper eyelid(s)

Ancillary Tests

It is important to begin evaluation of the patient with ptosis with a thorough history and physical examination. Uncovering various factors that cause ptosis helps direct the surgeon to proceed with the appropriate surgical procedure for repair.

Eyelid Measurements

Objective measurements may be obtained in the ptosis patient. These measurements provide an excellent source of information that will guide the surgeon in making an appropriate choice for surgical management. These measurements are recorded in millimeters:

MRD$_1$: upper eyelid margin to corneal light reflex distance in primary gaze
>   Normal: >3.5 mm
MRD$_2$: lower eyelid margin to corneal light reflex distance in primary gaze
>   Normal: 4.0 to 5.5 mm
LF (levator function): eyelid excursion from upgaze to downgaze
>   Normal: >10 to 12 mm

Various factors influence these numbers, including frontalis or brow function, the amount of eyelid skin, hypotropia, and so on. The measurements should be made with the patient upright, fully awake, and looking straight ahead (primary gaze). Often, eyebrow arching may occur in the presence of eyelid ptosis. The brow arching is an unconscious or conscious effort to open the eyelid. When obtaining lid measurements, brow lift should be isolated by placing a finger over the brow. This provides a more accurate measurement. If a large difference in eyelid position is present, the ptotic lid should be lifted and held with a finger to look for contralateral lid drop, which may result after surgical correction of unilateral ptosis.

Visual Fields

Ptosis has been demonstrated to reduce the peripheral visual fields. Visual field testing may be performed by various methods, including Goldmann, tangent screen, confrontation testing, or automated static perimetry testing. Several companies manufacture automated static perimetry machines, with specialized programs for ptosis field documentation. Most states now require testing to be done with the eyelids taped and untaped to simulate postoperative results and verify that surgery will improve any field loss.

Photographs

Photographic documentation has also been a method to provide documentation of the medical necessity for surgical repair of ptosis. Pictures document eyelid position and function. This information helps the surgeon during the surgical repair, helps provide documentation for reimbursement, and also helps demonstrate preoperative and postoperative eyelid positions. Consistent photographic technique provides the best documentation. Photographs are taken of both eyes in primary gaze and upgaze.

The Treatment

Repair of eyelid ptosis may be performed alone or may be combined with other eyelid procedures. The basic premise of repair is to reattach the disinserted levator aponeurosis to the tarsal plate. After the skin is incised, dissection is carried into the orbicularis to the level of the orbital septum. The septum is grasped, and a button-hole opening is made with scissors. Hemostasis is carefully controlled with handheld cautery or with bipolar forceps. Once opened, the septum should reveal preaponeurotic orbital fat. The levator complex is found under this layer of fat. At this point, the levator aponeurosis is identified and its attachment to the tarsal plate is evaluated. In the majority of cases, the levator will be disinserted. The pretarsal orbicularis is removed from the central tarsal plate. The aponeurosis is then advanced and reattached with suture to the tarsal plate. Once the levator complex is reattached to the tarsus, the patient is assisted into an upright position. By asking the patient to look in a variety of gazes, and by tightening the suture, the lid height can be adjusted. The final lid height is positioned 1 to 2 mm higher than the desired final lid position, as the lid invariably falls approximately this distance during healing. The skin is closed, and several deep suture bites are placed into the levator tissue to help reform the lid crease.

EYELID AND ADNEXAL LESIONS
Shoib Myint

ICD—9: 238.1

THE DISEASE

There are numerous benign and malignant eyelid neoplasms arising from the epidermis, dermis, and adnexal structures. The goal is to identify and appropriately diagnose these lesions. Although there are too many of these lesions to mention within the context of this chapter, only the most common types seen in clinical practice will be discussed. One should be aware of certain predisposing factors such as a history of skin cancer, excessive sun exposure, previous radiation therapy, smoking, and Celtic and Scandinavian ancestry. These offer clues regarding the likelihood of malignancy.

Benign Eyelid Lesions

Squamous papilloma (acrochordon, skin tag) is a frond-like projection of skin with a central vascular pedicle. It is the most common benign epithelial eyelid lesion. Histologically, these lesions will have increased thickness of the papillary dermis and redundancy of epithelial tissue. Patients will be asymptomatic but may be bothered by its appearance. The treatment is simple excision or cryotherapy.

Seborrheic keratosis occurs in the elderly population. These are benign basal epithelial cells with intradermal pseudocysts. These lesions appear "stuck on," oily pigmented, greasy, hyperkeratotic, and crust-like. There is a variant of this lesion called Dermatosis Papulosa Nigra occurring in African American patients with lesions on the eyelid and cheeks. The condition can be diagnosed with a shave biopsy. There is no risk of malignancy with seborrheic keratosis. The treatment for this is complete excision.

Pseudoepitheliomatous hyperplasia (PEH) is a disorder of the epidermis with rapid proliferation of epithelial or squamous cells. This can occur rapidly over several weeks, most commonly on the edges of burns, ulcers, and chronic inflammation and on the periphery of malignancies such as basal cell carcinoma and lymphoma. Sometimes, it can be induced by fungal infections. Clinically, they present with a hyperkeratotic nodule. The treatment is complete excision.

Verruca vulgaris (wart) occurs secondary to papillomaviruses VI or XI. This condition is seen as a pedunculated wart-like lesion. Histologically, the lesions have acanthosis, hyperkeratosis, and parakeratosis with vacuolated cells in the squamous layer. Treatment can be cryotherapy or simple complete excision.

Inverted follicular keratosis (cutaneous horn) is similar to verruca vulgaris. They may represent an irritated seborrheic keratosis. The lesions are composed of acanthosis lobules with proliferating basal and squamous cells. The treatment is complete excision.

Epidermal inclusion cyst is a slow-growing lesion that arises from the infundibulum of the hair follicle and is filled with keratin. They are the second most common benign lesions and can occur spontaneously or secondary to trauma. Patients present with a firm nodular lesion on the surface of the skin. Treatment is complete excision, marsupialization, or curettage.

Molluscum contagiosum appears as a waxy nodular lesion with central umbilication. Patients may complain of ocular irritation caused by follicular conjunctivitis. Treatment options include observation, excision, controlled cryotherapy, or curettage with treatment of the secondary conjunctivitis.

Xanthelasma are yellowish plaque-like lesions mostly occurring in the medial canthus. They represent lipid laden macrophages in the superficial dermis. Patients most often have normal cholesterol levels. If severe in the lower eyelid, they can result in cicatricial ectropion. Treatment is serial excision, carbon dioxide laser ablation, or topical dichloroacetic acid. They can recur, and patients should be informed of this.

Benign Adnexal Lesions

Acquired sebaceous gland hyperplasia appears as multiple well-circumscribed yellow nodules with an umbilicated center. They usually occur in the elderly secondary to chronic dermatitis and acne rosacea. Sometimes, patients can be prone to developing visceral malignancies and should be evaluated by an internist. These lesions can be destroyed by electrosurgery or excision.

Syringomas are the most common benign adnexal tumors. They appear as multiple waxy, pale, yellow papules near the eyelid margin in females during puberty. They are a benign proliferation of eccrine sweat glands. Carbon dioxide laser ablation or complete surgical excision has been successful in treating them.

Hydrocystoma is a translucent cyst of apocrine or eccrine origin. The eccrine type can appear as multiple lesions, especially during warmer climates. The apocrine type manifests as larger isolated lesions associated with the eyelashes. Both types arise from the glands of moll and can transilluminate. Treatment is usually marsupialization of the lesion.

Nevi are the third most common benign lesions of the eyelid and adnexa. The *junctional* type occurs mostly in children and involves the deeper dermis. The *compound* type appears in older children and younger adults and involves the junctional zone and dermis. The *intradermal* type occurs in the mature adult population and is the most common type encountered. They rarely transform into malignancy and can be treated with shave biopsy or complete excision.

Premalignant Epithelial Lesions

Actinic keratosis is hyperkeratotic, parakeratotic, with nuclear atypia and mitotic figures. They appear as flat, erythematous, scaly lesions in sun-exposed areas. There is a 12% chance these lesions will transform into squamous cell carcinoma, and therefore complete excision or cryodestruction is recommended.

Keratoacanthoma are fast-growing distinctive lesions with a central ulcer filled with keratin material. They most commonly appear in sun-exposed areas in the elderly and the immunosuppressed population. These lesions can resolve spontaneously in 4 to 6 months and have been viewed as low-grade squamous cell carcinomas. Complete excision is recommended.

Lentigo maligna melanoma occurs from lentigo maligna (Hutchinson's Freckle) and represents 10% of eyelid melanomas. They occur in sun-exposed areas and are solar induced. In suspecting a melanoma of the eyelid, the surgeon must take 5-mm wide surgical margins as frozen sections. These patients should be followed carefully, and a complete ocular exam is necessary to rule out any intraocular tumor.

Malignant Eyelid Lesions

Basal cell carcinoma is the most common eyelid malignancy, accounting for almost 90 to 95% of malignant tumors. The majority occur in the lower eyelid. Patients at the most risk usually have fair skin, blue eyes, red or blond hair, and English, Scandinavian, or Scottish descent. There is an increased risk of acquiring basal cell carcinoma with chronic sun exposure. Clinically, it presents as a pearly telangiectatic lesion on the eyelid margin, destroying the meibomian glands. Younger patients with a family history of basal cell carcinoma are prone to have Basal Cell Nevus syndrome (Gorlin syndrome) and Xeroderma Pigmentosum. The two distinctive types of basal cell are nodular and morpheaform, the latter being much more aggressive. Mortality from basal cell carcinoma is 3% because of canthal involvement, prior radiation therapy, or clinically neglected tumors. Treatment is directed toward complete wide margin excision. Radiation is palliative and not curative.

Squamous cell carcinoma is 40 times less common than basal cell carcinoma but much more aggressive and can be potentially lethal. It can occur spontaneously or secondary to actinic keratosis, immunosuppression, and human papillomavirus. Squamous cell can spread via lymphatics and blood and directly along nerve endings.

Sebaceous gland carcinoma arises from the meibomian gland, Zeiss gland, sebaceous gland caruncle, eyebrow, and facial skin and most commonly occurs in the upper eyelid. Most frequently present in females over age 50, it can destroy the meibomian glands, follicles, and cilia. Patients may present with chronic unilateral blepharitis not responding to typical medical therapy. Diagnosis is achieved by a full-thickness eyelid biopsy with wide excision because of its polycentricity. Radiation is inadequate because of its probability of recurring in 3 years. Muir Torre syndrome is a condition associated with sebaceous gland carcinoma and visceral malignancy, and a complete systemic evaluation should be performed by an internist.

Chapter 21

Pediatrics

AMBLYOPIA

Suzanne M. Wickum

ICD—9: 368.01—Amblyopia, strabismic
ICD—9: 368.02—Amblyopia, deprivation
ICD—9: 368.03—Amblyopia, refractive

THE DISEASE

Pathophysiology

Amblyopia is a unilateral or bilateral decrease in visual acuity, uncorrectable by optical means, without detectable anatomic damage in the eye or visual pathway. When form vision deprivation and/or abnormal binocular interaction occur during the critical or sensitive periods, amblyopia may develop.

Etiology

Amblyopia is a diagnosis of exclusion. In addition to ruling out ocular pathology, an amblyogenic factor must be present. There are four main etiologic categories of amblyopia.

Strabismic Amblyopia

- Abnormal binocular interaction secondary to constant or intermittent strabismus.
- Moderate to deep amblyopia is associated with constant, unilateral strabismus.
- Shallow amblyopia is possible with frequent intermittent, unilateral strabismus.

Refractive Amblyopia

- Isoametropic
  1. Bilateral visual disruption because of significant uncorrected ametropia.
  2. Bilateral hyperopia greater than 2 to 4D, myopia greater than 6 to 8D, and astigmatism greater than 1.50 to 2.50D can cause isoametropic amblyopia.
- Anisometropic
  1. Unilateral visual disruption because of significant uncorrected anisometropia.
  2. The greater the amount of anisometropia, the deeper the amblyopia.
  3. Uncorrected hyperopic anisometropia greater than 3.50D and myopic anisometropia greater than 6.50D leads to a 100% incidence of amblyopia.

4. Uncorrected hyperopic anisometropia of 2.00 to 3.50D and myopic anisometropia of 5.00 to 6.50D leads to a 50% incidence of amblyopia.
- Meridional
  1. Uncorrected astigmatism leads to meridional visual deprivation.
  2. Uncorrected astigmatism of 1.50 to 2.00D or more can be amblyogenic.

Combined Anisometropic-Strabismic Amblyopia
- Both anisometropia and strabismus are present.
- The strabismic eye is generally the more ametropic eye.

Deprivation Amblyopia
- Unilateral or bilateral visual deprivation because of the obstruction of the visual axis by ptosis, corneal opacity, cataracts, or other media opacities.
- May also be iatrogenic (e.g., patching).
- Often causes very deep amblyopia.

The Patient

Clinical Symptoms
- Decreased vision in one or both eyes.

Clinical Signs
- Reduced best corrected visual acuity in one or both eyes in the absence of ocular disease and in the presence of an amblyogenic factor.
- Abnormal contour interaction (crowding phenomenon) in the amblyopic eye.
- Eccentric fixation (usually associated with strabismic amblyopia).
- Decreased contrast sensitivity in the amblyopic eye.
- Binocular suppression of the amblyopic eye.
- Reduced accommodative response in the amblyopic eye.
- Mild afferent pupillary defects have also been reported in some amblyopic eyes.

Demographics

Amblyopia occurs in 1.4 to 5.6% of the general population. Amblyopia is the most common visual disability in children, with approximately 60,000 children diagnosed per year in the United States. Additionally, amblyopia is the leading cause of monocular vision loss in the 20- to 70-year age group.

Significant History
- A history of "lazy eye," misaligned eyes, uncorrected ametropia, extraocular muscle surgery, occlusion therapy, or other vision therapy may be elicited.

Ancillary Tests

A thorough eye examination is indicated with particular attention to best corrected visual acuity, binocularity, cycloplegic retinoscopy/refraction, and ocular health.

Visuoscopy is a useful ancillary test to determine the presence or absence of eccentric fixation.

The Treatment
Strabismic Amblyopia
- Optical correction of ametropia based on cycloplegic retinoscopy/refraction.
- Part-time, direct, full occlusion for 2 to 6 hours per day for mild to moderate amblyopia, with the possible need for increased hours for deep amblyopia.
- Full-time occlusion may be necessary when trying to break down and/or prevent binocular sensory anomalies (suppression, anomalous correspondence); however, care must be taken to prevent occlusion amblyopia. For patients 5 years and under, occlude the preferred eye the number of days equal to the child's age, and then occlude the amblyopic eye for 1 day.
- Penalization with 1% atropine may be used instead of traditional occlusion for mild to moderate amblyopia.
- Active monocular visual activities for 30 to 60 minutes per day.
- Follow up every 4 to 6 weeks.
- Manage the strabismus once the amblyopia treatment is completed or abandoned.

Isoametropic Amblyopia
- Optical correction of ametropia based on cycloplegic retinoscopy/refraction.
- Follow up in approximately 4 weeks.
- If necessary, make any changes to the prescription.
- Follow every 4 to 6 months to monitor acuity improvement.
- Patching or penalization are only necessary in cases of asymmetric aided acuity.

Anisometropic Amblyopia
- Optical correction of ametropia based on cycloplegic retinoscopy/refraction.
- Part-time, direct, full occlusion for 2 to 6 hours per day for mild to moderate amblyopia, with the possible need for increased hours for deep amblyopia.
- Penalization with 1% atropine may be used instead of traditional occlusion for mild to moderate amblyopia.
- Active monocular visual activities for 30 to 60 minutes per day. Once visual acuity in the amblyopic eye reaches 20/40–50, consider the addition of binocular vision therapy to break down remaining suppression.
- Follow up every 4 to 6 weeks.

Deprivation Amblyopia
- Remove the obstruction of the visual axis as soon as possible, ideally within 2 months of onset.
- Correct any significant ametropia or aphakia.
- Part-time, direct, full occlusion for 2 to 6 hours per day for mild to moderate amblyopia, with the possible need for increased hours for deep amblyopia.
- Penalization with 1% atropine may be used instead of traditional occlusion for mild to moderate amblyopia.

- Active monocular visual activities for 30 to 60 minutes per day.
- Follow-up every 4–6 weeks.

ESODEVIATIONS
Suzanne M. Wickum

ICD—9: 378.00—Esotropia, unspecified
ICD—9: 378.01—Esotropia, monocular
ICD—9: 378.02—Esotropia, monocular with 'A' pattern
ICD—9: 378.03—Esotropia, monocular with 'V' pattern
ICD—9: 378.04—Esotropia, monocular with other noncomitancy
ICD—9: 378.05—Esotropia, alternating
ICD—9: 378.06—Esotropia, alternating with 'A' pattern
ICD—9: 378.07—Esotropia, alternating with 'V' pattern
ICD—9: 378.08—Esotropia, alternating with other noncomitancy
ICD—9: 378.21—Esotropia, intermittent, unilateral
ICD—9: 378.22—Esotropia, intermittent, alternating
ICD—9: 378.35—Esotropia, with accommodative component

THE DISEASE
Pathophysiology

Esodeviations present with an inward eye turn, intermittently or constantly, resulting in convergent visual axes.

Etiology

Innervational, accommodative, genetic, and environmental factors play a role in the development of esotropia.

The Patient

Clinical Symptoms
- Patients may report diplopia, asthenopia, and/or blurred vision.

Esotropia Classification and Characteristics

Infantile Esotropia
- Clinical Characteristics: Onset occurs between birth and 6 months of age. The esotropia is constant, comitant (A or V patterns may be present), and moderate to large magnitude (30 to 70 prism diopters), and cross-fixation is common. The accommodative-convergence accommodation (AC/A) ratio is usually normal. The ametropia is skewed toward low hyperopia. Sensory adaptations are present in 35 to 72% of cases. Dissociated vertical deviation (DVD) is present in 50 to 75%

of cases. Overaction of the inferior oblique muscle is present in 68% of cases. Latent or manifest-latent nystagmus is found in 25 to 52% of cases.

Accommodative Esotropia
Refractive Accommodative Esotropia
- Clinical Characteristics: Onset is usually between 1 and 8 years of age with an average of 2.5 years. The deviation is typically moderate (20 to 40 prism diopters), variable, and intermittent with a gradual increase in frequency and duration over time. If the deviation becomes constant, sensory adaptations may develop. The deviation is typically comitant but A or V patterns may be found. The AC/A ratio is normal. The etiology is uncorrected hyperopia and insufficient fusional divergence. The ametropia is usually between +2D to +6D with an average of +4.75D.

Nonrefractive Accommodative Esotropia
- Clinical Characteristics: The characteristics are the same as refractive accommodative esotropia with a few exceptions. The AC/A ratio in this case is high, thus the near angle is larger than distance. The average ametropia is +2.25D, but any refractive error can be found. The etiology in this case is the high AC/A ratio; therefore, the esotropia typically responds to plus lenses at near.

Partially Accommodative Esotropia
- Clinical Characteristics: The characteristics are the same as refractive accommodative esotropia with a few exceptions. The esotropia is constant rather than intermittent, therefore sensory adaptations are likely. The AC/A ratio is normal or high. Typically, there is moderate to high hyperopia present. The esotropia magnitude decreases, but is not eliminated, with the hyperopic correction.

Nonaccommodative Acquired Esotropia
- Clinical Characteristics: Onset occurs after 6 months of age. The esotropia is typically constant, comitant (A or V patterns may be present), and moderate to large magnitude (20–70 prism diopters), and sensory adaptations may occur. Often, some amount of hyperopia is present. Causes include idiopathic, decompensated esophoria; disruption of fusion by occlusion; physical/emotional stress; and rarely CNS pathology.

Basic Esotropia
- This is the most common subcategory. The AC/A ratio is normal. The refractive error is usually insignificant.

Divergence Insufficiency Esotropia
- The AC/A ratio is low, thus the distance magnitude is greater than near. Divergence paralysis, which originates from a midbrain lesion, must be ruled out. Divergence paralysis initially presents as a noncomitant esotropia that may become comitant over time.

Acute Esotropia

- Diplopia is likely in these cases. Some patients may close or wink one eye to alleviate the diplopia.

Sensory Esotropia

- Onset may occur at any age. The deviation is constant, unilateral, and comitant, and the magnitude is often variable. The strabismus is secondary to significantly reduced visual acuity, resulting in a sensory obstacle to fusion. Visually depriving factors may include uncorrected anisometropia, ptosis, corneal opacities, cataracts, optic nerve lesions, or retinal lesions. Sensory esotropia is as frequent as sensory exotropia in children under 6 years of age; however, sensory exotropia predominates in older children and adults.

Microtropia
Clinical Characteristics

- Primary microtropia is likely present since birth, with no history of a larger angle of strabismus. Secondary microtropia is often the result of vision therapy or surgery for a larger deviation. Other causes may include aniseikonia, anisometropia, uncorrected vertical deviation, and foveal lesions. The deviation is usually constant and comitant, and the magnitude is between 1 to 10 prism diopters. Sensory adaptations are common and include anomalous correspondence, mild amblyopia, central suppression, and eccentric fixation. These patients have some peripheral fusion with anomalous vergence ranges and some local stereopsis, but no global stereopsis.

Incomitant Esotropia
Abducens Nerve Palsy

- A noncomitant esotropia with greatest magnitude in the affected muscle action field. The distance magnitude may be larger than near. An abduction deficit is present, with no restriction on forced duction testing. Patients typically report diplopia and may adopt a face turn toward the paretic eye in order to obtain fusion. (See Neuro-ophthalmic Disease.)

Duane Syndrome and Mobius Syndrome

- See Strabismus Syndromes later in this chapter.

Demographics

The prevalence of strabismus in the general population is between 2 and 6%. Esotropia occurs three times as often as exotropia. While most cases of esotropia have an accommodative component, 28 to 54% of esotropias are infantile.

Significant History

- Age and nature of onset
- Frequency of deviation
- Changes in the size or frequency of the deviation

- Associated symptoms (including diplopia)
- History of injury or illness
- History of neurologic, systemic, or developmental disorders
- History of ocular disease or reduced visual acuity
- History and outcome of prior treatment (occlusion, vision therapy, prism, surgery)
- Positive family history of strabismus

Ancillary Tests

A thorough ocular examination is indicated in all strabismic patients. Careful refractive error and visual acuity measurements should be performed to evaluate for amblyopia. Visuoscopy can be utilized to detect eccentric fixation. Measurement of the esotropia including frequency, laterality, magnitude, and comitancy is essential. Evaluation of ocular motility is necessary to rule out abducens palsy. In cases of intermittent esotropia, base-in (compensating) vergence ranges should be measured and sensory-motor fusion should be assessed (Worth-dot/stereopsis). Subjective assessment of the deviation is performed with tests such as Maddox rod and Bagolini lenses. The subjective angle of deviation is then compared to the objective angle of deviation in order to determine the presence/absence of anomalous correspondence. Cycloplegic retinoscopy/refraction is recommended in all strabismic patients. Lastly, a thorough ocular health examination is necessary to rule out causes for sensory deprivation.

The Treatment

- Treatment of infantile esotropia should start with correction of any significant refractive error. When amblyopia is present, it must be treated prior to surgical intervention. Once the patient can freely alternate fixation, strabismus surgery should be offered. Ideally, surgery should be performed within 1 year of onset of the esotropia for the best chance of establishing some form of binocularity.
- Treatment of refractive/accommodative acquired esotropia includes prescribing the full hyperopic correction. Consider giving an add for cases with a high AC/A ratio. Treat amblyopia and sensory-motor fusion as needed. If the esotropia is only partially accommodative, consider adding base-out prism when the residual esotropia is less than 15 to 20 prism diopters. If the residual esotropia is greater than 15 to 20 prism diopters, then strabismus surgery is recommended.
- Once the etiology of nonaccommodative acquired esotropia has been determined, treatment can begin. If amblyopia is present, it should be treated. For esotropia less than 15 to 20 prism diopters, base-out prism and/or vision therapy should be utilized. For deviations greater than 15 to 20 prism diopters, surgery should be considered as long as the deviation is stable.
- Microtropia treatment is often confined to best optical correction and treatment of amblyopia. When anomalous correspondence is present, binocular therapy is rarely undertaken; however, when normal correspondence is present, base-out prism and/or vision therapy can be utilized to obtain sensory-motor fusion.
- In the case of sensory esotropia, the underlying cause must be addressed first. Any significant ametropia should be corrected, and all patients should be given protective

glasses for full-time wear. If superimposed amblyopia is suspected, treatment should be implemented. If improved ocular alignment is desired, strabismus surgery may be performed.

EXODEVIATIONS
Suzanne M. Wickum

ICD—9: 378.10—Exotropia, unspecified
ICD—9: 378.11—Exotropia, monocular
ICD—9: 378.12—Exotropia, monocular with 'A' pattern
ICD—9: 378.13—Exotropia, monocular with 'V' pattern
ICD—9: 378.14—Exotropia, monocular with other noncomitancy
ICD—9: 378.15—Exotropia, alternating
ICD—9: 378.16—Exotropia, alternating with 'A' pattern
ICD—9: 378.17—Exotropia, alternating with 'V' pattern
ICD—9: 378.18—Exotropia, alternating with other noncomitancy
ICD—9: 378.23—Exotropia, intermittent, unilateral
ICD—9: 378.24—Exotropia, intermittent, alternating

THE DISEASE
Pathophysiology

Exodeviations present as an intermittent or constant outward eye turn resulting in divergent visual axes. The deviation often begins as an exophoria and over time becomes an intermittent exotropia. When left untreated, an intermittent exotropia may progress to a constant exotropia.

Etiology

Innervational, mechanical/anatomic, and multifactorial genetic inheritance patterns have all been implicated in the development of exotropia.

The Patient

Clinical Symptoms
- Patients may complain of asthenopia, squinting, photophobia, unilateral eye closure, diplopia, and/or blurred vision.

Exotropia Classification and Characteristics

Primary Comitant Exotropia
Clinical Characteristics
- Onset is usually between 6 months to 8 years of age. The exotopia is typically intermittent (80%) and comitant, although A or V patterns are found with overaction

of the superior or inferior oblique muscles. The deviation magnitude ranges from 20 to 70 prism diopters. Positive fusional vergence is insufficient. Sensory adaptations are minimal. Fatigue, illness, daydreaming, alcohol/sedatives, or going from dim to bright light ("dazzle effect") may decrease control of the exotropia.

- Subcategories of Primary Comitant Exotropia (based on Duane's categories):
  1. Basic Exotropia: Distance and near deviation magnitude are similar, yielding a normal AC/A ratio. The exotropia is manifest more often at distance than at near.
  2. Convergence Insufficiency Exotropia: Near deviation magnitude is greater than distance yielding a low AC/A ratio. The exotropia is typically at near and accompanied by a receded near point of convergence.
  3. True Divergence Excess Exotropia: Distance deviation magnitude is greater than near, yielding a high AC/A ratio. The exotropia is typically more frequent at distance.
  4. Pseudo-Divergence Excess Exotropia: Initial measurements look like divergence excess exotropia with the strabismus magnitude greatest at distance. These patients have increased tonic fusional convergence that is not broken down with a near cover test. With prolonged occlusion, or with +3.00D overcorrection, the magnitude of the near deviation is found to be similar to the distance deviation, resulting in a basic exotropia. Pseudo-divergence excess is more common than true divergence excess.

Infantile Exotropia
Clinical Characteristics
- A rare type of exotropia occurring in approximately 1/30,000 births. Onset occurs between birth to 6 months of age. The deviation is constant, moderate to large (30 to 90 prism diopters), and comitant with possible A or V patterns if superior or inferior oblique overactions are present. Sensory adaptations are likely. Infantile exotropia may occur in otherwise healthy infants but is typically associated with other ocular disorders, neurologic disease, craniofacial syndromes, and genetic syndromes.

Sensory Exotropia
Clinical Characteristics
- Onset may occur at any age. The deviation is constant, unilateral, and comitant, and the magnitude is often variable. The strabismus is secondary to significantly reduced visual acuity, resulting in a sensory obstacle to fusion. Visually depriving factors may include uncorrected anisometropia, ptosis, corneal opacities, cataracts, optic nerve lesions, or retinal lesions. Sensory exotropia is as frequent as sensory esotropia in children under 6 years of age; however, sensory exotropia predominates in older children and adults.

Oculomotor Nerve Palsy
Clinical Characteristics
- A large magnitude, noncomitant exotropia with hypotropia. Accompanied by limitation of elevation, depression, and adduction in the affected eye. A complete palsy also

presents with ptosis, loss of accommodation, and a dilated pupil. These findings are variable in the case of an incomplete palsy.

■ Refer to chapter 19, Neuro-ophthalmic Disease, for a complete description.

Demographics

The prevalence of strabismus in the general population is between 2 and 6%. Exodeviations occur less often than esodeviations in a 1:3 ratio. In addition, exodeviations occur more often in females than males. Approximately one-third of exodeviations are evident by two years of age.

Significant History

■ Age and nature of onset
■ Frequency of deviation
■ Changes in the size or frequency of the deviation
■ Associated symptoms (including diplopia)
■ History of injury or illness
■ History of neurologic, systemic, or developmental disorders
■ History of ocular disease or reduced visual acuity
■ History and outcome of prior treatment (occlusion, vision therapy, prism, surgery)
■ Positive family history of strabismus

Ancillary Tests

A thorough ocular examination is indicated in all strabismic patients. Careful refractive error and visual acuity measurements should be performed to evaluate for amblyopia. Visuoscopy can be utilized to measure eccentric fixation. Measurement of the exotropia including frequency, laterality, magnitude, and comitancy is essential. Evaluation of ocular motility and near point of convergence is necessary. In cases of intermittent exotropia, base-out (compensating) vergence ranges should be measured, and sensory-motor fusion should be assessed (Worth-dot/stereopsis). Subjective assessment of the deviation is performed with tests such as Maddox rod and Bagolini lenses. The subjective angle of deviation is then compared to the objective angle of deviation to determine the presence/absence of anomalous correspondence. Cycloplegic retinoscopy/refraction is recommended in all strabismic patients. A thorough ocular health examination is necessary to rule out causes of sensory deprivation.

The Treatment

■ For all classifications of exotropia, the initial treatment should include correcting significant refractive error and treating amblyopia.
■ Minus lenses may be used full-time as a passive therapy for young children or may be utilized during vision therapy sessions for older children and adults.
■ Relieving or correcting prism (base-in) may be used as an individual treatment or may be combined with vision therapy.

- Vision therapy can be utilized in some cases of exotropia. The therapy begins by increasing the patient's gross convergence ability, thus normalizing the near point of convergence. Next, sensory-motor fusion is trained with the goal of expanding the patient's positive fusional vergence range so as to compensate for the exotropia. Therapy techniques that enhance diplopia awareness and break suppression are recommended.
- Surgery is utilized in moderate- to large-angle exotropia. In cases of intermittent exotropia, many surgeons recommend that surgery be delayed until 4 years of age, unless the frequency of the exotropia is increasing. In the case of constant exotropia, surgery should be performed much earlier.
- Utilizing vision therapy before and/or after surgery improves the chances for functional binocular vision.

For cases of sensory exotropia, the treatment is different. First, the underlying cause of the reduced acuity must be addressed. Any significant ametropia should be corrected, and all patients should be given protective glasses for full-time wear. If superimposed amblyopia is suspected, treatment should be implemented. If improved ocular alignment is desired, strabismus surgery may be performed.

STRABISMUS SYNDROMES
Suzanne M. Wickum

ICD—9: 378.71—Duane's retraction syndrome
ICD—9: 378.61—Brown's syndrome
ICD—9: 352.6—Mobius syndrome
ICD—9: 378.62—Eye muscle fibrosis

DUANE RETRACTION SYNDROME (DRS)

THE DISEASE
Pathophysiology

Duane retraction syndrome is a congenital ocular motility disorder characterized by globe retraction and narrowing of the palpebral fissure in attempted adduction, frequent abduction deficiency, variable adduction deficiency, and often upshoots or downshoots upon attempted adduction.

Etiology

Although there have been many theories regarding the etiology of DRS, the most widely accepted theory involves innervational and central nervous system anomalies. It has been found that the abducens nucleus and nerve are absent or hypoplastic, resulting in limited or absent abduction. Additionally, there is anomalous innervation of the lateral rectus muscle by branches of the oculomotor nerve.

Most cases of DRS are sporadic; however, familial cases have been reported to occur in 5 to 23% of patients. The inheritance pattern is autosomal dominant with incomplete penetrance and variable expressivity. Since DRS is associated with a 10 to 20 times increase in frequency of other congenital ocular and nonocular anomalies, there is speculation that a teratogenic event may take place somewhere between the fourth and tenth week of gestation in sporadic cases.

The Patient

Clinical Symptoms
Because of the young age at diagnosis, the patient will not be symptomatic; however, the parents may complain that the child has an eye turn, an abnormal face turn, and/or abnormal eye movements.

Clinical Signs
DRS is divided into three categories. Each type has the common characteristics of globe retraction and narrowing of the palpebral fissure on adduction, as well as upshoots or downshoots on attempted adduction.

DRS type I characteristics: Esotropia or heterophoria are common in primary gaze, but exotropia is possible. There is marked limitation of abduction with no/minimal limitation of adduction. The child may adopt a face turn in the direction of the abduction deficit in order to maintain binocularity.

DRS type II characteristics: Exotropia is frequently observed in primary gaze. There is marked limitation of adduction with no/minimal limitation of abduction. The child may adopt a face turn in the direction of the adduction deficit in order to maintain binocularity.

DRS type III characteristics: Exotropia is frequently observed in primary gaze. There is combined limitation of abduction and adduction. Face turns are variable.

Demographics

Duane retraction syndrome is the most common of all congenital oculomotor anomalies and accounts for 1 to 4% of strabismus cases. While there is no racial predilection, there is a slight preponderance for females (55 to 60% of cases). The left eye is affected in approximately 60% of cases, the right eye in 22%, and bilateral in 18%. DRS type I is the most common (78%), followed by DRS type III (15%) and DRS type II (7%).

Significant History
- Age of onset
- Positive family history of ocular motility restriction/strabismus
- Presence of diplopia (DRS patients rarely report diplopia)

Ancillary Tests

Evaluation of ocular misalignment, abnormal face turn, range of extraocular motility, globe retraction, and palpebral fissure narrowing and observation of upshoots and downshoots are important. In difficult cases, forced ductions can be useful in differentiating between long-standing muscle problems with secondary fibrosis versus recently acquired cranial nerve palsies.

The Treatment

Surgery is utilized to improve unacceptable face turns, correct significant ocular misalignment in primary gaze, reduce severe globe retraction, and improve the appearance of upshoots and downshoots. It must be stressed that surgery may improve, but will not eliminate, the abnormal eye movements. For patients who are not good surgical candidates but who have asthenopia, vision therapy and/or prism can be beneficial.

BROWN SYNDROME

THE DISEASE

Pathophyslology

Brown syndrome is typically a congenital ocular motility disorder, although acquired forms are possible. The syndrome is primarily characterized by deficient elevation in adduction.

Etiology

In congenital Brown syndrome, the motility deficiency is constant and not likely to resolve. The motility deficiency is a result of a short or inelastic superior oblique tendon or because of a limitation of the tendon to slide through the pulley-like trochlea. Most cases of congenital Brown syndrome are sporadic; however, familial cases have been reported. The inheritance pattern is autosomal dominant with incomplete penetrance and variable expressivity.

In acquired Brown syndrome, the motility deficiency may be constant or intermittent and may resolve over time. This syndrome has been caused by surgical procedures including strabismus surgery, sinus surgery, blepharoplasty, and scleral buckling procedures. Brown syndrome is also associated with inflammatory disorders such as rheumatoid arthritis, sinusitis, and metastasis in the area of the trochlea. Direct, as well as indirect, trauma may also give rise to Brown syndrome.

The Patient

Clinical Symptoms

Patients may complain of pain or tenderness in between their eyes (in the area of the trochlea), especially during up gaze movements. Some patients may also report an audible "clicking" noise as they look up. Additionally, patients may complain of diplopia, particularly in up gaze.

Clinical Signs

There is limitation or absence of elevation in adduction with normal/near normal elevation in midline and abduction. Hypotropia of the involved eye may be found in primary gaze. Divergence occurs in up gaze, causing a V-pattern deviation. Downshoots on adduction are possible. There is minimal or no superior oblique overaction of the ipsilateral eye. Patients may adopt a compensatory chin-up head posture in order to preserve binocularity and/or eliminate diplopia.

Demographics

Brown syndrome occurs in less than 1% of strabismus patients. It has been estimated to occur in 1/20,000 live births. This condition does not show any gender or racial predilection. Brown syndrome is found unilaterally in 90% of cases and bilaterally in 10% of cases.

Significant History

- Age of onset
- Positive family history of ocular motility restriction/strabismus
- Presence of diplopia
- Recent history of strabismus surgery, sinus surgery, retinal surgery, or blepharoplasty
- History of inflammatory conditions like rheumatoid arthritis or sinusitis
- History of trauma

Ancillary Tests

Evaluation of ocular misalignment, abnormal head posture, and range of extraocular motility and observation of downshoots are important. Additionally, forced ductions are useful in confirming the restrictive nature of this syndrome.

The Treatment

In many cases of Brown syndrome, observation and patient/parent education are all that are necessary. This is particularly true in mild cases with preserved binocularity in primary gaze and without an anomalous head posture. Indications for surgical intervention in Brown syndrome include hypotropia present in primary gaze, significant anomalous head posture, and/or unacceptable downshoots of the involved eye. In cases that are inflammatory in nature, steroids administered orally or locally by injection are useful.

MOBIUS SYNDROME

THE DISEASE

Pathophysiology

Mobius syndrome consists of congenital facial diplegia and bilateral abducens nerve palsies. Systemic abnormalities and other cranial nerve palsies may also be present.

Etiology

The exact pathogenesis of Mobius syndrome is uncertain; however, the timing of the syndrome seems to be well defined. A pathologic insult takes place during the first trimester, typically between the fourth to sixth week of gestation, when the cranial nerve nuclei are undergoing rapid development. Trauma, illness, and maternal ingestion of certain medications have been associated with this syndrome. In more recent years, a vascular etiology of Mobius syndrome has been implicated. The vascular insult leads to hypoxia and ischemia of the cranial nerve nuclei.

While the majority of Mobius syndrome cases are sporadic, there have been case reports of pedigrees demonstrating autosomal dominant, autosomal recessive, and X-linked inheritance.

The Patient

Clinical Symptoms

Symptoms present in infancy and include difficulty sucking, excessive drooling, lack of facial expression, and lagophthalmos. Parents may also report crossed eyes and tracking problems.

Clinical Signs

Common ocular signs include esotropia, bilateral abduction deficits, lagophthalmos, and exposure keratitis. Additional ocular or orbital signs have been noted, including hypertelorism, epicanthal folds, small palpebral fissures, ptosis, and entropion. Abnormalities of the extremities, swallowing and speech difficulties, craniofacial abnormalities, defective brachial musculature, tongue hypoplasia, and mental retardation have all been reported as well.

Demographics

Mobius syndrome is very rare. No racial or gender predilections have been reported.

Significant History
- Trouble with sucking/feeding
- Eyes partially open when sleeping
- Presence of photophobia
- Problems with facial expression

Ancillary Tests

A complete eye exam is necessary, with special attention to eye alignment, extraocular motility, lagophthalmos, and exposure keratitis. When esotropia is present, one must also evaluate the patient for amblyopia. Because of the frequently associated systemic anomalies, the patient should also have a complete physical examination with a pediatrician.

The Treatment

Ocular management includes correcting any significant refractive error, providing therapy for amblyopia, considering strabismus surgery when significant esotropia is present, and treating keratitis associated with lagophthalmos. The patient's pediatrician should manage any associated systemic anomalies.

CONGENITAL FIBROSIS OF THE EXTRAOCULAR MUSCLES (CFEOM)

THE DISEASE

Pathophysiology

Congenital fibrosis of the extraocular muscles is a rare disorder characterized by congenital restrictive ophthalmoplegia.

Etiology

Congenital fibrosis of the extraocular muscles is typically a familial disorder inherited in an autosomal dominant pattern with significant variability in expression; however, cases of autosomal recessive inheritance as well as sporadic cases have been reported. Original reports describe CFEOM as having a myogenic origin. More recent reports indicate a primary neurogenic etiology that leads to subsequent degeneration of muscle fibers.

The Patient

Clinical Symptoms

Because of the young age at diagnosis, the patient will not be symptomatic; however, parents will report that the child has abnormal eye movements, abnormal eye alignment, ptosis, and/or an abnormal head posture.

Clinical Signs

Traditionally, this syndrome has been divided into five categories based on slight clinical differences. The *general fibrosis syndrome* is characterized by bilateral restriction of all of the extraocular muscles. The inferior rectus shows greatest involvement, thus causing the eyes to be fixed approximately 20 to 30 degrees below midline. As a result of the bilateral hypotropic eye position combined with bilateral ptosis, the patient will adopt a chin-up head position. *Congenital fibrosis of the inferior rectus with blepharoptosis* is a variant of CFEOM in which the inferior rectus is affected with little to no involvement of the other extraocular muscles. In cases of *strabismus fixus*, the eyes are fixed in either an esotropic or exotropic position with severe limitation of horizontal eye movements. The vertical eye movements are usually intact. In contrast, cases of *vertical retraction syndrome* demonstrate severely impaired vertical eye movements with relatively intact horizontal movements. Lastly, a unilateral fixed globe characterizes *congenital unilateral fibrosis*.

More recently, a revised classification has been proposed based on the identification of three CFEOM genetic loci. Patients with CFEOM1, mapped to chromosome 12, have the features of general fibrosis syndrome as listed above. Cases with CFEOM2, mapped to chromosome 11, present with exotropic strabismus fixus. Patients with CFEOM3, mapped to chromosome 16, present with variable expression of ptosis and restrictive ophthalmoplegia.

Demographics

Congenital fibrosis of the extraocular muscles is a rare disorder. The prevalence of CFEOM is relatively unknown, although one report from the United Kingdom estimates this condition to occur in 1 out of 230,000 people. There are no reports of racial or gender predilection.

Significant History
- Age of onset
- Positive family history of similar ocular motility restrictions and ptosis

Ancillary Tests

Forced duction testing is useful in confirming the restrictive nature of this condition. Orbital imaging such as computed tomography or magnetic resonance imaging might also be of benefit. Imaging studies may show extraocular muscle atrophy, abnormal insertion, or absence.

The Treatment

Treatment for CFEOM is primarily surgical, however, proper refractive correction and treatment of amblyopia should be done prior to surgical intervention.

LEUKOCORIA
Suzanne M. Wickum
ICD—9: 360.44

THE DISEASE
Pathophysiology

Leukocoria literally means white pupil. Leukocoria itself is not a specific diagnosis, but rather a clinical finding suggestive of intraocular pathology. When an ocular condition disrupts light from striking the retina, a whitish reflex will be evident at the pupil rather than the usual red reflex.

Etiology

- The most common cause of leukocoria in children is cataracts. These lens opacities may be unilateral or bilateral. With congenital cataracts, one-third are inherited, one-third are associated with systemic disorders or syndromes, and one-third are idiopathic. Diagnosis is typically made at birth or soon after. Acquired cataracts in children have a variety of causes including, but not limited to, trauma, uveitis, metabolic disorders, and drug induced.

- The most common primary malignant intraocular tumor in children is retinoblastoma. Leukocoria is the most common presenting sign. This tumor appears as a yellowish-white, nodular mass with overlying and/or intralesional vascularization. Strabismus, glaucoma, retinal detachment, vitreous seeding, vitreal hemorrhage, pseudohypopyon, hyphema, proptosis, and even orbital cellulitis may occur. The tumors may be unilateral or bilateral. The average age at diagnosis is between 12 and 21 months.

- Coats' disease is a sporadic retinal telangiectasis that may lead to exudative retinal detachments. Leukocoria in this case is because of the retinal detachment. This disease is predominantly found in males (80%) and is typically unilateral (90%). Onset is usually between 8 and 10 years of age, although presentation in infancy has been reported. Advanced cases of Coats' disease can be difficult to differentiate from retinoblastoma by clinical exam alone.

- Persistent hyperplastic primary vitreous (PHPV) is a congenital abnormality caused by failure of the primary vitreous to regress. This condition is typically unilateral (90%) and sporadic. PHPV presents as a white fibrovascular membrane or mass adherent to the back of the lens. Leukocoria can result from the retrolental opacity or from a secondary cataract. Other features of PHPV include microphthalmia, shallow anterior chamber, dilated iris vessels, elongated ciliary processes, retinal detachment, and secondary angle-closure glaucoma.

- Retinopathy of prematurity (ROP) is a vasoproliferative retinopathy that occurs in premature and low–birth weight infants. Infants at risk include those born at less than 32 weeks gestation and/or weighing less than 1500 to 2000 grams. Diagnosis is typically made at 4 to 6 weeks of age. Leukocoria is because of retinal detachment found in the advanced stages of ROP.

- Toxocariasis is caused by infection with the larvae of *Toxocara canis*. Toxocara is unilateral and found more frequently in males than females. Frequently, there is a history of contact with puppies, eating dirt, or playing in a sandbox. The mean age of presentation is 7 years. Characteristics of toxocariasis include a white retinal granuloma, vitreous cells and haze, vitreous traction bands attaching to the macula or optic nerve, and retinal detachment. Leukocoria may be secondary to the granuloma, endophthalmitis, and/or associated retinal detachment.

- Children with retinal detachments are often asymptomatic, and thus diagnosis may be delayed until clinical signs become evident. When a retinal detachment is central and/or large, leukocoria may be the presenting sign. Retinal detachments in children are associated with trauma, ROP, chorioretinal colobomas, high myopia, aphakia, optic nerve pits, Coats' disease, toxocariasis, and retinal or choroidal tumors.

- Coloboma of the Retina and Choroid. Colobomas are congenital abnormalities that result from the failure of normal closure of the embryonic fissure. Leukocoria is evident because of white sclera that is visible through the abnormal retina and choroid. Coloboma of the optic nerve, lens, or iris may also be found. Retinal detachments may occur due to breaks in the abnormal retinal tissue.

- Myelination of the optic nerve fibers does not normally extend anterior to the lamina cribrosa; however, in approximately 1% of the population, the myelination reaches the retina. This benign condition occurs slightly more often in males and tends to be unilateral. The typical appearance is a feathery white opacity adjacent to the optic nerve and, when dense myelination is present, leukocoria may be evident. Vision is typically normal, although in cases of dense myelination, a corresponding scotoma may be found.

The Patient

Clinical Symptoms
Clinical symptoms will vary based on the specific etiology. Parents and/or the patient will complain of a white pupil and possibly reduced vision and/or an eye turn.

Clinical Signs
The clinical signs will vary based on the specific etiology. (See characteristics described earlier.)

Significant History
- Age of onset
- Prematurity and/or low birth weight
- Metabolic disorders or other systemic disorders/syndromes
- Maternal infection during pregnancy
- Contact with puppies, eating dirt, or playing in a sandbox
- Positive family history of one of the conditions listed here

Ancillary Tests

A complete ocular examination is necessary and should include measurement of the corneal diameter (microphthalmia), careful examination of the iris for neovascularization (retinoblastoma) and dilated iris vessels (PHPV), examination of the anterior chamber, looking for hyphema or pseudohypopyon (retinoblastoma), evaluation of the lens (cataract, PHPV), and careful anterior vitreous and fundus examination (retinoblastoma, toxocariasis, PHPV, ROP, Coats' disease, retinal detachment, chorioretinal coloboma, or myelinated nerve fiber).

Additional tests that may be useful in diagnosis include:

- B-scan ultrasound (cataract, PHPV, retinoblastoma, RD)
- Serum ELISA test (toxocariasis)
- Anterior chamber paracentesis (toxocariasis)
- Fluorescein angiography (Coats' disease, retinoblastoma, ROP)
- CT scan and/or MRI of the orbits and brain (Coats' disease, retinoblastoma)
- Systemic examination (retinoblastoma, congenital cataract)

The Treatment

- Cataracts: Treat any underlying systemic/metabolic conditions. For visually significant cataracts, surgical intervention and aggressive visual rehabilitation should take place as early as possible.
- Retinoblastoma: Treatment options include enucleation, external-beam radiation, cryotherapy, laser photocoagulation, brachytherapy, thermotherapy, or chemotherapy.
- Coats' Disease: Laser photocoagulation and/or cryotherapy to the leaking vessels. Surgical intervention is necessary if a retinal detachment develops.
- PHPV: Treatment may include cataract extraction and possible fibrovascular vitreal membrane extraction. Aggressive visual rehabilitation should begin after surgery.
- ROP: Treatment options include laser photocoagulation and cryotherapy. Additional surgical intervention is necessary if a retinal detachment develops.
- Toxocariasis: Recommended treatment includes oral thiabendazole plus prednisone. Photocoagulation or cryocoagulation may be used to destroy the organism if it is outside the foveal area. Surgery is necessary if tractional retinal detachments occur.
- Retinal Detachment: Laser, cryotherapy, scleral buckling, or vitrectomy surgery is required.
- Coloboma of the Retina and Choroid: Specific treatment of the coloboma is not necessary; however, if a retinal detachment develops, surgical intervention is required.
- Myelinated Nerve Fiber: No treatment is needed for this benign condition.

RETINOPATHY OF PREMATURITY (ROP)
W. Craig Lannin

ICD—9: 362.21

THE DISEASE

Despite significant advances in our understanding and management of the disease over the past 15 years, there is much about retinopathy of prematurity that remains elusive. We still do not know many details as to its cause and prevention, and our treatments are less than optimal. That ROP can cause devastating vision loss at the very beginning of life underscores the importance of continued research and progress in the implementation of prevention strategies.

Pathophysiology

There are two main schools of thought regarding the pathogenesis of ROP. The older of these two theories holds that the cytotoxicity of oxygen to developing endothelial cells leads to vaso-obliteration and eventually to vasoproliferation. The vaso-obliteration results in retinal nonperfusion, and the subsequent hypoxia promotes the formation of a vasoproliferative factor, similar to the mechanism in diabetes and other ischemic retinovascular disease.

The other theory also subscribes to the cytotoxicity of oxygen but places the site of this action at differentiating mesenchymal cells. These primitive spindle cells are derived from the hyaloid artery and migrate outward in the retinal nerve fiber layer toward the ora serrata. During this migration, the spindle cells differentiate into endothelial cells and ultimately into new retinal vessels. Increased oxygenation presumably causes free radical formation, which interferes with normal differentiation. This leads to the development of abnormal endothelial cells and neovascular shunts. The fetal retina is particularly vulnerable to free radical–mediated cell membrane damage because of the lack of mature, protective antioxidant enzyme systems. In addition to the effect of oxygen, it is possible that light and other factors may also play a role in the generation of free radicals.

Etiology

The two most important risk factors for ROP are the birth weight and the degree of prematurity. Those infants with a birth weight <1250 gm and/or a gestational age of <36 weeks are at particular risk. However, ROP can and does occur in infants with higher values. Twin status also conveys increased risk. White infants appear to be at greater relative risk than are Black infants with otherwise similar risk profiles.

The subject of supplemental oxygen therapy is also an important issue. After the 1950s, when high oxygen levels were linked to ROP, the use of supplemental oxygen was severely restricted. Today, neonatologists generally use the lowest concentration of supplemental oxygen compatible with optimizing the infant's overall status. Interestingly, there may be some benefit to utilizing supplemental oxygen to retard the progression of ROP once it becomes advanced.

There seems to be a fine line between hyperoxia and hypoxia. Although hyperoxia initiates the events leading to ROP, hypoxia appears to be deleterious once the ROP has become well established.

The role of light exposure has also been investigated as a contributor to the development of ROP. Although the infant has left the complete darkness of the intrauterine environment into one with any level of illumination is probably important in switching on the retina, it is uncertain whether quantification of the amount of light exposure modulates the development of ROP.

The Patient

Clinical Signs

The initial clinical sign evident on indirect ophthalmoscopic examination is the presence of an avascular peripheral retina. Later, a ridge may develop at the demarcation between the vascularized and avascular zones. If the ROP progresses, extraretinal neovascularization may develop along the ridge. This may be accompanied by dilation and tortuosity of the posterior pole vasculature, referred to as Plus Disease. Further progression leads to vitreous hemorrhage and/or retinal detachment. Severe fibrovascular proliferation can cause leukocoria, which gave rise to ROP's earlier name, retrolental fibroplasia. Anterior segment signs include poor pupillary dilation with engorgement of iris vessels. Late signs, some of which are related to regression of the disease, include retinal/optic disc dragging and macular ectopia, lattice-like peripheral retinal degeneration, cataracts, glaucoma, myopia, decreased visual acuity, strabismus, and retinal detachment.

Infants with ROP often have other significant systemic problems, including hydrocephalus, interventricular hemorrhage, cerebral palsy, and mental retardation, as well as pulmonary disease and congenital cardiac defects.

Classification

The development of the International Classification of Retinopathy of Prematurity in the early 1980s was an important step in enabling progress in the understanding and management of ROP. The classification scheme involves assigning a stage indicative of the condition's severity, assigning a zone parameter determined by the distance of the vascular/avascular demarcation from the optic disc in order to denote its posterior extent (an important prognostic indicator), and recording the circumferential extent of any neovascularization in clock hours.

- Stage 1: Flat demarcation line separating vascularized and peripheral avascular retina
- Stage 2: Ridged (three-dimensional) demarcation line
- Stage 3: Ridge with extraretinal (projecting into the vitreous) neovascularization
- Stage 4:
  - A: Extrafoveal retinal detachment
  - B: Subtotal RD involving the macula (zone 1)
- Stage 5: Total, retinal detachment
  - Zone 1: Circle with radius of twice the disc-fovea distance, measured from disc (posterior pole)
  - Zone 2: Circle with radius from disc to nasal ora, excluding zone 1
  - Zone 3: Circle with radius from disc to temporal ora, excluding zones 1 and 2 (temporal crescent)
  - Extent: Number of clock hours of circumferential involvement (30° sectors)
  - Plus Disease: Presence or absence

Screening Protocol

As birth weight is the most consistent predictor of risk, this parameter is most frequently chosen as the screening criteria, with the value beneath which every infant is examined generally being somewhere between 1500 and 1750 gm. If hydrops is present, the infant's dry weight can be overestimated and ROP missed, if this is not kept in mind. At the neonatologist's discretion, other heavier-weight babies may need to be examined, particularly if they are doing poorly in general. Gestational age can also be used as the screening parameter, although it is less reliably measured.

The initial dilated retinal examination with scleral depression should be conducted at the age of 4 to 6 weeks, with follow-up exams every 1 to 3 weeks, depending on the initial determination of stage and zone, until retinal vascular maturity is reached. If threshold disease (stage 3 disease, with at least five contiguous clock hours or eight total clock hours of extraretinal neovascularization, in association with Plus Disease) is reached, treatment should preferably be performed within 72 hours.

The Treatment

Threshold Stage 3

The Cryo-ROP Study demonstrated the efficacy of cryotherapy in reducing unfavorable outcomes (defined by retinal folds and retinal detachment), when applied at the time of threshold neovascularization development. Treatment is applied in a confluent pattern to ablate all of the avascular retina. Because of limitations of cryotherapy, particularly when applied for zone 1 disease, there has been increased utilization of indirect ophthalmoscopic laser photocoagulation as an alternative means of achieving peripheral retinal ablation. Studies have thus far indicated that laser treatment is at least as effective as cryotherapy and probably superior to cryotherapy for zone 1 disease.

Retinal Detachment

The treatment of stage 4 and stage 5 ROP with surgical methods including scleral buckling, lensectomy/vitrectomy, and lens-sparing vitrectomy have been much more problematic, particularly from the standpoint of visual outcome. Although structural success statistics have shown significant gains with improved techniques, achievement of better visual results has lagged behind. Stage 5 disease has the worst prognosis, but ambulatory vision can be achieved in some cases.

Prevention

As mentioned earlier, supplemental oxygen therapy has been utilized in ROP, and its carefully selected use has reduced the incidence of severe disease in some studies. Vitamin E therapy has been employed as an antioxidant approach, but results have been less beneficial than had been hoped. Similarly, light reduction strategies have generally been disappointing. Several ongoing controlled clinical trials will hopefully provide more definitive information about these approaches. Newer pharmacologic therapies aimed at modulating vascular development and affecting the involution of blood vessels seem to show some promise.

RETINOBLASTOMA

Suzanne M. Wickum

ICD—9: 190.5

THE DISEASE

Pathophysiology

Retinoblastoma is the most common primary malignant intraocular tumor found in children, accounting for approximately 5% of childhood blindness. Retinoblastomas appear as yellowish-white, nodular retinal masses with overlying and/or intralesional vascularization. Intralesional calcification is practically pathognomonic of retinoblastoma. Three growth patterns are recognized: endophytic tumors grow forward into the vitreous cavity, exophytic tumors grow into the subretinal space, and diffuse infiltrating tumors grow within the retina. As the tumor becomes more advanced, leukocoria, sensory strabismus, glaucoma, pupil irregularity, hyphema, pseudohypopyon, vitreal haze (secondary to tumor seeding), vitreal hemorrhage, proptosis, and even orbital cellulitis may be found.

Etiology

Retinoblastoma is an undifferentiated malignant neuroblastic tumor that may appear as a single tumor in the retina, or may have multiple foci. The retinoblastoma gene (Rb or Rb1) is a tumor suppressor gene located on the long arm of chromosome 13 at the 13q14 segment. When both alleles of the Rb gene are absent or mutated, primitive retinal cells may replicate in an uncontrolled manner, leading to tumor formation.

Approximately 40% of retinoblastomas are inherited in an autosomal dominant pattern, while the other 60% arise spontaneously. Germline, hereditary retinoblastoma is usually bilateral and multifocal, with early onset and diagnosis at an average age of 12 months. Sporadic, nonhereditary cases are unilateral and monofocal and tend to be smaller, with relatively later onset and diagnosis at an average age of 21 months. Unilateral presentation does not rule out germline retinoblastoma, as 15 to 20% of unilateral cases are hereditary. Trilateral retinoblastoma refers to bilateral retinoblastoma associated with a pineal or suprasellar intracranial tumor.

The Patient

Clinical Symptoms
Because of the young age at diagnosis, the patient is not usually able to express symptoms; however, parents may report evidence of reduced visual acuity and in rare cases pain.

Clinical Signs
- Leukocoria—because of the tumor color and location
- Strabismus—because of vision loss
- Acute red eye—because of glaucoma or uveitis associated with tumor necrosis
- Pseudohypopyon—because of tumor seeding into anterior chamber
- Hyphema—because of iris neovascularization
- Vitreal hemorrhage
- Vitreal seeding
- Orbital cellulitis
- Nystagmus—because of significant visual acuity loss
- Pupil irregularity

Demographics

Retinoblastoma accounts for approximately 3% of all cancer in children less than 15 years of age. Retinoblastoma occurs in 1/15,000 to 1/20,000 live births in the United States. There is no gender or racial predilection. Because the tumor arises from primitive retinal cells, the majority of cases occur in children less than 4 years of age.

Seventy-five percent of patients present with unilateral involvement and 25% with bilateral involvement.

If left untreated, retinoblastoma is almost certainly fatal, but with early diagnosis and treatment, the survival rate is greater than 90%. If tumor cells extend into or beyond the lamina cribrosa, then the survival rate decreases to 60%. If tumor cells are present at the transection site after enucleation, the survival rate decreases to 10 to 20%. Death from retinoblastoma most commonly occurs as a result of intracranial extension; however, other locations of metastasis include bone marrow, the liver, lymph nodes, and, rarely, the lungs.

Significant History

- Age of onset of leukocoria. If present at birth, then a developmental anomaly is most likely the etiology rather than retinoblastoma.
- Positive family history of retinoblastoma.

Ancillary Tests

The diagnosis of retinoblastoma is often based on characteristic ophthalmoscopy findings; however, several other tests should be performed to confirm the diagnosis and rule out tumor extension and metastasis.

- Ultrasonography to look for calcifications characteristic of retinoblastoma
- CT of the orbits to confirm intralesional calcification and to evaluate the extent of the tumor and tissue invasion
- MRI of the orbits and brain to better evaluate possible optic nerve invasion/extension or intracranial involvement as a result of metastasis or trilateral disease
- Radionuclide bone scan, bone marrow exam, and lumbar puncture are utilized for evaluation of possible metastasis
- Aspiration needle biopsy of intraocular lesions is contraindicated because of the potential to disseminate malignant cells

The Treatment

The goals of treatment include patient survival, globe retention, and vision preservation. The patient's cancer team will decide which treatment options are best based on the tumor size, location, laterality, visual acuity, and tumor extension. Small intraocular tumors, either single or multiple, can be treated with local therapy such as laser photocoagulation, cryotherapy, thermotherapy, or plaque radiation (brachytherapy). Large intraocular tumors, or cases with vitreous seeding, are treated with chemotherapy followed by local treatment, if appropriate. External-beam radiation is used after failure of chemotherapy and local treatment in older children. Enucleation is typically reserved for cases with large, unilateral tumors with no useful vision, eyes with glaucoma secondary to the tumor, and eyes with tumors that have failed other treatments. Treatment options for extraocular retinoblastoma include palliative treatment with radiation and/or intrathecal chemotherapy for central nervous system disease plus supportive care. There is no clearly proven effective therapy for these cases, and prognosis for survival is poor.

Follow-up should occur every 2 to 4 weeks while on treatment. Once treatment is concluded, follow-up should occur every 2 to 4 months until 3 years of age and then every 4 to 6 months until 5 to 7 years of age. For patients with germline retinoblastoma, some protocols recommend that an MRI be performed every 3 months for the first year after diagnosis and at least twice a year for the next 3 years. Genetic counseling is also an important part of patient management in these cases.

Cataract and Refractive Surgery Comanagement

CATARACT SURGERY MANAGEMENT

Brian Chou

CATARACTS

ICD—9: 366.0—Infantile, juvenile, and presenile cataract

ICD—9: 366.1—Senile cataract

ICD—9: 366.2—Traumatic cataract

ICD—9: 366.3—Cataract secondary to ocular disorders

ICD—9: 366.4—Cataract associated with other disorders

ICD—9: 366.8—Other cataract

ICD—9: 366.9—Unspecified cataract

ICD—9: 743.3—Congenital cataract and lens anomalies

THE DISEASE

Cataracts are a clouding of the crystalline lens. They are the leading cause of blindness in the world according to the World Health Organization. Depending on the location of clouding in the crystalline lens, cataracts are categorized as capsular, cortical, or nuclear.

Etiology

Although cataracts can be congenital, the most common cause of cataracts is because of natural aging. Other cataracts are associated with ocular inflammation, systemic disease (e.g., diabetes, Wilson's disease), radiation exposure, trauma, and the prolonged use of corticosteroids and other medicines (e.g., phenothiazines).

The Patient

Clinical Symptoms

Patients with cataract may complain of reduced vision, glare while driving into oncoming headlights and sunlight, a dulling of colors, and double images.

Clinical Signs

- Reduced best spectacle-corrected visual acuity with variable refraction.
- Crystalline lens opacity noted with biomicroscopy. Dilated examination of the lens using an optic section and retroillumination assists in visualizing the affected portion of the crystalline lens.
- The practitioner's view of the posterior pole with fundoscopy is degraded proportionate to the density of the cataract.

Ancillary Tests

When a dense cataract obscures the practitioner's view of the posterior pole during fundoscopy, the following measurements are useful:

- Potential acuity meter (PAM). The PAM provides an estimate of the patient's achievable acuity following cataract surgery. A reduced PAM measurement may indicate that amblyopia or pathology other than cataract limits the success of cataract surgery.
- B-scan ultrasound. When a dense cataract or vitreous hemorrhage obscure the direct view of the fundus, a B-scan can image the internal eye anatomy and determine whether the retina is intact.

The traditional indication for cataract surgery has been a best spectacle-corrected visual acuity worse than 20/40. However, functional disability can occur even with acuity in the 20/25 to 20/30 range. When case history describes functional disability, cataract surgery can also be justified when the following measurements show visual reduction:

- Glare testing (e.g., Brightness Acuity Tester)
- Contrast sensitivity (e.g., Bailey-Lovie and Pelli-Robson charts)

The Treatment

Cataract extraction with intraocular lens implantation is appropriate if the cataract interferes with the patient's activities of daily living. Surgery is also indicated if the cataract is obstructing examination of the posterior pole—for example, when the patient is under management for glaucoma or diabetic retinopathy.

Prior to surgery, a dilated fundus examination is necessary to rule out ocular pathology, which may contribute to reduced vision, such as macular disease. A-scan ultrasonography and keratometry are also required for calculating the power of the intraocular lens implant. Specular microscopy is desirable for obtaining an endothelial cell count. An endothelial cell count of 1,000 cells/mm^2 or less is at moderate to high risk of developing postoperative corneal edema (see section later).

Phacoemulsification describes cataract removal by emulsifying the lens with ultrasonic energy. Also called "phaco," this technique requires a small incision at the corneal limbus followed by a capsulorhexis, or creation of an opening through the anterior capsule. These entries allow a small ultrasonic probe to contact the cloudy lens material, breaking it up into small pieces that are concurrently irrigated and aspirated from the capsular bag. In place of the cloudy lens, the surgeon places a folded intraocular lens (IOL) through the corneal incision into the capsular bag, where the IOL is unfolded and properly positioned. Sutures are not usually necessary to close the small incision.

Phacoemulsification is currently the preferred form of cataract removal and has essentially replaced the older technique of extracapsular cataract extraction (ECCE), where the entire crystalline lens (except for the capsule) was removed in one piece through a larger incision. The use of a small self-sealing incision in phacoemulsification allows for a faster recovery with less patient discomfort. Small incisions also minimize any change in corneal curvature, which could negatively affect the postoperative refractive outcome. In selected cases, however, ECCE is still appropriate over phacoemulsification, including congenital cataracts and extremely hard and dense cataracts.

Postoperative Cataract Management

For the uneventful cataract surgery, an acceptable course of postoperative management includes the following:

- Antibiotic drops (e.g., moxifloxacin HCl 0.5%, one drop four times a day for 1 week)
- Nonsteroidal anti-inflammatory drops (e.g., diclofenac sodium 0.1%, one drop four times a day for 1 week)
- Corticosteroid drops (e.g., prednisolone acetate 1.0%, one drop four times a day for 1 week, then one drop two times a day for 2 weeks)
- The patient should use nighttime protective goggles and avoid strenuous activity for 1 to 2 weeks following surgery. No hot tubs, saunas, or swimming for 2 weeks after surgery.

Although there is no universal postoperative schedule, the following represents the author's usual schedule and measurements performed at each:

- Postop 1 day. Unaided visual acuity, pinholed visual acuity, biomicroscopy, tonometry
- Postop 1 week. Unaided visual acuity, refraction, biomicroscopy, tonometry
- Postop 4 weeks. Unaided visual acuity, refraction, biomicroscopy, tonometry, prescribe eyewear
- Postop 3 months. Spectacle-corrected visual acuity, biomicroscopy, tonometry, dilated fundus examination, recheck in 3 to 6 months

---

POSTOPERATIVE CATARACT COMPLICATIONS
Brian Chou

UVEITIS
ICD—9: 364.23—Lens-induced iridocyclitis
ICD—9: 364.04—Secondary iridocyclitis, noninfections

THE DISEASE

Some inflammation in the anterior chamber is expected during the immediate postoperative recovery. However, an unusually severe degree of cell and flare early after surgery or the persistence of intraocular inflammation beyond 4 weeks is not typical and requires further investigation.

Etiology

There are multiple causes of abnormal intraocular inflammation following phacoemulsification. The differential diagnosis includes infectious endophthalmitis, phacoanaphylaxis to lens protein remnants, abrupt taper of corticosteroids, patient nonadherence in using corticosteroid drops, preexisting uveitis, epithelial down growth, use of prostaglandin-like ocular hypotensives, uveitis-glaucoma-hyphema (UGH) syndrome, and incarceration of vitreous or iris to the wound.

The Patient

Clinical Symptoms
The patient may complain of photosensitivity, eye pain, and blurred vision, each with a wide range of severity.

Clinical Signs
Biomicroscopy will show inflammatory cells and possibly flare (protein transudate) in the anterior chamber. Other findings may include keratic precipitates, ciliary injection, a miotic pupil, and an intraocular pressure that is lower in the affected eye. In severe cases, a hypopyon may be present with fibrin in the anterior chamber.

Ancillary Tests

If infectious endophthalmitis is suspected, perform cultures and sensitivities on samples of the aqueous and vitreous. Gonioscopy is sometimes useful for detecting vitreous or iris to the wound and detecting remnants of lens material in the anterior chamber.

The Treatment

Treatment is based on the suspected cause of postoperative uveitis. For infectious endophthalmitis, refer to page 660 of this chapter. For phacoanaphylaxis, refer to Chapter 10, pages 236 to 239. If case history indicates patient nonadherence in using the corticosteroid drops or an abrupt taper, use of the drops should be reinstituted, emphasizing the importance of compliance to the patient. For preexisting uveitis, refer to Chapter 10, pages 236–239. For epithelial down growth, the patient should undergo argon laser treatment of the affected areas. In the case of prostaglandin-analog–induced uveitis, switch the patient to another class of ocular hypotensive. With UGH syndrome, the patient should have the IOL explanted or reanchored to prevent further iris chafing. For vitreous to the wound or iris prolapse, the patient should be referred promptly to the cataract surgeon for surgical management.

CORNEAL EDEMA
ICD—9: 371.2—Corneal edema
ICD—9: 371.20—Corneal edema, unspecified
ICD—9: 371.22—Secondary corneal edema
ICD—9: 371.23—Bullous keratopathy

THE DISEASE

Pseudophakic bullous keratopathy (PBK) describes irreversible corneal edema following cataract surgery with IOL implantation. Surgical trauma and inflammation can damage the corneal endothelium, the layer of cells that regulates corneal hydration. The effect of mild corneal edema is limited to the stroma, while moderate to severe corneal edema also affects the epithelium. When the corneal epithelium is edematous, blisters or "bullae" form that substantially reduce vision.

Etiology

The corneal epithelium and endothelium are semipermeable membranes involved in regulating corneal hydration. The stroma lying in between contains proteoglycans that attract fluid into the collagen. Intraocular pressure also tends to drive fluid into the cornea. When the stroma imbibes fluid, the tissue swells. To prevent excess corneal swelling, the endothelium drives fluid out of the cornea by creating an osmotic gradient. If the endothelial pump is impaired by disease or trauma, steady-state hydration is lost, causing corneal edema.

The Patient

Clinical Symptoms
Blurry and cloudy vision results with epithelial edema. The rupture of the epithelial bullae can cause pain, foreign body sensation, and photophobia.

Clinical Signs
Biomicroscopy will show folds in the corneal stroma, areas of microcystic epithelial edema, and epithelial bullae. Chronic cases may have corneal neovascularization. Endothelial guttata may be observable in cases of pre-existing endothelial dystrophy (e.g., Fuchs).

Ancillary Tests

Although the clinical diagnosis of corneal edema is primarily made with biomicroscopy, specular microscopy, and pachymetry can assist in the diagnosis. These measurements are also useful preoperatively for assessing the risk of persistent postoperative corneal edema.

- Specular microscopy. Imaging the endothelial layer provides a method for obtaining endothelial cell density. Normal densities may range from 2,000 to 3,500 cells/mm^2 depending on the age of the patient. Densities of 1,000 cells/mm^2 or less present an increased risk of problematic postoperative corneal edema.
- Pachymetry. The average central corneal pachymetry is approximately 550 microns, but in an edematous cornea, the tissue can swell substantially and result in increased corneal thickness of over 600 microns. This measurement is not diagnostic alone, since some individuals without corneal edema have thick corneas. However, within an individual, serial pachymetry can indicate diurnal fluctuations in corneal hydration or show longer term changes in corneal hydration because of endothelial damage.

The Treatment

Medical therapy primarily involves topical hyperosmotics, including 2% and 5% NaCl drops and ointment. Topical hyperosmotics draw out excess fluid from the cornea. Hyperosmotic ointment is usually used at bedtime, while the drops are used 3 to 5 times daily in the morning. In some cases, ocular hypotensives can also minimize the degree of corneal edema.

When there is a rupture of epithelial bullae, a high dK bandage soft contact lens (e.g., lotrafilcon A) can control of the discomfort until reepithelialization. Since ruptured bullae create the potential for microbial entry, a broad spectrum antibiotic drop should be prescribed for prophylaxis (e.g., moxifloxacin 0.5% tid).

Corneal transplantation is reserved for severe corneal edema where hyperosmotics provide insufficient benefit.

INTRAOCULAR PRESSURE SPIKES
ICD—9: 365.04

THE DISEASE

Increased intraocular pressure is commonly detected in the early postoperative cataract recovery. While a nonglaucomatous eye can sustain an IOP into the mid-20s mm Hg for a short duration without damage, higher IOPs require clinical action.

Etiology

Intraocular pressure spikes may result from a variety of causes:

- Retained viscoelastic. Viscoelastic is the thick cushioning solution used to "inflate" the anterior chamber during surgery and to protect the endothelium from mechanical insult. In some individuals, viscoelastic can significantly impede aqueous outflow, causing an IOP spike.

- Inflammatory material, hyphema, and dispersed pigment. The trabecular meshwork can become clogged with any of these components, leading to an IOP spike. Retained cortical fragments can incite an inflammatory response in proportion to the amount of cortical remnants. Uncommonly, an intraocular lens may incarcerate an iris blood vessel causing hemorrhage or rub against the iris dispersing pigment granules.
- Pupillary block. Formation of synechiae between the iris, and IOL can disrupt aqueous outflow and increase IOP. Pupillary block is rare and is seen mostly with anterior chamber IOLs where an iridectomy was not performed.
- Malignant glaucoma. This rare condition results when aqueous is misdirected into the vitreous cavity causing the iris to bow forward, causing a shallow anterior chamber. Unlike pupillary block, a peripheral iridotomy does not resolve the increased IOP.

The Patient

Clinical Symptoms
Patient symptoms generally do not signal elevated IOP when under 25 mm Hg. However, an acute rise of IOP over 35 mm Hg, as can happen with in pupillary block of malignant glaucoma, can be accompanied with redness, pain, and photophobia. Nausea and vomiting may also occur.

Clinical Signs
Elevated IOP is the primary indicator. Depending on etiology, biomicroscopy may show a flat anterior chamber, cortical remnants, hyphema, and so on.

Ancillary Tests

Not applicable.

The Treatment

When prescribing topical ocular hypotensives postoperatively, β-blockers are the drugs of choice. Avoid prostaglandin analogs and epinephrine derivatives. Prostaglandin analogs can exacerbate intraocular inflammation, while epinephrine can lead to cystoid macular edema. Intraocular pressure may also be quickly reduced by "burping" the paracentesis site to release aqueous.

In the case of pupillary block, a laser peripheral iridotomy should be performed if the cornea is clear enough to allow the treatment. However, if the cornea is steamy, instill a topical mydriatic agent (e.g., 1% cyclopentolate) to try breaking the synechiae. If the intraocular pressure is still not controlled, prescribe a topical β-blocker, oral carbonic anhydrase inhibitor, and/or oral hyperosmotic. Prednisolone acetate 1% q1 h should also be instilled to control intraocular inflammation. As soon as the cornea clears, a peripheral iridotomy should be performed.

For the treatment of malignant glaucoma, see Chapter 18, pages 470–476.

INFECTIOUS ENDOPHTHALMITIS
ICD—9: 360.01

THE DISEASE

Infectious endophthalmitis is perhaps the most feared complication following cataract surgery. Despite an incidence of less than 0.1%, the condition can quickly and irreversibly devastate vision. Infectious endophthalmitis can present within the first few days after surgery or have a delayed onset, weeks to even years later.

Etiology

Several different microorganisms may cause infectious endophthalmitis. Acute infectious endophthalmitis is most commonly caused by *Staphylococcus epidermidis*. Delayed onset infectious endophthalmitis may be because of fungi (including *Aspergillus* and *Candida*) and *Proprionibacterium acnes*.

The Patient

Clinical Symptoms
Worsening redness, pain, photosensitivity, and decreasing vision.

Clinical Signs
Unusually severe intraocular inflammation postoperatively, which may include granulomatous keratic precipitates and hypopyon. Signs include lid edema, conjunctival injection, pronounced cell and flare in the anterior chamber, and vitritis.

Ancillary Tests

Lab testing for postoperative infectious endophthalmitis is given in Chapters 1 and 3.

The Treatment

Bacterial endophthalmitis is an ocular emergency that requires prompt treatment to minimize vision loss. Patients should receive intravitreal antibiotics (e.g., vancomycin 1.0 mg/0.1 mL for gram-positive coverage and ceftazidime 2.25 mg/0.1 mL for gram-negative coverage) at the time of vitreal biopsy. Also prescribe topical fluoroquinolone (e.g., moxifloxacin 0.5% q1 h), corticosteroid (e.g., prednisolone acetate 1.0% q1 h), and a cycloplegic (e.g., homatropine 5% bid). Monitor the clinical outcome carefully every 4 to 8 hours until improvement is noted.

Although bacterial endophthalmitis was previously treated with systemic antibiotics, the results of the Endophthalmitis Vitrectomy Study (EVS) found no difference in final visual acuity or media clarity whether or not systemic antibiotics were employed. The EVS also found that patients presenting with hand-motion vision or better do not require an immediate pars plana vitrectomy, but patients presenting with only light perception have the best visual outcome when they undergo an immediate vitrectomy.

With fungal endophthalmitis, administer intravitreal amphotericin B (5 to 10 micrograms) at the time of vitreal biopsy. Therapeutic vitrectomy can be considered as well. Broad-spectrum antifungal therapy includes natamycin 5% suspension q1 h, flucytosine 37.5 mg/kg po q6 hs, and amphotericin B 0.25 to 0.3 mg/kg/day intravenously initially, then increased to 0.75 to 1.0 mg/kg/day in divided doses.

CYSTOID MACULAR EDEMA
ICD—9: 362.53

THE DISEASE

Cystoid macular edema (CME) refers to thickening of the retina around the fovea with or without small fluid-filled cysts. CME can occur in diabetic retinopathy, retinal vein occlusions, and many other conditions. When it occurs after cataract surgery, the condition is also referred to as Irvine-Gass syndrome. Approximately 3% of patients undergoing cataract surgery experience vision loss as a result of CME within the first postoperative year. The peak incidence occurs 6 to 10 weeks following surgery.

Etiology

Cystoid macular edema results from leaky perifoveal capillaries. There are several specific elements that may cause these capillaries to leak after cataract surgery:

- Intraocular inflammation where inflammatory mediators including prostaglandins cause vasodilation of the perifoveal capillaries
- Vitreal-retinal traction because of surgery or vitreal prolapse
- Use of epinephrine (or the prodrug, dipivefrin) eye drops
- Ultraviolet light

The Patient

Clinical Symptoms
Gradual and painless decrease in vision.

Clinical Signs
Using a 78 diopter or similar lens while viewing with an optic section will show retinal thickening and fluid cysts using an optic section. Resolution of the edema is best using a contact lens to view the macula.

Ancillary Tests

Fluorescein angiography shows leakage of the perifoveal capillaries during the early phase and a petal-shaped hyperfluorescence over the macula during the late phase. Optical coherence tomography (OCT) has been demonstrated to detect retinal thickening even before angiographic evidence of CME.

The Treatment

Postoperative CME often resolves spontaneously within 6 months. However, resolution can be hastened with a topical nonsteroidal anti-inflammatory (NSAID, e.g., diclofenac sodium 0.1% qid for 1 to 3 months). By inhibiting the cyclooxygenase pathway, prostaglandin synthesis is disrupted, which in turn is thought to reduce the perifoveal capillary leakage. There are also anecdotal reports that carbonic anhydrase inhibitors (e.g., acetazolamide, 250 mg p.o. bid) help clear macular edema. About 90% of pseudophakic CME with posterior chamber IOLs eventually regain acuity of 20/40 or better.

POSTERIOR CAPSULE OPACIFICATION (PCO)

ICD—9: 366.5—After-cataract
ICD—9: 366.50—After-cataract, unspecified
ICD—9: 366.52—Other after-cataract, not obscuring vision
ICD—9: 366.53—After-cataract, obscuring vision

THE DISEASE

Posterior capsule opacification is the most common complication following cataract surgery. A 1998 meta-analysis found that the rate of PCO after extracapsular cataract surgery with IOL implantation was 11.8% after 1 year, 20.7% after 3 years, and 28.4% after 5 years.

Etiology

PCO is characterized by a proliferation of equatorial lens epithelial cells along the posterior capsular surface. The result is thickening and clouding of the posterior capsule.

The Patient

Clinical Symptoms
Patients complain of decreased vision and glare.

Clinical Signs
Biomicroscopy shows a fibrotic membrane over the posterior capsule, most easily seen with the pupil dilated.

Ancillary Tests

Not applicable.

The Treatment

When PCO causes visual impairment, Nd:YAG (neodymium: yttrium-aluminum-garnet) capsulotomy is indicated. YAG treatment creates an opening in the posterior capsule by photodisrupting the opaque membrane. This procedure is routine and relatively safe. However, potential complications include intraocular inflammation, cystoid macular edema, IOP spikes, and retinal detachment.

Recent studies show that the incidence of PCO can be minimized through surgical techniques with capsular tension rings (CTRs) and square-edge intraocular lens implants.

RETINAL DETACHMENT
ICD—9: 361.0

THE DISEASE

The incidence of rhegmatogenous retinal detachment after uncomplicated cataract surgery is estimated at 0 to 3%, with approximately half of cases occurring within the first year of surgery. Loss of vitreous during the surgery is a significant risk factor because of resulting vitreo-retinal traction. There are conflicting reports on whether YAG capsulotomy increases the risk of retinal detachment.

(For Etiology, Clinical Symptoms, Clinical Signs, Ancillary Tests, The Treatment, see Chapter 17.)

WOUND LEAK
ICD—9: 360.3

THE DISEASE

Ocular hypotony refers to an abnormally low IOP, generally 5 mm Hg or less. One possible cause of postoperative hypotony is wound leak.

Etiology

Wound leak occurs when aqueous leaks from the anterior chamber to the globe's exterior.

The Patient

Clinical Symptoms
The patient may be asymptomatic or complain of eye pain and reduced vision.

Clinical Signs
Low IOP, positive Seidel's test, shallow anterior chamber, corneal folds.

Ancillary Tests

B-scan ultrasound is useful if the fundus is not easily viewed because of media opacity. In these cases, the B-scan can rule out causes of hypotony besides wound leak, including cyclodialysis and choroidal detachment.

The Treatment

In small leaks where the anterior chamber is still formed, place a bandage contact lens (e.g., lotrafilcon A), and prescribe a broad-spectrum antibiotic (e.g., moxifloxacin 0.5% qid) for prophylaxis. Recheck in 24 hours, as the wound can seal spontaneously. In larger wounds, consider applying cynoacrylate with a bandage contact lens on top. Large wounds require suturing.

LASIK MANAGEMENT
Brian Chou

THE PROCEDURE

LASIK, laser-assisted in situ keratomileusis, is the most widely performed refractive surgery. It is used to treat varying degrees of myopia and hyperopia either with or without astigmatism. During the procedure, the surgeon creates a hinged corneal flap, which is reflected back. The exposed stromal bed is then ablated with an excimer laser. The corneal flap is repositioned over the stromal bed, where the flap assumes a new curvature from the underlying ablation and then adheres without the need for sutures. Visual recovery is rapid, with most patients achieving functional vision by the next day.

Since the first LASIK procedure in 1991, the technique has evolved with improvements in microkeratectomy and the excimer laser ablation. An increasing number of surgeons are embracing femtosecond lasers in place of traditional blade technology to create the corneal tissue flap. In addition, most excimer platforms are FDA approved to attempt correcting higher order wavefront aberrations including coma, trefoil, secondary astigmatism, spherical aberration, and quadrafoil. The continuing refinements in LASIK technology should further improve safety and visual outcomes.

PREOPERATIVE EVALUATION

Candidates for LASIK should meet the following major criteria:

- Age 18 or older with stable refractive error. LASIK surgery on minors is controversial. Refractive stability is generally accepted as 0.50 diopters or less of change in any meridian during the past 6 months.
- Good general health. Systemic disease such as hypertension and diabetes should be well controlled before undergoing LASIK. Autoimmune diseases including rheumatoid arthritis and lupus generally preclude LASIK candidacy because of the risk of abnormal healing.

- Good eye health. The patient should not have uncontrolled or progressive eye disease such as cataracts, glaucoma, or macular degeneration. Contraindications for LASIK include keratoconus, pellucid marginal degeneration, Sjögren's syndrome, epithelial basement membrane dystrophy, and herpetic keratitis.
- Not pregnant or lactating. Hormonal changes during pregnancy and breast-feeding are documented to change refractive error in some individuals. Refractive fluctuations can interfere with determining the attempted correction and measuring the postoperative outcome.
- Realistic expectations. Arguably the most important factor in determining the patient's satisfaction with LASIK is whether the patient has realistic expectations. Individuals that expect perfect vision should not have LASIK, as they will probably be dissatisfied with most reasonable outcomes. A key point of understanding for patients is that corrective lenses are still required by the vast majority of those after LASIK to achieve the best vision. Of course, dependency of corrective lenses is usually reduced dramatically. Aside from dispelling unrealistic hopes and expectations, the clinician should make sure the patient does not harbor unrealistic fears about LASIK.

ROUTINE POSTOPERATIVE LASIK MANAGEMENT

For the uneventful LASIK surgery, an acceptable course of postoperative management includes the following:

- Antibiotic drops (e.g., moxifloxacin HCl 0.5%, one drop four times a day for 1 week)
- Corticosteroid drops (e.g., prednisolone acetate 1.0%, one drop four times a day for 1 week)
- The patient should use nighttime protective goggles and avoid strenuous activity for 1 to 2 weeks following surgery. No hot-tubs, saunas, or swimming for 2 weeks after surgery. Eye rubbing is not allowed for 4 weeks.

Although the schedule of postoperative visits varies from clinic to clinic, it is common to have progress checks at 1 day, 1 week, 4 weeks, 3 months, 6 months, and 12 months following the surgery.

COMMON POSTOPERATIVE LASIK COMPLAINTS

Most patient complaints following LASIK are not because of serious complications, such as flap dislodgement or infectious keratitis. Rather, many of the symptoms are just expected changes during the immediate postoperative recovery, for example, blurred and fluctuating vision, dryness symptoms, nighttime "glare and halos," and light sensitivity. All patients should be educated about these symptoms *before* their surgery so that they do not mistakenly conclude that they are experiencing a complication. However, when the aforementioned symptoms persist beyond the early recovery, action is necessary to prevent these clinical nuisances from becoming complications in the mind of the patient.

- Blurry vision because of residual refractive error. Although the excimer laser has submicron ablation precision, corneal healing and the biomechanical response lead to variable visual outcomes. The cornea may over- or underrespond to the LASIK treatment and result in residual refractive error. Treatment includes glasses and contact lenses, usually for part-time use. Surgical enhancement is also a possibility if refractive stability is achieved following the primary procedure (usually 3 months postoperative) and there is enough corneal thickness.

- Night vision disturbances. "Glare and halos" are common during the first few weeks after LASIK because of flap edema and remodeling of the stromal architecture. Lingering night vision problems beyond this time have several other causes, of which the most common is uncorrected spherical-cylindrical refractive error. Glasses for nighttime use is the primary treatment in such cases. Other causes of nighttime visual disturbances include irregular astigmatism, the pupil enlarging beyond the functional optical zone, and media opacity. Treatment is dictated on etiology. For a pupil enlarging beyond the functional optical zone, a common treatment is brimonidine tartrate 0.15% prn. While brimonidine is best known as an ocular hypotensive, it also has a miotic effect with generally favorable patient tolerance.

- Dryness symptoms. Dry eye is frequent after LASIK, especially in patients who were symptomatic before the procedure. The neurotrophic hypothesis states that post-LASIK dry eye occurs when the microkeratome severs nerves essential for lacrimation. These nerves can take months to regenerate, causing superficial punctate epitheliopathy and a poor tear film in the interim. Severe cases may show filamentary keratitis. Interestingly, some patients who show these signs do not complain of dryness, possibly because of sensory denervation. Other patients without clinical signs of dry eye complain of pronounced dryness symptoms, which can be explained by spontaneous firing of severed sensory nerves. Ocular lubricants are the cornerstone of therapy. Punctal plugs may also provide relief. In cases where there is a pre-existing inflammatory component to the dry eye, topical corticosteroids (e.g., 0.2% loteprednol bid) and immunosuppresives (e.g., cyclosporine 0.05% bid) can help. An often overlooked cause of dryness symptoms is meibomian gland dysfunction. Patients are warned not to rub their eyes after LASIK, which is conducive to causing meibomian gland inspissation. Normal flora on the eyelid metabolize the sebum into fatty acids, which are toxic to the corneal surface and produce symptoms of burning and dryness. Because lid hygiene may disturb the corneal flap soon after LASIK, oral doxycycline 100 mg bid is a more appropriate treatment in these cases.

POST-LASIK COMPLICATIONS

To be sure, the overwhelming number of LASIK surgeries proceed uneventfully, and the patients are happy with the outcomes. Yet as with any type of surgery, potential risks come as part of the territory. Patients should understand that the postoperative visits are important for catching problems before they become serious. The visits are also important for monitoring the healing and response to treatment. The key point of patient education is that LASIK is not an isolated event that takes 15 to 20 minutes in the surgical suite but that it is a *process* that also requires appropriate professional care before and after the procedure.

- Epithelial defects result in 1.6% of LASIK cases after microkeratectomy, with greater frequency in older patients. Epithelial membrane basement dystrophy (EBMD) and a history of corneal abrasion are also risk factors for epithelial defects after LASIK. A bandage contact lens is placed in these cases to improve patient comfort while the epithelial defect closes, usually within 48 hours. Pressure patching is contraindicated because of the risk of flap dislodgement. Frequent ocular lubricants are necessary to facilitate adherence of the epithelium and to prevent recurrent corneal erosion. If the epithelium overlying the defect is raised and irregular, prescribe 5% NaCl solution qid and nighttime ointment. Any surface irregularity may take weeks to months to smooth out and in the meantime can disturb vision, especially if it is located within the visual axis. The presence of epithelial defects after LASIK is a documented risk factor for epithelial ingrowth and diffuse lamellar keratitis.

- Epithelial ingrowth refers to the migration of epithelium underneath the flap edge. Epithelial ingrowth exists to some degree in 10 to 30% of cases after LASIK. However, only a fragment of these cases are clinically where vision is threatened and surgical removal is necessary. Epithelial ingrowth cannot be diagnosed the day after LASIK. However, potential areas of ingrowth are detectable at postop day 1 by instilling fluorescein to show areas of the flap gutter that have not "zippered" to prevent migration of epithelium under the flap. Epithelial ingrowth is generally detectable days to weeks after LASIK. In mild presentations where epithelial migration is less than 1.0 mm under the flap edge, biomicroscopy will show a thin sheet in the interface between the stromal bed and corneal flap. These mild cases are often easiest to detect with biomicroscopy using indirect illumination. If follow-up shows the mild ingrowth is stable, no treatment is necessary. However, progressive epithelial ingrowth beyond 1.0 mm from the flap edge can impede nutrient diffusion and lead to keratolysis if not removed promptly by the surgeon. In these severe cases, the epithelium will form opaque, cyst-like nests. Removal requires relifting the flap.

- Also called "Sands of the Sahara" to describe its clinical appearance, diffuse lamellar keratitis (DLK) is characterized by a sterile accumulation of inflammatory cells in the interface between the stromal bed and corneal flap. DLK is usually noted the day after LASIK during biomicroscopy. The inflammatory cells originate from the limbal vasculature and spread centrally. Mild cases are estimated to occur in 1 of every 25 LASIK cases. Severe, vision-threatening DLK is estimated to occur in 1 of every 5,000 LASIK cases. Patients with DLK are usually asymptomatic, presenting with a white and quiet eye. Sometimes, they may complain of light sensitivity and foreign body sensation. While the cause of DLK is mysterious, a multifactorial etiology is likely. Proposed culprits include bacterial endotoxins, blood, talc from gloves, dust, and residual chemicals from the microkeratome. It is also noteworthy that epithelial defects are associated with a 13 times greater incidence of DLK and that there are reports of late-onset DLK secondary to corneal trauma. Mild cases of DLK generally resolve just with the usual postoperative course of corticosteroids. Moderate cases require an increased dosing of corticosteroids (e.g., prednisolone acetate 1% q1 h) with follow-up each day until there is improvement. Florid presentations necessitate immediate referral to the surgeon for flap lifting and interface irrigation. If severe DLK is untreated, the inflammatory cells can release keratolytic enzymes, leading to permanent vision loss.

- The incidence of post-LASIK infectious keratitis is estimated at 1 in every 3,000 LASIK cases. Unlike DLK, post-LASIK infectious keratitis is accompanied by symptoms of redness, aching pain, and photosensitivity. Most cases of infectious keratitis present during the first week after surgery. Slit-lamp findings include conjunctival injection and the presence of infiltrate (often with an associated epithelialopathy) and inflammatory cells in the surrounding interface in a more focal pattern. In severe cases, cell and flare are present in the anterior chamber. When infectious keratitis is suspected, immediate referral to the surgeon is appropriate for flap lifting and culturing. Empiric therapy is not recommended, as most of the organisms are opportunistic and not responsive to conventional therapy. In one study, the most common organisms cultured in post-LASIK infectious keratitis were atypical mycobacterium and staphylococci.

- Folds in the corneal flap are most commonly introduced after high myopic ablations, when the flap conforms to the ablated stromal bed. Less frequently, striae occur after trauma displaces the flap. Crinkles in Bowman's membrane usually do not significantly impair visual quality. In contrast, a true fold in the flap can decrease vision, especially when within the visual axis. Visually significant folds are present in about 1% of all LASIK procedures. These cases are treated by surgically relifting the flap to stretch and smooth out the undulation. Removal of striae is most effective when done early. Removal becomes progressively more difficult after weeks to months elapse.

- Irregular astigmatism can occur from ablation and healing abnormalities. Categories of irregular astigmatism include iatrogenic keratectasia, central islands, peninsulas, and decentered optical zones. Clinicians can lower the incidence of iatrogenic keratectasia by preoperatively excluding patients who have asymmetric corneal topographies, less than 500 microns of central corneal thickness, and a calculated posterior stroma of less than 250 microns following microkeratectomy and ablation. New excimer technologies with eye-tracking and scanning, small-area ablations have reduced the incidence of central islands, peninsulas, and decentered optical zones. Significant irregular astigmatism may lead patients to complain of poor visual quality even when looking through the best spherical-cylindrical overrefraction. Visual acuity will improve with pinhole. Irregular astigmatism is manifested by manual keratometry as mire distortion. Corneal topography will show asymmetrical steep and flat areas. Wavefront aberrometry can measure the magnitude of higher order aberrations. Soft contact lenses can sufficiently mask mild irregular astigmatism. However, with moderate to severe irregular astigmatism, rigid gas permeable contact lenses are the primary treatment for restoring good vision. Keratoconus lens designs are usually necessary for iatrogenic keratectasia, while reverse geometry designs are typically required for central islands, peninsulas, and decentered optical zones. Intracorneal ring implantation (i.e., Intacs™, Addition Technologies, Inc.) is under investigation for post-LASIK ectasia. Wavefront and topographically driven excimer lasers are under investigation for "touch-up" surgeries to fix central islands, peninsulas, and decentered optical zones.

- Interface debris may include fibers, blood, implanted epithelium, meibomian gland secretions, talc from gloves, and metallic blade remnants. In most cases, the sequestration of these substances underneath the corneal flap is not clinically significant, and they may be left alone. However, when vision may be reduced, flap lifting and irrigation/removal is appropriate. For example, implanted epithelium lying within the entrance pupil should be removed. Even though epithelial ingrowth does not result in these cases, the implanted epithelium can cause a local inflammation and result in surrounding opacification. Another instance where removal is indicated is when fiber debris extends outside the flap edge. A jutting fiber can serve as an entry point for microbial infection underneath the flap. In most cases, these fibers can be removed behind the slit lamp without lifting the flap by using topical anesthesia and a surgical spear or forceps.

KERATOCONUS

Brian Chou

ICD—9: 371.60—Keratoconus, unspecified
ICD—9: 371.61—Keratoconus, stable condition
ICD—9: 371.62—Keratoconus, acute hydrops

THE DISEASE

Pathophysiology

Keratoconus is a noninflammatory, progressive corneal ectasia. Inferior and irregular corneal steepening is typical. Keratoconus is generally accepted as a bilateral condition, although the severity of corneal distortion is often asymmetric between the two eyes.

While corneal perforation is rare in keratoconus, acute corneal hydrops occurs in some cases. Hydrops describes a rupture of Descemet's membrane followed by aqueous being imbibed into the corneal stroma.

Etiology

The cause of keratoconus is not completely understood. A genetic predisposition is known, however. Individuals with keratoconus are more likely to have another family member with the same disease. In the Collaborative Longitudinal Evaluation of Keratoconus (CLEK), 13.5% of the 1,209 keratoconic subjects reported a blood relative also with the condition.

External factors, including eye rubbing and gas permeable (GP) contact lens wear, may also have a role in the pathophysiology. In CLEK and other studies, at least half of the keratoconus subjects studied reported significant eye rubbing. Despite the strong association, it is not known whether eye rubbing actually causes keratoconus. Additionally, there are reports of "normal" patients undergoing hard contact or GP lens wear, whereupon discontinuation of contact lens wear, keratoconus was diagnosed. Although the implication is that hard or GP contact lens wear can cause keratoconus, this is difficult (if not impossible) to prove because a disproportionate number of these contact lens wearers may have undiagnosed keratoconus.

One unifying hypothesis is that corneal microtrauma, whether from eye rubbing or contact lens wear, can cause the up regulation of degradative enzymes in the cornea of genetically predisposed individuals. The degradative enzymes can lead to focal thinning and distortion of the cornea. Future studies will test the validity of this hypothesis.

The Patient

Clinical Symptoms

Despite the best spectacle lenses or soft contacts, the keratoconus patient may complain of a poor quality of vision with multiple images. Vision may fluctuate. Less common complaints include photophobia and foreign body sensation.

Acute hydrops causes sudden blurred vision, redness, photophobia, and discomfort.

Clinical Signs

Advanced keratoconus is relatively easy to diagnose, whereas diagnosis of early keratoconus and subclinical "forme-fruste" disease is often difficult. In cases of suspected keratoconus, you may need to monitor several of the following clinical signs over time to make a definitive diagnosis.

- External evaluation. Advanced cases will demonstrate Munson's sign: When the patient looks downward, the apex of corneal distortion will displace the lower eyelid margin.
- Keratometry. Keratometry values that are steep (e.g., over 48.00 diopters K) in conjunction with mire distortion are common. To extend the range of the manual keratometer, tape a +1.25 diopter trial lens on the side that faces the patient. Add 8.00 diopters K to the drum reading that you measure.
- Corneal topography. The classic topographical pattern shows asymmetric inferior corneal steepening.
- Retinoscopy. The retinoscopic reflex is frequently irregular, with a swirling or scissoring motion.
- Manifest refraction. The refraction end-point is often variable. High myopia and astigmatism are common. Visual acuity is frequently reduced but can improve with pinhole.
- Biomicroscopy. The most common slit-lamp finding is a Fleischer's ring (present in 86% of keratoconus patients), a deposition of iron that may form a partial or complete ring around the cone's base. The cobalt blue filter can enhance the visualization of a Fleischer's ring. Corneal folds at the level of Descemet's membrane, called Vogt's striae, are present in 65% of keratoconus patients. These folds are usually vertical, running parallel to the steep meridian of the cornea. Vogt's striae temporarily disappear when intraocular pressure is raised by gentle pressure on the globe. Apical scarring is present in 53% of keratoconus patients. The scarring may result from the disease itself or a contact lens that causes mechanical trauma.

Demographics

Keratoconus affects approximately 1 in 2,000 individuals. There is no known gender or racial prediction.

Onset is typically during adolescence and is followed by progressive corneal thinning and distortion. Keratoconus usually arrests on its own and stabilizes during the third to fourth decade of life.

Several clinicians have noted that few older keratoconus patients are seen in the office. This has led to the suggestion the life expectancy of keratoconus is reduced. One study has shown, that their life expectancy does not significantly differ from that of the normal population. Rather, it appears that older keratoconus patients do not seek eyecare as frequently.

Some early literature suggested a link between keratoconus and certain collagen-vascular disorders, such as Ehlers-Danlos syndrome, Marfan's syndrome, and osteogenesis imperfecta. More recent data questions the existence of these associations.

Ancillary Tests

- Pachymetry. Central corneal thickness below 450 microns may suggest keratoconus. Abnormal midperipheral and peripheral pachymetry may also assist in diagnosis.
- Posterior corneal topography. Keratoconus patients typically have abnormalities on the posterior corneal surface in addition to the anterior surface. The Orbscan II (Bausch & Lomb) provides the posterior corneal topography readings.
- Wavefront aberrometry. Although the role for diagnosis is still emerging, studies already show that keratoconus demonstrates a relatively large amount of higher order aberrations, including coma.

The Treatment

Supportive

Prescribe a mast-cell stabilizer and antihistamine combination (e.g., Patanol) to minimize eye rubbing and to increase ocular comfort. Advise the patient that LASIK is contraindicated. Recommend that family members have their eyes examined because of an increased likelihood that they also have keratoconus. Direct patients to nonprofit information resources such as Center for Keratoconus (www.Kcenter.org) and the National Keratoconus Foundation (www.NKCF.org).

Visual Rehabilitation

For mild cases, spectacles and soft contact lenses can provide functional vision. For most with keratoconus, specialty GP contacts remain the principal treatment for providing good vision. GP contacts provide a smooth optical surface to effectively address most of the aberrations in keratoconus. GP contacts do not retard the natural progression of keratoconus. Popular GP lenses for keratoconus include nonproprietary designs (e.g., Soper and McGuire designs) and proprietary designs (e.g., Rose-K, ComfortKone, Ni-Cone, etc.). Although there is some evidence that GP lenses may cause keratoconic progression, no reasonable practitioner should withhold prescribing them to give functional vision.

For patients intolerant of even optimally prescribed GP lenses, consider piggyback systems (e.g., Flexlens Piggyback), large diameter GP lenses (e.g., Dyna-Intralimbal, Macrolens), and hybrid lenses (Softperm). Patients that fail all contact lens modalities, even after any ocular surface disease is managed, may be candidates for intracorneal ring implantation (Intacs).

Intacs surgery for keratoconus was first performed in 1997. Intacs are approved by the FDA for keratoconus under a Humanitarian Device Exemption. One study showed improvement of unaided visual acuity by four lines and improvement of best spectacle-corrected acuity by two lines. The vast majority of keratoconus patients undergoing Intacs still require postoperative visual correction. The goal of Intacs for keratoconus is to offer the GP-intolerant patient adequate vision in soft contacts and glasses and to avoid penetrating keratoplasty. The long-term consequences of Intacs on the natural disease process, if any, are unknown.

The end-of-the-line treatment for keratoconus is penetrating keratoplasty (PKP). The predominant indication is when corneal scarring within the visual axis limits vision even with an optimally prescribed contact lens. Some 10 to 25% of keratoconus patients will undergo PKP. It is a highly successful type of surgery, with about 95% of patients achieving an optically clear donor cornea. However, most will still require visual correction. One study found that up to 30% require spectacles and 47% require contact lenses following the procedure.

Acute Corneal Hydrops

Hydrops is treated with hyperosmotics (5% NaCl gtts qid) and cycloplegia. Nevertheless, the corneal swelling can persist for weeks to months. When the hydrops resolves at least some scarring is left behind. In some cases, the scarring can flatten the corneal shape, making vision better than before. Because of the possibility of improved vision after resolution, acute hydrops is not an emergent indication for PKP.

Ophthalmic Abbreviations

A	assessment	AZT	azidothymidine
AC	anterior chamber	BAT	brightness acuity test
ac	before meals	BCC	basal cell carcinoma
AC/A	accommodative convergence/accommodation ratio	BCG	Bacille de Calmette-Guerin
		BD	base-down prism
ACE	angiotensin-converting enzyme	BI	base-in prism
		bid	two times a day
ACG	angle-closure glaucoma	BO	base-out prism
ACT	alternate cover test	BRAO	branch retinal artery occlusion
ACIOL	anterior chamber intraocular lens	BRVO	branch retinal vein occlusion
AION	anterior ischemic optic neuropathy	BSS	balanced salt solution
ALK	automated lamellar keratoplasty	BU	base-up prism
		Bx	biopsy
ALK-E	automated lamellar keratoplasty-Excimer	CAI	carbonic anhydrase inhibitor
ALL	allergies	CB(B)	ciliary body (band)
ALP	argon laser photocoagulation	CBC	complete blood count
		CC	chief complaint or chief concern
ALT	argon laser trabeculoplasty (or trabeculopexy)	cc	with correction (cum correctio)
AMPPE	acute multifocal placoid pigment epitheliopathy	ccl	with contact lenses
		CCT	central corneal thickness
ANA	antinuclear antibodies	C/D	cup-to-disc ratio
APD	afferent pupillary defect (see RAPD)	CDCR	conjunctivodacryocysto-rhinostomy
APON	acquired pit of the optic nerve	C&F	cell and flare
		CF	confrontation field or count fingers vision
AR	autorefraction		
ARC	abnormal or anomalous retinal correspondence	CL	contact lens
		CME	cystoid macular edema
ARMD	age-related macular degeneration	CMV	cytomegalovirus
		CNV	choroidal neovascularization
ASC	anterior subcapsular cataract	COAG	chronic open-angle glaucoma
A/V	artery to vein ratio		

CPEO	chronic progressive external ophthalmoplegia	ESR	erythrocyte sedimentation rate
CR	cycloplegic refraction	ET	esotropia
CRAO	central retinal artery occlusion	ET′	esotropia at near
		E(T)	intermittent esotropia
CRVO	central retinal vein occlusion	EUA	exam under anesthesia
		EWCL	extended-wear contact lens
CS	contrast sensitivity	FA	fluorescein angiography
CSF	cerebrospinal fluid	FB	foreign body
CSM	central, steady, and maintained fixation	FH	family history
		FTA-ABS	fluorescent treponemal antibody absorption test
CSME	clinically significant macular edema		
CSR	central serous retinopathy	FTFC	full to finger counting (confrontation visual fields)
CT	cover test or center thickness (contact or spectacle lens) or computed tomography		
		Fx	fracture
		GBE	ginkgo biloba extract
		GCA	giant cell arteritis
		GO	Graves' ophthalmopathy
CVA	cerebrovascular accident	GPC	giant papillary conjunctivitis
Cyl	cylinder	gt	drop (gutta)
D	diopter	gtt	drops (guttae)
DCG	dacryocystography	H	hypophoria
DCR	dacryocystorhinostomy	HA	headache
dd	disc diameter	HADM	hemorrhage at the disc margin
D&I	dilation and irrigation		
DS	diopter sphere	HCL	hard contact lens
DVD	dissociated vertical deviation	HEMA	hydroxyethylmethacrylate
DWCL	daily wear contact lens	HLA	human leukocyte antigen
Dx	diagnosis		
E	esophoria	HM	hand motion (or movement)
E′	esophoria at near		
ECCE	extracapsular cataract extraction	HPI	history of present illness
		HRR	Hardy-Rand-Ritter color vision plates
EKC	epidemic keratoconjunctivitis		
		HRT	Heidelberg retina tomograph
ELISA	enzyme-linked immunosorbent assay		
		HSV	herpes simplex virus
EOG	electro-oculogram	HT	hypertropia
EOM	extraocular muscles	HTN	hypertension
EPI	epinephrine	Hx	history
ERG	electroretinogram	HZV	herpes zoster virus

ICCE	intracapsular cataract extraction		Lproj	light projection
ICE	iridocorneal epithelial syndrome		LR	lateral rectus muscle
			MCT	medial canthal tendon
ICG	indocyanine green		MEDS	medications
IDDM	insulin-dependent diabetes mellitus		MEWDS	multiple evanescent white dot syndrome
IDU	idoxuridine		MG	myasthenia gravis or Marcus-Gunn pupil
IK	interstitial keratitis		MHA-TP	microhemaglutination test for *Treponema pallidium test*
INH	isoniazid			
INO	internuclear ophthalmoplegia			
			MLF	medial longitudinal fasciculus
IO	inferior oblique muscle			
IOFB	intraocular foreign body		mm Hg	millimeters of mercury
IOL	intraocular lens		MKM	myopic keratomileusis
ION	ischemic optic neuropathy		MR	medial rectus muscle or manifest refraction or Maddox rod
IOP	intraocular pressure			
IPC	intermediate posterior curve		MRA	magnetic resonance angiogram
IR	inferior rectus		MRI	magnetic resonance imaging
IRMA	intraretinal microvascular abnormalities		MS	multiple sclerosis
			MTMT	maximum tolerated medical therapy
IVFA	intravenous fluorescein angiography		N	nasal
JXG	juvenile xanthogranuloma		NaFl	sodium fluorescein
			NAG	narrow-angle glaucoma
KM	keratomileusis		NCT	noncontact tonometer
KP	keratic precipitates		Nd	neodymium
K's	keratometric readings		NFL	nerve fiber layer
KCS	keratoconjunctivitis sicca		NFLA	nerve fiber layer analyzer
			NIPH	no improvement with pinhole
LCT	laser coherence tomography or lateral canthal tendon			
			NKDA	no known drug allergies
			NLD	nasolacrimal duct
LASEK	laser epithelial keratomileusis		NLP	no light perception; total blindness
LASIK	laser in situ keratomileusis		NPA	near point of accommodation
LI	laser interferometry		NPC	near point of convergence
LKP	lamellar keratoplasty			
LL	lower lid		NPDR	nonproliferative diabetic retinopathy
LLLL	lids, lashes, lacrimals, lymphatics			
			NRC	normal retinal correspondence
LP	light perception			

NS	nuclear sclerosis	PCO	posterior capsular opacification
NSAID	nonsteroidal anti-inflammatory drug	PD	prism diopter (symbol: Δ) or pupillary distance
NVD	neovascularization of the disc	PDR	proliferative diabetic retinopathy
NVE	neovascularization-elsewhere	PDT	photodynamic therapy
NVG	neovascular glaucoma	PE	pigment epithelium
NVI	neovascularization of the iris	PED	pigment epithelial detachment
O	objective	PEK	punctate epithelial keratopathy
OA (OAD)	overall diameter of contact lens	PERRLA	pupils equal, round, reactive to light and accommodation
OAG	open-angle glaucoma		
OCT	ocular coherence tomography	PET	positive emission tomograph
OD	right eye (oculus dexter)		
ODM	ophthalmodynamometry	PH	pinhole visual acuity
OHT	ocular hypertension	PHM	posterior hyaloid membrane
OKN	optokinetic nystagmus		
ON	optic nerve	PHN	postherpetic neuralgia
ONH	optic nerve head	PHPV	persistent hyperplastic primary vitreous
OPG	oculopneumoplethysmo-graphy	PI	peripheral iridectomy or iridotomy
OR	overrefraction		
OS	left eye (ocular sinister)	PKP	penetrating keratoplasty
OU	both eyes (oculi unitas) or each eye (oculi uterque)	pl	plano lens
		PL	preferential looking
		PMMA	polymethyl methacrylate
OWS	overwear syndrome	PMH	past medical history
OZ	optical zone of a contact lens	po	by mouth (orally)
		POAG	primary open-angle glaucoma
P	plan		
PAM	potential acuity meter	POH	past ocular history
PAR	posterior apical radius	POHS	presumed ocular histoplasmosis syndrome
PAS	peripheral anterior synechia or periodic-acid Schiff		
		PP	perfusion pressure
PC	peripheral curve on a contact lens or posterior chamber	PPRF	pontine paramedian reticular formation
		prn	as needed
pc	after meals	PRP	pan-retinal photocoagulation
PCF	pharyngoconjunctival fever	PRK	photorefractive keratectomy (or keratoplasty)
PCIOL	posterior chamber intraocular lens		

PSC	posterior subcapsular cataract	sc	without correction *(sine correctio)*
PSP	progressive supranuclear palsy	SCC	squamous cell carcinoma
PTC	pseudotumor cerebri	SCL	soft contact lens
PTG	pneumatonograph	SH	social history
PTK	phototherapeutic keratectomy	SL	Schwalbe's line
		SLE	slit-lamp examination or systemic lupus erythematosus
PVD	posterior vitreous detachment		
PVR	proliferative vitreoretinopathy	SLK	superior limbic keratoconjunctivitis
PXE	pseudoxanthoma elasticum	SLO	scanning laser ophthalmoscope
PXF	pseudoexfoliation	SLT	selective laser trabeculoplasty
q	every		
qd	one time per day	SO	superior oblique muscle
qh	every hour	S&P	sharp and pink
qhs	at bedtime	SPK	superficial punctate keratopathy (or keratitis)
qid	four times a day		
RAPD	relative afferent pupillary defect	Sph	sphere
RB	rose bengal stain	SR	superior rectus muscle
RCE	recurrent corneal erosion	SRNVM	subretinal neovascular membrane
RD	retinal detachment	SS	scleral spur
RGP	rigid gas permeable contact lenses	STS	serological test for syphilis
RK	radial keratotomy	SVP	spontaneous venous pulsation
RLF	retrolental fibroplasia		
ROP	retinopathy of prematurity	SWAP	short wavelength automated perimetry
ROS	review of systems	T	temporal
RP	retinitis pigmentosa	TA	temporal arteritis
RPR	rapid plasma reagin	Tap	applanation tonometry
RPE	retinal pigment epithelium	TBUT	tear breakup time
		TED	thyroid eye disease
R&R	recess-resect	TIA	transient ischemic attack
RTA	retinal thickness analyzer		
		tid	three times a day
RTC	return to clinic	TKP	thermal keratoplasty
S	subjective	TLS	tight lens syndrome
SBV	single binocular vision	TM	trabecular meshwork
		TTT	transpupillary thermal therapy
SC	secondary curve on a contact lens	Tx	treatment

UGH	uveitis-glaucoma-hyphema syndrome	VER	visual-evoked response
		VF	visual fields
UL	upper lid	X	exophoria
ung	ointment	X′	exophoria at near
VA	visual acuity	XT	exotropia
VDRL	venereal disease research laboratory test	XT′	exotropia at near
		X(T)	intermittent exotropia
		YAG	yttrium-aluminum-garnet laser
VEP	visual-evoked potential		

Vertex Conversion Chart/ Dioptic Conversion Chart

▶ **TABLE B.1** Vertex Conversion Chart

Spectacle Lens Power	Plus Lenses		(+)		Vertex Distance/mm			
	8	9	10	11	12	13	14	15
4.00	4.12	4.12	4.12	4.12	4.25	4.25	4.25	4.25
4.50	4.62	4.75	4.75	4.75	4.75	4.75	4.75	4.87
5.00	5.25	5.25	5.25	5.25	5.25	5.37	5.37	5.37
5.50	5.75	5.75	5.75	5.87	5.87	5.87	6.00	6.00
6.00	6.25	6.37	6.37	6.37	6.50	6.50	6.50	6.62
6.50	6.87	6.87	7.00	7.00	7.00	7.12	7.12	7.25
7.00	7.37	7.50	7.50	7.62	7.62	7.75	7.75	7.75
7.50	8.00	8.00	8.12	8.12	8.25	8.25	8.37	8.50
8.00	8.50	8.62	8.75	8.75	8.87	8.87	9.00	9.12
8.50	9.12	9.25	9.25	9.37	9.50	9.50	9.62	9.75
9.00	9.75	9.75	9.87	10.00	10.12	10.25	10.37	10.37
9.50	10.25	10.37	10.50	10.62	10.75	10.87	11.00	11.12
10.00	10.87	11.00	11.12	11.25	11.37	11.50	11.62	11.75
10.50	11.50	11.62	11.75	11.87	12.00	12.12	12.25	12.50
11.00	12.00	12.25	12.37	12.50	12.75	12.87	13.00	13.12
11.50	12.62	12.87	13.00	13.12	13.37	13.50	13.75	13.87
12.00	13.25	13.50	13.62	13.87	14.00	14.25	14.50	14.62
12.50	13.87	14.12	14.25	14.50	14.75	15.00	15.25	15.37
13.00	14.50	14.75	15.00	15.25	15.50	15.62	16.00	16.12
13.50	15.12	15.37	15.62	15.87	16.12	16.37	16.62	16.87
14.00	15.75	16.00	16.25	16.50	16.75	17.12	17.50	17.75
14.50	16.50	16.75	17.00	17.25	17.50	17.87	18.25	18.50
15.00	17.00	17.37	17.75	18.00	18.25	18.62	19.00	19.37
15.50	17.75	18.00	18.25	18.75	19.00	19.37	19.75	20.25
16.00	18.25	18.75	19.00	19.37	19.75	20.25	20.50	21.00
16.50	19.00	19.37	19.75	20.25	20.50	21.00	21.50	21.87
17.00	19.75	20.25	20.50	21.00	21.50	22.00	22.25	22.87
17.50	20.50	20.75	21.25	21.75	22.25	22.75	23.25	23.75
18.00	21.00	21.50	22.00	22.50	23.00	23.50	24.00	24.62
18.50	21.75	22.25	22.75	23.25	23.75	24.50	25.00	25.62
19.00	22.50	23.00	23.50	24.00	24.75	25.25	26.00	26.50

(continued)

▶ **TABLE B.1** Vertex Conversion Chart (Continued)

Spectacle Lens Power	Minus Lenses		(—)		Vertex Distance/mm			
	8	9	10	11	12	13	14	15
4.00	3.87	3.87	3.87	3.87	3.87	3.75	3.75	3.75
4.50	4.37	4.37	4.25	4.25	4.25	4.25	4.25	4.25
5.00	4.75	4.75	4.75	4.75	4.75	4.75	4.62	4.62
5.50	5.25	5.25	5.25	5.12	5.12	5.12	5.12	5.12
6.00	5.75	5.62	5.62	5.62	5.62	5.50	5.50	5.50
6.50	6.12	6.12	6.12	6.00	6.00	6.00	6.00	5.87
7.00	6.62	6.62	6.50	6.50	6.50	6.37	6.37	6.37
7.50	7.12	7.00	7.00	6.87	6.87	6.87	6.75	6.75
8.00	7.50	7.50	7.37	7.37	7.25	7.25	7.25	7.25
8.50	8.00	7.87	7.87	7.75	7.75	7.62	7.62	7.50
9.00	8.37	8.37	8.25	8.25	8.12	8.00	8.00	8.00
9.50	8.87	8.75	8.62	8.62	8.50	8.50	8.37	8.37
10.00	9.25	9.12	9.12	9.00	8.87	8.87	8.75	8.75
10.50	9.62	9.62	9.50	9.37	9.37	9.25	9.12	9.12
11.00	10.12	10.00	9.87	9.75	9.75	9.62	9.50	9.50
11.50	10.50	10.37	10.37	10.25	10.12	10.00	9.87	9.87
12.00	11.00	10.87	10.75	10.62	10.50	10.37	10.25	10.12
12.50	11.37	11.25	11.12	11.00	10.87	10.75	10.62	10.50
13.00	11.75	11.62	11.50	11.37	11.25	11.12	11.00	10.87
13.50	12.25	12.00	11.87	11.75	11.62	11.50	11.37	11.25
14.00	12.62	12.50	12.25	12.12	12.00	11.87	11.75	11.50
14.50	13.00	12.75	12.62	12.50	12.37	12.25	12.00	11.87
15.00	13.37	13.25	13.00	12.87	12.75	12.50	12.37	12.25
15.50	13.75	13.62	13.50	13.25	13.00	12.87	12.75	12.62
16.00	14.25	14.00	13.75	13.62	13.50	13.25	13.00	12.87
16.50	14.50	14.37	14.12	14.00	13.75	13.62	13.50	13.25
17.00	15.00	14.75	14.50	14.25	14.12	14.00	13.75	13.50
17.50	15.37	15.12	14.87	14.75	14.50	14.25	14.00	13.87
18.00	15.75	15.50	15.25	15.00	14.75	14.62	14.37	14.12
18.50	16.12	15.87	15.62	15.37	15.12	14.87	14.75	14.50
19.00	16.50	16.25	16.00	15.75	15.50	15.25	15.00	14.75

▶ **TABLE B.2** Diopter Conversion Chart

Diopters	mm	Diopters	mm	Diopters	mm	Diopters	mm
20.00	16.875	39.00	8.653	45.00	7.500	51.00	6.617
22.00	15.340	39.12	8.627	45.12	7.480	51.12	6.602
24.00	14.062	39.25	8.598	45.25	7.458	51.25	6.585
26.00	12.980	39.37	8.572	45.37	7.438	51.37	6.569
27.00	12.500	39.50	8.544	45.50	7.417	51.50	6.553
28.00	12.053	39.62	8.518	45.62	7.398	51.62	6.538
29.00	11.638	39.75	8.490	45.75	7.377	51.75	6.521
29.50	11.441	39.87	8.465	45.87	7.357	51.87	6.506
30.00	11.250	40.00	8.437	46.00	7.336	52.00	6.490
30.50	11.065	40.12	8.412	46.12	7.317	52.12	6.475
31.00	10.887	40.25	8.385	46.25	7.297	52.25	6.459
31.50	10.714	40.37	8.360	46.37	7.278	52.37	6.444
32.00	10.547	40.50	8.333	46.50	7.258	52.50	6.428
32.50	10.385	40.62	8.308	46.62	7.239	52.62	6.413
33.00	10.227	40.75	8.282	46.75	7.219	52.75	6.398
33.50	10.075	40.87	8.257	46.87	7.200	52.87	6.383
34.00	9.926	41.00	8.231	47.00	7.180	53.00	6.367
34.25	9.854	41.12	8.207	47.12	7.162	53.12	6.353
34.50	9.783	41.25	8.181	47.25	7.142	53.25	6.338
34.75	9.712	41.37	8.158	47.37	7.124	53.37	6.323
35.00	9.643	41.50	8.132	47.50	7.105	53.50	6.308
35.25	9.574	41.62	8.109	47.62	7.087	53.62	6.294
35.50	9.507	41.75	8.083	47.75	7.068	53.75	6.279
35.75	9.440	41.87	8.060	47.87	7.050	53.87	6.265
36.00	9.375	42.00	8.035	48.00	7.031	54.00	6.250
36.12	9.343	42.12	8.012	48.12	7.013	54.12	6.236
36.25	9.310	42.25	7.988	48.25	6.994	54.25	6.221
36.37	9.279	42.37	7.965	48.37	6.977	54.37	6.207
36.50	9.246	42.50	7.941	48.50	6.958	54.50	6.192
36.62	9.216	42.62	7.918	48.62	6.941	54.62	6.179
36.75	9.183	42.75	7.894	48.75	6.923	54.75	6.164
36.87	9.153	42.87	7.872	48.87	6.906	54.87	6.150
37.00	9.121	43.00	7.848	49.00	6.887	55.00	6.136
37.12	9.092	43.12	7.826	49.12	6.870	55.12	6.123
37.25	9.060	43.25	7.803	49.25	6.852	55.25	6.108
37.37	9.031	43.37	7.781	49.37	6.836	55.37	6.095
37.50	9.000	43.50	7.758	49.50	6.818	55.50	6.081
37.62	8.971	43.62	7.737	49.62	6.801	55.62	6.068
37.75	8.940	43.75	7.714	49.75	6.783	55.75	6.054
37.87	8.912	43.87	7.693	49.87	6.767	55.87	6.041
38.00	8.881	44.00	7.670	50.00	6.750	56.00	6.027
38.12	8.853	44.12	7.649	50.12	6.733	56.50	5.973
38.25	8.823	44.25	7.627	50.25	6.716	57.00	5.921
38.37	8.795	44.37	7.606	50.37	6.700	57.50	5.869
38.50	8.766	44.50	7.584	50.50	6.683	58.00	5.819
38.62	8.738	44.62	7.563	50.62	6.667	58.50	5.769
38.75	8.708	44.75	7.541	50.75	6.650	59.00	5.720
38.87	8.682	44.87	7.521	50.87	6.634	60.00	5.625

Extended Range Keratometry Chart

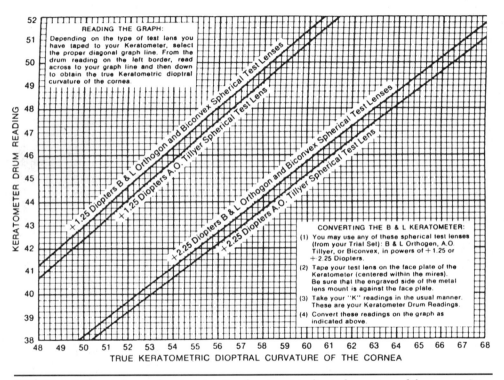

FIGURE C.1. Extended range keratometry: True keratometric dioptral curvature of the cornea. Steep corneas beyond the normal range of the B & L Keratometer can be easily measured by using an auxiliary lens and this graph. Follow the directions for converting your keratometer and for reading the graph.

Grand Rounds and Case Report Sheets

Grand Rounds and Case Reports

Patient	Medical Record Number	Date of Exam	Diagnosis

Grand Rounds and Case Reports

Patient	Medical Record Number	Date of Exam	Diagnosis

Grand Rounds and Case Reports

Patient	Medical Record Number	Date of Exam	Diagnosis

Grand Rounds and Case Reports

Patient	Medical Record Number	Date of Exam	Diagnosis

Telephone Numbers

Contact Lenses

Family Practice

Low Vision

Medical Eye Service

Pediatrics & Binocular Vision

External Clinics

Admitting

Anesthesia

Bacteriology

Chemistry

CT

Cytology

Electrodiagnostics

Emergency Room

Hematology

ICU

Library

Medical Records

Nursing

On-Call Service

Operating Room

Pathology

Pharmacy

Radiology

Recovery Room

Security

Others

INDEX

Page numbers followed by f indicate a figure; t following a page number indicates tabular material